Sports Medicine

FITNESS • TRAINING • INJURIES

Third Edition

Sports Medicine

FITNESS · TRAINING · INJURIES

Third Edition

Edited by

Otto Appenzeller, M.D., Ph.D.

University of New Mexico
School of Medicine
Albuquerque

Urban & Schwarzenberg
Baltimore-Munich

Urban & Schwarzenberg, Inc.
7 E. Redwood Street
Baltimore, Maryland 21202
USA

Urban & Schwarzenberg
Pettenkoferstrasse 18
D-8000 München 2
West Germany

Printed in the United States of America

Second Printing—August 1989

Notices

The Editor (or Author(s)) and the Publisher of this work have made
every effort to ensure that the drug dosage schedules herein are accurate and in accord with the standards accepted at the time of publication. The reader is strongly advised, however, to check the product information sheet included in the package of each drug he or she plans to
administer to be certain that changes have not been made in the recommended dose or in the contraindications for administration.

The Publishers have made an extensive effort to trace original
copyright holders for permission to use borrowed material. If any have
been overlooked, it will be corrected at the first reprint.

Library of Congress Cataloging-in-Publication Data

Sports medicine.

Includes bibliographies and index.
1. Sports medicine.   2. Physical fitness.   3. Physical education
and training.   I. Appenzeller, Otto.
[DNLM: 1. Athletic Injuries.   2. Exertion.   3. Physical Education
and Training.   4. Sports Medicine.
QT 260 S7703]
RC1210.S686   1988   617'.1027   88-10689
ISBN 0-8067-0143-9
ISBN 0-8067-0133-1 (pbk.)

Compositor: Brushwood Graphics Inc., Baltimore, MD
Printer: Arcata Graphics, Kingsport, TN
Production and design: Stony Run Publishing Services, Baltimore, MD

Paperback
ISBN 0-8067-0133-1 Baltimore
ISBN 3-541-70133-1 Munich

Hardcover
ISBN 0-8067-0143-9 Baltimore
ISBN 0-541-70143-9 Munich

Dedicated
to the Memory of
Papa (1899–1980)
Who Inspired Us
by Example
and to the Memory of
Glenn T. Peake, M.D. (1937–1987)
Who Encouraged Much of the
Work Reported Herein as
Director of the
University of New Mexico
Clinical Research Center

Contents

1   **Introduction**
     Ernst Jokl

Section 1
The Nervous System
and Sports

     Otto Appenzeller

     Otto Appenzeller

     Robert Kellner

Section 2
Nutritional and Gastrointestinal
Aspects of Sports

     Otto Appenzeller

     Nicholas A. Volpicelli and Monroe H. Spector

     Neil Kaminsky

Section 3
Sports and Hormones,
Fluids, and Electrolytes

     Maire T. Buckman and Glenn T. Peake

Contributors

Bob Anderson
P.O. Box 767
Palmer Lake, Colorado 80133

Otto Appenzeller, M.D., Ph.D.
Department of Neurology
University of New Mexico
　　School of Medicine
Albuquerque, New Mexico 87131

Maire T. Buckman, M.D.
Department of Medicine
University of New Mexico
　　School of Medicine
Albuquerque, New Mexico 87131

Karen Carlberg, Ph.D.
Department of Biology
Eastern Washington University
Cherey, Washington 99004

Thomas W. Chick, M.D.
Pulmonary Division
Veteran's Administration Medical Center
Albuquerque, New Mexico 87108

Stephen F. Crouse, Ph.D.
Department of Health and Physical
　　Education
Texas A&M University
College Station, Texas 77840

Kenneth D. Gardner, Jr., M.D.
Department of Medicine/Nephrology
University of New Mexico
　　School of Medicine
Albuquerque, New Mexico 87131

Jerome E. Goss, M.D.
1001 Coal S.E.
Albuquerque, New Mexico 87106

Vivian H. Heyward, Ph.D.
Department of Health, Physical
　　Education, and Recreation
University of New Mexico
Albuquerque, New Mexico 87131

William B. Hobbins, M.D.
Thermal Image Analysis, Inc.
5510 Medical Circle
Suite B
Madison, Wisconsin 53719

Philip L. Hooper, M.D.
1808 Boise Avenue
Loveland, Colorado 80537

Ernst Jokl, M.D., Ph.D.
Departments of Neurology and Exercise
　　Physiology
University of Kentucky
340 Kingsway
Lexington, Kentucky 40502

Neil Kaminsky, M.D.
Encino Medical Plaza
717 Encino Place, N.E.
Suite 9
Albuquerque, New Mexico 87102

Robert Kellner, M.D., Ph.D.
Department of Psychiatry
University of New Mexico
　　School of Medicine
Albuquerque, New Mexico 87131

Carol Kresge, MsT.
Take Care
238 E. 5th
Tallahassee, Florida 32303

Stephen R. Loane
Sugar Tree Club
Sugar Loaf/USA
Carrabassett Valley, Maine 04947

Laurel Traeger Mackinnon, Ph.D.
Roswell Park Memorial Cancer Institute
Buffalo, New York 14263

Barry R. Maron, M.D.
New Mexico Orthopaedic Specialists,
　　Ltd.
6100 Pan American Freeway, N.E.

Suite 130
Albuquerque, New Mexico 87109

William J. O'Brien, Ph.D.
% New Mexico Physical Therapy, Inc.
2607 Wyoming, N.E.
Suites A & B
Albuquerque, New Mexico 87112

Robert M. Parks, D.P.M.
Albuquerque Associated Podiatrists
121 Sycamore Street, N.E.
Albuquerque, New Mexico 87106

Glenn T. Peake, M.D.*
Department of Medicine
University of New Mexico
   School of Medicine
Albuquerque, New Mexico 87131

Jonathan M. Samet, M.D.
Department of Medicine
University of New Mexico
   School of Medicine
Albuquerque, New Mexico 87131

David S. Schade, M.D.
Department of Medicine
University of New Mexico
   School of Medicine
Albuquerque, New Mexico 87131

William R. Schiller, M.D.
8401 North 74th Place
Scottsdale, Arizona 85258

**William Selezinka, M.D., M.S.,
   F.A.C.S.**
Department of Ophthalmology
University of California, San Diego
La Jolla, California 92161

Neal Shadoff, M.D.
Albuquerque Cardiovascular Associates,
   Ltd.
201 Cedar, S.E.
Suite 604
Albuquerque, New Mexico 87106

Toby L. Simon, M.D.
Department of Pathology
University of New Mexico
   School of Medicine
Albuquerque, New Mexico 87131

John E. Smialek, M.D.
Chief Medical Examiner
State of Maryland
111 Penn Street
Baltimore, MD 21201

Monroe H. Spector, M.D.
717 Encino Place, N.E.
Albuquerque, New Mexico 87102

Thomas B. Tomasi, M.D.
Roswell Park Memorial Cancer Institute
Buffalo, New York 14263

Nicholas A. Volpicelli, M.D.
Presbyterian Professional Building
201 Cedar, S.E.
Suite 409
Albuquerque, New Mexico 87106

Stephen C. Wood, Ph.D.
Lovelace Medical Foundation
Albuquerque, New Mexico 87108

*Deceased.

Preface to
the Third Edition

The future of sports medicine depends on clinical research because human sporting activity can best be assessed by a searching scrutiny of performing subjects. Clinical scientists and sports medicine enthusiasts are incurably optimistic but clinical research is a delicate flower requiring continuous care and attention. Two things are vital to assure the future of sports medicine: adaptability to changing circumstances and the ability to reproduce. Clinical science has demonstrated its remarkable adaptability, but does the clinical sports medicine community reproduce? Others have coined memorable phrases on this subject, for instance "we need the young upon our shoulders and should not trample them under our feet" and "it is for sports medicine elders to lead and for teachers to encourage an inquisitive frame of mind which fosters clinical research." The third edition of this book may help young recruits to clinical sports medicine and we should give them the support needed and freedom to pursue their work without hinderance.

This new edition extends to the furthest reaches of sports medicine, from the nervous system and its ubiquitous influence to immunology and of course to the expanding therapeutic alternatives. This diversity will encourage converts to the discipline, foster clinical research, and help legions of active men and women in their quest for a more meaningful, satisfying, and productive life.

This edition has been extensively revised and restructured to keep pace with the burgeoning field and to incorporate other disciplines that impinge upon the field. Hematology, immunology, and forensic medicine have made their contributions and are included in an expanded or new format. New methods of therapy have been added because they have proven their value (and limitations) and qualify for mention in a text that strives for completeness and timeliness.

Most clinicians need to separate knowledge, convictions, and the beliefs to which they are emotionally attached. The guiding principal of inviting contributors to the third edition was their capacity to detach their beliefs and emotions and write dispassionately about current knowledge.

Spring 1988   Otto Appenzeller

Preface to
the Second Edition

When King George III confronted the historian Gibbon, who had just completed another book, he remarked, "Scribble, scribble, scribble, eh, Mr. Gibbon? Another fat book, eh, Mr. Gibbon?" What are the justifications for continuously adding to the already gigantic piles of books in print? Is it possible that one is attempting to intrude into libraries without first asking permission to enter? But, publishers are not in the charitable business, and new editions appear because old ones have sold out or have become obsolete. Sports medicine is rapidly evolving, and interest in this country in providing training in this all-embracing discipline has quickened with the advent of participant rather than observational athletic activities. Justification for the Second Edition lies in the success of the first and in heeding the constructive criticism from many quarters which has been incorporated into the new version. The contributors to the new edition attest to the holistic nature of sports medicine and should make this volume more useful for students and practitioners who have little contact with other than the medical aspects of sports.

The importance and limitation of sports medicine must be reassessed in order to appreciate the value of this clinical branch of medicine in promoting a desirable lifestyle, in preventing disease, and in enhancement of ethical values, particularly as they pertain to the training of physicians and of athletes themselves. It is important to document the value of exercise and athletics not only for the young, as it was done in the past, but also its possible implication in maintenance of health in large segments of our aged, but otherwise healthy, population.

These as yet not widely recognized influences of sports medicine have led to the inclusion of new chapters into this volume in the hope that those for whom this book is intended will find it all-encompassing and a source of existing knowledge supported by adequate scientific investigation and of hypotheses which might stimulate further research in this important new field.

The editors share the enthusiastic interest of the contributors for the physiologic and clinical effects of athletic endeavors, but sports will also have an important impact on the quality of life to which physicians and others working in the field of health maintenance have contributed in the past and hopefully will continue to do so in the future.

Spring 1983   Otto Appenzeller
                                                                                                      Ruth Atkinson

Acknowledgments

The editor could not have produced this volume without the devoted cooperation of his staff and publisher. Many of those who provided assistance must remain anonymous, but mention must be made of those who did more than their share to bring this Third Edition to fruition. They include Carol Cameron and the Department of Medical Illustrations at the University of New Mexico School of Medicine and its director, Mike Norviel. The generous support of the Clinical Research Center, University of New Mexico School of Medicine is gratefully acknowledged (Grant #DRR, NIH 5 MO1 RR00997 9-12).

We gratefully acknowledge the assistance of Flexi-Therm who supported the production of the color thermograms.

•1•

Introduction
Medicine, Science, and Sports

Ernst Jokl

To understand the explosive development of the international sports movement, consideration must be given to a number of historically unique changes that occurred during the past century. Some of these changes are of a social nature; others were engendered by the revolutionary advancements of science and technology. The result is the establishment of standards of growth, health, and fitness that never before existed.

CHILD LABOR

Until the end of the last century, child labor was prevalent throughout Europe. This problem was particularly severe during the Industrial Revolution, when hordes of workless, starving vagrants flocked from the countryside into the towns. Children were driven by the poverty of their parents into factories and mines. Child-slaves, orphaned and friendless, were supplied in droves by the workhouses to employers. Children as young as even 3 years of age spent 12 hours at a time in the darkness of the mines.

Lord Shaftesbury was among the most active proponents of reforms. "Never," he said in a parliamentary debate on child labor in the House of Commons, "have I seen such a display of selfishness, frigidity to every human sentiment, such ready and happy self-delusion."

In 1859, children less than 10 years old and girls and women were excluded altogether from the mines, but it was not until 1875 that employment of boy chimney sweeps was prohibited. The 1870s saw compulsory free education established throughout Great Britain, and thus a barrier was interposed between children and the factories. In the same decade the first kindergartens were introduced. The Society for the Prevention of Cruelty to Children, founded in 1872, took the initiative in promulgating progressive social legislation. It goes without saying that children until then had been in poor health, neither willing nor able to engage in sport.

LEISURE

To understand why, during the past decades, sports have become one of the major leisure pursuits of human beings, it must be realized that the concepts of both leisure and sport have only recently assumed their present meaning. The idea that time for leisure would be available to the ordinary individual sounded revolutionary not so long ago, when the worker, unless he or she was working, rested to recuperate from and gather new strength for work. The boys and girls who slaved in coal mines and textile mills around the middle of the 19th century had neither the time nor the strength to play. Their situation, as well as that of their elders, was incomparably worse than the conditions prevailing during the preceding millennium, in the relatively stable, predominantly rural village environment throughout Western Europe.

HEALTH

That medicine would ever become a science was beyond imagination only a few centuries ago. For example, consider the gorgeous portrait of Louis XIV (1638–1715) by Hyacinthe Rigaud. It shows the grand monarch in his ermine-lined robes of state, scepter in hand, arm on hip, gazing out on the world with affable condescension and consummate poise. We see the epitome of majesty: grace, dignity, command. It is disillusioning to turn to the king's private life, as described by his doctors. A new and disconcertingly human figure emerges, a man plagued by chronic infirmities of all kinds, pestered by doctors and surgeons, subjected to incredible purges, enemas, and emetics. The health of even the humblest citizen today is infinitely better protected than was that of "The Sun King" 300 years ago. Throughout his reign Louis XIV was attended by three "premier médicins" who kept a *Journal de la Santé du Roi*. It describes the illnesses of the royal patient: "rheumatism, vapors, humors, fistula, insomnia, indigestion, fluxes, headaches, chronic fevers, anthrax, melancholy, urinary difficulties, night sweats, vertigo, erysipelas, colds, colic, bile, acid mouth, chronic toothaches," and inevitably, "a great deal of gout." It is not difficult to understand why, as his biographer Philippe Ariés mentions, "Louis XIV showed a marked lack of enthusiasm for tennis."

MILITARY RECRUITS 1790–1819

To assess the extent to which physique, strength, and fitness of the present generation of youths in the United States and Europe have benefitted from the advancements of science and technology, one must evaluate the status of young people two centuries ago. A book entitled *The Enlistings, Discharging and Pensioning of Soldiers During the Years 1790–1819*, published in 1839 by Henry Marshall, Deputy Inspector-General of British Army Hospitals, describes that the 100,000 men who during that period enlisted on a long service contract of 21 years were a miserable lot: For a regiment, recruited in 1797 at Cork for embarkation to Buenos Aires, minimum weight was 116 lb 9 oz (52 kg), minimum height 5 ft 5½ in (1.66 m). Every recruit who complied with these standards was accepted, irrespective of his age. In the French Army, minimum weight was 110 lb (50 kg), minimum height 5 ft 2 in (1.575 m). (In the United States today, many schoolchildren 12 years of age would thus have qualified for acceptance!) At that time, every conceivable disease — epilepsy, palsy, insanity, rheumatism, hernia, blindness, ulcerations, etc. — was either simulated or intentionally reproduced in attempts to avoid army service. Nor did lashes deter malingerers from their set purpose. Hernias were produced by incising the scrotum, inserting the stem of a clay pipe, and with the assistance of a pal, blowing until the skin was as tight as a drum. Men were quite prepared to lose the sight of one eye if it could get them their discharge. This was done by the application of a caustic, by scraping the surface of the cornea, or by piercing it with a sharp needle and scratching the lens to cause cataracts.

NUTRITION

The means to conquer hunger and malnutrition is but a recent triumph of science. The role of vitamins as essential elements of a good diet was unknown until the beginning of this century. In 1913 Sir John Boyd Orr assessed the incidence of rickets in Glasgow, Scotland: 40% of the city's school population was afflicted. In a repeat survey in 1936, only 10% of the children in Glasgow had rickets. Vitamin D had been identified by Adolf Windaus of Goettingen who was awarded a Nobel Prize in 1928. The Glasgow study was repeated once more in 1965, when not a single case of rickets was found among children born in Glasgow. However, the incidence of rickets among Asian immigrants to England today is comparable to that found in Glasgow in 1913. Malnutrition is still widespread in Asia and Africa, whereas in affluent societies obesity has become a major health problem.

INFECTIOUS DISEASES

The greatest single contribution of medical research to society is that it has brought infectious diseases under control. In 1900, infectious diseases were responsible for most deaths in the United States. Throughout the preceding centuries no family was spared the sorrow of children dying from "fevers." In his Johann Sebastian Bach Memorial Lecture delivered at Hamburg in 1950, Paul Hindemith mentioned that Bach lost 11 children. Today, few children die during infancy. The chief causes of death in the United States are no longer infectious diseases but cardiovascular afflictions, malignant tumors, accidents, and crime. The average length of life has increased from 48 years in 1898 to 73 years today. Whooping cough, diphtheria, smallpox, and poliomyelitis were brought under control only after World War II.

ACCELERATION OF GROWTH

Against the background of such changes as the foregoing, the favorable status of children today must be assessed. Today's boys and girls are taller and stronger than their parents and grandparents. An average-sized high-school boy aged 17 does not fit into the armor of Elizabethan knights in the Tower of London. There has been a steady acceleration of growth and maturation over the centuries, with a noticeable spurt during the past decades. One manifestation of this spurt is the appearance today of children and adolescents in sports such as swimming, gymnastics, ice-skating, and other athletic disciplines. Children now run the 26-mile marathon, climb the highest mountains, and participate in long-distance ski races. In 1979, two 12-year-old boys swam the English Channel; at the Pan African Track and Field Games in Nairobi in July, 1979, a 12-year-old girl won the 1500 m final against adult competition.

The corresponding opposite to the acceleration of growth is a deceleration of aging, a phenomenon representing the physiologic basis for the participation of large numbers of senior men and women in a great variety of sporting events. At the Montreal Olympic Games in 1976, more than 400 athletes over 40 years of age entered the competitions, several of them with conspicuous success. At both Moscow (in 1980) and Los Angeles (in 1984), the number of senior Olympians was even greater.

WOMEN IN SPORTS

The athletic status of women reflects the far-reaching changes that have taken place in the Western world during this century. The unfolding of the "power potential of the Second Sex" is still in progress, even though scientific evidence on women's physical performance capacities was available long before it was applied in practice.

"A horse sweats, a man perspires, but a lady only glows." This statement illustrates the general attitude toward exercise and athletics for females during the Victorian age. Since then, social attitudes have changed profoundly. During the past 50 years, millions of women have indulged in sports, gymnastics, and games; competed in swimming, track and field events, and horseback riding; climbed many of the highest mountains; and swum through thousands of rivers and lakes. Participation in such activities has given women some of the most valuable experiences of their lives. All the evils of which they had been warned have been conspicuous by their absence. The women have not developed a masculine appearance; most of them marry and have children. None suffer physical damage or "overstrain" from muscular exertion; their hearts have not been "weakened through athletics"; and most of them attain a ripe old age.

That the present generation of women grows stronger, that their physical maturation is better balanced and their appearance more attractive, that the health of young mothers and their children today is superior, that physically active women no longer look old at the age of 30, and that many schoolgirls play on the same team as their mothers—all these facts are, at least in part, the result of the interest now taken in the physical education of girls. Sports and games and athletics for women are significant elements of that which many consider best in contemporary culture.

The role of women in sport was discussed in antiquity. In Plato's *Republic,* Socrates raises the question whether "females should guard the flock and hunt with males and take a share in all they do, or be kept within doors as fit for no more than bearing and feeding their children while all the hard work is left to the males." Socrates' brother, Glaucon, agreed that "women are expected to take their full share, except that we must treat them as not quite so strong." The two disputants concurred that both men and women ought to receive the same upbringing and education. Such a system, Socrates remarked, would at first appear revolutionary, but he pointed out that "it is not so long since the Greeks thought it ridiculous as well as shameful for men to be seen naked in the gymnasium. When gymnastic exercises were first introduced in Crete and later in Sparta, the cynics had their chance to make fun of them." But, he observed, "a new attitude was soon accepted and it will be the same once women are given equal access to physical education."

However, Plato was concerned with the education of an elite, a selected group of leaders of proven excellence of character, mind, and body. Thus, he argued logically that once the principle of selection is recognized and the wide scope of individual differences among men and women accepted, a distinction beween the educational systems for boys and girls is no longer justified.

The fact that well-trained women athletes are superior to untrained men in all branches of sport signifies a revolutionary change in society's attitude toward the female. Views held until recently, that menstruation, pregnancy, childbearing, and menopause prohibit females from participation in sports, were shown to be false.

In several athletic disciplines, women's average levels of performance equal those of men. In terms of aesthetic criteria, women athletes rank above men in such sports as gymnastics and figure skating. The physical educability of women is much greater than was assumed until recently; for instance, a young woman won the Washington State weightlifting championship in the flyweight class (52 kg), winning the title against male competitors. Few, if any, men could have beaten Olga Korbut and Nadja Comaneci on the uneven parallel bars or balance beam in the 1972 and 1976 Olympics. The women's 400 m record of 47.60 sec, established by Marita Koch in 1985, is remarkable. At some marathon races in the U.S., more than 1,000 women started; on average, 96% of them finished. The current women's world record for the marathon, 2:21:06, is equal to or faster than most of the Olympic winning times for men prior to World War II. Most of the best female athletes in 1987 would have won the men's competitions in their respective events at Olympic Games a few decades ago: Marita Koch (400 m, 47.60 sec); Marina Stepanova (400 m hurdles, 52.94 sec); Yordanka Donkova (100 m hurdles, 12.26 sec); Stefka Kostadinova (high jump, 2.09 m); Fatima Whitbread (discus, 254 ft 1 in, 77.45 m); and Petra Felke (javelin, 274 ft 4 in, 83.62 m).

ATHLETIC RECORDS

The chief elements from which all physical performances are synthesized have been identified through scientific analyses of athletic records. The world's best performances in sport have been documented since the beginning of this century, some of them longer. It has thus been possible to construct growth curves of world records for all sports events, including those held at Olympic Games. From them, the magnitude of the performance explosion during the past decades in all branches of sport can be assessed. However, rates of performance growth differ for different athletic disciplines. In swimming, performance growth continues, whereas in short- and middle-distance track, the steep ascent of record growth curves is about to come to an end. In a few events, terminal positions may be in sight; for instance, the probability is not great that Bob Beamon's long-jump record of 29 ft 2.5 in (8.90 m) established in Mexico City in 1968 will be improved by much. Altogether, it is not generally realized that "the expanding athletic universe" is bound to reach its limits.

UNEXPLORED RESOURCES

As to the future of athletic records, it must be taken into account that the advancements of science and technology which in many areas of the world have eradicated hunger and controlled infectious diseases have not yet benefitted more than a quarter of the human race. The medical status of most populations of Asia and Africa today is no better than it was in Europe during the Middle Ages. The extent to which infectious diseases affect the physical status of entire ethnic groups became evident during the past 30 years in East Africa, where smallpox was eradicated through the introduction of vaccination. Only then did Hamitic athletes from Tanzania, Ethiopia, and Kenya appear on the international athletic scene. Their conspicuous successes at the 1968 Olympic Games established their countries as major track and field powers. Their status will continue to gain as further public health measures are effective. A worldwide upgrading of all sports performances is bound to occur when the results of preventive and curative measures that are currently being introduced by the World Health Organization throughout the Third World become effective. The issue has wide implications.

Generally held beliefs that medical science has conquered most of our great killer diseases are fallacious. In the *Listener* of August 9, 1979, Brian J. Ford pointed out:

We cannot yet reliably cure any virus disease and know next to nothing of the cause or cure of a host of major scourges, from cancer and coronary heart attacks to schizophrenia, arthritis, strokes and the degenerative diseases, from cystic fibrosis to Huntington's chorea. The tropical diseases alone, from schistosomiasis and river blindness to an array of worm parasites and the trypanosomes which waste the body, afflict hundreds of millions of people.

During the next two decades, public health measures are likely to reduce the incidence of disease everywhere. A worldwide advancement in growth and development should thus occur and from it further improvements of all athletic records. Considering the achievements of medical research so far, such forecasts seem justified.

Technologic innovations will continue to play an important role in the athletic performance explosion of the twentieth century. The introduction of Tartan tracks, newly designed javelins and discuses, fiberglass poles, and foam rubber mats has noticeably altered the entire track and field scene. The temperature control of swimming pools, improved filtration systems, and establishment of smooth water surfaces through vertical lane markers have facilitated achievement of new swimming records. The availability of large indoor facilities, such as the air-conditioned Astrodome in Houston and the Louisiana Superdome in New Orleans, has opened vistas not yet fully explored, e.g., that of creating optimal temperatures and other advantageous environmental conditions for individual athletic events throughout the year.

Last but not least, the fact that numbers of participants in all sports are continually increasing throughout the world renders probable the appearance from time to time of "athletic geniuses" and thus the establishment of extraordinary records—the phenomenon of Bob Beamon is likely to recur, at some future date, in other athletic disciplines.

THE FIELDS BEYOND

Once the limits of physical performance growth are reached, a chief objective of athletics will be to explore the aesthetic possibilities that are inherent in sports—possibilities derived from the inexhaustible choice of designs of expression and communication of human movements.

In a few decades from now, the athletic situation will be comparable to that of oil painting in the middle of the 17th century, of the ballet prior to World War I, and of piano music during the 1920s.

The development of oil painting extended over the better part of two centuries, starting in the 15th century with Jan van Eyck's search for a varnish that would dry without being put in the sun; his discovery was subsequently elaborated by Giovanni Bellini from whom Albrecht Dürer learned the technique he applied in his masterpiece *The Four Apostles*. Oil painting reached a zenith with Diego Velazquez, Jan Breughel, and Peter Paul Rubens.

The technical possibilities of the ballet were explored during the early years of the twentieth century when Serge Diaghilev presented his Ballet Russe in Paris, with Michel Fokine as choreographer; Vaslav Nijinsky, Anna Pavlova, and Tamara Karsavina as dancers; and Picasso, Derain, and Benois as "decorators." From it emerged Émile Jaques-Dalcroze's *Musical Calisthenics,* Claude Achille Debussy's *Dance Plays,* Richard Strauss's *Joseph's Legende,* and, more recently, John Cranko's *Stuttgart Ballet.*

Piano technique as we know it started with Beethoven's use of the hammerklavier and its exploration through his pupil, Carl Czerny, who became the teacher of Franz Liszt. To Liszt's Weimar school belonged Eugen d'Albert and Ferruccio Busoni, under whose direction Egon Petri acquired a level of keyboard mastery equaled but not surpassed by today's great pianists, not even Vladimir Horowitz, Rudolf Serkin, Sviatoslav Richter, or Benedetti Michelangeli.

When the history of gymnastics is written, the names of Olga Korbut, Nadja Comaneci, Nelli Kim, and their teachers will rank in the chronology of the subject like those to whom the arts are indebted for the technical perfection of painting, dancing, and music.

Through the unprecedented differentiation of the motor system that physical performance in all its manifestations is able to accomplish, sport is destined to reveal its powers of experience and communication and thus create a new culture—the third, if one considers the humanities and the natural sciences first and second.

The number of those who will take full advantage of this "third culture" will remain limited, just as the number of those who realize the aesthetic and intellectual possibilities of the arts and sciences remains limited. The pursuit of excellence in all its forms has always been entrusted to an elite in the sense defined by Lord Kenneth Clark:

> If you don't have an elite in some sense of the word—and it does not mean a class elite—and some people of superior mind and character guiding the people then it all falls into barbarism. The general rough-and-tumble of uneducated people is not going to produce a civilization.

The Nervous System and Sports

•2•

Temperature Regulation and Sports

Otto Appenzeller

The recent evolution of the thermoregulatory system has made it a recurrent subject of physiological investigation. Moreover, sporting activities, induced by environmental heat or excessive heat loads due to physical activity, may cause serious and sometimes lasting disorders in well- or less well-trained individuals.

The term *homeothermy* implies the maintenance of body temperature within certain limits and normal functioning of the thermoregulatory systems, but the nature of the regulatory mechanism, or set point, how it adjusts to external heat loads and internal heat production, and the way it responds to pyrogens are matters of debate. Considerable evidence now shows that thermosensitive neurons in the anterior and preoptic hypothalamus respond to blood temperature changes, and that these same neurons are also activated by impulses from the periphery and cervical spinal cord. Various systems concerned with heat loss or preservation are brought into play. These include behavioral changes, which are important in conscious thermoregulation. Neurons participating in thermoregulation release a number of transmitters at their terminals. The thermoregulatory set point has been thought of in biochemical terms without much consideration of control theory. For example, a balanced release of neurotransmitters or a balance in calcium or sodium in the immediate neuronal environment probably maintains body temperature, but this does not explain how neurotransmitters are released or ionic balance comes about, thus addressing components of the system but not its operational principles.

The study of environmental and internal temperatures and their relationship to thermoregulation suggests that a simple neuronal connection exists between thermosensors and thermoeffectors. In humans, heat production, heat loss effectors, and their set point could be based entirely upon (neuronal) signals generated in the central nervous system (CNS). The injection of norepinephrine, 5-hydroxytryptamine, and the cholinomimetic substance carbamylcholine into the cerebral ventricles of a variety of animals shows that their thermoregulatory effects are the same as those obtained from disturbance-response analyses.

Increased heat storage from increased heat production or increased peripheral vasomotor tone with inhibition of heat loss from sweating occurs during fever and during heat stroke associated with physical exertion. Fever is caused by a pyrogen, which increases heat production and decreases heat loss. Such a pyrogen might act between cold sensors and the crossing inhibitory influences on evaporative heat loss, a hypothesis that has been tested in animals. Present evidence suggests that bacterial endotoxins or prostaglandin E_1, both pyrogens, act on cold sensors or pathways from them. This occurs prior to activation of inhibitory influences on heat loss processes. Numerous animal studies implicate aspartate, acetylcholine, carbamylcholine, dopamine, γ-aminobutyric acid, histamine, 5-hydroxy-tryptamine, indoleamine, prostaglandin E_1, and taurine in normal temperature regulation. Marked species differences in response to intraventricular injection of these agents and to agonist or antagonist drugs have been noted. It is uncertain how many and in what capacity these substances are involved in human temperature regulation (Bligh [1]).

TEMPERATURE REGULATION AND EXERCISE

During physical activity, several organs share the demand for increased blood supply. The heart must supply adequate blood to its own contracting muscle and to the skin for transfer of the excessive heat produced from muscular contraction.

Cardiac Output

In thermally neutral conditions during exercise, cardiac output increases in proportion to the rate of oxygen uptake. Increased cardiac output is associated with increased muscular blood flow.

It is not clear, however, whether a simple relationship exists between cardiac output and oxygen uptake when skin perfusion demand is high. Cutaneous blood flow is determined largely by body temperature, but reflex vasoconstriction of skin vessels occurs during hypotension. Nevertheless, at the onset of exercise, metabolic heat increases at a rate directly proportional to exercise intensity and is far in excess of heat dissipation.

Because of this imbalance, body temperature rises until heat loss through the skin by increased blood flow and sweating equals heat production. When this is achieved, a new set point at a higher steady internal body temperature or homeothermy occurs and is maintained until either further heat loads change the set point upward or decreased work load lowers body temperature again. The combined circulatory demands of muscles and skin are determined not only by body temperature, but also in part by average skin temperature, which is, in turn, closely related to environmental temperature. Therefore, when exercise intensity is great and ambient temperature high, the circulatory demands are considerably increased. The heart must then provide sufficient blood flow to both muscles and skin or compromise delivery of blood to one or the other.

If heavy exercise occurs in very hot environments, contracting muscles demand a disproportionately large segment of the cardiac output, which is shifted away from the skin; this, in turn, limits heat dissipation from the body core to the skin. Core temperature increases and ultimately leads to progressive hyperthermia, which eventually limits exercise. If, on the other hand, adequate blood flow to the skin is maintained at the expense of contracting muscles, anaerobic work occurs and adenosine triphosphate (ATP) synthesis is decreased along with the ability to maintain continuing muscle contraction.

Compromised Blood Flow   To prevent compromised blood flow to muscles, skin, or any other tissue during exercise, particularly in the heat, cardiac output must increase continuously. Recent experiments on treadmills in neutral and hot environments suggest that splanchnic blood flow is progressively reduced with increasing exercise intensity and is further reduced during exercise in heat, compared to the same work performed in cooler conditions. This might, in part, compensate for additional demands of the skin, but in extreme conditions of both exercise and heat, the body is prevented from maintaining both skin and muscle circulatory homeothermy.

Skin and Muscle Competition for Blood   The competition between skin and muscle blood flow during exercise in maintenance of homeothermy is further complicated by increased cutaneous venous volume during elevated body temperature. This increase is thought to be due, in part, to vasodilation of the skin veins because of their high compliance and reduced tone, which may result from an increased thermoregulatory drive. Increased venous blood in the skin permits additional heat transfer because of decreased velocity of flow and increased time for heat exchange between the blood and skin. However, increased peripheral blood volume reduces central volume, which, in turn, reduces the cardiac filling, thus potentially compromising cardiac stroke volume. If reduction in stroke volume occurs, compensatory increase in heart rate is necessary to maintain cardiac output. A further complicating factor that decreases the central blood volume during exercise is the loss of plasma water to the extravascular compartment. Many investigators report significant fluid losses from the intravascular compartment during relatively short or prolonged exercise. The cause of the movement from the intravascular to the extravascular compartment is thought to be the relative tissue hyperosmolality that occurs in active muscles. This transcapillary movement of fluid, however, could also result from increased filtration pressure in active muscles. The absolute fluid loss for the intravascular compartment during exercise seems most closely related to the intensity of exercise rather than to the ambient temperature.

Body Fluid Loss   Another factor leading to central volume depletion and, therefore, fall in cardiac filling, is body fluid loss through sweating, which is directly related to ambient temperature and intensity of exercise. The sweat rate may exceed 1–1.5 L/hr during prolonged exertion in a hot environment. Eventually, progressive reduction in central blood volume causes decreased cardiac filling, reduced stroke volume, and failure of appropriate perfusion for a given level of physical activity. As the systemic pressure drops, maintenance of cardiac output becomes more dependent upon increased heart rate brought about by activation of baroreceptor reflexes. These same reflexes also increase the force of ventricular contraction and the ejection fraction, but in healthy individuals this is not adequate to maintain cardiac output, particularly during high heart rates and short cardiac filling times.

Cutaneous Vasoconstriction

When near-maximal heart rates are attained and the cardiac output is falling as a result of reduced filling pressure, cutaneous vasoconstriction occurs in spite of the firmly established vasodilator drive. This, in turn, decreases an already marginal heat transfer from the core to the surface, resulting in heat storage, but helps maintain arterial blood pressure, cardiac filling, and thus, indirectly, muscle perfusion. Vasoconstriction during falling systemic blood pressure is activated by baroreflexes, which override thermoregulatory activity. It is not clear, however, whether cutaneous vasoconstriction is initiated by critical decrease in blood volume, increased internal body temperature, a specific level of peripheral flood flow, or, perhaps, critical reduction in the cardiac output (Nadel et al. [2]). During cycle ergometer exercise for 20–25 min at 40–70% of maximal aerobic power at different ambient temperatures, fit, non-endurance-trained subjects were able to maintain constant thermal and circulatory levels in all but heavy exertion in the heat. Thermal regulation was impaired during exercise in the heat (36°C). The esophageal temperature (an approximation of central temperature) at the termination of heavy exercise averaged almost 38.1°C during performance in comfortable ambient temperatures, but at an ambient temperature of 36°C the esophageal temperature reached almost 39°C. The cardiac output in the steady state exercise was appropriate to the oxygen uptake, but was significantly higher during exercise in the heat, and this was entirely due to increased heart rate. Thus, under varying increased ambient temperatures with moderate exercise, the cardiac output can be elevated above that found under cool conditions, in order to deliver the appropriate amount of blood to both muscles and skin. During heavy exercise in the heat, however, it becomes more and more difficult to increase cardiac output because the heart rate is approaching maximum levels for a given individual, and stroke volume is, therefore, limited. Under those conditions, cardiac output is maintained as in cooler ambient temperatures but is achieved only with a relative cutaneous vasoconstriction superimposed upon the heat-induced vasodilation.

Stroke Volume and Plasma Volume Cutaneous vasoconstriction occurred when stroke volume and plasma volumes began to decrease. Skin vasoconstriction, therefore, presumably prevented further reduction in stroke volume and stabilized central circulation. The price of stabilization by skin vasoconstriction is, of course, decreased heat transfer from the core to the surface, and central body temperature rises after 20 min of exercise. Therefore, in subjects who are not endurance-trained or heat-acclimated, circulatory regulation takes precedence over temperature homeostasis.

Body Position There is some evidence that cutaneous vasoconstriction during exercise in heat is influenced by body position. Vasoconstriction is greater in the upright position than when the subject is semi-upright on a bicycle ergometer. Evidence that this vasoconstriction is produced by activation of cardiopulmonary baroreflexes has now been found (Roberts and Wenger [3]). The absence of this cutaneous constrictor response at a critical level of exercise in the heat may cause a precipitous fall in stroke volume and, therefore, of cardiac output, forcing termination of exercise and collapse of the athlete. Furthermore, if peripheral venous hydrostatic pressure due to upright posture is abolished by supine exercise, which increases venous return from the periphery to the heart, then the cutaneous vasoconstriction is abolished because, at least with moderate exercise duration, cardiac output is not impaired (Nadel [4]).

HYDRATION, EXERCISE, AND THERMOREGULATION

It has been known empirically for some time that dehydration profoundly affects body temperature and circulation during heating or prolonged submaximal exercise or both. Experimentally, core temperatures were higher in dehydrated subjects at a given intensity of work than when the same subjects were normally hydrated, and similar observations were made in dehydrated subjects at rest. Reduced sweating and forearm blood flow under conditions of dehydration have been attributed to higher internal body temperature and inadequate temperature regulation. The mechanism by which the thermoregulatory system is modified by hydration, however, is still controversial. It is not, for example, clear whether dehydration changes the thermoregulatory activity of central nervous system neurons or whether it decreases the activity of thermoregulatory effector systems in response to certain central signals.

Blood Volume Effect

Some investigators have found that impaired cardiac output during exercise while one is dehydrated must result from dependence, at least to some extent, upon the initial blood volume. It seems, therefore, if one accepts this interpretation, that during exercise with a high initial blood volume, exercise-induced decrease in plasma volume is less likely to cause circulatory strain than if the same plasma volume were lost with a low initial blood volume. Therefore, in hypovolemia, circulatory adjustments must occur more quickly if physical activity is to continue. This, however, does not indicate whether peripheral circulation is impaired in order to maintain muscular perfusion during dehydration; nor does it examine how cutaneous blood flow is affected if the muscles are adequately perfused during dehydration-association exercise.

Attempts to answer these questions were made in subjects who were exercised in a normally hydrated, dehydrated (approximately 5% of body weight loss), or overhydrated condition. Again, these subjects were fit but had not been trained for endurance. They exercised for a relatively short time in a semi-upright position on a cycle ergometer at 60–70% of maximum oxygen uptake in the heat (36°C). During these experiments the thresholds for cutaneous vasodilation were considerably higher in dehydrated subjects, but once vasodilation occurred, the relationship between central temperature and blood flow was similar to that in normally hydrated subjects.

From this it may be concluded that heat transfer of the cutaneous circulatory bed is as responsive per unit of central temperature change in hypovolemic as in normovolemic individuals. Surprisingly, however, the vasoconstrictor influence was superimposed upon the heat-induced cutaneous vasodilatation at very much reduced blood flows during dehydration. The differences in blood flow between control and hyperhydrated subjects were not significant.

Results of Dehydration or Hypovolemia   The consequences of dehydration are that the increased central temperature threshold for vasodilation and the relative vasoconstriction at higher internal temperature in hypovolemic subjects cause much greater elevation in body temperature than in well-hydrated exercising individuals, even though total heat production is the same. The notion, therefore, that maintenance of adequate circulation takes precedence over temperature regulation in conditions of high demand upon multiple systems suggests that the sparing of circulation varies between an initial hypovolemic state and progressive decrease in blood volume during heavy exercise.

During dehydration or initial hypovolemia, the vasodilator threshold shift to the right implies that the central nervous system is responsible for this phenomenon because a change in the gain of the thermal detector does not occur. When normal hydration prevails, however, the central nervous system increases the vasoconstrictor drive to the periphery during progressive fluid loss with exercise. Experiments on subjects with mild hyperosmolality have shown that central nervous osmoreceptors are also involved in the control of the peripheral circulation. They, however, seem to be subordinate to the "volume receptors" because the hypovolemic vasodilatory shift appears without an increase in plasma osmolality.

Muscular Activity   Muscular activity places a burden on both thermoregulatory and skin vasomotor systems by creating a thermal load proportional to exercise intensity and causes a reduction in central blood volume that is also related to the amount of work performed.

When extreme heat or dehydration prevails, compromises in cutaneous circulation and thermoregulation are made. Increased body temperature, attributed to increased metabolism of the exercising muscles, is perceived in the central nervous system. A central temperature threshold for vasodilatation in the cutaneous vascular bed exists, which allows increased blood flow proportional to the increased temperature.

When skin blood flow is high, venous return and cardiac filling are reduced. Egress of fluid from the vasculature during exercise also decreases plasma volume. At that point, cutaneous vasoconstriction occurs, and this redirects some of the blood to the heart. In turn, heat transfer is reduced from the core to the surface. If, under these circumstances, cardiac filling improves, as may occur with recumbent posture, cutaneous vasoconstriction is immediately abolished and the core-to-skin transfer of heat is improved.

When relative dehydration is present at the beginning of exercise, the threshold for cutaneous vasodilation shifts to higher central temperatures, suggesting the presence of centrally generated inhibition of the vasodilator drive. How this occurs is not clear. Nevertheless, answers to these questions and elucidation of the mechanisms of temperature regulation operative in endurance-trained and heat-acclimated subjects may give an insight into physical capabilities and ways of improving performance during heat stress in athletes.

Effects of Heat

The effect of a desert environment (dry heat) on work and cardiac output during rest and during exercise has been examined in young and old subjects (Myhre et al. [5]). Surprisingly, during short-term exercise, cardiac output was unchanged, irrespective of whether activity was in a comfortable, cool environment or in the desert sun. During short-term exercise the metabolic rate is, apparently, the sole factor that determines cardiac output and not the environmental heat stress. Therefore, short-term exercise in dry heat can be sustained, provided the heart rate increases to compensate for the reduced stroke volume.

An increased heart rate, however, is not the case for endurance events in which maximum heart rate occurs during exercise requiring less than maximum oxygen consumption. One subject in this study, who had been examined 50 years earlier and again under similar conditions at age 85, showed no change in his ability to cope with the dry heat of the desert during short-term exercise. The changes in his performance were attributable to decreased muscle mass and strength and decreased respiratory and cardiovascular reserve. No changes were observed in the thermoregulatory system.

Comparisons of the work capacity of acclimatized and unacclimatized subjects and of acclimatized fit subjects in the desert environment heat have also been made (Wells et al. [6]). Prior observations showed that trained, unacclimatized runners are heat-tolerant to the extent that exercise hyperthermia with training at any environmental temperature may "pre-acclimatize" them to perform better in hot ambient temperatures. Intensive running may improve capacity for heat acclimatization so that a highly trained, unacclimatized person may not actually exist. It has been reported that training in humid heat improves heat tolerance during subsequent performance in moderate ambient temperatures. Moreover, anecdotal reports from the Honolulu marathon, staged in hot and humid conditions, suggest that Hawaiian runners perform better than those from the mainland.

Significance of Physical Fitness

Subsequent studies on work performance of subjects of varying physical fitness in dry heat with significant solar exposure also show that acclimatization both of those who are fit and those who are average nonfit persons offers definite cardiovascular advantages for work in heat. In the acclimatized subjects, heart rates were lower during equal work, and rectal temperatures of acclimatized, fit subjects performing higher work loads did not reflect any greater metabolic heat load than those of unacclimatized subjects in the heat. Moreover, the better cardiovascular function of endurance-trained members of the study during work in the heat also suggested larger stroke volumes.

In unacclimatized subjects, even though evaporative rates did not differ from those of acclimatized subjects, skin temperatures were very much higher, a result suggesting that unacclimatized persons must have greater cutaneous blood flow. This may constitute a disadvantage, since the higher peripheral flow lowers stroke volume and increases heart rate to maintain cardiac output. If one assumes that the central temperature is the main drive for an increasing cutaneous blood flow with work, then those who were acclimatized and particularly those who were endurance-trained had less cardiovascular strain during work in the heat.

Endurance training probably does not increase sweating, but endurance-trained subjects may sweat at lower central temperatures, and continuous aerobic activity may enhance sweating sensitivity. Because heat acclimatization in both fit and physically untrained subjects causes lower central temperatures for a given amount of work in hot ambient conditions, a smaller fraction of the cardiac output need go to the skin to maintain temperature homeostasis. This might result from increased sweating sensitivity after acclimatization.

One may conclude, therefore, that heat acclimatization decreases work strain in hot environments and that endurance training 1) offers an added advantage when continuously high metabolic heat loads, preferably with an additional external heat load, are used; 2) further improves the performance; and 3) decreases cardiovascular and homeothermic regulatory stress. It is clear that heat- and exercise-acclimatized subjects dissipate thermal loads more efficiently, thus decreasing peripheral circulatory demands, with the result that cardiovascular performance is improved (Wells et al. [6]).

Plasma Volume Expansion   One aspect of natural or artificial acclimatization to heat is a 10–25% expansion of plasma volume. In addition, isotonic expansion of the interstitial fluid also occurs. A close correlation has been observed between increased plasma volume and the thermoregulatory and cardiovascular adaptations to heat. Increased plasma volume presumably enhances heat tolerance and improves physical performance during high ambient temperatures by decreasing core body temperature and heart strain. In addition, endurance training also increases blood volume, mainly as a result of increased plasma volume.

Hypervolemia is associated with decreased heart rate, increased stroke volume during both rest and exercise, and a reduced hematocrit. All of these are associated with increased maximum oxygen uptake and cardiac output. There are, therefore, close similarities between thermoregulatory adaptive responses to a hot environment and those to exercise training—namely, an increased sweat rate, decreased heat storage, and decreased core temperature at certain work loads.

Plasma volume expansion during heat acclimatization is a thermoregulatory adaptive response, but most studies employed exercise in addition to heat exposure. Therefore, it is unclear whether the hypervolemia after exercise training is primarily the result of thermal stress or is induced by endurance training with its associated increased metabolic demands and internal heat loads. Nevertheless, a recent study suggested that exercise-induced hypervolemia is associated with 40% thermal factors and 60% nonthermal factors. The nonthermal exercise-induced factors were a twofold increase in plasma osmotic and vasopressor forces during exercise and a fivefold increase in resting plasma protein, all of which contribute to the hypervolemia. Two groups of subjects were exposed to either exercise training or heat, each of which raised rectal temperatures to the same levels. Plasma volume increased more during exercise training in a cool environment than during testing in a hot environment, a finding that supports the proposition that metabolic factors, in addition to external heat loads, are important in raising plasma volume during endurance training in either hot or cool ambient temperatures.

The hypothesis, therefore, that increased metabolism or other factors induced by exercise in the heat are necessary for maximal expansion of plasma volume and maximal performance under hot environmental temperature is further supported. The question has also been addressed as to how often thermoregulatory and metabolic systems need to be stressed in order to maintain the adaptive responses induced by heat and exercise training for expansion of plasma volume. Studies suggest that chronic intermittent exercise and heat exposure should be applied at least at 4-day intervals and that the adaptive plasma volume expansion diminishes significantly within a week when no further stresses are applied.

The studies of plasma proteins and their relations to hypervolemia during exercise and heat exposure suggest that exercise rather than environmental body heating was the main stimulus to hyperproteinemia. The cause of the increase in plasma proteins, however, with the associated hypervolemia, is not clear. Whether the additional protein is derived entirely from cutaneous interstitial spaces by means of a "flushing action" on the lymphatics or is the result of increased synthesis or decreased degradation has not been established.

The relationships of plasma electrolyte osmotic and endocrine responses to the hypervolemia in the experimental conditions of exercise alone or heat exposure without exercise are complex and not fully understood. Angiotensin and vasopressin increase more during exercise than during heat exposure alone, and this rise is accompanied by increased plasma osmolality. The hyperosmolality associated with prolonged exercise seems to be the dominant stimulus for the release of angiotensin and vasopressin. The hypervolemia also occurring during exercise is a secondary stimulus.

Surprisingly, the increase in vasopressin during exercise did not stimulate an appropriate increase in plasma renin. This result implies that plasma renin was at an optimal level to produce maximum sodium retention and protect against stress-induced plasma volume loss. It seems, then, that reduced plasma volume during exercise training, exposure to heat, and increased plasma renin were not primary factors accounting for the increased plasma volume.

The changes in the angiotensin-vasopressin system and the increased plasma osmolality during exercise training were closely related to the chronic hypervolemia. Therefore, during either heat acclimatization or endurance training, elevated plasma renin enhances sodium retention, which, in turn, increases plasma osmolality and vasopressin and thus promotes fluid retention. Whether sufficient stimuli are left after intermittent exposure to stress to account for the progressive chronic hypervolemia of either endurance training or heat acclimatization or both, is not clear. However, the fluid balance seems to be restored after stress in direct proportion to the length of exposure and the level of dehydration that occurred. Exercise depletes intracellular water more than does rest in a hot environment. Therefore, it is possible that depletion of intracellular fluid is more important than depletion of extracellular fluid volume in the production of chronic hypervolemia of heat adaptation and endurance training (Convertino et al. [7]).

The sauna has been used by some for heat acclimatization, particularly if ambient conditions are not suitable for this. Exercise on bicycle ergometers in saunas has been used for this purpose. It is also not uncommon to take a sauna after strenuous exercise. The exposure to the high temperatures places stress on the homeothermy and cardiovascular adaptive mechanisms.

Peripheral vasodilatation, which occurs during heat load in the sauna, is evidenced by increased heart rates and great variability in systolic and diastolic blood pressures. Myocardial ischemia and associated electrocardiographic changes during sauna exposure have been reported (Taggart et al. [8]).

The response of the normal person to additional heat in the sauna after heavy exercise and its metabolic heat load is not known. A recent study compared aspects of exposure to a sauna environment during recovery from heavy exercise with recovery in a comfortable environment (Paolone et al. [9]). Electrical repolarization of the cardiac conducting system differed during recovery following heat exposure from that during recovery in comfortable conditions; specifically, increased J-point displacement, prolongation of the QT interval, and loss of T-wave amplitude were noted.

These changes were associated with decreased diastolic blood pressure, elevated central body temperature, and greater myocardial oxygen demand. The J-point displacement seen during the final periods of exercise was attributed to the increased heart rate, and recovery in the hot environment was much delayed. The decrease in T-wave amplitudes in intense heat is well recognized and is probably due to the decreased stroke volume that accompanies heat exposure. The clinical significance of the prolonged QT interval in hot ambient conditions after exercise is not fully appreciated. It may be a secondary response to the discrepancy between oxygen supply and demand and perhaps signifies impending ischemic ST change.

From this study it was clear that the putative reduction in myocardial oxygen supply did not produce ischemic ST segment changes in normal subjects. This was interpreted to show that the low myocardial oxygen demand in the healthy person at rest, even in the sauna, does not lead to myocardial ischemia, despite increased heart rate. Although a number of electrocardiographic changes during sauna exposure after heavy physical exercise occurred in normal subjects, it seems that these do not pose an undue risk to those who are clinically normal and wish to engage in this post-exercise activity.

DECONDITIONING AND TEMPERATURE REGULATION

Although we have some understanding of the basic mechanisms of adaptation to chronic intermittent exercise in normal subjects, the mechanism of deconditioning during bed rest is less understood. During the Apollo missions, following bed rest and after prolonged water immersion, decreased maximal oxygen intake, reduced plasma volume, and loss of cardiovascular tolerance to tilting were found. Exercise, either prior to or during exposure to weightlessness or to bed rest provided some protection from the deconditioning effects.

Deconditioning seems to result from, or at least seems to be associated with, reduced hydrostatic pressure on the cardiovascular system from recumbency and the elimination of longitudinal pressure on bones and muscles, together with reduced daily energy output as a result of decreased physical activity. The physiologic changes that occur during deconditioning include diuresis, reduced plasma volume, decreased red blood cell mass, and lower body weight. There is also decreased heart volume, impaired vasomotor tone, and changed carbohydrate metabolism, all of which may contribute to the decreased maximum oxygen uptake and changes in orthostatic and acceleration tolerances.

Moreover, the hypovolemia and impaired vasomotor tone could clearly affect thermoregulatory responses. The effect of bed rest deconditioning on temperature regulation is not well known. Most data on temperature before, during, and after bed rest were derived from non-exercising subjects who felt chilly, especially in the legs, at normally comfortable ambient temperatures and humidities after the second month of a 4-month bed-rest study. The time taken for the rectal temperature to return to control levels after elevation from arm immersion in hot water was increased during bed rest, but the time to onset of sweating in response to progressively increased ambient temperatures was significantly shortened and occurred at lower skin temperatures after 14 days of bed rest. After prolonged bed rest, auditory canal temperatures decreased in humans. In animals exercised to exhaustion after prolonged confinement, rectal temperatures rose more rapidly. Therefore, the evidence, though still fragmentary, indicates that impairment of body temperature regulation exists after deconditioning.

The question of whether bed rest changes thermoregulatory responses during rest and exercise, and if so, whether this can be influenced by isometric exercise during bed rest, was studied. Rectal and mean skin temperatures and sweating responses were measured in 7 men during 70 min of submaximal supine exercise while ambulatory and after three 2-week bed-rest periods separated by 3 weeks of normal ambulation. During each of the three bed-rest periods, isometric or isotonic exercises for 1 hr per day, or no exercise, were carried out. The results of this study suggest that the excessive rise in rectal temperature during submaximal exercise after bed-rest deconditioning is influenced by changes in skin heat conductance and that there is also a relative inhibition of sweating, which may be a factor in the increased core temperature. The mechanism, however, for the hyperthermic response is not definitively established, although decreased plasma volume found during all three bed-rest periods could account for the excessive increases in rectal temperature.

In ambulatory subjects, such a decrease in plasma volume would be accounted for by inhibition of sweating. The impaired peripheral vascular function during prolonged bed rest could also account for the feeling of coldness in the extremities. The maximum oxygen uptake decreased after bed rest and, in the experiments reported here, the work load given in the exercise experiments did cause a constant absolute oxygen uptake; subjects were, therefore, working at a greater load after the rest period. It is not clear whether this greater load, evidenced by relatively submaximal heart rates, could also have played a role in the hyperthermic response to exercise after bed rest. Fragmentary evidence suggests that greater skin conductance of heat is associated with lower rectal temperature and vice versa, implying variable heat transfer from the core to the periphery. Evidence so far on this aspect of temperature control in relation to deconditioning is incomplete, but it does suggest that the excessively increased rectal temperatures during exercise after various periods of bed rest might be, at least in part, due to changes in skin conductance of heat and also to increased sweating sensitivity and evaporative heat loss (Greenleaf and Reese [10]).

The influence of heat acclimatization combined with exercise at 50% of maximum oxygen uptake on the deconditioning responses after 8 hr of water immersion was examined (Schvarz et al. [11]). The question addressed whether or not heat acclimatization prevents deconditioning after water immersion and is superior to exercise training in a cool environment. Heat acclimatization, together with exercise in a hot environment, results in improved exercise tolerance after water immersion. This is attributed to increased stroke and plasma volumes, known to occur during heat acclimatization. In the acclimated group, the changes in maximum oxygen-carrying capacity, maximal heart rate, and decreased exercise tolerance were distinctly minor compared to the changes in the control group, whose members were not heat acclimatized before water immersion. The acclimated group started water-immersion periods with higher plasma volumes than those of the controls, but water immersion, known to result in decreased plasma volume, was in fact associated with an excessive loss in the experimental group so that the postimmersion plasma volumes in the control and heat-acclimated subjects were equal.

It is interesting that the increased stroke volume, evidenced by decreased resting heart rate after acclimatization, was maintained after water immersion, but this increase in stroke volume did not occur in the control group. This might partly explain the better exercise tolerance with heat acclimatization after deconditioning. One effect of water immersion is diuresis, but this was equal in the two groups. The diuresis may reflect sodium levels during water immersion and decreases in norepinephrine excretion. The latter may have been more marked in the control group than in those acclimated to heat, because acclimatization can cause sodium conservation. Impaired sympathetic nervous system activity may have unfavorably affected the exercise tolerance in controls.

It is clear, of course, that strenuous training in cool ambient conditions is superior to heat acclimatization without exercise in improving maximum oxygen-carrying capacity, cardiac output, and oxygen delivery to the working muscles. Nevertheless, heat-acclimated subjects tested in temperate environments do have better thermoregulation than those who are trained without heat exposure. Heat acclimation may prevent the adverse effects of water-immersion deconditioning on exercise capabilities to some extent. Whether exercise capacity can be maintained by heat acclimation alone during prolonged periods of bed rest or water immersion deconditioning has not been determined (Schvarz et al. [11]).

PERIODIC THERMOREGULATION

Athletes are well aware of fluctuations in their performance that occur at different times of the day or night. This variation in physical capacity is often attributed to nonspecific causes such as diet, environmental conditions, winds, temperature, or just not feeling right. Body temperature also fluctuates over time and has been extensively studied, and the current views are summarized by Feldberg [12] and Benzinger [13]. Numerous endogenous biologic rhythms with periodicities that approximate 24 hr (circadian) or longer (infradian), or shorter than 24 hr (ultradian) occur in animals and man. Ultradian rhythms may either occur every few milliseconds or be recurrent every 90 min or so.

Rhythmic fluctuations in temperature have also been noted for many years, and the autonomic effectors of human skin have ultradian cycles with periods of several minutes. Variations in normal temperature control in homeothermic animals often are linked to periodicities of critical temperature fluctuations controlled by the thermostat, but the extent of variations in the periodicity of normal rather than critical temperature has not been extensively investigated.

An influence of biologic clocks upon perceptual phenomena has been found. For example, experiments on human subjects with visual perception measured by critical flicker fusion thresholds show a spontaneous endogenous rhythm of ultradian periodicity. Similar results have been found in subjects performing maximal speed tapping; again, an ultradian periodicity in performance has been found. These two perceptual tasks show the same ultradian periodicities and this, of course, suggests consistencies in quantitative aspects of perceptions. Therefore, any change in perceptual acuity might act as a *Zeitgeber* (time signal) in the regulation of perceptual clocks. An obvious *Zeitgeber* is, of course, the onset of sleep, at which time a change in body temperature occurs. Sleep onset is also, perhaps, accompanied by slowing of perceptual clocks. In a large number of healthy subjects, skin temperature was recorded every 60 sec, in both the awake and sleeping state. The rhythms were significantly longer during sleep than waking, in a subsequent study using autocorrelation analysis of the results. The ultradian periodicities of temperature were similar on the hand, in the axilla, and on the tympanic membrane. It is, therefore, suggested that hypothalamic temperature oscillations of ultradian periodicity may be the source of these temperature rhythms (Lovett-Doust [14]).

Blood flow in small capillaries of the skin is fluctuant rather than random. Periodic capillary flow may be necessary to ensure adequate oxygenation of small capillaries, particularly those with diameters smaller than red blood cells. Furthermore, it has been suggested that an animal's body weight, rather than its surface area, governs rhythmic fluctuations of temperature, blood flow, oxygen consumption, and heart rate (Iberall [15]). From the extensive studies of the ultradian perceptual clock, it is known that its properties include endogenous rhythm and dependency upon neural integrity; it can be entrained by damage to the nervous system; it is capable of phase shifts by single perturbations; it has a small variance; and moreover, it seems to be independent of environmental and relatively free from chemical or hormonal influences. This perceptual clock maintains the foregoing characteristics independently of intercurrent events or reactive feeling states in humans. Skin temperatures in ordinary subjects at rest in a pleasant ambient environment are controlled by mechanisms that emit ultradian pulsations. The periodicity of these mechanisms is related to the subject's state of alertness and is much longer during sleep. It may be that body temperature and ultradian variation in alertness are responsible for the differential performance of individuals at different times of the 24-hr cycle. Whether endurance training with its profound effect upon homeothermic mechanisms influences the ultradian periodicity of temperature has not been established. In some highly abnormal states, as in schizophrenia during abnormal perception, the ultradian temperature fluctuations are prolonged, a finding that suggests that at least in humans, a change in the periodicities of temperature and perhaps ultradian rhythms in perception occurs in certain pathologic conditions (Lovett-Doust [16]).

TEMPERATURE REGULATION AND THE MARATHON

Some regulatory responses during long-duration sporting events have been measured. The performance of athletes in such events depends to a great extent upon their capacity to lose the excess metabolic heat produced during long exertion. The transfer of heat from the core to the surface and dissipation through convection, radiation, and sweating become important in these circumstances. Anything that reduces blood flow to the skin or sweat evaporation markedly decreases efficiency of temperature regulation and increases the risk of overheating and cardiovascular collapse. Core temperatures in marathoners may reach 40°C or higher, even in cool weather.

During long-term athletic performances, such as marathon races, body temperature depends upon metabolic rate, and this, in turn, is affected by work load and body weight. Therefore, heavier athletes have higher rectal temperatures than do lighter competitors, even when performing at the same pace. In order to maintain body temperature, large evaporative sweat losses occur during prolonged competition. Those with unsuitable hydration prior to competition may, therefore, be at a disadvantage and have inordinate increases in body temperature, thus seriously limiting performance and increasing the risk of hyperthermia.

Animals that run at very high speeds can increase heat production to 60 times above resting values but will refuse to continue running, unlike human beings, if their central temperature reaches a certain level. The distance, therefore, over which they are conditioned to pursue prey is limited only by the rise of body temperature. Human beings, on the other hand, continue physical work in spite of high body temperatures until collapse or other serious consequences occur.

HEAT ILLNESS

There are four varieties of heat illness: 1) heat stroke, or high body temperature in a setting of impaired consciousness, delirium, and convulsions; 2) heat hyperpyrexia, a condition in which none of the clinical features of heat stroke occurs, except for body temperature greater than 41°C associated with excessive heat load or abnormalities in thermoregulation; 3) anhidrotic heat exhaustion, the absence of sweating because of sweat gland abnormalities and hot environment, causing abnormally high body temperatures; and 4) acute anhidrotic heat exhaustion, associated with mild infections in hot and humid climates.

In the fourth condition, the first symptom of infection may be failure of sweating in hot ambient temperatures rather than the usual chill, rigor, and fever. Such patients may also notice sudden cessation of sweating during exertion, associated with headache, anorexia, confusion, and mild ataxia. In this condition, the skin is hot and dry but otherwise normal, and normal thermoregulation, including sweating, will return within a day or two with recovery, if cooling is accomplished and exertion is temporarily curtailed.

Heat Stroke

When rectal temperatures reach 41°–43°C and are associated with disturbed consciousness, mortality ranges from 50% to 70%. This situation can occur during excessive heat storage generated by working muscle during a marathon run, particularly in adverse conditions that make heat dissipation difficult or impossible. An understanding of the pathogenesis of heat stroke makes it preventable and should reduce mortality during heat waves, which claim 4000 lives per year in cities around the United States.

Preventive measures include education of those exposed to heat and humidity because of ambient conditions, and in particular, education of athletes to avoid excessive heat loads by limiting physical work. Close attention to hydration and adequate, but not excessive, salt intake during physical work may also help prevent heat stroke, a condition that is not confined to the healthy and young athlete or military recruit in training in hot and humid climates, but also occurs in the elderly during heat waves.

In the elderly, heat stroke is often associated with preexisting disease, such as atherosclerotic heart disease, diabetes mellitus, or alcoholism. The use of phenothiazines, anticholinergic drugs, sedatives, or diuretics predisposes to heat stroke by action upon the thermoregulatory effector system.

Deaths from all causes during the July 1980 heat wave in St. Louis and Kansas City, Missouri, increased by 57% in St. Louis and 64% in Kansas City. While deaths in the predominantly rural areas of Missouri increased by only 10%, one of every 1000 residents in the two cities was hospitalized for or died from heat-related illness during the heat wave. The incidence rates of documented hyperthermia were 26.5% in St. Louis and 17.6% in Kansas City, and those for persons over 65 years of age were 12 times higher than for younger individuals (Jones et al. [17]).

Assessment of risk factors for heat stroke in the same heat wave indicated that, apart from air conditioning and shaded residences, those who were able to care for themselves and engaged in vigorous physical activity, but reduced their activity during the heat wave and took extra fluids, were less at risk for heat stroke than those who were less able or normally less inclined to physical effort (Kilbourne et al. [18]).

Symptoms Heat stroke is a medical emergency, and delay in diagnosis and treatment may lead to death or irreversible damage. It should be suspected in any person whose behavior or mental status changes during heat stress.

The criteria of diagnosis include high environmental temperatures and humidity, high rectal temperature, sometimes (though not always) hot, dry skin, and cardiovascular and central nervous system disturbances leading to clouded consciousness and collapse.

In exercise-associated heat stroke, the hemodynamic changes are those that occur normally during adaptation to heat with exercise; that is, increased heart rate and cardiac output, and decreased systemic vascular resistance and appropriate responses of effector organs that increase heat dissipation. These hemodynamic changes occur in impending heat stroke in young or older individuals in whom exercise results in excessive circulatory loads.

In contrast, elderly patients suffering from heat stroke unassociated with exertion have decreased cardiac output and increased peripheral resistance. The exact mechanism of this response in the elderly is not fully understood, but may be related to their inability to counter ambient heat loads with tachycardia and cutaneous vasodilation during increasing body temperature.

Hypovolemia is present in exercise-associated heat stroke in the young or in disease-associated heat stroke in the elderly, and correction of this with large amounts of intravenous fluids does not seem to result in pulmonary edema, perhaps because of the inappropriately low cardiac output.

A hyperventilatory response to extreme heat occurs, but patients with heat stroke continue to hyperventilate and develop respiratory alkalosis. In addition, because of the hypovolemia and hypotension, the increased metabolic demands cannot be met and lactic acidosis often is also present, so that combined respiratory alkalosis and metabolic acidosis coexist.

Temperature correction of arterial blood gas measurements is necessary for accurate assessment of the metabolic respiratory changes in patients with heat stroke. Though the heat stroke patient may appear to have respiratory alkalosis and hypoxemia, correction for the increased temperature may show metabolic acidosis without hypoxemia. Therapeutic decisions based on the metabolic status of patients should be made only after temperature conversion of the blood gas results.

Hypokalemia, hypocalcemia, and hypophosphatemia are common, and rhabdomyolysis may occur in exertion-induced heat stroke, but the latter is rarely seen in those who did not exercise prior to the hyperthermia. In addition, hypoglycemia is a feature of exertion-induced heat stroke, whereas hyperglycemia is the rule in other patients.

Heat stroke is the second cause of death among athletes in this country, despite the fact that it is preventable, and, in addition, it affects a significant proportion of people over the age of 50. It is important to avoid heat stroke, whenever possible, by heat acclimatization, adequate hydration, and endurance training, which, as mentioned earlier, improves the capacity of the homeothermic system to dissipate heat.

Abnormalities of nervous system function in heat stroke include loss of consciousness or a sense of impending doom, headache, dizziness, confusion, and weakness. On occasion, euphoria may precede coma. Agitated delirium can appear, once the patient is stuporous, and extensor plantar responses, abnormalities in pupillary reactions to light, and seizures have also been observed. Occasionally, in severe cases, hemiplegia, incontinence, and decorticate posturing occur.

With cooling, consciousness returns promptly if the hyperpyrexia has not persisted for too long. If unconsciousness persists for 24 hr or longer and seizures are present, recovery is rarely full, and neurologic deficits of varying degree may be found some time after clinical improvement. In such patients, cerebellar function is particularly affected and the cerebellar deficits may be permanent.

On examination of the circulatory system of patients with heat stroke, the rapid pulse and wide pulse pressures are striking, and ST segment depression and T-wave changes, often with supraventricular tachycardias, may be seen. Although the cardiac output falls eventually, survival depends upon an increased cardiac output to meet the excessive circulatory demands. In addition, blood flow is high in skin and muscles, particularly in heat stroke associated with exercise, a result of a decreased vascular resistance, but splanchnic blood flow is reduced. Even when body temperature is restored to normal, the cardiac output remains high and the peripheral resistance low for hours, a condition not dissimilar to that seen after trauma or during severe infection.

Myocardial injury and sometimes increased pulmonary vascular resistance are the causes of heart failure in heat stroke. In addition, the petechiae and often large hemorrhages that occur, together with consumptive coagulopathy, have been attributed to heat-induced vascular endothelial damage, which has been identified by electron microscopy. Dehydration and electrolyte imbalances are seen most often and are most severe in cases associated with sports, particularly marathon running. Acute tubular necrosis occurs in 10–35% of heat stroke patients and is related to direct injury to the tubules by heat, circulating blood pigments, and reduced renal blood flow.

In some patients, histologic evidence of liver damage includes central lobular necrosis and extensive cholestasis, findings particularly prominent in liver biopsies from gold miners after heart stroke. In these subjects, heat exposure, exertion, and dehydration must have been present. Occasionally in marathon runners with severe heat stroke, transient malabsorption syndromes have occurred, but these abnormalities did not persist for longer than 3 months. Perhaps heat damage to the ileal mucosa with subsequent regeneration accounts for the clinical course of this disorder.

Treatment of Heat Stroke   There are two principles of treatment of heat stroke. First, the body should be cooled, and second, vital systems should be supported. Clothing should be removed and the patient placed in an ice-cold bath or cooling blanket if available. Naturally, in the field, substitution of these cooling methods by wet clothing and increased air circulation, together with shading, may be the only modalities available. Massage of the extremities promotes cooling because it counteracts the cutaneous circulatory stasis.

Once the body temperature falls, the patient should be removed from the cold environment. Reflex shivering, which tends to raise body temperature, sometimes occurs concurrently with a precipitous drop in core temperature, together with a cold stimulus on the skin. Phenothiazines may be used during the continued cooling to avoid this occurrence.

Support of the cardiovascular system to ensure continuous high cardiac output by correction of dehydration, hypovolemia, and acid-base disturbances should be prominent on the list, particularly for heat stroke associated with exertion, such as marathon runs. Intravenous fluid (1400 ml) is usually recommended in the first hour of treatment, but more, of course, needs to be given to those patients in whom heat stroke occurred after prolonged exertion.

Urine output must be carefully monitored at hourly intervals through a catheter, and if necessary, mannitol should be given to promote diuresis. Digitalis for heart failure, when it appears, can improve myocardial contractility, but because of the occasional respiratory alkalosis, digitalis toxicity may occur. Sometimes β-adrenergic stimulation by isoproterenol can increase cardiac output to its necessary level, but α-adrenergic drugs should not be used, because they decrease skin perfusion and, therefore, impede heat exchange. If oxygen tension falls, oxygen may be given, though hypoxemia and shunting of blood through the lungs is not common in heat stroke. The therapy of disseminated intravascular coagulation with heparin in a dose of 7500 units every 4 hr is also useful. If coma persists in spite of normal body temperatures and normal kidney function, diuretics and urea or other dehydrating agents to reduce brain edema are necessary. For seizures, anticonvulsants are used in the usual manner. Most patients recover in a few hours if cooling, maintenance of the circulation, and hydration are prompt.

Heat Stroke During Marathon Running

The explosive growth of interest in long-distance running has led to serious problems in many endurance events during climatic conditions favoring heat stroke when sufficient precautions are not taken. The well-trained, heat-acclimated athlete may compete under conditions that would ordinarily cause heat stroke in the poorly trained or those trained in cold environments.

There are several climatic and situational factors that may lead to heat stroke, even in relatively cool ambient conditions, under continuous and high endogenous heat production such as that seen during marathon or ultramarathon competition. These factors are as follows:

1.   At the beginning of a race, running speed is usually fast and large amounts of blood are shunted from the skin and other organs to active muscles.
2.   Increased body temperature normally accompanies strenuous muscular activity and leads to sweating.

3. If the environment is hot or, particularly, humid and windless, decreased evaporative heat loss from sweating by convection and radiation from the skin occurs. Moreover, the decreased blood flow through the skin at a time when cardiac output must be maintained to sustain continuous muscular activity contributes to decreased convection and radiation and, therefore, considerable reduction in heat transfer from the body core to the surface.
4. The normally high sweat rates contribute to dehydration.
5. Once dehydration appears, the high cardiac output cannot be maintained, and skin blood flow is further reduced because of decreased intravascular volume and the overriding need to supply adequate blood to active muscles.

This is the vicious cycle that leads to heat stroke. Once this cycle occurs, sudden decrease in sweating heralds impending heat stroke and should be the signal for competitors to abandon further exertion. The decreased sweat rate is due to progressive dehydration and once this appears, body temperature increases rapidly and collapse ensues. Warning signs need to be heeded.

Impending heat stroke is associated with decreased capacity for continuous physical performance, clouding of consciousness, ataxia, and decreased sweat rate in spite of continuous muscular activity. It is imperative that preventive and restorative measures be taken at this stage rather than after collapse, when restoration of homeothermy may be difficult and the high body temperature is dangerous to a variety of organs.

Nonexertional Heat Stroke

Two million or more people from 80 different nations gather annually for the Makkah Hajj. This traditional 7-day pilgrimage to Mecca is a gigantic recurring experiment in human temperature regulation. The large number of people squeezed into a small area at high ambient temperatures (dry bulb 35°–50°C) and the rites of pilgrimage involving unaccustomed exertion further stress participants' heat-dissipating mechanisms. In one pilgrimage week in September 1982, a review of 172 heat stroke patients from Mina and Arafat treatment centers showed that 85% were comatose and 69% had constricted pupils (Al-Khalwashki et al. [19]). The pathogenesis of coma in severe heat stroke is unknown, and although a variety of hypotheses have been proposed, none has been confirmed in humans.

Endogenous opioids are secreted during physical and emotional stress (Thompson [20]). Both exogenous opiates and endogenous opioids modulate thermoregulation and constrict pupils. In certain diseases, coma is reversible by naloxone and high levels of opiods are measurable in the brain and cerebrospinal fluid. Endocrine responses in this unique setting (measurements of "stress hormones" including immunoactive β-endorphin secreted by the pituitary and adrenal glands) during heat stroke and after recovery in previously healthy pilgrims have been reported (Appenzeller et al. [21]). The plasma levels of each of the four "stress hormones" were significantly elevated during acute heat stroke in comparison with the convalescence. And an analysis of variance for comparison of mean percentage changes in β-endorphin levels with those of stress hormones showed significant differences (Fig. 2-1).

While emotional stress during the Makkah Hajj is presumed, it is neither uniform nor measurable (Khogali [22]). The severity of heat stress, on the other hand, can be quantified and the hormonal responses to ambient heat, while possibly a nonspecific reaction to stress, suggest nevertheless that hormonal secretion during hyperthermia is distinct from that found in response to other stressors such as physical exercise, hypoglycemia, or even hypnotic suggestion of hyperthermia (Vigas [23]; Adlercreutz et al. [24]). Such earlier studies have identified rises in growth hormone prolactin and cortisol during hyperthermia, but

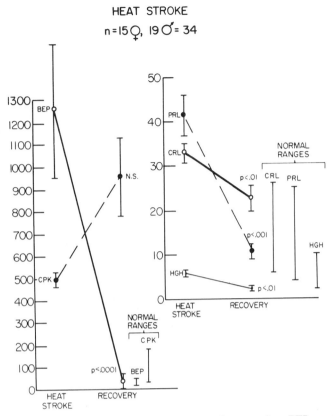

2-1 Endocrine response during and after spontaneous heat stroke. BEP = β-endorphin–β-lipotropin; CPK = creatine phosphokinase; PRL = prolactin; CRL = cortisol; HGH = growth hormone.

plasma β-endorphin–β-lipotropin values have not hitherto been reported in heat stroke patients. While the Makkah Hajj victims of 1982 were a unique group, the results are nevertheless similar to descriptions of sauna-induced hormone secretion (Leppaluoto et al. [25]), which have identified rises in growth hormone, prolactin, and cortisol during hyperthermia. The importance of circulating (pituitary) β-endorphin in heat adaptation is reinforced by animal studies in which hypophysectomy diminished naloxone hyperthermia during acute heat exposure (Holaday et al. [26]), and the normal rise in body temperature with exercise in humans is abolished by naloxone (DeMeirler et al. [27]).

The effectiveness of naloxone in reversing certain forms of shock and coma apparently results from its normalization of the sympathetic-parasympathetic balance. This balance may also be deranged during heat stroke, as suggested by the characteristically dry skin and miosis and by precipitation of experimental heat stroke by atropine (Hubbard et al. [28]). Though deaths of heat stroke victims during the Makkah Hajj have been reduced by expert supportive treatment and sophisticated cooling, these findings suggest a therapeutic potential for opioid antagonists in the management of such patients and also in heat stroke occurring during athletic events (Appenzeller et al. [21]).

Head Coverings and Face Fanning in the
Prevention of Central Nervous System Hyperthermia

In many animal species, selective brain cooling during hyperthermia prevents an inordinate increase in central nervous system temperature. In humans, a selective cooling mechanism of the brain also exists (Cabanac [29]). For example, the sweat secreted on the face evaporates and cools the blood in the capillary bed of the skin, which is maximally vasodilated. In hyperthermia, the blood of the face is collected and flows to the angular veins and on from the face to the brain, whereas during hypothermia the flow is reversed from the brain to the face (Caputa et al. [30]). In one study, 9 male trained subjects were exerted on a treadmill at increasing speed and slope until exhaustion with fanning of the face conducted throughout both the exercise and postexercise periods. A similar period of exertion was again attempted by the subjects but with fanning of the face ending with exercise cessation. It was found that continual fanning reduced the initial elevation in body temperature as measured on the tympanic membrane and decreased this temperature much faster after cessation of exercise. However, an increase of nearly 0.5°C occurred when fanning was stopped after the cessation of exercise.

High rectal temperatures sometimes recorded in heat stroke may not reflect temperature in the brain. Actual brain temperatures may be much lower than trunk or core temperatures, which are the most common measurements of temperature. Since it appears that selective brain cooling through fanning is a useful mechanism of defense against high brain temperatures even in humans, this may be an important factor during prolonged exertion and it is similar to the protection provided by running or bicycling (Carbanac [29]). These studies suggest that running without head covers might be important in reducing the risk of central hyperthermia during hot ambient conditions. A head cover is therefore also important in the maintenance of central homeothermy in cold conditions. Moreover, sweating seems to be preserved during dehydration (often the case at the end of a marathon) on the scalp and face. The increase in sweating on the face and head reported by many runners at the end of a run is due to the decrease in convection leading to a transient increase in central temperature after stopping. It is therefore recommended that in most ambient conditions and during prolonged exertion, head covering be omitted to ensure preservation of brain temperature within acceptable limits. Moreover, in heat stroke when intensive cooling is not readily available in the field, the face should be moistened and fanned to improve cooling of the brain.

HYPOTHERMIA

The popularity of physical activity in relatively cold environments where participants might be scantily clad is increasing. Moreover, sudden worsening in the weather, increasing winds, and wet clothing make the risk of hypothermia unpredictable and often lead to fatal outcomes. It should be stressed that clinical hypothermia may occur in persons exposed to relatively mild temperatures if prolonged exertion, dehydration, and relative lack of food, with consequent hypoglycemia, are also present. Deterioration in the judgment and strength of the exposed person with impending hypothermia is often an early sign that needs to be recognized. Hypothermia can occur with great rapidity, leading to death if preventive measures are not instituted.

When the rectal temperature falls below 30.2°C, clouding of consciousness and soon restless stupor occur. Slurring of speech, ataxia, and occasionally involuntary movements develop. Pallor, cyanosis, sometimes edema of the face, slow cerebration, and a croaky voice may suggest the presence of hypothyroidism. The body is characteristically cold; the cold is not confined to the extremities but extends to covered portions, particularly the axillae and groins. The pupils may be abnormally dilated or pinpoint and react sluggishly to light. Muscle tone is increased and the patient may have generalized rigidity and neck stiffness.

At this stage, shivering is absent. When shivering occurs, particularly in those who have completed prolonged endurance events, it is a sign of impending hypothermia, and rewarming measures should be instituted by bystanders because the subject is unusually incapable of correct judgment. During hypothermia, deep tendon reflexes are decreased, and delayed relaxation of the ankle jerk, as in myxedema, may be seen. The plantar responses are often extensor but revert to normal with rewarming. Hypotension, compensatory tachycardia, slow atrial fibrillation, or sinus bradycardia are commonly present. The occasional occurrence of gangrene of the toes has been attributed to intense vasoconstriction. Slow, sighing respirations are characteristic, but occasionally Cheyne-Stokes respirations occur. With respiratory depression, hypoxia and acidosis are seen.

Occasionally, pancreatitis has been documented by elevated serum amylase and also at necropsy. The abdomen may be distended as a result of decreased peristalsis, bowel sounds are commonly absent, and sometimes gastric dilatation with vomiting occurs. Massive hepatic necrosis has been reported, but it is uncommon. Decreased renal blood flow reduces creatinine clearance, and in spite of diminished glomerular filtration, diuresis usually occurs because of decreased secretion and responsiveness of tubular cells to antidiuretic hormones. Eventually, dehydration and continued fall in renal blood flow produce oliguria. Renal failure from acute tubular necrosis may occur.

Investigation of Hypothermic Subjects

Emergency investigation of hypothermic individuals must include X rays of the chest to detect infection and of the abdomen to show gastric dilatation, possibly to avoid the danger of inhalation pneumonia. Continuous electrocardiographic monitoring is necessary to reveal episodic severe bradycardia, which might necessitate intracardiac pacing, and to recognize ventricular asystole or fibrillation. To gauge fluid and electrolyte needs, biochemical monitoring is necessary, and this must include urea and creatinine, electrolytes, glucose, amylase, and arterial blood gasses. Platelet counts and plasma cryocrit should be done. If antibiotic treatment is indicated, anaerobic and aerobic blood cultures should be taken prior to the administration of these drugs.

Hypothermia in the Elderly Person

Accidental hypothermia is not confined to healthy athletes exposed to adverse climatic conditions, but also occurs in elderly persons in whom the clinical picture may be slightly different. Though elderly people may have low body temperatures and symptoms or complaints of cold, those with accidental hypothermia do show decreasing alertness with the decrease in body temperature. The patient, therefore, may not detect the problem. The incidence of accidental hypothermia in those involved in outdoor activities is increasing because of larger numbers of participants. Accidental hypothermia in the elderly seems also to be a large problem, but exact estimates of its incidence are not available. Most studies have been done in Great Britain. Hypothermia does not leave diagnostic postmortem findings, so that in the elderly, death from this condition is often erroneously attributed to concomitant disease.

Accidental hypothermia out of doors and also in the elderly is often complicated by the ingestion of drugs that interfere with thermoregulatory mechanisms or accelerate heat loss during inclement weather. Alcohol, particularly, has been implicated as a cause, and yet is often used in the treatment of accidental hypothermia. A number of controlled investigations, however, involving cold water immersion, showed no difference in heat loss in those taking alcohol as compared to controls (Ledingham and Mone [31]). Furthermore, one report indicated decreased heat loss after alcohol ingestion, and it was concluded that alcohol intake could be beneficial because it reduced the discomfort and anxiety of cold exposure.

Alcohol-Induced Hypothermia

Alcohol-induced hypothermia causes hypoglycemia, and the reduced core temperature may interfere with hepatic detoxification of alcohol. Moreover, alcohol may inhibit hepatic gluconeogenesis independently. Thus, hypoglycemia, apart from occurring in those who exercise for prolonged periods, may be additionally aggravated by alcohol ingestion. In a study of water immersion that examined the rate of cooling before and for 24 min at room temperature after removal of the subject from the water, a rapid decline in core temperature continued after standing without drying for 24 min. When alcohol was given prior to immersion, central body temperature declined faster, and recovery of normal temperature after removal from the water was delayed. Shivering under those conditions was considerably decreased.

In spite of the lower core temperature and decreased shivering, the subjects ingesting alcohol perceived less cold and judged the environment warmer than did those who did not ingest the alcohol. Thus, exposure to cold (water immersion) plus alcohol ingestion may seriously reduce central body temperature. Alcohol intake during or after sporting events in cold weather is dangerous and may accelerate the fall in central body temperature, causing serious complications. In addition, alcohol potentiates exercise-induced cutaneous vasodilatation, with consequent increased heat loss from the extremities. Barbiturates and other psychotherapeutic drugs in question have also been associated with accidental hypothermia. In such persons, the prognosis is related to the disorder for which the drugs were taken and to the degree of the hypothermia.

Preexisting Diseases

Hypothermia may mask preexisting disease. Severe infections may be concealed by depressed consciousness, hypertension, variable leukocyte counts, and the absence of fever. Neurologic lesions might escape clinical detection because of the generalized nervous system depression during hypothermia. Elevated enzymes from hypothermia or pressure necrosis of muscles related to unconsciousness, plus the electrocardiographic abnormalities that occur in both hypothermia and myocardial infarction, make the diagnosis of myocardial infarction difficult.

The usual criteria for brain death are not applicable in hypothermic patients. Patients may be deeply comatose, without reflexes and with fixed dilated pupils and slow, deep, sighing respirations, marked bradycardia, and severe hypotension and yet make complete recovery. Whether or not this is the result of decreased oxygen requirements during hypothermia is not known. Disorders resulting from hypothermia are potentially fully recoverable even though clinical examination suggests the contrary.

Accidental Hypothermia

Accidental hypothermia from water immersion after shipwreck is uncommon. The main cause of low body temperatures in such subjects with normal thermoregulation is exposure to cold water. In spite of theoretic considerations and popular belief, exercise during cold water immersion accelerates heat loss irrespective of clothing, initial temperature, or amount of adipose tissue. The survival time, however, rarely longer than 7 hr in 15°C water, varies with the amount of body fat. Thick subcutaneous fat reduces heat loss. Moreover, long-distance swimmers, particularly those who brave the English Channel, are about the only athletes whose performances are improved by increased body fat.

Diagnosis of Hypothermia

The diagnosis of hypothermia depends upon accurate measurement of body temperature. In normal subjects, variations in temperature exist among different body parts. Skin temperature of the extremities, for example, varies considerably with changes in the surrounding temperatures. In accidental hypothermia, extremity temperature may be much lower, as a result of vasoconstriction, than temperature in other parts of the body.

Because hypothermia poses a threat only if core temperatures are low, it is necessary to obtain a reasonable estimate of the central temperature for accurate diagnosis. Mouth or rectal temperature does not adequately measure the rapid changes in hypothalamic temperature that are closely related to thermoregulation in both animals and humans. Rectal temperature reflects central temperature changes but sometimes is fallacious. For example, if warm saline is infused intravenously or one limb is immersed in warm water, little change in rectal temperature occurs, but oral temperature rises strikingly. Oral temperature measurement reflects arterial blood temperature changes better than rectal measurement and does not merely indicate changes in oral or pharyngeal blood flow.

Central temperature recorded from the external auditory meatus is satisfactory for experimental and clinical situations. In fever, when slow temperature changes occur, and perhaps also in accidental hypothermia, rectal temperature measurement is adequate and is not liable to many technical errors. Because thermometers are geared to measure fever rather than hypothermia, they are rarely shaken down below 37°C. It must, therefore, be remembered that this instrument measures temperatures only above the level to which it is shaken down. When central temperatures are low, a thermometer that registers appropriately should be used. Hypothermia is present if the central body temperature is below 35°C. Between 35°C and 32.2°C, shivering and behavioral thermoregulation prevent further hypothermia, provided consciousness is not impaired and other physical disabilities do not exist. If the central temperature falls below 32.2°C, depression of tissue metabolism with progressive clouding of consciousness occurs, and below 24°C death from ventricular fibrillation is usual. Mechanisms that prevent core-temperature drop, such as vasoconstriction and shivering, usually fail at these low temperatures. The body then loses heat like an inanimate object.

Treatment of Hypothermia

The therapy of hypothermia consists of immediately stopping heat loss by insulating the subject and adequate and effective rewarming (equal or greater than 0.5°C/hr). Spontaneous rewarming if heat loss is stopped is adequate, and active means depend greatly on available resources. Tissue perfusion and oxygenation must be maintained. Dopamine can be given to counter hypotension, and high concentration of oxygen by face mask should be given to all subjects, at least initially, if possible. Some need intubation and ventilation before hypoxemia can be improved. Hypoglycemia, if present, should be corrected and thiamine should be given, particularly if accidental hypothermia is suspected to be associated with alcohol intake. In such patients, even circumstantial evidence of alcohol ingestion should lead to the exclusion of possible intracranial trauma by appropriate radiologic studies. Subdural hematomas may remain silent until active rewarming has restored brain volume and only then become symptomatic, usually with disastrous results.

It should be noted that intravenous fluids should be given only after careful monitoring of electrolytes and renal function, and fluids must be prewarmed. It may be dangerous to give intravenous fluids to those who have had prolonged hypothermia, but raised serum potassium levels must be corrected because of the increased risk of ventricular fibrillation.

If asystolic cardiac arrest occurs or ventricular fibrillation is present, intracardiac pacing or direct current shock should be attempted.

No heparin, dextran, or plasma protein solutions should ever be given in the presence of cryofibrinogenemia, because these drugs cause polymerization of the cryofibrinogen. There is no place for steroids, thyroid hormones, or cardioactive or vasoactive drugs in routine management of hypothermia.

Although in nonathletes intercurrent disorders (alcoholism, subdural hematoma, old age) dominate the clinical picture and dictate additional manipulations and therapeutic attempts, accidental hypothermia in athletes is usually of good prognosis, unlike that which occurs with intercurrent illness. It requires usually nothing more than slow passive rather than active rewarming, best achieved by insulation and exposure to normal room temperature.

If cryofibrinogen levels are increased, serious hazards are present because of increased blood viscosity. If abrupt exposure to even superficial cold occurs after the subject has become hypothermic, it can cause cryofibrinogens to gel, and this can drastically increase viscosity, with a marked and serious reduction of the microcirculation, no longer sustainable under those circumstances. It should be stressed, however, that hypothermia in association with exercise is not commonly associated with cryofibrinogenemia. Rather, the presence of cryofibrinogen in the blood is more a feature of complicated hypothermia, particularly infection with Escherichia coli of the urinary tract, malignancy, or diabetes. In folate deficiency (occasionally seen in athletes, malnourished elderly, and those with thrombotic tendencies) cryofibrinogenemia is particularly common. Extensive purpura or bruising should lead to the suspicion of cryofibrinogenemia. This results from occlusion of cutaneous vessels from gelling of the cryofibrinogen. Careful attention to the situation in which athletes were found hypothermic must be given because falls and bruises associated with athletic performances may, in hypothermic athletes, be misleading.

Some very hypothermic athletes do well even without intensive medical management or active rewarming, and most recover. Intercurrent disease or associated injuries sustained during falls, in mountain accidents in particular, determine the outcome and may change the usually good prognosis. It should also be clearly recognized that the ordinary signs of brain death are not reliable in hypothermia; some subjects have recovered when all other evidence suggested that they may have died. Cerebral death, therefore, should not be assessed until body temperature has returned to near normal (MacLean [32]).

REFERENCES

1. Bligh, J. 1980. Central neurology of homeothermy and fever. In: Lipton, J.M. (ed): Fever. Raven Press, New York, pp 81–89.
2. Nadel, E.R., et al. 1979. Circulatory regulation during exercise in different ambient temperatures. J Appl Physiol 46:430–437.
3. Roberts, M.F., Wenger, B.C. 1980. Control of skin blood flow during exercise by thermal reflexes and baroreflexes. J Appl Physiol 48:717–723.
4. Nadel, E.R. 1980. Circulatory and thermal regulations during exercise. Fed Proc 39:1491–1497.
5. Myhre, L.G., et al. 1979. Cardiac output during rest and exercise in desert heat.

Med Sci Sports 11:234–238.
6. Wells, C.L., et al. 1980. Training and acclimatization: effects on responses to exercise in a desert environment. Aviat Space Environ Med 51:105–112.
7. Convertino, V.A., et al. 1980. Role of thermal and exercise factors in the mechanism of hypervolemia. J Appl Physiol 48:657–664.
8. Taggart, P., et al. 1972. Cardiac responses to thermal and emotional stress. Br Med J 3:71–76.
9. Paolone, A.M., et al. 1980. Effects of post-exercise sauna both on ECG pattern and other physiologic variables. Aviat Space Environ Med 51:224–229.
10. Greenleaf, J.E., Reese, R.D. 1980. Ex-

ercise thermoregulation after 14 days of bed rest. J Appl Physiol 48:72–78.

11. Schvarz, E., et al. 1979. Deconditioning-induced exercise responses as influenced by heat acclimation. Aviat Space Environ Med 50:893–897.

12. Feldberg, W. 1974. Body temperature and fever: changes in our views during the last decade. The Ferrier Lecture. Proc R Soc London [Biol] 191:199–229.

13. Benzinger, T.H. 1977. Temperature: I. Arts and Concepts. II. Thermal Homeostasis. Dowden, Hutchinson and Ross, Inc. Stroudsburg, Pennsylvania.

14. Lovett-Doust, J.W. 1979. An ultradian periodic servo-system of thermoregulation in man. J Interdiscipl Cycle Res 10:95–103.

15. Iberall, A.S. 1972. Blood flow and oxygen uptake in mammals. Ann Biomed Eng 1:1–8.

16. Lovett-Doust, J.W. 1962. Consciousness in schizophrenia as a function of the peripheral microcirculation. In: Roessler, W., Greenfield, D.A. (eds): Physiological Correlates of Psychological Disorder. Wisconsin Press, Madison, pp 61–69.

17. Jones, T.S., Liang, A.P., et al. 1982. Morbidity and mortality associated with the July 1980 heatwave in St. Louis and Kansas City, Missouri. JAMA 247: 3327–3331.

18. Kilbourne, E.M., Choi, K., et al. 1982. Risk factors for heat stroke. JAMA 247:3332–3336.

19. Al-Khalwashki, M.I., et al. 1983. Clinical presentation of 172 heat stroke cases seen at Mina and Arafat—September 1982. In: Khogali M., Hales J.R.S. (eds): Heat Stroke and Temperature Regulation. Academic Press, Sydney, pp 99–108.

20. Thompson, J.W. 1984. Opioid peptides. Brit Med J 288:259–260.

21. Appenzeller, O., Khogali, M., et al. 1986. Makkah Hajj: heat stroke and endocrine responses. Ann Sports Med 3:30–32.

22. Khogali, M. 1983. Epidemiology of heat illness during the Makkah pilgrimages in Saudi Arabia. Int J Epid 12:267–273.

23. Vigas, M. 1984. Problems of definition of stress stimulus and specificity of stress response. In: Usdin, E., et al. (eds): Stress: The Role of Catecholamines and Other Neurotransmitters. Gordon and Beach, New York, pp 919–927.

24. Adlercreutz, H., Kvopposalmi, K., et al. 1982. Use of hypnosis in studies of the effect of stress on cardiovascular function and hormones. Acta Med Scand (Suppl) 660:84–94.

25. Leppaluoto, J., Ranta, T., et al. 1975. Strong heat exposure and adenohypophyseal hormone secretion in man. Horm Metab Res 7:439–440.

26. Holaday, J.W., Wei, E., et al. 1978. Endorphins may function in heat adaptation. Proc Natl Acad Sci USA 75:2923–2927.

27. DeMeirler, K., Arentz, T., et al. 1985. The role of endogenous opiates in thermal regulation of the body during exercise. Brit Med J 290:739–740.

28. Hubbard, R.W., Matthew, C.B., et al. 1982. Heat stressed rat: effect of atropine desalivation or restraint. J Appl Physiol 53:1171–1174.

29. Cabanac, M. 1983. Face fanning: a possible way to prevent or cure brain hyperthermia. In: Khogali, M., Hales, J.R.S. (eds): Heat Stroke and Temperature Regulation Academic Press, Sydney, pp 213–221.

30. Caputa, M., Perrin, M., et al. 1978. Ecoulement sanguin reversible dans la veine ophtalmique: mecamisme de refroidissment selectif du cerveau humain. C R Acad Sci 287:1011–1014.

31. Ledingham, I., Mone, J.G. 1980. Treatment of accidental hypothermia: a prospective clinical study. Br Med J 1: 1102–1104.

32. MacLean, D. 1986. Emergency management of accidental hypothermia: a review. J Royal Soc Med 79:528–531.

• 3 •

Neurology of Endurance Training

Otto Appenzeller

There is an active lobby seeking to shift the focus of medical care from the relief of suffering to the prevention of disease. An increasing number of enthusiasts are urging that we adopt cheap public health measures as a way of avoiding expensive health maintenance. Numerous recipes to ensure a reduction in medical care costs by the prevention of disease include aerobic training achieved through sports such as running, cross-country skiing, bicycling, and long-distance swimming. Even psychiatrists are sometimes urging endurance training as a cure for a variety of mental diseases. Anecdotal and usually inadequate studies support the notion that physical activity promotes a sense of well-being and influences nervous system and other bodily functions. Exercise seems to have acquired a mystical quality that renews and revitalizes, but a solid scientific basis for this claim is not at hand as yet. Limited studies that have been carried out to measure exercise benefits for the relief of anxiety, depression, and other mental disorders have usually adopted questionary scores, scales, and inventories that largely depend on the cooperativeness of respondents. The answers of enthusiastic exercisers before and after exertion or endurance training provide eloquent and statistically valid evidence of improvement and benefit in central nervous system function. But these responses are incomplete measures because they depend on language that itself is not easily quantified (Appenzeller [1]).

Controversy about the role of physical fitness in prevention of heart disease continues. Studies since the early 1950s have shown that, in large populations who are physically active, exercise or physical work is one of the main factors in preventing overt heart disease. While those who engage in regular aerobic or endurance activities seem to live longer, have fewer illnesses, and function better, the evidence for these statements remains incomplete. Nevertheless, a sedentary lifestyle is increasingly recognized as a major risk factor that can easily be modified. Those who engage in regular aerobic activity are more likely to abandon habits detrimental to physical well-being, such as smoking, overeating, and excessive alcohol intake, all known to predispose to incurable diseases. Although exercise seems to be beneficial, it remains a complex set of activities that needs to be prescribed on an individual basis. It must be approached in a safe way to make it rewarding for the participant, and it is clear that physicians and other health professionals have a great deal to offer to make the choice easy and to promote physical well-being (Appenzeller and Atkinson [2]).

Marathoning, ultra-long-distance running, triathloning, and adventure runs have for some individuals replaced religious services. They certainly occupy as much or more time, they are pursued with equal fervor, and persuasion is used to convince friends and aquaintances of the righteousness of such activity. Many long-distance runners also show withdrawal symptoms and guilt if they miss training. It is therefore necessary to gain insight into the benefits of aerobic training and to assess its possible contribution to the prevention as opposed to the cure of many degenerative diseases. While a considerable body of evidence has accumulated to show the effects of training on the cardiovascular and musculoskeletal systems, the nervous system has in general been neglected, even though it is the final orchestrator for adaptation to physical and mental stress, both of which abound during the various stages of endurance training.

In this chapter, the author attempts to place in perspective what is known of the effects of endurance training on the nervous system and on the age-related changes in nervous system function. While the convert is often exposed to ridicule by those who sit, eat, and make merry, it is nevertheless pretty much the case of the person who is laughing being the one who has not heard the bad news.

The chief function of the central nervous system is to send messages to the muscles which will make the body move effectively as a whole. This, of course, is true of animals also, but only man has a mind to enable him to do things with cognition and intent, which are qualities different from those attainable by animals. Whereas a great deal has been learned about muscle strength, the interactions of muscular activity, mood, and behavior remain elusive. Reflex movement, which forms an elementary unit of the nervous system's activity, cannot explain the complex behavioral sequences that induce millions to exercise daily, which until recently was considered bizarre behavior. Moreover, the effects of such behavior on nervous system function and dysfunction remain important issues needing further study.

EXERCISE AND SKELETAL MUSCLES

The modern fascination with physical fitness and athletic performance has changed the care of athletes from being exclusively the concern of orthopaedic surgeons to being in the domain of physicians of a variety of specialties, including neurology. Though neurologists have had a long-standing interest in normal muscle physiology and muscle diseases, the role of exercise in changing muscle physiology is a comparatively recent neurologic preoccupation.

Historical Aspects

Galvani pursued the subject of normal muscle contraction, and in the latter part of the 19th century muscle contraction was first described in humans (Landouzy and Dejerine [3]). But the biochemical study of muscle disease and normal muscle contraction has greatly advanced since the 1950s to include the physiologic implications of glycogen storage for continued and transient physical activity and the abnormalities in storage of this substance (McArdle [4]). Absent lactate production during ischemic forearm exercise in a patient who presented with muscle cramps after exercise led the way for the recognition of the enzyme defect in McArdle's syndrome (absence of myophosphorylase).

Electromyographic and histochemical studies of healthy and abnormal muscles and the study of the effect of exercise on muscle fiber types have increased knowledge of muscle adaptation. The muscle's nerve supply determines its functional characteristics, which suggests that adaptation to certain athletic disciplines ultimately depends on muscle fiber types. Because exercise affects the blood supply to muscles and this in turn depends partly on the autonomic innervation of muscle vessels, it is possible that normal adaptation to exercise and muscle degeneration and regeneration result from alterations in the circulation and/or the innervation of muscle blood vessels (Appenzeller and Ogin [5]).

Clinical Aspects

Prolonged muscle contraction as it is found in exercise is associated with increased strength and endurance occasionally without change in total muscle bulk. Sometimes weakness follows excessive and prolonged training; this is recognized clinically when the force produced by muscle contraction falls below the expected value for age, stature, and sex of an individual. It is of interest that most patients with muscle disease do not complain of weakness but more often notice inability to perform certain tasks and may be weak at rest, while athletes usually have normal resting strengths but may complain of abnormal fatigability or of excessive premature "exhaustion after accustomed exertion." Other clinical manifestations include cramps or episodic weakness and sudden loss of muscle tone lasting only seconds. These are often difficult to categorize and are sometimes thought to be due to anxiety, to hysteria, or, when they appear in otherwise well balanced athletes, to excessive pressure of competition. They certainly can interfere with performance.

Weakness and Strength   The force produced by any muscle is directly proportional to the cross-sectional area of contractile muscle proteins. Muscle fiber hypertrophy or atrophy can be associated with increasing or decreasing strength or force. In athletes, muscle weakness is always proportional to the loss of contractile tissue. This may result from muscle fiber damage during exertion and consequent destruction of muscle fibers. After prolonged immobilization or lack of training because of athletic injury, shrinkage and atrophy of muscle fibers may occur. Atrophic fibers, however, do not disappear altogether. Under such circumstances, the cross-sectional area of contractile protein tissue decreases. It may be that the slender muscle seen in successful long-distance runners unassociated with weakness results from gradual and repeated breakdown of muscle tissue or a minimally destructive myopathy associated with prolonged and continued training.

Fatigue   Fatigue is a common complaint of many athletes in training and its physiologic basis has been extensively discussed by Wiles et al. [6]. The definition of fatigue is descriptive because its true genesis is not understood. In general, athletes complaining of fatigue do so because of failure to reach or maintain the desired power or force generated by muscle contraction. Subjects with decreased muscle bulk from whatever cause produce proportionally less force in a given period of time and tire more rapidly. There are athletes with normal or even hypertrophied muscles who also fatigue rapidly or more quickly than they are accustomed to. In an athletic population, this is usually due to some change in muscle energy metabolism, such as depletion of energy stores by prolonged training, rather than from myasthenia gravis, as is often suspected by neurologists. Abnormal muscle metabolism or depletion of metabolic substrates for contraction does not always result in fatigue, however. Patients with hypothyroidism have decreased muscle adenosine 5-triphosphate (ATP) turnover but can maintain isometric contractions for longer periods than can euthyroid persons.

Myoglobinemia and Myoglobinuria   When muscle breaks down (rhabdomyolysis) myoglobin is released into the circulation. This can occur after crush injuries during athletic accidents, but more often it results from prolonged exertion in otherwise healthy athletes. It can be a symptom of metabolic muscle disease, of course, such as carnitine palmityl transferase or myophosphorylase deficiency. Myoglobinuria and myoglobinemia also occur in subjects who are hypothermic but at rest, for example, victims of mountaineering accidents. Myoglobin excretion in the urine can seriously affect renal function, and hemodialysis for renal failure may be required.

INVESTIGATIONS OF EXERCISE-ASSOCIATED MUSCLE SORENESS

Athletes referred for investigation of muscle soreness are often treated as though they have muscular disease, which is not usually the case.

Clinical History and Examination

The first part of this essential step is the routine history taking and the description of symptoms, particularly in relation to exercise. Attention is paid to family history of similar symptoms that might hint at a genetic basis for the complaint, though this is rarely found. The physical examination is directed toward demonstrating impaired performance due to weakness of particular muscle groups. Attention should be paid also to posture and to the shape of the spine, which may be changed by weakness, and length of the legs, inequality of leg length being a cause of overuse problems in muscle groups of the lower limbs. Weakness is often associated with characteristic gait changes and postural adaptations. Skeletal abnormalities may cause muscle pain associated with exertion but do not necessarily preclude championship athletic performance, as demonstrated by Harold Connolly, gold medalist in the hammer throw in the 1956 Melbourne Olympic Games who had a left brachial plexus birth injury.

Laboratory Investigations

Plasma electrolyte and thyroid function studies, full blood count and erythrocyte sedimentation rate, plasma protein, immunoglobulin, and serum creatine kinase (CK) are often indicated. Some athletes give a history of pigmenturia; in these cases myoglobin levels in the serum should be measured. The possibility of hypo- and hyperkalemia associated with episodic paralysis and changes in muscle function should be excluded.

An abnormally high serum calcium can cause weakness, and an elevated sedimentation rate points to inflammatory disease. These tests are useful to eliminate the possibility of bone disease or inflammatory myopathy. Normal plasma proteins and immunoglobins exclude the presence of autoimmune states that may cause muscle dysfunction. The plasma CK activity is the most widely used index of muscle breakdown because it is released from muscle in several pathologic conditions. Increased CK activity is an indicator of active disease in nonathletes only. Otherwise, normal habitual exercisers who spend many hours in training often show remarkable elevation in CK activity (see below).

Electromyography

Electromyography is a tool for differentiating muscle disease from neuropathic processes. In the investigation of athletes, however, it is rarely used and then only in patients who complain of acute symptoms related to certain muscle groups. In these cases, electromyography may identify a primary abnormality in muscle or nerve function. Muscle fiber irritability is increased for some time after prolonged muscle contraction, and myotonic discharges may also occur. Therefore the timing of the electromyography is of importance in the interpretation of the results. The use of spectral analyses that give quantitative information about interference patterns is mainly confined to study of muscle fatigue and is, at present, a research tool not generally used in the management of athletic problems (Adrian and Bryant [7]; Ballantyne and Hansen [8]).

Recording of single muscle fiber activity and intraneural microneurographic techniques, respectively, have been used to study muscle activity and autonomic discharges to muscle blood vessels. Athletes have participated in these endeavors in an effort to delineate differences in sympathetic vascular tone between trained and untrained muscles (Wallin [9]).

Muscle Biopsy

The examination of muscle biopsies is the most important diagnostic tool for recognizing muscle disease. However, biopsies in athletes are usually used for research purposes only in the study of metabolic substrate and enzyme content at rest, during competition, and after competition. Many muscle disease centers advocate open muscle biopsy, but athletes are usually studied by needle biopsy that allows adequate histochemical and biochemical examination of the tissues (Edwards et al. [10]).

Nuclear Magnetic Resonance

Nuclear magnetic resonance (NMR) is a minimally invasive technique and is used for the study of chemical changes in the nervous system and in intact muscles (Dawson et al. [11]). Newer machines allow measurement of muscle constituents, and new techniques may improve the study of chemical and metabolic aspects of muscle contraction in health and disease. This technique is also promising for assessing metabolic changes induced by dietary manipulation in athletes and may place the numerous anecdotal testimonials on more scientific ground.

Ultrasound

Ultrasound can be used to determine the cross-sectional area of muscles in order to measure changes produced by strength or endurance training. With this technique, a clear distinction can be made between muscles and subcutaneous fat and between muscle and bone. Ultrasound is unreliable, however, when muscle is replaced by fat and connective tissue. On the other hand, if wasting occurs, for example after fracture of a limb when the muscle is not replaced by fat because it is not directly injured, ultrasound can measure the efficacy of rehabilitation in restoring muscle bulk and strength.

Computerized Tomography

Computerized tomography has been used for cross-sectional visualization of muscle and distinguishes between muscle and bone. It can be used for diagnosing muscle swelling that may occur after athletic performance and recognizes the extravasation of blood into ruptured muscles.

Tests of Muscle Function

Tests of muscle function should be properly evaluated, and it is desirable to combine them with metabolic studies of the muscles tested. For this purpose, it is useful to test the quadriceps muscle, since it is sometimes weak in athletes, particularly long-distance runners, who have trained excessively. This muscle is also load bearing and is important in many other types of athletic performance. The quadriceps is comparatively free of large blood vessels and nerves so that needle biopsy, if indicated, can be taken easily and can be repeated at intervals after treatment or after changes in training techniques have been in effect. The best way of testing force at maximum voluntary contraction is the use of the commercial Cybex machine that helps determine force velocity characteristics and also the fiber type composition of the muscle (Amphlett et al. [12]). In ordinary clinical practice it is assumed that for most body sizes, the maximum quadriceps strength is directly related to body weight. This is not necessarily true, however, in athletes who may normally have excessive strength by these criteria or normal strength that may represent weakness for an individual who is seeking advice about declining performance. In nonathletes, the force that can be generated at the ankle during isometric maximum contraction is about 75% of body weight.

A well-known clinical phenomenon in athletes is slowing of muscle relaxation after prolonged activity. This also occurs in animals under experimental conditions and has been investigated in humans (Edwards et al. [13]). Relaxation may be influenced by the rate of cross-bridge turnover. The slowing of ATP turnover that occurs in slowly relaxing muscles supports this interpretation (Edwards et al. [14]). With the use of phosphorus NMR, however, no change was found in ATP turnover in frog muscles. A decreased rate of calcium reuptake by the sarcoplasmic reticulum is a possible explanation for the slowed muscle relaxation (Edwards et al. [15]). It is, however, generally agreed that the slowing of relaxation after prolonged contraction is associated with decreased muscle phosphagen (ATP plus phosphocreatine) and relaxation rates recover with a similar time course to that of phosphocreatine synthesis (Wiles [16]).

Heavy or ischemic exercise changes the shape of the force frequency curve. Force is depressed at lower frequencies of stimulation relative to the force at higher frequencies. It may take several hours and occasionally as long as 24 hr after exercise for full recovery. The so-called low frequency fatigue may actually result from muscle cell membrane damage and new protein synthesis, and the repair of the cell membrane may be required before recovery. Whether this is the cause of the muscle enzyme leakage and of myoglobinuria in prolonged exertion in otherwise normal athletes is not clear.

The rate of perceived exertion (RPE) or the perception of physical effort can be measured, and this influences the development of central fatigue. If RPE is excessive, it becomes more difficult to complete a given task. It is not known whether the cessation of effort arises centrally or peripherally, but RPE is closely related to heart rate and peripheral lactate accumulation. Perception of efferent motor drive to muscles and peripheral sensory input from muscle tendons and joints to the brain during activity may contribute to RPE, and a change in RPE may be one cause for unusual fatigability. This may be assessed by comparing voluntary and electrically stimulated contraction in appropriate muscles. Central fatigue is often an important cause of loss of quadriceps strength in normal persons near the end of prolonged maximal voluntary contraction. Rate of perceived exertion for a given amount of work may be decreased by training at high altitudes, a beneficial factor when competition later will be at sea level.

ATROPHY AND HYPERTROPHY

Inactivity and immobilization result in overuse injuries when activity is resumed. More serious athletic accidents can cause atrophy, and conversely increased activity when associated with strength training causes hypertrophy. Submaximal prolonged activity improves muscle fiber oxidative capacity by induction of mitochondrial oxidative enzymes and also causes changes in the volume densities of mitochondria (Howald et al. [17]). There is also a significant increase in the volume density of intracellular lysosomes in Type 2 fibers and it seems that endurance training leads to an enhancement of the oxidative capacity in all muscle fiber types. Resistive exercises are capable of increasing muscle strength and mass. Two mechanisms are proposed for the growth of muscles: a) an increase in size of cells (hypertrophy) and b) an increase in the number of muscle cells (hyperplasia). In human muscles, however, changes result from either a decrease or an increase in cell size rather than a change in cell numbers. In destructive myopathies, muscle fiber splitting occurs that suggests a potential for hyperplasia in humans under abnormal conditions (Swash et al. [18]). This is not an important mechanism for muscle growth in athletes and normal subjects and most likely represents evidence of muscle damage.

Endurance exercise leads to characteristic adaptations within the trained muscle tissue. Increased capillarization and an increase in mitochondrial enzyme activities or mitochondrial volume densities enhance the capacity for oxygen transport in trained muscles. Adaptation of the muscle to increased aerobic capacity and cardiovascular adaptations have been thought to account for the increased maximal oxygen uptake rate after endurance training. Surprisingly, however, an increased oxygen uptake is also observed during work with untrained muscles, for example arm cranking after bicycle endurance training. While this transfer effect has been attributed to cardiovascular adaptation, other evidence suggests that an increase in the net oxidation of lactate might also account for the observed increase in oxygen uptake of untrained muscles (Rosler et al. [19]). To understand the mechanism of muscle hypertrophy and atrophy, knowledge of normal growth and maintenance of cellular proteins in muscle is required. Muscle fiber protein content depends on the balance between synthesis and breakdown. Hypertrophy or atrophy of muscles results from either increased or decreased protein degradation if synthesis is constant. In some situations, however, muscle protein is increased and accompanied by an increased rate of protein catabolism. An example of this occurs during rapid growth with weight gain (Maruyama et al. [20]). It may also occur in adult muscles and can be monitored by urinary 3-methylhistidine levels.

There is no good explanation as yet for the differential susceptibility to atrophy of Type 2 faster contracting fibers more prone to this change than Type 1 fibers. A differential protein turnover between the two fiber types is, however, found in animal studies.

Insulin, thyroid hormones and corticosteroids affect muscle growth in animals and humans. Thyroid hormones augment protein turnover and maintain proteins in normal animals. Reduced protein synthesis and degradation occur after thyroidectomy; replacement therapy restores turnover rates to normal (Millward et al. [21]). Insulin stimulates protein synthesis both in vivo and in vitro. Fractional synthesis rates of skeletal muscle protein are reduced by one third or one half of normal, and RNA content is considerably decreased in muscles of diabetic animals; these changes can be reversed by the administration of insulin. Insulin does increase transport of amino acids into muscle and may be the cause of increased protein synthesis after insulin administration. It may be that protein synthesis is also influenced by other actions of insulin. Insulin may directly influence intracellular protein through an as yet unrecognized "second messenger."

Glucocorticoids affect muscle protein turnover and growth in a way opposite to that of insulin. Corticosteroids presumably bind receptor proteins and thus influence gene expression, and they may inhibit glucose uptake by muscle fibers. Overall, these hormones induce muscle wasting by supressing protein synthesis and have little influence on protein breakdown. When high doses of glucocorticoids are used for whatever clinical reason, increased degradation of protein occurs (DuBois and Almon [22]). Other evidence suggests that glucocorticoids bind to specific high-affinity cytosolic receptors and that the number of activated or transformed receptor complexes available for binding to the nuclear chromatin determines their cellular effects. High hormone levels increase binding, but also the number of receptors is increased in the cytosol. This situation occurs in denervated muscles and may account for denervation atrophy. It may also be present after severe athletic injury and disuse, a situation in which atrophy may be excessive and muscle bulk is never returned to normal even after successful strength rehabilitation.

Although molecular mechanisms responsible for denervation atrophy have been investigated extensively, definitive answers for this phenomenon are not yet in hand. Microscopically, denervated muscle is similar to skeletal muscle that has been exposed to excessive glucocorticoids (Cushing's disease or from therapeutic administration of large doses of glucocorticoids). The fast-twitch glycolytic (Type 2B) muscle fibers are more susceptible and shrink more than do the slow-twitch oxidative (Type 1) fiber so that the explosive element rather than the prolonged performance in athletic events is predominantly affected in both denervation and glucocorticoid-induced atrophy. Because of these similarities, it may be that denervation atrophy is mediated by endogenous glucocorticoids via increased numbers of specific cytosolic binding sites. It is of particular significance in athletic medicine that in disuse atrophy, induced by experimental immobilization of the knee and ankle joints for 8 days, significant up-regulation of glucocorticoid receptors occurs (DuBois and Almon [22]). Prolonged excess of glucocorticoids produces, in addition to changes in receptors and atrophy of skeletal muscles, a focal increase in glycogen and clustering of mitochondria. Dilation of the lateral cisternae of the sarcoplasmic reticulum and increased lipid globules are also seen. Gluconeogenesis and UDPG-glycogen synthetase activity cause increased glycogen content of the skeletal muscle fibers. In addition, calcium uptake into the fragmented sarcoplasmic reticulum is reduced and changes in oxidation of glucose, long-chain fatty acids, and ketone bodies occur in cultured myotubes. If these features are mediated through glucocorticoid receptors, it is still unclear why they occur in immobilized muscles and are not found in denervated muscles that were not simply immobilized.

The mode of entry of glucocorticoids into the target tissue is not understood. Entry may occur through passive diffusion through the surface membrane, and once the hormone is in the cytosol it rapidly attaches to its receptors forming an activated receptor–hormone complex. These complexes may then penetrate the nuclear membrane and attach to some component of the nuclear chromatin. This attachment to the proposed regulatory sites of the genome alters the production of specific messenger RNA (mRNA), which in turn influences the synthesis of the appropriate proteins. It has been proposed that the regulation either upward or downward of specific mRNA by glucocorticoids is the key to the cellular effects of these hormones, but this has not been studied in skeletal muscles. It is reasonable to suggest that endogenous steroids have a role in denervation and disuse atrophy of skeletal muscles, that their influence is mediated through specific mRNA synthesis, and that this in turn translates messages for myofibrillar proteins and other mRNA that regulates catabolic enzymes. In support of this interpretation is the well-known up-regulation of nicotine acetylcholine receptors in extrajunctional plasma membranes after muscle fiber denervation. Therefore, because of immobilization after athletic injury, the associated emotional and physical stress, and the related augmented release of endogenous glucocorticoids, disuse atrophy in athletes is more pronounced than in nonathletes. This excess atrophy is mediated through glucocorticoid effects on skeletal muscle fibers (Karpati [23]).

Muscle growth is affected by growth hormone, but the mode of action is not clear. The effects of growth hormone are not separable from its effect on insulin and on food intake. Growth hormone may stimulate protein synthesis in muscle through the intermediate action of somatomedins. Purified somatomedin administration enhances amino acid incorporation into isolated muscle. It may be that both somatomedins and insulin heighten muscle protein turnover by activating the same or similar receptor sites.

ABNORMAL FATIGABILITY IN ATHLETES

Muscle fatigue is common in nonathletic individuals and in athletes. Some athletes have profound unaccustomed fatigability that limits athletic performance. The investigation of such individuals is difficult because their perception of symptoms is often greater than the objective changes. Fatigue can result from changes in the central nervous system, the neuromuscular junction, or the muscle itself. Before identifying the cause of excessive fatigability in athletes, it is necessary to consider mechanisms of fatigue in nonathletic normal subjects. The "law of fatigue" was first defined by Kennelly in 1906 (24), who found a mathematical relationship between power output in running and that in endurance time in several species. Finger flexors fatigue in humans was investigated by Mosso (1981) (25) with an ergograph. He observed the effects of exercise, altitude, and emotional stress on force generated in a series of brief contractions and concluded that fatigue was central in origin because the motor drive from the central nervous system failed before muscle contraction declined. This interpretation of his results was accepted after it was noted that the presence of fatigue in voluntary contractions did not affect the force of electrically stimulated contractions. This assessment was challenged when it was shown that fatigue in the adductor pollicis muscle was accompanied by failure of muscle contraction. Fatigue accompanied by loss of force may therefore occur from neuromuscular junction failure (Stephens and Taylor [26]). While abnormalities in neuromuscular transmission are an important cause of fatigue in patients with myasthenia gravis, they are not important in otherwise healthy but fatigued athletes. Fatigue occurring at rest is a feature of effort syndromes and may be related to postural hypotension due to deconditioning.

Energy Metabolism and Exertion

Most patients with defects in muscle metabolism have normal or almost normal strength when rested, but their exercise capacity is limited. Such individuals are not usually athletes, but because of exercise limitation, may present in sports medicine clinics. Defects in glycolytic pathways present with complaints of painful contracture of the exercised muscles that are electrically silent. Mytochondrial disorders produce limited exercise tolerance, usually associated with blood lactate levels far above those expected for a given amount of work, suggesting ischemic or partially ischemic exercise.

The common genetic defects of muscle energy metabolism include glycolytic pathway disorders, mitochondrial enzyme abnormalities with defective pyruvate and fatty acid metabolism and the abnormalities of the cytochrome components of the electron transport chain. All of these conditions interfere with the secondary energy supply to the muscle after the prime reserves of phosphocreatine are depleted. Defects in actomyosin ATP or in muscle CK function have not been described, perhaps because they are lethal in utero.

Acquired glycolytic defects may occur in patients with chronic alcoholism where reduced glycolysis has been found (Perkoff et al. [27]), and this perhaps accounts for the limited exercise tolerance of such individuals. In patients with hypothyroidism, reduced muscle phosphorylase may in part result from the predominance of Type 1 fibers in this disease. Impaired glycolysis was found in serial samples of the quadriceps muscle of hypothyroid patients during sustained isometric contractions of the muscle (Wiles et al. [28]). The overall decrease in anaerobic glycolysis during ischemic contractions was reversed after appropriate treatment for the thyroid disorder. Paradoxically, circulating lactate decreases during dynamic exercise in hypothyroid patients attributed to reduced oxygen supply to working muscles, secondary to decreased cardiac output in such subjects. A reduction in acid maltase is also found in hypothyroid patients, and enzyme activity returns to normal with replacement therapy.

Impairment of the lactate response to ischemic exercise also occurs in alcoholic myopathy, myasthenia gravis, polymyositis, steroid myopathy, and some spinal muscular atrophies. Patients with these diseases may engage in athletic endeavors that then are seriously interfered with by the disease-induced impairment of the lactate response. They complain of sudden fatigability and impaired performance.

In a review of fat metabolism and its relationship to muscle contraction, DiMauro et al. (29) highlight the importance of weakness, exercise intolerance, muscle stiffness, and pain sometimes accompanied by myoglobinuria. Because symptoms are most troublesome when the main substrates for muscle energy metabolism are free fatty acids, the problem is most likely to occur during endurance events in which exercise in a relatively fasting state is common.

The observation of excessive accumulation of lipid in some muscle biopsies and subsequent metabolic studies of human muscle (Engel et al. [30]) hinted at the existence of disorders of lipid metabolism. Fat accumulates around muscle fibers in Duchenne muscular dystrophy, but uniform distribution of fat droplets within muscle fibers is pathognomonic of disorders of fat metabolism. Two diseases described in the early 1970s were muscle carnitine deficiency and carnitine palmityl transferase deficiency (CPT) (Engel and Angelini [31]; DiMauro and DiMauro [32]). Carnitine and CPT function in a shuttle mechanism for transfering free fatty acids into the mitochondria, a step necessary for the beta-oxidation of free fatty acids. Two tranferases are postulated to be located on the mitochondrial membrane: CPT1 on the outer surface and CPT2 on the inner surface. Carnitine is actively taken up into muscle after synthesis in liver and transported via the blood to the tissues. Carnitine deficiency symptoms may occur because of failure of synthesis or carnitine uptake by muscles. Both of these conditions have been recognized in humans, and though clinically indistinguishable, they can be differentiated by laboratory means. Normal serum carnitine, as reported in a number of patients, suggests normal hepatic synthesis but failure of muscle uptake. Patients with both reduced serum and liver carnitine levels have also been found (Karpati et al. [33]).

The exercise tolerance of patients with carnitine deficiency secondary to hepatic involvement can be improved markedly by oral administration of carnitine. Some clinical improvement may occur also in those with a defect in muscle carnitine transport after oral carnitine even though the muscle carnitine level is not changed by the treatment (Karpati et al. [33]).

An acquired partial carnitine deficiency in muscle may occur in patients on chronic renal dialysis, in septic patients, in those with malnutrition or liver disease, and in those with a dietary deficiency of lysine or methionine. The postdiphtheritic myocardial degeneration in experimental or human infections may be associated with carnitine deficiency also. The normal metabolism of carnitine and factors that influence its metabolic activity are not fully understood; nevertheless, it may be that in some elite athletes with associated anorexia nervosa, the ultimate breakdown of exercise tolerance results from partial acquired carnitine deficiency (Fleischmann and Siegel [34]).

Deficiency of CPT is more common in males and is characterized clinically by recurrent pain and myoglobinuria often precipitated and aggravated by fasting and prolonged exercise. Symptoms are preceded by increased plasma CK activity indicating muscle damage. Weakness is not present except during episodes of pain and myoglobinuria. The lipid accumulation in muscle is less pronounced than in carnitine deficiency, and muscle carnitine content may in fact be increased (Engel et al. [30]). Oxidation of palmitate requires CPT1 and CPT2, but oxidation of palmityl carnitine depends only on CPT2, that is, the enzyme on the inner surface of membranes. Leukocytes (Layzer [35]), platelets, and cultured fibroblasts are also deficient in CPT in affected patients (DiDonato et al. [36]).

Disorders of muscle fat metabolism can be distinguished on clinical grounds. Patients who have carnitine deficiency are weak, and those who have absent or impaired CPT activity have reasonably normal strength at rest but are symptomatic and have raised plasma CK and myoglobinuria after fasting or exercise. It is assumed that metabolic pathways of these two disorders are similarly affected, but the explanation for the clinical difference is not at hand. The understanding of the use and storage of lipids by muscle and possible damage caused by free fatty acids is a challenge for further investigation in sports neurology.

Changes in skeletal muscle mitochondria can be found within one or a few hours of continuous muscle stimulation (Schmid et al. [37]). The distribution of mitochondria in skeletal muscle immediately after an extended bout of endurance exercise has also been examined. An extensive study of a group of 7 well-trained long distance runners has been carried out by Oberholzer et al. (38). In this study, needle biopsies of the vastus lateralis were collected 1 month prior to a 100-km race, and a second sample was obtained from these same men 15–30 min after completion of the race. The time taken to run the 100-km in this group ranged from 7 to 10 hr of continued exercise. Reevaluation of these samples showed that capillary density and mean interfibrillar mitochondrial volume density were significantly correlated with running time in this race. The volume densities of lipid droplets and interfibrillar glycogen decreased significantly after the race. Volume density of interfibrillar mitochondria before the race was highest near the fiber border and decreased progressively with increasing distance toward the muscle fiber center. After the race, density of interfibrillar mitochondria remained unchanged at the fiber border but was significantly high in the center of the fiber. This increase in mitochondrial volume density was thought to be due to shrinkage of the fibers from consumption of energy stores expended during the race, which was relatively greater for interfibrillar glycogen than for subsarcolemmal glycogen. The primary effect of this prolonged exertion in highly trained individuals was a complete depletion of the interfibrillar glycogen and of lipids, but there was no evidence of a redistribution of mitochondria after such prolonged exertion (Kayar et al. [39]).

Myotonia and Athletics

Myotonia is characterized by slow and often delayed muscle relaxation that differs from the relaxation delay in hypothyroidism or in fatigued muscle because it is accompanied by continuing electrical activity. Myotonia is affected by exertion and must therefore be briefly mentioned here. It occurs in a number of muscle disorders and can be produced experimentally; it has many different causes. The most widely studied of human myotonic conditions, myotonia congenita, or Thomsen's disease, usually has autosomal dominant inheritance, but recessive cases have been reported, often with more severe symptomatology. In this disease, unlike most other primary muscle disorders, true muscle hypertrophy occurs that must be distinguished from pseudohypertrophy in which muscle enlargement is due to replacement of the tissue with fat. The myotonic stiffness affects limb muscles, and patients often have difficulty in letting go after a strong grip. Cold aggravates the condition, and athletes with myotonia congenita, of which there are quite a few (usually weight-lifters or throwers), may have trouble performing during cold weather. The diagnostic features of myotonia are contraction on percussion of the muscles, particularly the thenar or tongue muscles, and absence of persistent weakness. Undue fatigue after prolonged exertion may also be a feature that can be demonstrated during tetanic stimulation.

The study of myotonia has been facilitated by the use of myotonic goats. These animals have muscle stiffness and rigidity after sudden movements and assume bizarre postures when startled. They are unable to jump fences and were bred for this important attribute in the southern United States. The animal's symptoms are similar to those of human myotonia congenita. An unexplained feature both in goats and humans is the relief of myotonia by dehydration, a peculiarity that has allowed a number of myotonic individuals to perform better during long-distance events, gaining, as it were, a second wind toward the end of a marathon when dehydration becomes a problem for ordinary athletes. Electromyography shows that the slow relaxation in myotonia is associated with electrical activity (Brown and Harvey [40]). Moreover, myotonia induced by muscle percussion persists after nerve section and/or curarization. Myotonic muscle is abnormally sensitive to intra-arterial acetylcholine or potassium chloride, suggesting that the disorder is a primary myopathy. Similar experiments in humans using nerve blockade have led to the conclusion that myotonia congenita is a disorder of muscle (Floyd et al. [41]).

Theoretically, a primary muscle membrane defect might account for the myotonic syndromes. In support of this is the observation that, in myotonia congenita, renal concentrating capacity is reduced, suggesting that the proposed membrane disorder might be generalized and affect other tissues in which chloride permeability is also important.

Paramyotonia Congenita   Paramyotonia congenita is an autosomal dominantly inherited condition with symptoms similar to those of myotonia congenita, except that they are often more pronounced in the cold, and transitory weakness, particularly after prolonged exercise, often occurs. The following is a case study.

A 31-year-old man had suffered from paramyotonia congenita; his 12-month-old daughter was also affected. When rested and warm he was entirely normal. The father's first serious manifestation of the disease occurred at the age of 8. While walking through a field in summer, his legs gradually became weak and were eventually paralyzed before he was able to return home. His paralysis lasted for 3 days. Numerous similar attacks during exercise occurred after that time, with predominant involvement of the legs and more often after unusual exertion. Though the paralytic episodes were more common during the colder months, they also occurred during the summer. A frequent and daily occurrence was progressive weakness of jaw muscles toward the end of a meal—the patient could no longer close his mouth. This was often accompanied by diplopia, particularly in the evening, when he had to turn his head in order to see from side to side. Long conversations induced hoarseness and slurring of speech. During work he had frequent weakness, particularly of his thumbs, which he used continuously. Stiffness and inability to relax, aggravated by cold, were present. The patient's face and eyelids were stiff and he could not open his eyes for some seconds after several blinks. Quinine helped the stiffness, but did not affect the episodic paralysis that had increased in frequency with increasing age.

Examination in a warm environment showed no hypertrophy or wasting but paradoxic myotonia of the eyelids with inability to open them after several blinks (the reverse of that usually found in myotonia congenita). A "myotonic lid lag" was present, and extraoccular muscles were paradoxically myotonic. The hands showed marked paradoxic and percussion myotonia in the thenar muscles, tongue, and shoulder girdle. Weakness was not present. Paradoxic myotonia increased with cold exposure. Glucose and insulin infusion produced a paraparesis and marked weakness of all muscles tested, evident only after several muscular contractions. The right leg became completely paralyzed after strength testing; concomitantly, the untested left leg could still resist gravity. His hands became paralyzed only toward the end of dressing; the jaw was paretic after a few bites of a meal. Conjugate eye movements were not possible after a few side-to-side saccades. His weakness improved 24 hr after the infusion but persisted to some extent for 48 hr. Afterwards, generalized muscle soreness was present. Action potential amplitudes did not decrease after repetitive nerve stimulation. Myotonic potentials occurred after voluntary effort and muscle percussion. Fibrillation-like potentials were occasionally seen. Action potentials on voluntary effort showed a normal interference pattern and were predominantly of normal amplitude duration and configuration. No myastenic reaction was demonstrable with or without glucose and insulin infusion.

Laboratory tests showed a normal serum potassium and thyroid function. An increased CK and urinary creatinine were found.

The disorder in this family is unique because it is distinguishable from myotonia congenita by the episodic paralysis associated with exercise, from paramyotonia congenita by the presence of paralysis independent of myotonia and cold exposure, and from paralysis periodica paramyotonica because of involvement of extraoccular muscles and the induction of paralysis by glucose and insulin infusion. It can be distinguished from adynamia episodica hereditaria because of the normal resting serum potassium and low potassium during induced attacks and from myotonic dystrophy by the absence of dystrophic signs. The disorder is probably dominantly inherited though this has not been ascertained (Appenzeller and Amick [42]).

Periodic Paralyses

Periodic paralyses are attacks of weakness. There are two types, with similar symptoms but separate causes. Hypokalemic periodic paralysis is an autosomal dominantly inherited condition that sometimes is associated with thyrotoxicosis. The attacks of weakness are often nocturnal and are precipitated by carbohydrate meals, especially if taken after exercise. Most of the skeletal muscles are involved in severe attacks, and flaccid paralysis occurs that may impair speech and coughing. Insulin provokes attacks of paralysis, but regardless of how attacks are induced, they can be aborted by the oral administration of 10–15 g of potassium chloride or potassium citrate. Exercise of affected muscles may help reduce the duration of attacks. Serum potassium characteristically falls either with onset of weakness or prior to weakness, and muscle strength can return to normal before serum potassium normalizes. Serum potassium is not lost from the body but moves into muscle cells. Between attacks, muscle potassium is low and intracellular sodium is elevated. Histologically, muscle fibers contain vacuoles. These may be a swollen T system or sarcoplasmic reticulum. Early in the disease course, muscle strength is normal between attacks but with repeated paralyses, the vacuoles in muscles become persistent, in association with myofibrillar loss and clinically persistent weakness. Muscle excitability is absent with direct or indirect electrical stimulation during attacks. The paralysis is accompanied by depolarization of the muscle membrane, and the relief of weakness with oral potassium chloride is associated with repolarization (Riecker and Bolter [43]).

When normal human intercostal muscle is tested in a low external potassium medium and with insulin in the presence of normal potassium, only slight changes in excitability are found. If muscles from patients, however, are similarly tested, a large depolarization leading to inexcitability occurs. In familial periodic paralysis, if the muscle is exposed to a potassium-free medium, the addition of insulin causes repolarization. Repolarization also occurs in muscle samples from patients with familial periodic paralysis with reduction of sodium conductance (by adding procaine or replacing sodium with choline) in a low-potassium medium.

Weakness often occurs in patients with hyperkalemic periodic paralysis in the first decade of life. It is provoked by potassium and relieved by glucose and insulin. The situation is therefore the reverse of that in hypokalemic periodic paralysis. The level of serum potassium is variable during attacks of weakness attributed to movement of potassium out of muscle cells and perhaps other tissues into the circulation. The chronic changes in hyperkalemic periodic paralysis are similar to those found in hypokalemic periodic paralysis although the circumstances that provoke weakness are different. Muscle sodium increases and muscle potassium decreases during attacks and abnormalities of ionic concentrations are present during attack-free periods. Morphologically, vacuolation of muscle fibers similar to that in hypokalemic periodic paralysis is characteristic of affected skeletal muscles when muscles are studied by electron microscopy. This condition, though closely linked to paramyotonia, is not characterized by myotonic discharges. The resting membrane potentials measured by microelectrodes are low between attacks, but large depolarizations occur during an attack. Weakness often occurs before serum potassium increases, and it may be that hyperkalemia results from muscle depolarization (Engel and Angelini [31]). The cause of depolarization of muscles in hyperkalemic periodic paralysis remains unknown. It has been suggested that during development of depolarization the electrical potentials approach threshold, resulting in membrane hyperexcitability and myotonic responses of the muscle. As depolarization continues, the muscle becomes inexcitable and paralyzed.

Exercise in patients with periodic paralyses is difficult, though many participate in athletics, particularly during their earlier years before evidence of permanent muscle damage occurs.

MALIGNANT HYPERTHERMIA

This condition can occur in healthy and athletic individuals. It is associated with anesthesia and results in alarming and often fatal hyperpyrexia. During anesthesia induction, muscle tone and plasma lactate levels increase. Body temperature rises rapidly and eventually cardiac failure ensues. Renal damage due to myoglobinuria complicates the condition, and prognosis is poor unless treatment is instituted early. Use of the anesthetic halothane and/or of muscle relaxants such as suxamethonium chloride precipitates malignant hyperpyrexia. The condition is hereditary (autosomal dominant); more males than females are affected. Muscle biopsies of clinically athletic and healthy persons who are genetically at risk for this problem are abnormal histologically. Internal nuclei, target fibers, small angular fibers and "moth eaten fibers," are seen. Ultrastructural examination shows disruption of sarcomeres and Z-band streaming (Isaacs [44]). If the condition is suspected, diagnosis can be made prior to surgery by the in vitro examination of a muscle specimen that shows a greater tendency to contract when caffeine is added to the medium (Nelson et al. [45]). Active muscle phosphorylase is elevated in susceptible individuals (Willner et al. [46]). A similar condition, characterized by rigidity, acidosis, and hyperkalemia, occurs in certain strains of pigs when they are stressed, not necessarily by anesthesia. These animals eventually die from heart failure.

CRAMPS, CONTRACTURES, AND MUSCLE PAIN

Unaccustomed physical activity or muscle contraction over and above usual training often results in discomfort. The cause of pain so induced is not understood, but it might be due to muscle injury. Ischemia causes pain, and this may be exaggerated by other factors in excessively exercised muscles if preceded by prolonged ischemia. However, pain does not occur earlier with exercise preceded by experimental ischemia. Therefore, a simple relationship of pain to lack of oxygen does not exist, nor is there a direct connection between muscle pain and accumulation of metabolic products such as lactic acid. It may be that muscle contraction is associated with the release of pain-producing substances that excite nociceptive nerve fibers. Bradykinin, prostaglandin, histamine, ATP, or increased hydrogen ion concentration due to anaerobic glycolysis are candidates for such pain-producing substances. Sympathetic activity to muscle blood vessels is increased during isometric contractions. When the limb is then made ischemic, though the muscles are no longer contracting, the sympathetic activity continues to increase concomitantly with the pain, suggesting that the sympathetic nervous system may also be involved with continued pain from unaccustomed exertion through the perivascular nerve plexuses, which contain nociceptive afferents.

Individual muscle fibers, single motor units, or several groups of motor units may contract involuntarily and cause cramps. The dysfunction can arise in the central nervous system, in peripheral motor nerves, or in muscles themselves. Cramps are associated with electrical activity that distinguishes them from contractures associated with electrical silence. Such contractures are seen in patients with metabolic disorders who exercise, for example, myophosphorylase deficiency.

Drug-Induced Muscle Weakness

The administration of some drugs sometimes results in weakness. Some destroy muscles through unknown mechanisms, other affect contractile properties. In the latter category are drugs causing hypokalemia. Pain and weakness characterize drug-induced myopathies. Clorfibrate, salbutamol, some cytotoxic drugs, and isoetharine produce a cramp-like discomfort without weakness. Such minor but still painful myopathies are unexplained, and the symptoms and signs usually disappear when the drug is withdrawn. Unfortunately, no simple relationship exists between the severity of muscle disease and/or pain. In steroid myopathies, weak and wasted muscles are usually painless. Megavitamins and vitamin E, often ingested by some athletes and claimed to improve performance, may produce proximal leg weakness. Biopsies have not been done in affected individuals though, and the morphology or genesis of this transient myopathy remains unknown. Anabolic steroids are widely used by throwers and lifters to improve strength. This is not sanctioned by official athletic organizations, and efforts are being made to curb their use. The administration of these drugs illegally to endurance athletes has also been reported. Anabolic steroids (17-ethyl, 19-nortestosterone) administration increases creatine excretion in normal subjects, probably from increased muscle synthesis, but it may produce several major and minor abnormalities in humans, including the induction of liver cancer.

EXERCISE AND STRESS

Opioids and Endurance Training

Advances in opioid research have kindled interest in their function in humans. They are important in pain modulation, sleep, respiration, thermoregulation, sexual function, and endocrine secretion. The actual and hypothetical influence of these substances continues to expand. The relationship between a given opioid level and modification of physiologic function including exercise tolerance and behavior is not known, and there is no recognized correlation between different opioid or hormone levels and athletic performance. Nevertheless, endurance training has been advocated for a number of diseases, and countless healthy persons participate in strenuous sports in an attempt to improve their physical appearance and to stave off the ravages of age. Adaptive phenomena to sustained high-energy expenditure during training and long distance competition include changes in the plasma and possibly in the cerebrospinal fluid (CSF) levels of opioids. Studies show increased plasma β-endorphin and β-lipotropin at various times during athletic performances, particularly in long distance running (Fig. 3-1). However, the run-induced elevation of plasma β-endorphin and β-lipotropin seems to be reduced at the end of later races in runners who participated in the same events over several years (Fig. 3-2). β-Endorphin and β-lipotropin are released together with other stress hormones (cortisol, growth hormone, and prolactin) during muscular exertion. Another measure of stress that may have changed with continued running was needed to exclude the possibility that better and longer training accounted for a decrease in stress with repeated competition, thus decreasing the stress-induced outpouring of opioids. Serum myoglobin in the same participants, however, was increased at the end of the race compared with previous years so that exertion during the race, at least as measured by the increase in myoglobin was, if anything, more severe (Fig. 3-3). The transient acute exercise-induced rises in plasma β-endorphin and β-lipotropin or their removal from the circulation at the finish are altered by continued training.

It may be that training-associated heat loads change the blood–brain barrier to circulating β-endorphin and β-lipotropin and allow entry into the CSF, thus decreasing peripheral levels also. Animal studies support this interpretation. Exploration of the link between β-endorphin in blood and CSF during endotoxin stress suggests that reflux of plasma β-endorphin into the CSF occurs and may be secondary to the endotoxin-induced fever. Body temperature rises with training and racing. A breakdown of the blood–brain barrier by high body temperature during a race might therefore contribute to the remarkable decrease in the exercise-induced elevation of plasma opioid levels seen with continued training (Appenzeller et al. [47]).

Exercise in Hemiparetic Patients

Ultrastructural examination of paretic muscles in patients with hemiplegia due to upper motor neuron lesions shows altered mitochondria. Their numbers are reduced and both outer and inner mitochondrial membranes are changed (Ahlquist et al. [48]). Succinate

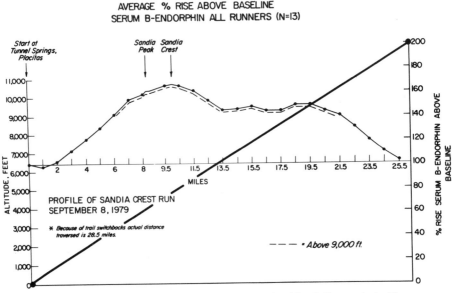

3-1 Average increase above baseline in circulating β-endorphin–β-lipotropin in 13 runners participating in prolonged trail running at altitude (average time for completion of race 5 hr).

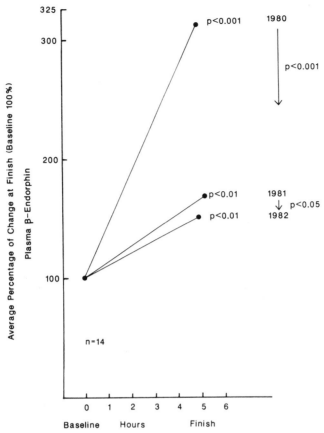

3-2 Longitudinal study of plasma beta-endorphin showing a significant decrease in run-induced outpouring of opioids. Same runners each year. (Reproduced from Appenzeller et al. [47].)

dehydrogenase in the inner mitochondrial membrane of hemiplegic muscles is low also (Saltin et al. [49]).

Examination of paretic muscles during rhythmic median-nerve-stimulation-induced exercise shows an abnormally increased lactate production and reduced ability to oxidize free fatty acids. Electrical stimulation results in recruitment that involves both Type 1 and Type 2 fibers (true with normal contractions also). Muscle metabolism during exercise in partially paretic patients with upper motor neuron lesions has been examined. When both legs (the paretic and nonparetic one) were exercised simultaneously, oxygen uptake on the partially paralyzed side was significantly lower than on the healthy side. Similarly, glucose uptake was less and there was no net exchange for lactate on the paretic side. Judged by strength of contractions, the paretic leg did less work than the healthy side. During exercise of the paretic leg, only oxygen and glucose uptakes of the working and resting legs were similar, but lactate release was significantly greater on the paretic side. Glycogen depletion patterns indicate that mainly Type 2 fibers were activated during exercise on the paretic side and mainly Type 1 fibers were activated during exercise on the normal side. Blood flow was reduced, lactate production increased, and the capacity to oxidize free fatty acids decreased in the hemiparetic leg that was capable of some work. These changes can be attributed to Type 2 muscle fibers and perhaps to a mitochondrial change in the muscle. Circulatory and metabolic changes suggest that exercising one leg at a time in hemiparesis is preferable to exercising both legs simultaneously in such patients (Landin et al. [50]).

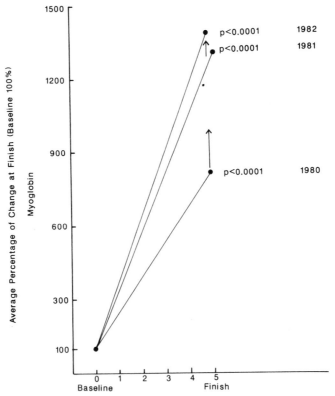

3-3 Longitudinal study of serum myoglobin showing a significant increase in run-induced release into the circulation. Same runners (Fig. 3-2) each year. (Reproduced from Appenzeller et al. [47].)

In healthy humans, passive limb movement causes a significant increase in pulmonary ventilation. This increase is partly due to an augmented breathing frequency while mean tidal volume remains unchanged. The effect of passive limb movement in hemiparetic patients with a flaccid hemiplegia was also studied and showed that hyperventilation induced by passive limb movement was abolished in the hemiplegic patients when the flaccid limbs were passively moved, but there was also a reduction in the passive-limb-movement-induced pulmonary hyperventilation when the healthy side was moved. Because all patients had evidence of cortical or capsular lesions, it was concluded that the integrity of the cortical spinal pathway is necessary to obtain the ventilatory response to passive limb motion. The decreased responses from the healthy side are attributed to impairment of chest wall and diaphragmatic function on the hemiplegic side (Sandrini et al. [51]).

Atrial Natriuretic Factor

The regulation and maintenance of blood volume is under control of several factors such as aldosterone, the antidiuretic hormone arginine-vasopressin (AVP), and other hormones. Low-pressure sensors in the heart (in the atria and also, perhaps, in the ventricles) have been implicated as the most important sense organs to assess the fullness of the blood stream (Genest and Cantin [52]).

Some cells in the atria of the heart have been found to contain secretory granules that release their contents (atrial natriuretic factor, or ANF) when the atrial walls are stretched. The stretch may occur when perfusion pressure or expanded blood volume is the stimulus. Release of ANF also occurs with stress.

Isolation of ANF and its chemical characterization has led to extensive studies on its effects on renal excretion and on water and sodium balance. The actions of ANF are multifactorial and often related to its vasorelaxation on renal arteries and arterioles. It also causes an increase in glomerilar filtration rate and filtration fraction, leading to an increased excreted fraction of filtered sodium. In addition, kaliuresis is found (Goldsmith [53]).

Atrial natriuretic peptide has antihypertensive effects. This is most likely the result of vasorelaxation rather than its effect on sodium loss and subsequent falls in extracellular fluid volume.

Plasma AVP (antidiuretic hormone) decreases considerably during the intravenous administration of ANF so that a fall in AVP may contribute to the ANF-induced diuresis.

Specific binding sites for ANF have been found in renal glomeruli in the zona glomerulosa of the adrenal gland, the posterior pituitary, and the vascular endothelium. Similar binding sites have been identified by immunofluorescent techniques in the rat brain, particularly in the area postrema, the nucleus tractus solitarius, the subfornical organ, and the anteroventral third ventricular region, all areas of the brain that are intimately connected to the regulation of water homeostasis and blood pressure.

In patients who have polyuria associated with elevated atrial pressures during paroxysmal atrial tachycardia, significant increases in plasma ANF have been found; similar increases occur in congestive heart failure. Moreover, distension of the human atrium is reported to increase the release of ANF into the circulation (Singer et al. [54]). Studies on the effects of central venous pressure on the release of human ANF were carried out in normal individuals by passive leg raising to 60° and head-up whole body tilt at 60°. The effect of these maneuvers on ANF levels suggests that secretion is regulated physiologically by changes in central venous pressure (Ogihara et al. [55]).

Immobilization stress for 4 hr stimulates a 5- to 20-fold increase in ANF levels, and in animals with hereditary cardiomyopathies or congestive heart failure tremendous increases in ANF levels can also be found.

Fluid volume regulation during exercise has been a topic of considerable interest for many years. With the increase in exercise and health awareness throughout the world, consideration of problems pertaining to fluid volume depletion and repletion have received renewed scrutiny. Endocrine regulation of fluids and salts have been investigated and attention has been paid to changes in aldosterone, AVP, and catecholamines, but ANF has been neglected. Exercise usually results in volume depletion, which in turn should cause a reduced plasma level of ANF. However, prolonged exertion constitutes a severe physical stress, albeit quite unlike immobilization stress in animals. For these reasons, the authors' group decided to measure plasma concentrations of ANF in marathon runners.

A report on the effects of short bouts of exercise in untrained subjects suggested that such exertion causes an increase in plasma ANF concentration (Tanaka et al. [56]). Our studies, on the other hand, were related to high- and moderate-altitude running during a city and mountain marathon and the effect of such prolonged exertion on ANF and AVP levels in well-trained endurance athletes. Significant increases in ANF and marked increases in AVP were found after each race (Table 3-1).

A number of variables could change plasma ANF levels during exercise. Secretion of ANF could be triggered by an increase in venous return, believed by some to be the normal mechanism for increasing ANF secretion. Plasma ANF could also be increased by exercise-associated tachycardia, by autonomic discharges, by AVP release, and by the stress of the exertion. On the other hand, ANF release should be inhibited by the run-associated volume depletion, but secretion of ANF inhibits release of AVP and aldosterone, two hormones also of interest in exercise physiology.

Endurance training causes an increase in blood volume at rest, but this may be markedly altered immediately after prolonged races because of the run-associated dehydration.

Table 3-1 Atrial Natriuretic Factor (ANF) Before (Baseline) and After (Postrun) a Marathon and Wilderness (Mountain) Run

	Baseline (pg/ml)	Postrun (pg/ml)
Marathon Run (42 km) N=15	185.8 ± 16.9	262.1 ± 20 .7*
Mountain Run (46 km) N=23	207.6 ± 9.2	269.1 ± 11.0**
Arginine-Vasopressin(AVP) (pg/ml)		
Mountain Run (46 km) N=16	3.28 ± 0.79	23.9 ± 5.5***

Arginine-vasopressin from the same runners over the same terrain (obtained 1 year earlier).
*p < .001
**p < .02
*** p< .01

Under normal conditions, a reciprocal relationship between levels of ANF and AVP is found and ANF suppression of AVP secretion would enhance volume loss. In our study, however, both AVP and ANF increased in the same subjects with the stress of the mountain run.

Vasopressor agonists such as vasopressin, phenylephrine and angiotensin II increase plasma ANF in animals. In humans, acute volume expansion and oral water loading or high salt intake causes an increase in plasma ANF levels. Head-out total body water immersion also causes a marked increase in plasma ANF, which is correlated with the increase in urine volume in such experimental subjects. Plasma ANF concentration in recipients of cardiac transplants without cardiac failure or evidence of rejection also showed significant increases in the circulating ANF levels but the mechanism underlying this phenomenon, just like the increase in ANF levels in endurance-trained subjects, remains obscure. Nevertheless, this finding suggests that denervated transplanted atria may secrete ANF.

Fluid homeostasis in response to hypoxia (found during our mountain race) is complex and not fully understood. Acute mountain sickness with peripheral edema, antidiuresis, and pulmonary edema has led to the evaluation of plasma renin, aldosterone, and arginine vasopressin levels in humans during hypobaric hypoxia. The many conflicting results probably reflect the varied conditions and exercise intensities, the different altitudes and temperatures, the duration of exposure, the age of the study subjects, and also salt and water balance. Moreover, it has been suggested that different vasopressin levels during hypoxia reflected varying changes in circulating plasma volume rather than the effect of hypoxia per se. Studies in untrained individuals during 6 hr of mild exertion on a treadmill in a hypobaric hypoxic environment caused a lower mean arterial pressure and yet failed to elevate plasma renin, aldosterone and AVP (Meehan [57]). These subjects, however, were nonacclimated and untrained, quite different from participants in the mountain run. In such subjects, a clear increase in both AVP and ANF was seen both after the marathon race (1700-m altitude) and after the mountain crossing (reaching an altitude of 3300 m).

A decrease in peripheral vascular resistance, particularly in muscle blood vessels, occurs during exercise to ensure proper perfusion of contracting tissues. A similar decrease in peripheral vascular resistance occurs during hypoxia, which could facilitate nonosmotic release of AVP. But if hydration is maintained, the slight fall in mean arterial pressure associated with mild exercise in untrained males does not change AVP levels, unlike the very marked increases found in our study (Table 3-1). Animal data suggest that hypoxia stimulates the release of AVP with resultant antidiuresis if blood volume is not altered. But marked individual variations have also been found in AVP release in humans in hypoxic environments without exercise. An increase in AVP in subjects with lower mean arterial pressure and symptoms of acute mountain sickness has been reported and symptomatic subjects have even greater AVP levels. On the other hand, some altitude sojourners may become ill without an increase in AVP. When carbon dioxide is administered to hypoxic subjects, the AVP increase can be prevented, even though acute mountain sickness is aggravated by this procedure. It is concluded from these studies that a rise in AVP is not a prerequisite for developing acute mountain sickness. None of the runners had altitude-related symptoms suggestive of mountain sickness in spite of having very high AVP levels.

Catecholamine-induced release of AVP can, in turn, cause secretion of ANF in vitro. We have previously shown that during our city marathon race, significant increases in catecholamines occurred. It is well known that systolic ventricular pressures and pulmonary artery pressures increase during the early parts of exertion and that this increase is linearly related to workload. Altitude is also known to increase pulmonary artery pressures. Thus hemodynamic changes during exercise both in the city marathon and in the high-altitude race may have caused distention of atria and stimulated ANF release.

The increase in heart rate during both races may have contributed to the enhanced ANF levels also. In hypertensive patients, exercise is said to cause a reduction of blood pressure and a decrease in extracellular fluid volume, but this occurs only if blood lactate thresholds have not been reached during the workloads. It is possible that an increase in ANF with exertion is also important in the therapeutic lowering of blood pressure in some hypertensive exercisers.

In animals, profound analgesia related to the release of endogenous opioids can be produced by inescapable stressful electric shocks to the feet. This is antagonized by naloxone (a specific opioid antagonist) only if the shocks are intermittent, producing rhythmic movements. Stress-induced analgesia is not antagonized by this drug when the shocks are continuous, causing prolonged muscle spasm. It seems, therefore, that rhythmic muscle contractions can be associated with analgesia and that the afferent stimulus for this opioid-dependent stress-induced analgesia may be neurogenic and perhaps arise from the rhythmically contracting muscles. Heretofore the release of ANF and AVP had been attributed to changes in atrial pressures in blood volume and fluid and electrolyte homeostasis. It is possible, however, that the increases in ANF and AVP in our city and mountain runs may have been due to neurogenic afferent stimuli arising in the rhythmically contracting skeletal muscles in the enduranced-trained subjects.

During both city and mountain runs, the exercise-associated volume depletion would promote an inhibition of release of ANF. The observed increase in ANF in the runners could be misread as a signal that blood volume had actually increased, but it remains uncertain what the consequences of this missignaling might be.

If stress was the predominant factor in causing increased ANF secretion in subjects, then the marathon at 1700-m altitude was a maximal stimulus, because the mountain run (reaching 3300 m) did not produce a larger increase in ANF levels. However, it remains for sea level races to be studied to support this unlikely interpretation.

DISEASES OF MUSCLES, MUSCLE PAIN, AND FATIGUE IN SPORTS PARTICIPANTS

Athletes with muscular disease are uncommon; they usually do not do well in competition. However, the exercise boom has spread to nonathletic individuals and has led to the appearance of amateur athletes with muscular disease. They may complain of excessive fatigue or weakness during exercise over and above their usual levels. This is increasingly important, because with proper management such patients may continue to be active sports participants, and in some cases this may have salutary effects on maintaining independent existence for longer periods of time.

Muscle aches and cramps normally accompany excessive exercise, pregnancy, and dehydration. However, cramps may also be the first symptoms of myopathic disorders related to thyroid dysfunction, uremia, electrolyte abnormalities such as hypomagnesemia, intermittent claudication of the legs or spinal cord, or caudaequina. In amytrophic lateral sclerosis it may be the first manifestation of disease and may also be a feature of hyper- and hypoparathyroidism. Fatigue, severe cramps, and weakness are the hallmarks of muscle disease that is part of a generalized disorder and are more common in such conditions than in primary myopathies. Weakness, painful cramps, and fatigue occur in inflammatory myopathies such as dermatomyositis, polymyositis, polymyalgia rheumatica, myopathy associated with hypokalemia, alcoholic myopathies, and muscle disorders due to drugs such as lithium, amphetamine, clofibrate, tolbutamide, and numerous other toxic agents. Metabolic bone disease may be accompanied by a myopathy, and a predominantly proximal weakness occurs in either primary or secondary hyperparathyroidism, in hypophosphatemia, in renal tubular dysfunction, and in intoxication with anticonvulsants. Patients with these disorders rarely participate in competitive events or begin athletic activities. Still, established athletes may succumb to these diseases and develop fatigue, cramps, and weakness, and therefore these possibilities should be kept in mind.

Muscle enzyme levels in athletes should be interpreted with caution. Serum CK is increased, particularly just after competition and for some days thereafter. This is well documented and is attributed to increased or abnormal permeability of muscle membranes, perhaps because of inadequate oxygen supply during contraction. This is found even in highly trained athletes and often after relatively minor exertion in nonathletes. Ultrastructural examination of muscles of athletes has not shown tissue damage, even though CK levels have been high. Serum CK and other muscle enzyme levels after vigorous exercise are determined by training prior to exertion. Even in the same individuals, if untrained muscles are exercised (for example, the arms in a runner) CK levels are higher than when well-trained muscles are exercised to similar levels (legs in a trained runner). Evaluation of resting plasma muscle enzyme levels in athletes demands abstention from training for at least 10 days before representative resting levels can be expected.

Creatinine kinase and MB isoenzyme (CK-MB) is thought to be a sensitive and specific marker of myocardial injury. However, this enzyme is also released into the circulation in athletes and correlates with serum myoglobin. It may be that it is a sensitive marker for exertional rhabdomyolysis. Plasma CK-MB levels in male marathon runners during training and after competitive events were similar to those in patients after myocardial necrosis. However, examination of the hearts of the marathoners by Tc-99m-pyrophosphate scanning showed no evidence of myocardial infarction. Other clinical evidence of myocardial damage was not found in highly trained marathon runners with elevated CK-MB isoenzymes. The enzyme probably enters the circulation from skeletal muscles also.

Advice to Patients with Myotonia

Patients with primary myotonias, including myotonia congenita, paramyotonia congenita, and Isaac's syndrome (cramps, stiffness, continuous muscle fiber activity, occasionally with hyperhidrosis), can be helped to improve exercise performance with appropriate counseling, and some are successful athletes. In such individuals, the myotonia stiffness is worse initially and improves with continued effort. Continuous low-level activity prior to athletic events or training is therefore beneficial in achieving muscle relaxation. Such handicapped athletes should avoid rest and indulge in extended warm-ups of rather low intensity.

Similar advice is also useful to novice normal individuals who embark upon athletics. Because warmth improves suppleness of muscles and decreases myotonia, patients should dress warmly prior to exertion. Increasing doses of oral quinine in the morning and a high carbohydrate intake prior to competition facilitates prolonged activity and improves myotonia. High-carbohydrate diet improves exercise capacity in such individuals by decreasing plasma potassium with its well-known deleterious effects on myotonia. Carbohydrate-induced insulin release allows both glucose and potassium to enter the muscle cell and decreases myotonia.

Muscle Pain and Its Investigation

Exercise often produces pain in normal muscles, but muscle pain occurs commonly in a variety of pathologic conditions also. It may be the presenting symptom of many disorders of muscles and nerves, and though the diagnoses may be clear (rheumatoid diseases, severe depression) a number of patients with myalgia remain who present diagnostic and management problems. If a definitive diagnosis cannot be made, the management of pain in muscles that may be generalized or local becomes difficult. Analgesics, mechanical vibration, hot or cold compresses, antidepressants, and/or transcutaneous nerve stimulation may be tried. When considering the use of drugs for treatment of postexertional myalgia, one must take into account that athletes, particularly during competitive years, are likely to become dependent on even mild analgesics and certainly on narcotics. This will interfere with performance and with official recognition of athletic achievement in local, national, and international competitive events.

Several reviews concerning muscle pain have been published (Serratrice et al. [58]; Mills and Edwards [59]). The following scheme has been proposed for the investigation of such puzzling patients: strength and exercise testing, because symptoms often appear only with exercise; electromyography; needle muscle biopsy; plasma CK erythrocyte sedimentation rate (ESR); and electrolytes. In spite of such tests and even in centers for the diagnosis of muscle disease, there are many cases in which no further diagnosis can be made. Many such patients are depressed and somatization of their depression is in the form of myalgia. A significant number have abnormal muscle structure or function that does not fall into any known category of muscle diseases. Since this is found mainly in young people, particularly in women, perhaps such patients have an unusual propensity to damage of muscle with exercise or have an as yet unrecognized enzyme deficit. It is best, however, to regard these abnormalities as nonspecific since morphologic changes on biopsy usually do not indicate a specific known disease and elevated CK levels might simply reflect unaccustomed exertion in the days prior to the examination. Urine should be tested for myoglobinuria, and mitochondrial enzyme abnormalities should be considered in appropriate patients.

All pain from muscles must ultimately activate pain receptors in the muscles or in muscle attachments. The existence of such nociceptors in humans is not well established, but in cats pain is produced by tension, and increases in lactate, potassium, histamine, bradykinin, serotonin, and other substances. In inflammatory muscle disease, it is postulated that pain is mediated by kinins released from inflammatory cells. Ischemic muscular pain or muscle pain induced by exhaustion of energy substrates may be caused by potassium or phosphate accumulation or by increased lactate. High lactate levels, however, are not the cause of muscular pain in myophosphorylase deficiency. Exacerbation of pain is often related to contraction of the muscles. The role of tension receptors in muscle pain and their interaction with signals due to metabolic changes have not been delineated.

Eccentric muscle contraction or lengthening of a muscle simultaneously with contraction has been associated with pain and often causes discomfort after unaccustomed exertion. Repeated eccentric contractions in normal individuals causes fatigue (Newham et al. [60]). In such individuals, a rise in CK and damage to Z-lines together with sarcomere disruption occur.

Extensive analysis of the most useful test in patients presenting with myalgia has shown muscle biopsy to be the best indicator of organic disease; the least sensitive for organic disease of muscles is the sedimentation rate. Many patients with muscle pain remain without specific diagnosis. The most nonspecific test should therefore be used first, and that is the ESR. If normal, this separates patients in whom a tissue diagnosis will not be made. Initially, an ESR and CK are estimated, and muscle biopsy, electromyography, and strength and exercise testings are done later if the initial tests are abnormal. In those in whom no abnormality is found on the two initial screening tests yet muscle disease is still suspected, biopsy and electromyography are the most productive subsequent tests.

THE NERVOUS SYSTEM

Human adaptation to endurance training and athletic activity is not fully understood; recent studies point to the large gaps in knowledge of the effects of physical activity on the normal and the diseased nervous system. Several examples may be useful. The effect of vigorous exercise on cerebral oxygen consumption remains controversial. One study suggests that oxygen consumption is increased; others contend that it remains unchanged (Greenhouse [61]). Glucose utilization by the brain also seems to remain unaffected by exercise. In animals, brain stem and hypothalamic monoamines decrease with acute exertion and serotonin increases in the same area, but the net result of this change is not known. Positron emission tomography (PET) of the human brain may provide useful insights into brain metabolism neurotransmitter physiology and show focal alterations in these functions produced by exercise. Moreover, manipulations of athletic performance may become correlated with changes in PET scans. It is already known that cerebral blood flow and metabolism may change focally in appropriate areas in response to motor or sensory activation, but blood flow to the whole brain does not change with exercise. Extensive studies of cerebral blood flow in endurance-trained subjects, however, have not been carried out with PET, nor has the effect of exercise at altitude been studied with this technique.

Repetitive stimuli in the peripheral and perhaps in the central nervous system alter function of nerves and the brain. It remains controversial, however, whether the repetitive stimulation of prolonged exertion affects central or peripheral nervous system function. While it is generally assumed that fatigue originates in the muscles, it is clear that the central nervous system plays an important role in this area, since incentive, stress, temperature, and other psychologic factors affect fatigue. Moreover, some studies suggest that centrally acting drugs may affect fatigue even in nervous system disease such as multiple sclerosis (Rosenberg et al. [62]). The RPE (discussed earlier in this chapter) is grossly abnormal in severe depression or schizophrenia. However, measurements of brain and peripheral nerve electrical activity suggest that these functions are unaffected by fatigue. Visual evoked responses, somatosensory evoked responses and brain stem auditory evoked responses remain unaffected. While it has been proposed that peripheral nerve conduction velocities also show no change with fatigue, tibial nerve conduction before and after a 46-km mountain race when corrected for temperature changes showed a significant slowing of the conduction attributed to a "steel phenomenon" when blood was shunted away from the nerve to the exercising muscles (Berger and Appenzeller [63]).

The autononomic nervous system is important in adaptation to exercise and stress. Parasympathetic overactivity leads to bradycardia of endurance-trained subjects, and blockade of the sympathetic nervous system causes impaired exertional performance. Moreover, mobilization of free fatty acids, glycogen utilization, and catecholamine secretion (all related to sympathetic activation) are important adaptive responses to meet exertional demands.

Tests of autonomic function in endurance-trained subjects have shown different responses from those expected in normal nontrained individuals. For example, the diving response, normally consisting of bradycardia and hypertension, shows a significant bradycardia but no hypertension in individuals trained for endurance. The cold pressor test, consisting of an increase in blood pressure and cardiac output with cold immersion of a limb, is found to be markedly blunted at rest and converted to a hypotensive response after exercise (Appenzeller et al. [64, 65]). Telemetric electroencephalographic (EEG) recording during exercise shows an influence of exertion on alpha rhythm. The amount of alpha activity in the EEG is usually related to alertness and alpha "reactivity"; that is, blocking of alpha rhythm by attention, eye opening, and mental activity is also altered. Nevertheless, extensive telemetric studies in endurance-trained subjects during prolonged exertion have not been carried out. Preliminary investigations in some but not all well-trained subjects suggest an absence of alpha rhythm during eye closure at rest intervals during prolonged exertion for runs of 16 km or more at racing speed (Appenzeller [66]). In epileptic patients, the interictal epileptiform activity is markedly decreased with exercise and fatigue, and inactivity has the opposite effect.

The influence of exercise on EEG recorded sleep stages is controversial, primarily because of the diversity of subjects studied. In endurance-trained individuals, deep sleep seems to be increased after a marathon. Altitude and exertion also influence sleep stages, depending on the subject's level of training, the duration of altitude exposure, the degree of exertion, and subject sex. In general, endurance-trained subjects and those who are altitude acclimated have more deep sleep after exertion at altitude than do those who are less adapted to this additional stress.

Intellectual performance is decreased by fatigue, but endurance training in disturbed children improves behavior, perhaps by lessening fatigability. Exercised subjects can perform better on specific cognitive tests, but in these studies only mild exertion was used, so that the effect of endurance training on cognitive performance remains controversial. Nevertheless, academic achievement improves with sustained training. Whether this results from the training or the personality traits that contribute to the initiation and maintenance of a conditioning program is not clear. It has been shown that endurance-trained subjects are self-sufficient, intelligent, sober, shy, imaginative, conceited, and reserved. This might account for the suggestion that psychologic aging is slowed by a higher level of physical training if it is maintained for some time. Effects on intellectual capacity of factors such as dietary modification, cessation of smoking, and changes in alcohol intake, which frequently accompany endurance training, have not been studied.

Little is known of the nervous system's role in the acquisition of athletic skills and selection of athletic disciplines. Training unquestionably influences the establishment of appropriate motor and sensory circuits and causes adaptation of muscle fiber contractile properties for specific events. In addition, learning plays a major role in the development of skills and adaptation of proper nerve circuits in the central and peripheral nervous systems. However, genetic factors are important in achieving excellence in sports because of the advantage offered by body size, limb length, and weight. Whether a less obvious genetically determined nervous system role exists that makes it advantageous for persons to pursue certain athletic disciplines is not known. Could specific synapses in one or the other hemisphere cause one individual to excel in track and field, swimming, tennis, or other sports and another to excel in language skills or mathematical prowess?

Endurance Training and Aging

Participation in athletics by age groups has led to eager anticipation of entry in to the next-older age bracket by weekend competitors and others, in the hope that performance will not decline but will, even if static, be comparatively better than in the just-departed 5-year segment. The anticipation of competing in an older age bracket and performing better in comparison with other members of that group seems to remove the sense of passing time and the sadness of old age. The flattery commonly addressed to elderly joggers ("You look wonderful") motivates those who frequent parks and promenades. It also encourages the old to exercise regularly.

All measurable functions of the nervous system deteriorate with age. Visual evoked responses, brain stem auditory evoked responses, somatosensory evoked response, and peripheral nerve conduction velocities fall in that category. Investigations of endurance-trained elderly individuals show shortened visual evoked response times and faster peripheral nerve conduction velocities at rest compared with values for age-matched non-endurance-trained subjects. Peroneal nerve conduction velocities and tibial nerve conduction velocities unquestionably show a decrease or absence of the age-related decay in peripheral nerve function in endurance-trained elderly subjects. Many more studies, however, are necessary to fully appreciate the effect of training on the aging of the nervous system. For example, temperature regulation, or the capacity to maintain constant body temperatures with cold or heat exposure and exercise loads, deteriorates with advancing years. This has not been studied in endurance-trained individuals. Similarly, baroreceptor function progressively fails in old age. Endurance exercise affects autonomic function, but definitive studies on baroreflex activity of trained individuals and the age-related deterioration of baroreflexes are only now being contemplated. Preliminary results of Valsalva's maneuver and the changes of blood pressure with sustained handgrip in persons trained for endurance suggest differences in young and older endurance-trained subjects compared with sedentary subjects.

Coordination, which can in part be assessed by posturography, has shown some alterations in the maintenance of posture of endurance-trained subjects (Seelinger and Appenzeller [67]). Even more remarkable, when world marathon records are considered, between the ages of 30 and 70 only a minor deterioration in performance occurs per decade. This, of course, refers to record times in various age groups, but it must depend, among many other things, on adaptation of the nervous system to stress and relative preservation of bodily function by endurance training (Fries [68]).

Altitude and Performance

Increased physical activity at altitudes at which humans formerly sojourned for only short periods of time is now common. Although permanent inhabitants do exist between 1500 and 4600 m, considerable populations are not found at that altitude. Very few venture much beyond 5500 m, and even fewer perform physical tasks at such altitudes. The adaptive mechanisms that occur in those who are acclimated to high altitude are numerous but beyond the scope of this section.

Acute Mountain Sickness The commonest manifestation of maladapted sojourners is acute mountain sickness. The important clinical manifestations of acute mountain sickness are severe, often pounding, headache; nausea; dimmed vision; restlessness; palpitation; anorexia; sleeplessness; and anxiety. Rapid ascent increases chances of developing acute mountain sickness.

High-Altitude Pulmonary Edema Rapid ascent may also be associated with high-altitude pulmonary edema in a minority of sojourners. Pulmonary edema occurs in a setting of increased thoracic intravascular volume and consequent extravascular fluid accumulation, especially in the peribronchial spaces and lung edema. If pulmonary edema is present, there is almost always an additional increased vascular permeability in other tissues. In the brain this may manifest itself as cerebral edema; retinopathy and increased intraoccular pressure, including peripheral edema, may be present. Though hypoxia is the assumed underlying cause, rapid ascent and low barometric pressure may also be important. The delay in onset of symptoms after arrival in a hypoxic environment suggests that secondary or tertiary factors are the actual triggers of altitude illness. Fluid retention occurs in all subjects on altitude exposure along with an increased sodium excretion. Those with altitude illness retain relatively more sodium than do those who are not affected by the problem. The cause of the fluid retention in this situation is not known.

High-Altitude Cerebral Edema   Although a complication of altitude exposure, high-altitude cerebral edema usually is seen at rather higher altitudes than acute mountain sickness and in those who are unacclimatized. The manifestations of altitude cerebral edema are the same as those of cerebral edema occurring at sea level: retinal hemorrhages, papilledema, clouded consciousness, confusion, and eventually coma. Nevertheless, judging from logs of Himalayan expeditions of acclimatized mountaineers, mental function sufficient to record at least metereologic data is adequate at altitudes up to 8500 m and, experimentally, at altitudes of up to 5500 m no measurable impairment of cerebral metabolism has been found.

Doppler flow velocymmetry in endurance-trained subjects at altitude showed a direct relationship among increasing altitude, common carotid, and temporal artery bloodflows, suggesting that cerebral and scalp flows are increased in endurance-trained subjects without evidence of central nervous system dysfunction in this particular study group (Appenzeller et al. [69]).

Treatment and Prevention of Altitude Illness

The best preventive measure against altitude illnesses is slow acclimation to increasing altitude. The current recommendations include a sojourn of 3 days per 1000-ft ascent over and above 10,000 ft. However, in practice this is rarely achieved, and altitude illness is a frequent occurrence in recreational altitude sojourners. The oral use of acetazolamide for 2 or 3 days prior to ascent is protective against acute mountain sickness and perhaps, though to a lesser extent, high altitude pulmonary edema. The treatment of the latter requires oxygen administration and, most important, immediate evacuation to lower altitudes. Once acute mountain sickness or high-altitude pulmonary edema is well developed, the use of diuretics, morphine, or other drugs is not effective. Acute mountain sickness alone can be treated with aspirin, cold fluids, and carbohydrate-containing food, which alleviates the condition until acclimatation has occurred. High-altitude pulmonary and cerebral edemas, however, should not be managed at altitude; evacuation to lower levels is essential. Endurance training may provide some protection from altitude illness but good evidence for this is not available. Once a person has had high-altitude pulmonary or cerebral edema, these conditions are likely to recur on reexposure to appropriate altitudes.

Anecdotal accounts exist that well acclimatized persons not suffering from mountain sickness experience personality changes that may affect the success or failure of an expedition. Whether these personality alterations are the result of hypoxia or changes in brain neurotransmitters with altitude exposure has not been determined. Neuropsychologic effects of high-altitude sojourn show certain similarities between mountaineer sojourners and those who are mildly intoxicated with alcohol. There is an increased vigilance, often manifested by difficulty in sleeping rather than in performance tests. Electroencephalograms recorded at 5500 m may show arousal patterns and decreased mean alpha frequency. Occasionally the normal suppression of alpha rhythms with eye opening did not occur and EEG signs of sleep were present in individuals who had, in fact, their eyes open. Subjects were aroused easily from deep sleep, and they experienced multiple arousal during an all-night EEG recording at altitudes of 4300 m. Visual and somatosensory evoked responses showed either no change or lengthening or shortening of latencies. It is clear, however, that brain function and the EEG are altered with altitude exposure. Other effects include somnolence, withdrawal, inattention, lethargy, fatigue, frequent desire to sleep but inability to fall asleep, Cheyne-Stokes respirations, and occasionally drowsiness. Psychomotor skills and decision making are variably affected in different individuals by altitude exposure. The intellectual changes that are associated with high altitude are similar to the impairment and slowing of mental function of advancing age. Reports of perseveration, difficulty with calculations, faulty judgment, and unpredictable emotional outbursts have appeared. Because unimpaired judgment is often critical to survival and success of mountaineering expeditions, this has been an area of interest, but comparatively little changes have been found in the ability to perform skillful tasks at altitudes below 5500 m.

The light sensitivity of the visual system is impaired, acuity is decreased, and critical flicker fusion (which depends on the metabolic rate of retinal ganglion cells) becomes impaired between 3000 and 3500 m and above. Intraocular pressure increases, particularly with exercise at altitude, but it has not reached pathologic levels in those in whom it was measured (Carlow and Appenzeller [70]). Decreased central visual acuity attributed to retinal arteriolar hemorrhage and hypoxia of ganglion cells may occur at altitudes above 5500 m. Previous high-altitude exposure to about 5000 m, even though the subject may no longer be altitude acclimated, seems to protect against visual disturbances and particularly against retinal hemorrhages upon reexposure to altitude. Recovery from retinal hemorrhages, except for those that involved the macula, is usually complete. Scotomata from macular hemorrhage may persist indefinitely, while the rest of the visual impairment sustained because of altitude exposure recovers completely.

Incoordination occurs at about 5500 m: Subjects are unsteady upon standing and are unable to stand on one leg or with eyes closed. Truncal ataxia may be so severe that support during motion is required. This usually improves with cessation of physical activity and disappears when lower altitudes are reached. Drop attacks and tetraplegia to the extent that communication is possible only by facial grimacing and with the aid of neck muscles have been reported. Tendon reflexes decrease in amplitude above 4500 m and increase again at about 6100 m and higher. This has been attributed to cerebral and brain stem hypoxia. In general, no altitude-related effects on the sensory system have been found except in those who in addition to altitude, also suffer from cold injury, which is common and affects limb sensation preferentially.

Permanent neurologic deficits after high altitude exposure have been reported (West [71]). But the evidence for this extends only to about 1 year after exposure and refers to finger-tapping speed. This has been gleaned from mountaineers who, in general, are not endurance trained.

Exercise at Altitude

Altitude adaptation increases performance in high altitudes but the capacity to perform work is still less at altitude than at sea level for a given adapted individual. Oxygen is less available to muscles and vital capacity decreases. Nevertheless, transient efforts lasting no more than a few minutes may be enhanced by altitude because of decreased air resistance. Athletic events requiring more than a few minutes for completion are considerably altered by altitude and performance is worse. This applies to acclimatized and unacclimatized athletes, though acclimatization and training at high altitude may improve performance significantly for endurance events.

While altitude illness is present, subjects should not participate in athletic events or excessive exertion because muscular work accentuates hypoxia. It is also important to realize that oxygen consumption for a given amount of work at high altitude is greater than that for the same amount of work at lower elevations, and thus mountain sickness is aggravated with even minor exertion. Efficiency of muscle contraction is also reduced and cardio-pulmonary recovery is prolonged at altitude.

Acclimatization improves oxygen delivery to tissues by its effect on the hematocrit tissue capillary density and 2,3-diphosphoglycerate, all further improved by training at altitude. Three or more weeks of altitude training are necessary before all physiologic adjustments can be expected and the maximum exercise potential for a given altitude obtained. Performance is always worse in an individual athlete at altitude if effort duration is more than a few minutes. The methods of training at altitude to achieve optimum and speedy acclimatization have not been fully investigated, and athletes not suffering from mountain sickness can engage in athletic activity at maximum effort without harm. Speed and short-duration efforts might be emphasized in order to build power and coordination because of prolonged recovery periods at high altitude.

Occasional disorders of nervous system function may be affected by altitude sojourn. If properly treated, epilepsy, hypertension, and diabetes mellitus seem not to be adversely affected by physical activity at altitude. No one knows how many epileptic individuals are successful climbers, and accidents during climbs have not been attributed to seizures. Some anticonvulsants protect the central nervous system from ischemic or hypoxic damage. Whether they are also protective against the ill effects of high altitude on nervous system function is not certain. Cerebral vascular and heart disease can be aggravated by hypoxia superimposed on an already compromised circulation; however, serious accidents have not been reported from altitude exposure of patients with established disease, although strokes in elderly climbers have occurred while exposed to altitude.

Even well-controlled myasthenia gravis and multiple sclerosis in remission may be affected adversely by altitude exposure, and weakness, ataxia, and spasticity can be aggravated or brought on by travel to elevations above 3000 m.

Tolerance to alcohol and sedative drugs is decreased at altitude. This may be related to the similarity of effects of altitude and alcohol on central nervous system function. The effect of sedative drugs might be compounded by the respiratory depression in a setting of hypoxia. Migraine is precipitated by altitude exposure in some sufferers (Appenzeller [72]). Nonneurologic conditions influenced by high altitude include sickle-cell disease, in which crises leading to vascular occlusion and splenic infarcts may occur at altitudes above 2300 m. There is also an increased propensity toward cold injury associated with decreased judgment and the physiologic stress of altitude exposure in all individuals, but this may also in part be related to changes in circulation and the altitude polycytemia, which increases blood viscosity.

Eyes and exposed skin should be protected from ultraviolet radiation, which is increased by the thin atmosphere and reflection from snow. When combined with hypoxia, ultraviolet radiation may severely injure these organs (Petajan [73]).

NEUROLOGIC HANDICAP AND REHABILITATION THROUGH SPORTS

Handicapped individuals have special biomechanical requirements for performance in certain sports. For example, wheelchair ping-pong is quite different from ordinary games of this type. But the biomechanics of wheelchair archery are not much different from the traditional variety. Recreational and athletic competition is available for poliomyelitis patients, paraplegics, and amputees, and Special Olympics are offered for the physically and mentally handicapped. Careful analysis of weakness and spasticity of force velocities, motion, and electromyographic kinesiology in those with neurologic handicaps helps with special modification of physical activities and adaptation of exercises to patients. It is important to recognize functional rather than diagnostic categories of neurologic deficits. The recognition of spasticity alone is insufficient because a description of the speed of muscle activation, the delay between intent and movement, and tension and strength of a particular limb are all important. Delays in relaxation occur and influence athletic activity also. Mirror movements and overflow of purposeful activity to other limbs, particularly in patients with cerebral palsy, may interfere with athletic activity. Respiratory control is all-important in performance of such patients. Many also have problems with visual tracking, particularly those with extrapyramidal lesions, and this affects sports that require good visual coordination.

Some patients with neurologic disease have associated cardiac involvement. An example of this is Friedreich's ataxia and some muscular dystrophies. To be cognizant of this is important in some nonprogressive muscular dystrophies that may improve with endurance training and may increase exercise tolerance in patients, including the usefulness of minimally or noninvolved muscles.

Each patient must have a modified exercise testing protocol to adapt to his or her neurologic handicap. For example, bicycle ergometer or treadmill testing, usually used for nonhandicapped individuals, is not appropriate for some types of neurologically impaired subjects.

Finally, psychologic aspects of sports and training must be considered, because self-respect and satisfaction are derived from participation in athletics. It is often thought that the psychologic advantages arising from competition or athletic activity in the neurologically handicapped far outweigh any possible risks inherent in such pursuits. Therefore, in the long run, reckless abandon is more advantageous than cautious restriction when advice is given to patients with neurologic handicaps (Challenor [74]).

Sports in the Wheelchair

Basketball, tennis, sprinting slalom that involves maneuvering wheelchairs around obstacles and ramps, weight-lifting, table tennis, archery, javelin throwing, bowling, and shot putting from a wheelchair are all disciplines accessible to paraplegics. Many of these sports have international competitive standards, and although they were originally developed for patients with posttraumatic spinal cord disorders, paraplegics with other lesions are now also included. Roughly equal handicaps that can be classified allow patients to compete against each other in the same handicap class. In international competition, different divisions ensure fair competition based on residual function.

Sophisticated modifications of wheelchairs for competitive events are available. The largest event in the wheelchair division is the marathon, which necessitates competitors to be sent off before the actual start of the footrace.

Creditable athletic performances by amputees have been recorded. The role of the nervous system in adaptation of skills after limb amputation is best illustrated by the achievement of Karoly Takacs, the Hungarian who ranked among the top pistol shooters in the world when he participated in the 1936 Olympic games. In 1938 Takacs's right arm was accidentally amputated midway between the elbow and wrist. He then retrained his nervous system, including his eye, in order to shoot the pistol with his left hand. Takacs became world pistol shot champion in 1939, a year after the amputation, and won gold medals in the Olympic games in London in 1948 and in Helsinki in 1952.

Sports and Cerebral Palsy

Deficits in patients with cerebral palsy are related to timing, sequencing, and isolation of movements. Motor performance is distorted and movements overflow to other parts of the body. Stress is known to magnify spasticity, athetosis, and ataxia, and competition even in handicapped categories is usually too much for children with cerebral palsy. Nevertheless, participation in adaptive ball games in which special balls that travel slower than normally and weigh less are used is within their capacity. Rarely, cerebral palsy children may participate in volleyball games. Motor-handicapped children may swim freely, and competition is against the patient's own previous performance rather than against other individuals. Similar consideration to motor deficits must be entertained for respiratory muscles. Therefore, endurance events much beyond 400 m are usually difficult for spastics. Activities requiring agility and rapid movements are also not within their capabilities.

Blindness and Physical Activity

Many athletic events are open to blind persons, either with a guide or with devices that emit auditory signals. Blind children who participate in sports develop more self-reliance and security in moving about their environment. Advice from international and national sports organizations for the handicapped is available to blind persons who wish to train in a variety of different sports disciplines. Mentally retarded persons may participate in the Special Olympics program established by the Joseph P. Kennedy, Jr. foundation. Moreover, the United States Olympics program has a committee devoted to sports for the handicapped that promotes national and international competition for disabled persons. There are other organizations that deal with sports for deaf, blind, and paraplegic persons separately. The neurologically handicapped should be encouraged to participate in athletics without the necessity to compete.

Stroke, Transient Ischemic Attack, Multiple Sclerosis, and Degenerative Central and Peripheral Nervous System Diseases

Patients with completed strokes and progressive central nervous system disease have completed marathons and even ultramarathons. However, in general, those with transient ischemic attacks (TIA) should not exercise since TIAs may result from emboli to the cerebral circulation, and exercise may increase the risk.

Patients with multiple sclerosis in remission have participated in games and even in endurance training. Increased environmental and body temperatures may, however, aggravate existing symptoms in such patients or bring new ones to the neurologist's attention. Clearly, patients who are sensitive to heat should not participate in activities that tend to raise body temperature. Many multiple sclerosis patients with stable disease find that exercise improves strength and dexterity of affected parts and decreases fatigability. These patients particularly like and should be encouraged to swim. Some evidence suggests that rhythmic movement associated with exercise in multiple sclerosis patients may improve fatigability because of the release of endogenous opioids into the circulation (Rosenberg et al. [62]).

Exercise-Induced Syncope   Syncope is the result of global cerebral ischemia due to failure of cerebral perfusion. Perfusion failure in athletes during or at the end of an athletic event may be related to hyperthermia associated with a drop in cardiac output, alcohol intake after prolonged exertion, or an activation of the diving response associated with bradycardia but absence of blood pressure increase. During prolonged exertion, blood vessels to the muscles are maximally dilated and those to the skin maximally constricted. Alcohol ingestion causes vasodilation of skin vessels through its direct vasodilator effect. Cutaneous vasodilation while muscle blood vessels are still dilated compromises cardiac output to the extent that it is no longer sufficient to perfuse the brain, and syncope may result.

The treatment of syncopal episodes is directed at the cause: volume replacement and cooling for hyperthermia, horizontal positioning, and cessation of alcohol intake to allow cardiac output to recover sufficiently to maintain brain perfusion.

HEADACHE

"One should be able to recognize those who have headache from gymnastic exercises or running or walking or hunting or any other unseasonable labor or from immoderate venery." This was Hippocrates's view. Many exercise-related symptoms, including headache, have appeared with the mushrooming of participation in sports (Atkinson and Appenzeller [75]). Until not long ago, exercise-induced headaches were worthy of reporting. Now this is a frequent complaint, though definitive figures on its incidence are not available. Acute headache associated with exercise, straining, coughing, sneezing, laughing, or stooping can be a symptom of life-threatening intracranial disorders, or it may result more frequently from poorly understood benign causes related to exercise. Exertional headache must be distinguished from the more common aggravation by exercise of an established headache. Exercise aggravates vascular headache of the migrainous type, but it is useful in aborting, in some patients, attacks of cluster headache. Premenstrual symptoms, including headache, improve in some instances with endurance training, placing such activity into the therapeutic armamentarium for this condition. Benign exertional headache is more common in men than in women and is more frequent in older individuals. Organic lesions associated with exertional headache are rare but include Arnold-Chiari deformities, platybasia, basilar impression, chronic and subacute subdural hematoma, hemangioendothelioma, gliomas, and frontal meningiomas, particularly in the vicinity of the optic nerves. In such conditions, the type of exercise is not specific, but the severity of the headache is related to the degree of effort, and in some patients, the headache, which is often pulsatile and associated with visual phenomena (particularly in meningomas) may easily be mistaken for attacks of migraine induced by exertion. Headache onset in any particular site is not characteristic of a specific lesion, but in exertional headache unassociated with organic intracranial disease the pain may be bilateral, frontal, occipital, or generalized. Benign exertional headache is usually abrupt in onset; is often severe; may be sharp, stabbing, or pulsatile; and lasts for minutes or may outlast the exercise for a time. The etiology of benign exertional headache in nonathletes is obscure. Scalp tenderness is not present, and the pain is not influenced by pressure on the scalp or extracranial vessels. In brain tumors, the associated headaches are only rarely exertional. Similarly, in subdural hematomas, exertional headache is rare. The treatment of exertional headache associated with recognizable pathology is that of the primary disease. Benign exertional headache unassociated with intracranial lesions in nonathletes has been treated, without much success, with sedatives, analgesics, and ergot preparations alone or in combination. In nonathletes with benign exertional headache, 75 mg/day of indomethacin is occasionally helpful. Rare brain tumors associated with exertional headache are sometimes characterized by headache induced by changes in position or precipitated by other effort. This occurs rarely, but when it does it is characteristically in intermittent obstruction of the CSF pathways in the third or fourth venticle, usually due to a colloid cyst. This type of headache is frontal or frontal occipital and can be bilateral or unilateral. The headache is sometimes relieved by sudden changes in position opposite to the position that triggered it. Vomiting may be present at the height of the pain, and visual disturbances, impaired mental function, tinnitus, and decreased alertness, often intermittent, have been reported. Significant hemorrhage into previously unrecognized brain tumors has occurred in two joggers. These may have been related to the rise in blood pressure (usually proportional to physical fitness) during the first few minutes of exercise and to the fragility of blood vessels within the tumors.

Effort Migraine

Migrainous attacks after athletic effort of any kind can occur but tend to be more frequent at high altitude. During Olympic competitions in Mexico City (altitude 2375 m), effort migraine was frequent and recurrent in some athletes engaged in repeated competition. Many effort migraine attacks have only part of the syndrome. Scotomata, which usually occur immediately after exertion, may be the only manifestation. Hyperventilation, nausea, and severe pulsatile retro-orbital unilateral pain indistinguishable from classic migraine may occur. This is rare in well-trained athletes. It is common in poorly trained individuals in appropriate settings, and it may be precipitated by dehydration, excessive heat, hypoglycemia, and unaccustomed altitude. The pain is intense and throbbing and may be occipital or frontal. Focal neurologic deficits other than scatomata are not seen, though threatening intracranial disorders are often feared. Headaches of this type are generally benign and are not apt to recur with repeated exertion, provided physical fitness improves and other precipitating factors are avoided.

Altitude may also precipitate serious and sometimes life-threatening intracranial catastrophies that, early on, may mimic migrainous attacks. A case in point is the 25-year-old healthy man who arrived from sea level at an altitude of about 4000 m during a skiing holiday and on his first ascent to the summit of the ski area developed a severe right-sided retro-orbital and temple pulsatile headache with left hemiparesis. This was initially thought to be his first migrainous attack, until further investigations showed severe right hemisphere edema and occlusion of the intracranial portion (syphon) of the internal carotid artery. This altitude-associated and arteriographically proven occlusion of the intracranial carotid artery was attributed to dissection, and 2 weeks later complete recanalization of the artery had occurred (Fig. 3-4). Similar exercise-associated cases have been reported, but the pathogenesis of this disorder remains unclear. It perhaps is related to the altitude-associated increase in intracranial blood flow. Fortunately, such cases are extremely rare, but nevertheless an important consideration when confronted with unilateral headaches and focal neurologic deficits. These should not be glibly attributed to relatively benign altitude-induced migrainous attacks.

Other Exercise-Associated Headaches

Occasional would-be athletes who are inexperienced and untrained have exertional headache at low levels of activity. Such people complain of occipital throbbing headaches accompanied by nausea. Focal neurologic symptoms or signs are not present, and the pain is aggravated by increasing effort and neck movement. Such pain may persist for hours after cessation of exertion, and support of neck muscles and analgesics taken before exertion often prevent attacks.

Ischemic muscular exercise can be associated with excruciating headaches. This has been reported in patients with occlusion of the aorta below the origin of renal vessels and also in subjects who performed treadmill exercise while circulation to the legs was experimentally occluded. With ischemic work, blood pressure rises to levels comparable to those found during hypertensive crises, and the height of the blood pressure is related to the degree of ischemia. The reflex increase in blood pressure presumably causes the headache.

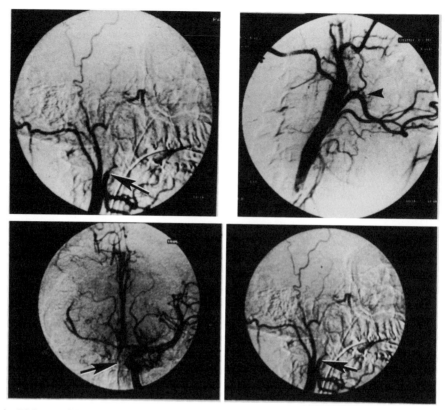

3-4 Right carotid arteriogram, internal carotid occlusion in the syphon (arrows), and complete re-canalization 2 weeks later (arrowhead).

Paroxysmal neurogenic hypertension in quadriplegic individuals is accompanied by elevated plasma catecholamines. However, norepinephrine levels achieved by infusion must be 21 times higher than those found in quadriplegic individuals in order to raise the blood pressure to similar heights. Therefore, the plasma norepinephrine per se is probably not the cause of the neurogenic hypertension and headache in paraplegic individuals or in those performing ischemic exercise. The pathogenetic importance of catecholamines in the genesis of headache associated with physical activity, in autonomic hyperreflexia, or in coital headache (all conditions in which increases in plasma catecholamine have been documented) has not been assessed.

Pressure headache, caused by athletic equipment (for example from pressure on frontal nerves by goggles) or pressure on spinal roots (weight lifter's headache) can be treated by appropriate manipulation or changes in exercise techniques.

CONCLUSIONS

Exercise and training improve performance and have profound effects on nervous system function, including adaptive changes in muscle and autonomic activity. Prolonged training seems to delay the age-related decay in nervous system function and changes mood and behavior. Millions of active exercisers are spending considerable time in an inexpensive public health measure (exercise) that may avoid expensive health maintenance. However, continued exertion for many years may have its dangers and certainly many complications that detract from its benefits. The extent of the modification by chronic exercise of nervous system function and the influence of chronic exercise on other bodily functions in health and disease need to be carefully assessed with long-term studies before this activity can be generally recommended as the cure and prevention of many ills. The slogan "exercise is medicine" has, as yet, no thorough scientific support.

REFERENCES

1. Appenzeller, O. 1982. A symposium: Mental health and illness. Exercise and mental health. In: Bernstein, E. (ed): 1983 Medical and Health Annual, Encyclopedia Brittanica, Inc. Chicago, pp 134–141.
2. Appenzeller, O., Atkinson, R. (eds). 1978. Health Aspects of Endurance Training Medicine and Sport. S. Karger, New York, vol 12.
3. Landouzy, L., Dejerine, J. 1884. De la myopathie atrophique progressive (myopathie hereditative) debutant, dans l'enfance par la face, sans alteration du systeme nerveux. C R Acad Sci 98:53–55.
4. McArdle, B. 1951. Myopathy due to a defect in muscle glycogen breakdown. Clin Sci 10:13–25.
5. Appenzeller, O., Ogin, G. 1975. Hypothesis: pathogenesis of muscular dystrophies: sympathetic neurovascular components. Arch Neurol 32:2–4.
6. Wiles, C.M., Jones, D.A., et al. 1981. Fatigue in human metabolic myopathy. In: Porter, R., Whelan, J. (eds): Human Muscle Fatigue: Physiological Mechanisms. Pitman Medical Publishing, London, pp 264–282.
7. Adrian, R.H., Bryant, S.H. 1974. On the repetitive discharge in myotonic muscle fibres. J Physiol (London) 240:505–515.
8. Ballantyne, J.P., Hansen, S. 1978. Neurogenic influence in muscular dystrophies. In: Rowland, L.P. (ed): Pathogenesis of Human Muscular Dystrophies. Excerpta Medica, Amsterdam, pp 187–199.
9. Wallin, G. 1983. Intraneural recording and autonomic function in man. In: Bannister, R. (ed): Autonomic Failure. Oxford University Press, Oxford, pp 36–51.
10. Edwards, R.H.T., Round, J.M., et al. 1983. Needle biopsy of skeletal muscle: a review of 10 years' experience. Muscle and Nerve 6:676–683m.
11. Dawson, M.J., Gadian, D.G., et al. 1980. Mechanical relaxation rate and metabolism studied in fatigued muscle by NMR. J Physiol (London) 299:465–484.
12. Amphlett, G.W., Perry, S.U., et al. 1975. Cross innervation and the regulatory protein system of rabbit soleus muscle. Nature 257:602–604.
13. Edwards, R.H.T., Hill, D.K., et al. 1972. Effect of fatigue on the time course of relaxation from isometric contractions of skeletal muscle in man. J Physiol (London) 227:26P–27P.
14. Edwards, R.H.T., Hill, D.K., et al. 1975. Metabolic changes associated with slow relaxation in fatigued mouse muscle. J Physiol (London) 251:287–301.
15. Edwards, R.H.T., Hill, D.K., et al. 1977. Fatigue of long duration in human skeletal muscle after exercise. J Physiol (London) 272:769–778.
16. Wiles, C.M. 1980. The determinants of the relaxation rate of human muscle in vivo. Doctoral dissertation, University of London, 1980.
17. Howald, H., Hoppeler, H., et al. 1985. Influences of endurance training on the ultrastructural composition of the different muscle fiber types in humans. Pflugers Arch 403:369–376.
18. Swash, M., Schwartz, M.S., et al. 1978. Pathogenesis of longitudinal splitting of muscle fibers in neurogenic disorders and in polymyositis. Neuropathol Appl Neurobiol 4:99–115.
19. Rosler, K., Hoppeler, H., et al. 1985. Transfer effects in endurance exercise: adaptations in trained and untrained muscles. Eur J Appl Physiol 54:355–362.
20. Maruyama, K., Sunde, M.L., et al. 1978. Growth and muscle protein turnover in the chick. Biochem J 176:573–582.
21. Millward, D.J., Bates, P.C., et al. 1980. Quantitative importance of non-skeletal muscle sources of N_2-methylhistidine in urine. Biochem J 90:225–228.
22. DuBois, D., Almon, R.R. 1980. Disuse atrophy of skeletal muscle is associated with an increase in number of glucocorticoid receptors. Endocrinology 107:1649–1651.
23. Karpati, G. 1984. Denervation and disuse atrophy of skeletal muscles—involvement of endogenous glucocorticoid hormones. TINS 7:61–62.
24. Kennelly, A.E. 1906. An approximate law of fatigue in the speeds of racing ani-

mals. Proc Am Acad Arts Sci 42:275–331.

25. Mosso, A. 1981. Fatigue. Translated by Drummond, M., Drummond, W.G. Allen and Unwin, London, pp 78–80.

26. Stephens, J.A., Taylor, A. 1972. Fatigue of maintained voluntary muscle contraction in man. J Physiol (London) 220:1–18.

27. Perkoff, G.T., Hardy, P., et al. 1986. Reversible acute muscular syndrome in chronic alcoholism. N Engl J Med 274:1277–1285.

28. Wiles, C.M., Young, A., et al. 1979. Muscle relaxation rate, fibre-type composition and energy turnover in hyper- and hypothyroid patients. Clin Sci 57:375–384.

29. DiMauro, S., Trevisan, O., et al. 1980. Disorders of lipid metabolism in muscle. Muscle and Nerve 3:369–388.

30. Engel, W.K., Vick, N.A., et al. 1970. A skeletal muscle disorder associated with intermittent symptoms and a possible defect of lipid metabolism. N Engl J Med 282:697–704.

31. Engel, A.G., Angelini, G. 1973. Carnitine deficiency of human skeletal muscle with associated lipid storage myopathy: a new syndrome. Science 179:899–902.

32. DiMauro, S., DiMauro, P.M.M. 1973. Muscle carnitine palmital transferase deficiency and myoglobinuria. Science 182:929–931.

33. Karpati, G., Carpenter, S., et al. 1975. The syndrome of systemic carnitine deficiency. Clinical, morphologic, biochemical and pathophysiologic features. Neurology 25:16–24.

34. Fleischmann, K., Siegel, A.J. 1983. For debate: Are some compulsive runners really closet anorexics: Dieting to run or running to starve? Ann Sports Med 1:98–99.

35. Layzer, R.B. 1977. Glycolysis and glycogens. In: Rowland, L.P. (ed): Pathogenesis of Human Muscular Dystrophies (International Congress Series 404). Excerpta Medica, Amsterdam, pp 395–403.

36. DiDonato, S., Cornelio, F., et al. 1978. Muscle carnitine palmitaltransferase deficiency: a case with enzyme deficiency in culture fibroblasts. Ann Neurol 4:465–467.

37. Schmid, P., Simmler, M., et al. 1983. Mitochondrial reaction in skeletal muscle to induced activity. Int J Sports Med 4:116–118.

38. Oberholzer, F., Claasen, H., et al. 1976. Ultrastrukturelle, biochemische und energetische Analyse einer extremen Dauerleistung (100km.—Lauf). Schweiz Z Sportmed 24:71–98.

39. Kayar, S.R., Hoppeler, H., et al. 1986. Acute effects of endurance exercise on mitochondrial distribution and skeletal muscle morphology. Eur J Appl Physiol 54:578–584.

40. Brown, G.L., Harvey, A.M. 1939. Congenital myotonia in the goat. Brain 62:341–363.

41. Floyd, W.F., Kent, P., et al. 1955. An electromyographic study of myotonia. Electroenceph Clin Neurophysiol 7:621–630.

42. Appenzeller, O., Amick, L. 1972. Paralysis with paradoxic myotonia. Trans Amer Neurol Assn 97:245–247.

43. Riecker, G., Bolter, H.D., Membran Potenziale einzelner Skeletmusscelzellen bei hypokalamischer periodischer Muskel paralyse. Klin Wochenschr 44:804–807.

44. Isaacs, H. 1978. Myopathy and malignant hyperthermia. In: Aldreta J.A., Britt, B.A. (eds): International Symposium on Malignant Hyperthermia: 2nd Proceedings. Grune and Stratton, New York, pp 89–102.

45. Nelson, T.E., Jones, E.W., et al. 1972. Malignant hyperthermia of Poland China swine: studies of myogenic etiology. Anesthesiol 36:52–56.

46. Willner, J.H., Wood, D.S., et al. 1980. Increased myophosphorylase in malignant hyperthermia. N Engl J Med 303:138–140.

47. Appenzeller, O., Appenzeller, J., et al. 1985. Opioids and endurance training: longitudinal study. Ann Sports Med 2:22–25.

48. Ahlquist, G., Landin, S., et al. 1975. Ultrastructure of skeletal muscle in patients with Parkinson's disease and upper motor lesions. Lab Invest 31:673–679.

49. Saltin, B., Nazar, K., et al. 1976. The nature of the training response: peripheral and central adaptations of one-legged exercise. Acta Physiol Scand 96:289–305.

50. Landin, S., Hagenzeldt, L., et al. 1977. Muscle metabolism during exercise in hemiparetic patients. Clin Sci Molecular Med 53:257–269.

51. Sandrini, G., Aquilani, R., et al. 1984. Ventilatory responses to passive limb movement: effect of hemiplegia. Ann Sports Med 2:11–15.

52. Genest, J., Cantin, M. 1986. Regulation

of body fluid volume: the atrial natriuretic factor. News in Physiological Sciences 3:5.

53. Goldsmith, M.F. 1987. Atrial peptide study proceeds apace. JAMA 257:287.

54. Singer, D.R.J., Buckley, M.G., et al. 1986. Raised concentrations of plasma atrial natriuretic peptides in cardiac transplant recipients. Br Med J 293: 1391–1392.

55. Ogihara, T., Shima, J., et al. 1986. Changes in human plasma atrial natriuretic polypeptide concentration in normal subjects during passive leg raising and whole-body tilting. Clin Sci 71:147–150.

56. Tanaka, H., Shindo, M., et al. 1986. Life Sci 39:1685–1693.

57. Meehan, R.T. 1986. Renin aldosterone and vasopressin responses to hypoxia during six hours of mild exercise. Aviation, Space and Environmental Medicine 57:960–965.

58. Serratrice, G., Gastaut, J.L., et al. 1980. Serum and muscle activities (glycolitic and transferase) in human cortisone myopathies. Sem Hop (Paris) 56:1241–1244.

59. Mills, K.R., Edwards, R.H.T. 1983. Investigative strategies for muscle pain. J Neurol Sci 58:73–88.

60. Newham, D.J., Mills, K.R., et al. 1983. Pain and fatigue after concentric and excentric muscle contractions. Clin Sci 64:55–62.

61. Greenhouse, A.H. 1981. The relation of physical activity to disorders of neurologic function. Semin Neurol 1:237–241.

62. Rosenberg, G., Appenzeller, O., et al. 1987. Multiple sclerosis, fatigue, and amantadine. Neurology 39:108.

63. Berger, G., Appenzeller, O. 1988. Tibial nerve conduction velocities: effect of age, training and competition. Neurology, in press.

64. Appenzeller, O., Spar, J., et al. 1986. Diving response: effects of endurance training. Ann Sports Med 3:19–21.

65. Appenzeller, O., Hudson, T., et al. 1986. Parasympathetic function: endurance training mimics severe diabetic vagal neuropathy? Muscle and Nerve Suppl. 55:240.

66. Appenzeller, O. In press. Maximal speed running: absence of alpha rhythm during short rest intervals. Ann Sports Med.

67. Seelinger, D., Appenzeller, O. Posturography before and after a prolonged run.

68. Fries, J.F. 1980. Aging, natural death and the compression of morbidity. N Engl J Med 302:130–135.

69. Appenzeller, O., Greene, E.R., et al. 1985. Doppler common carotid and pre-auricular blood flows and resistances at altitude: a study of endurance-trained subjects. Ann Sports Med 2:120–124.

70. Carlow, T.J., Appenzeller, O. 1983. Neurology of endurance training. In: Appenzeller, O., Atkinson, R. (eds.): Sports Medicine: Training, Fitness, Injuries. Urban and Schwarzenberg, Baltimore, MD, pp 35–42.

71. West, D. 1986. Neurologic deficits effect of extreme altitude. Personal communication.

72. Appenzeller, O. 1986. Barogenic headache. In: Vinken, P.J., Bruyn, G.W., et al. (eds): Handbook of Clinical Neurology: 4. Headache. Elsevier, Amsterdam, pp 395–404.

73. Petajan, J.H. 1981. The effects of high altitude on the nervous system and athletic performance. Semin Neurol 1:253–262.

74. Challenor, Y.B. 1981. Exercise and the handicapped child. Semin Neurol 1:358–364.

75. Atkinson, R., Appenzeller, O. 1981. Headache in Sports. Semin Neurol 1:334–344.

.4.

Physical Health,
Mental Health,
and Exercise

Robert Kellner

PHYSICAL DISEASE AND MENTAL DISORDERS

The notion that a healthy mind resides in a healthy body has been shared by physicians and laypersons since antiquity. Unlike numerous cherished beliefs such as the wandering womb, ailments of organs in the hypochondrium, and the benefits of bleeding and purging, the belief that a diseased body can cause the mind to be ill has stood the test of time as well as that of research.

Several studies have shown that psychiatric illness is more common in patients who have physical diseases, and among psychiatric patients physical disease is substantially more common than in people who have no mental illness. There is also substantial evidence that successful treatment of physical disease improves mood as well as psychologic functioning. The causes for these associations are numerous: Metabolic disturbances and endocrine diseases can cause profound changes in mood, brain damage and brain disease can cause organic brain syndromes, and diseases that cause chronic pain are a source of continuous suffering leading to demoralization and depression. Conversely, patients with serious psychiatric illness tend to neglect themselves, do not take adequate precautions, and are less likely to comply with recommended treatments. One can argue that successful treatment and prevention of disease will, at least to a small extent, enhance mental health.

However, a substantial proportion of people who are physically healthy suffer from psychiatric ill health and from psychophysiologic disturbances. For example, somatic symptoms are exceedingly common and only a small proportion are caused by physical disease (Kellner [1]). Minor psychiatric illnesses, such as brief adjustment disorders with anxiety or depression, are so common that statistically they belong to normal experiences. The results of two studies in strikingly different sociocultural settings are similar: In midtown Manhattan and in a rural community in Nova Scotia only 13 and 18% of people, respectively, were free of emotional symptoms and regarded themselves well on any one day (Srole et al. [2]; Leighton et al. [3]).

PHYSICAL FITNESS AND MENTAL HEALTH

While the evidence for the link between physical disease and psychiatric illness has accumulated in this century, the knowledge that mood and psychologic functioning can be improved in physically healthy individuals by improving their physical fitness has been acquired mainly in the last two decades (Sachs and Buffone [4]). In view of the high prevalence of mental ill health and the suffering and cost it entails, any treatment that has only a few risks and side effects and is inexpensive merits scrutiny by physicians. A case can be made that vigorous physical exercise is such a treatment, and the research on this topic is examined in this chapter.

There is extensive literature on the psychologic effects of exercise (Sachs and Buffone [4]), and the literature is growing each year. The studies for this chapter were selected because they either were representative of their kind, or, conversely, had some unusual features. Some of the findings are evaluated and some of the methodologic obstacles that could lead to misleading conclusions are discussed. All published controlled studies of the effects of exercise in depression are briefly discussed because of their implications for treatment. Finally, the trends that are emerging from the better-designed studies are discussed.

Conflicting Findings

Numerous studies show that people who exercise vigorously tend to rate themselves less distressed on self-rating scales of anxiety or depression, tend to show a better self-concept, and score higher on scales of adjustment than do those who do not exercise.

However, a few studies have yielded discordant results. For example, Colt et al. [5] found among nonelite runners a higher prevalence of primary affective disorders than among a group of orthopedic patients who had been rated by other investigators using the same interview schedule.

Some other studies suggest that the deliberate pursuit of vigorous exercise may have only small effects on changes in personality and adjustment. Werner and Gottheil [6] administered the Cattell 16 Personality Factor test (16PF) to more than 500 cadets entering the United States Military Academy. More than 300 of the cadets had one previous sports letter award and were classified as athletes; more than 100 who had not participated in an athletic sport at least shortly before entering the academy were labeled as nonathletes. Athletes showed significantly more favorable personality traits, and were described as being, among other things, more sociable, dominant, enthusiastic, and adventurous. During their stay in the academy all cadets participated in athletics. The authors had assumed that after regular exercise the nonathletes would begin to resemble the college athletes; however, this did not occur. The personality differences between the two remained largely unchanged in spite of participation by all in a vigorous athletic program.

Another study in which improvement in physical fitness did not lead to substantial improvement in psychologic adjustment was reported by Tillman [7]. The author examined 386 junior and senior boys in a high school and selected boys from the upper and lower 15th percentiles in performance on physical fitness tests for participation in the study. The physically unfit showed significantly poorer psychologic adjustment on the Cattell 16PF. The low-physical-fitness group was divided into an experimental and control group ($n = 16$ and 24, respectively). After nine months of participation in the physical fitness program the experimental groups' physical fitness had improved significantly, but changes in psychologic tests were only small.

Uncontrolled Studies

Several uncontrolled studies have yielded impressive results regarding the effects of exercise on mental health. Among these, a study by Shoenfeld et al. [8] stands out. The authors examined the effects of vigorous exercise on neurocirculatory asthenia (NCA). The term *neurocirculatory asthenia* has become obsolete, largely because it is now regarded as a variant of anxiety neurosis with predominantly cardiovascular symptoms. Other names for the disorder have been soldier's heart, cardiac neurosis, and da Costa's syndrome. The predominant symptoms are pain in the chest in the region of the pericardium, palpitations, fatigue often associated with anxiety, tension, and mild depression.

The authors classified subjects as having "somatotype NCA" (these patients complained about somatic symptoms such as palpitation, dyspnea, chest pain, and dizziness during or at the end of an effort) or "neurotic NCA" (in addition to having somatic symptoms these patients suffered from psychiatric symptoms such as anxiety, nervousness, and insomnia). The subjects with somatotype NCA participated in an exercise program that lasted for 3 weeks and consisted of various activities, such as calisthenics, ball games, running, and physical work for at least 4 hr daily and increased to 6 hr daily later. The assessment of symptoms was based on an interview before and after the exercise program. At the end of training all the symptoms of the typical NCA syndrome had vanished. Although this is an uncontrolled study and the program was limited to somatoform NCAs, the result is striking because none of the previous studies with NCAs treated with a variety of methods had reported improvement of this order (Cohen and White [9]).

Prospective Controlled Studies

The results of controlled studies tend to differ with the populations studied. Folkins et al. [10] compared junior college students enrolled in a jogging course to those enrolled in archery and golf courses at the beginning and at the end of the semester. There was an improvement both in physical fitness and in scores of psychologic inventories and self-rating scales at the end of the semester in the jogging group, and in women there was also a significant correlation between measures of physical fitness and decrease in depression, increase in self-confidence, and improved adjustment. There were no significant changes in the other group.

Short et al. [11] examined the effects of exercise in 45 metropolitan policemen who were considered overweight. Both randomly selected groups had lectures on diet and exercise; one half continued with their routine program, and the other half participated also in an aerobic conditioning program. The participants were administered subscales of the Tennessee Self-Concept Scale before and after the program. Both groups improved, but the group that participated in physical exercise improved significantly more on the physical self and self-satisfaction subscales of the self-concept scale.

Studies of Depression

There are many uncontrolled studies in the literature that examine the effects of vigorous exercise on depression, as well as a few controlled studies; these have been reviewed by Simons et al. [12]. Most of the studies consisted of the measurement of self-ratings of depression in nonpatient volunteers, including normal individuals, and some others examined the effects of exercise in depressed psychiatric patients. Five controlled studies are summarized here, four of which dealt with depressed psychiatric patients and one of which studied female college students who scored high on a self-rating scale of depression.

Greist et al. [13] compared running ($n = 10$), time-limited psychotherapy ($n = 6$), and psychotherapy without time limits ($n = 12$) in young patients who had minor depression according to research diagnostic criteria. The depression scale of the Hopkins Symptom Checklist (SCL-90) scores improved to the same degree in the running group as in the psychotherapy groups.

Doyne et al. [14] compared three treatments in 41 women who met research diagnostic criteria for major and minor depression. The treatments compared were running, weight training, and being on the waiting list (control). Each treatment lasted for 8 weeks, 4 times a week for 30 min. In both exercise groups there was a significant reduction on the Beck Depression Inventory and on the Hamilton Rating Scale for Depression, and there was no change in the control group.

Greist [15] compared the outcome of treatment in patients who met Research Diagnostic Criteria for minor and major depression. The three treatments compared were exercise (walking and jogging 3 times a week), meditation, and psychotherapy once a week. All treatments lasted for 12 weeks. At the end of the study depression scores for exercise and meditation had improved significantly more than those for psychotherapy.

Martinsen [16] examined the effects of exercise in depressed psychiatric patients who had routine psychiatric care. Nineteen patients were subdivided into a group that participated in vigorous physical exercise at 50 to 70% of maximum aerobic capacity or a control group that continued with routine psychiatric treatment. Patients in both groups were given tricyclic antidepressant drugs. The exercise group improved significantly more on the Beck Depression Inventory and the Comprehensive Psychopathological Rating Scale.

Finally, McCann and Holmes [17] examined the effect of exercise in female college students who scored high on the Beck Depression Inventory. Sixty students were divided into a group that had vigorous aerobic exercise several times a week, a second group that combined relaxation training with short walks, and a third group that received no treatment. At the end of the study, the Beck Depression scores had improved in all three groups, but improvement was significantly greater in the group with aerobic exercise.

Studies in the Elderly

There have been several studies on the elderly in which changes in mood, behavior, and cognitive performance were compared before and after exercise. For example, Powell [18] compared the effects of an exercise treatment program in geriatric patients to those of conventional social therapy in a control group. Thirty geriatric patients participated for 12 weeks. Results on two of three cognitive tests improved significantly more in the exercise group than in the other two; there were no differences on the two behavioral scales. Dustman et al. [19] compared the effects of an aerobic exercise program in 50- to 70-year-old sedentary subjects. There were two control groups: flexibility exercise without aerobic conditioning and a nonexercise control group. The measures included a battery of neuropsychologic tests, sensory threshold, visual acuity, and two depression self-rating scales. Subjects who had aerobic training performed significantly better on the neuropsychologic test battery than did the control groups. The other measures, including depression self-rating, did not change.

Physiologic and Psychologic Correlates of Exercise

Vigorous exercise has been shown in many studies to effect substantial physiologic changes, for example, stress hormone responses (Schade [20]), the secretion of β-endorphins (Carr et al. [21]; Farrell et al. [22]), and changes in neurologic functioning (Carlow and Appenzeller [23]). Other possible mechanisms by which exercise could exert beneficial effects on psychologic functioning have been discussed by several authors, for example, Simons et al. [12] and Appenzeller [24]. A detailed description of these changes lies beyond the scope of this chapter; the changes are complex and interrelated, and by themselves are adequate to explain some of the changes in mood and psychologic functioning.

Regarding psychologic mechanisms that could contribute to improve mood and adjustment, several have been proposed by various authors. Greist et al. [13] described several phenomena they had observed: mastery—individuals who were runners developed a sense of success; generalization—some people described a new positive image of themselves and stated that this change helped them feel capable of becoming competent in other areas; distraction—subjects noticed new bodily sensations that distracted them from preoccupations with minor, but annoying physical symptoms; and positive habit—many subjects recognized running as a positive activity and seemed to substitute it consciously for more negative defenses and habits.

Zeiss et al. [25] discussed nonspecific effects in the treatments for depression and argued that any treatment is beneficial that includes a rationale, a training in new skills, the feasibility of using these skills independently, and patient attribution of improvement to having acquired these skills. Regular exercise has these features, and they are likely to contribute to the observed psychologic changes.

Risks of Exercise

It is beyond the scope of this chapter to enumerate the physical risks of exercise. The psychologic risks, however, appear to be few and small. Three have been mentioned by several authors: the athletic personality, vigorous exercise as a disguise for anorexia nervosa, and the compulsion to exercise.

Little [26] observed that neurotic patients who had an "athletic personality" had different causes for their breakdowns than did other neurotic patients. In former athletes, severe injuries or disease appear to have precipitated the neurosis. In other words, their athletic activities were suddenly interrupted. In other neurotic patients the causes appeared to be different, for example marital disruption, the illness of a family member, and rigid attitudes toward work. It appears that personal physical illness or injury can act as a precipitant for a neurosis in a few athletes, particularly when such an injury ends a successful career. In professional sportsmen this can entail a total change in lifestyle: Suddenly a successful, wealthy, and admired person may become unemployed and poor. It takes an unusually psychologically robust and resilient individual to be able to cope successfully with such a loss. Even in successful amateurs, achievement and fitness can become overvalued ideas, and ending their cherished activity because of disease or injury can be demoralizing, particularly if fitness and athletic achievement were important sources of self-esteem. Fortunately, however, psychiatric clinics are not teeming with former athletes. It appears that most manage to adjust to the loss of the excitement of competition, the prestige, and the adulation that accompany excellence in sports and find other sources of gratification.

It has been suggested that in many individuals vigorous exercise, including running, is a disguise of anorexia nervosa or is its analog. To the author's knowledge, only one study has addressed this issue. Blumenthal et al. [27] compared scores on the Minnesota Multiphasic Personality Inventory (MMPI) of runners and patients with anorexia nervosa. Runners scored generally within the normal range, whereas anorectic patients had higher scores of psychopathology on eight of the MMPI subscales. At present it appears that some anorectics exercise vigorously and that some other people who are not anorectic try to maintain a low body weight by various methods, including regular exercise. However, there appear to be profound differences between the two: Patients with anorexia nervosa are dissatisfied with their appearance until they achieve pathological thinness and use various methods to achieve this. In contrast, individuals who participate in regular vigorous exercise do not attempt to starve themselves once they have achieved a body weight which they regard as desirable, which in most cases is well within the statistically normal range for their height.

No sound research evidence is available on the topic of compulsion to exercise. There are no reports that suggest that vigorous exercise could be a manifestation of obsessive–compulsive neurosis, the symptoms of which include intrusive thoughts and images and characteristic compulsive acts. Somatic as well as emotional symptoms have been described in athletes who are deprived of exercise, such as a feeling of restlessness, missing the exhilaration of running, and paradoxically, feeling more fatigue than usual. The physiologic as well as psychologic symptoms that are associated with the sudden lack of exercise could make a person long to resume training. There are some people who tend to have obsessive traits who may let vigorous exercise become a duty that, if neglected, creates a feeling of unworthiness and having failed. This appears to be similar to their need to pursue other desirable pursuits to extremes, for example, to work long hours. The *reported* compulsion to exercise appears to be in some the need to recapture the feeling of well-being and in others a manifestation of a personality trait of conscientiousness and extreme dedication to worthy causes.

COMMENTS

The findings from epidemiologic studies and from uncontrolled prospective studies of the psychologic effects of exercise on mental health share several results: An association between physical fitness on one hand, and better psychologic functioning, better adjustment, and lower anxiety and lower depression on the other. In these studies it is not possible to determine the causes for the associations. Good adjustment could be a consequence of the benefits of exercise; conversely, exercise could be chosen by people who are on the average better adjusted. Although prospective controlled studies tend to show that exercise has beneficial effects, the findings are not uniform and there may be several other causes for this association.

Among the uncontrolled studies, there are a few that are impressive. For example, the results of treatment of somatotype neurasthenia as reported by Shoenfeld et al. [8] are superior to any other results of treatment of neurasthenia. In this study, as well as in the study reported by Gondola and Tuckman [28], there was a substantial improvement in functional somatic symptoms. It may be that the effects of vigorous exercise in psychophysiologic disorders may be as good, if not greater, than in the treatment of emotional maladjustment or minor psychiatric disorders. These will have to be confirmed in controlled studies.

Uncontrolled studies can be misleading, because improvement occurs virtually with all interventions, including placebo, reassurance, and merely attending a clinic (Kellner and Sheffield [29]; Thomas [30]). The reasons for this trend are complex: The majority of emotional and psychologic disorders tend to improve with the passage of time (albeit with the risk of recurrences at a later date), and any intervention that includes interests, attention, and investigations appears to have a reassuring and apparently beneficial psychologic effect.

There are a few discrepant results in epidemiological studies. For example, in the study by Colt et al. [5] the proportion of persons with primary affective disorder was higher in a group of nonelite runners than in a group of orthopedic patients. The authors comment that it is possible that the runners, who were better educated than average, were likely to discover an inexpensive nonpharmacologic treatment for depression, so that in any group that chooses to exercise vigorously there are likely to be a few who have done so for the purposes of self-treatment.

The controlled studies on the effects of exercise are also not uniform; for example Werner and Gottheil's [6] study with college athletes and nonathletes who entered the military academy found that even after an athletic program for both, the difference between former college athletes and nonathletes did not diminish. If vigorous exercise alone would have had beneficial effects, the psychologic difference between athletes and nonathletes should have become smaller. This might suggest that better psychologic adjustment helped the athlete to excel in sports, or perhaps the rewards for being successful in sports contributed to better adjustment of the athletes. In the study with high school students (Tillman [7]), an exercise program did not improve psychologic adjustment. It may be that in adolescence the nature of maladjustment differs from that of adults, and exercise may not be adequate to deal with unhappiness and conflicts at that age. Conversely, in sedentary old people exercise was found to have beneficial effects on neuropsychologic functioning, including cognitive performance, but there was no conspicuous improvement in mood.

Among the causes of the association between good adjustment and regular exercise are that psychologic well-being appears to be one of the consequences of vigorous exercise and, conversely, exercise could be chosen by people who are on the average better adjusted. And, of course, both could play a part. Those who excel in sports can have also other advantages, such as popularity and a higher self-esteem, that may contribute to greater contentment.

The results of controlled studies with adults who suffer from at least minor depression show that exercise has an antidepressant effect, and the published studies so far suggest these are as good or even better than psychotherapy. However, the studies comparing running to psychotherapy included only a small number of patients, and psychotherapy was of too brief a duration to have specific effects. Moreover, the specific effects of psychotherapy are mediated in a substantially different way and are probably of a different kind.

The results of the effect of vigorous exercise on psychologic fitness appear to be conflicting, yet they show a pattern that is common to studies in therapeutics when the effective treatment is only a small part of the total variance. For example, several controlled drug trials show the tested drug to be superior to placebo, whereas in an equal number of trials no such differences could be found. This in itself suggests that the drug is effective, because when an ineffective drug is being tested the distribution of results is entirely different: Most studies show no difference between treatment and controls, a few might show the treatment better than placebo, but in an equal number of studies placebo is better than the drug. This is clearly not the pattern found in the controlled studies of the psychologic effects of exercise. In a few studies, exercise was no better than control treatments, in others exercise was superior, but to this author's knowledge there are no prospective controlled studies with an adequate number of subjects in which the control group showed a better psychologic adjustment than the exercise group. The failure to demonstrate the psychologic benefits of exercise is caused in part by faults in design of the studies. When the effect of one variable is relatively small, then certain conditions need to be fulfilled (Kellner [31]) for the small tail to wag the statistical dog (Meehl [32]).

CONCLUSIONS

There is an association between physical and mental health: Patients with physical disease are more likely to have emotional disturbances and psychiatric patients have a larger proportion of physical diseases than people without psychiatric illness. Although this association is consistent, there are, of course, numerous people with severe disease who show remarkable adjustment and cope with their ordeal with determination and courage and, conversely, numerous patients with psychiatric disorders who are physically healthy. There is also an association in healthy people between regular vigorous physical exercise and good psychologic adjustment. However, the effects of physical fitness are only a small proportion of the total variance. There is some evidence to suggest that the effects of exercise vary between emotional disorders, and there appear to be also large differences between its benefits on individuals with the same disorder. In some disorders, such as somatoform neurocirculatory asthenia and perhaps some other psychophysiologic disorders, vigorous exercise might be the most suitable treatment. It can be recommended also as an appropriate treatment for minor depressive disorders and probably several others. Although vigorous exercise is a feasible treatment only in a few, it is important to bear in mind that it is a treatment that confers physical benefits, contributes to emotional well-being, has only trivial side effects and few risks, and is less expensive than most of the treatments physicians can offer.

REFERENCES

1. Kellner, R. 1986. Somatization and Hypochondriasis. Praeger-Greewood, Inc., Westport, CT.

2. Srole, L., Langner, S.T., et al. 1962. Mental Health in the Metropolis: The Midtown Manhattan Study. McGraw-Hill, New York.

3. Leighton, D.C., Harding, J.S., et al. 1963. Psychiatric findings of the Stirling County study. Am J Psychiatry 119:1021–1027.

4. Sachs, M.L., Buffone, G.W. 1982. Psychological Considerations in Exercise, Including Exercise as Psychotherapy, Exercise Addiction, and the Psychology of Running. Department of Science and Physical Activity, University of Quebec at Three Rivers, Quebec, Canada.

5. Colt, E.W.D., Dunner, D.L., et al. 1981. A high prevalence of affective disorders in runners. In: Sacks, M.H., Sachs, M.L. (eds): Psychology of Running. Human Kinetics Publishers, Champaign, IL, pp 234–248.

6. Werner, A.C., Gottheil, E. 1966. Personality development and participation in college athletics. Res Q 37:126–131.

7. Tillman, K. 1965. Relationship between physical fitness and selected personality traits. Res Q 36:483–489.

8. Shoenfeld, Y., Shapiro, Y., et al. 1978. Rehabilitation of patients with NCA (neurocirculatory asthenia) through a short-term training program. Am J Phys Med 57:1–8.

9. Cohen, M.E., White, P.D. 1951. Life situations, emotions and neurocirculatory asthenia. Psychosom Med 13:335–357.

10. Folkins, C.H., Lynch, S., et al. 1972. Psychological fitness as a function of physical fitness. Arch Phys Med Rehabil 53:503–508.

11. Short, M.A., Dicarlo, S., et al. 1984. Effects of physical conditioning on self-concept of adult obese males. Phys Ther 64:194–198.

12. Simons, A.D., McGowan, C.R., et al. In press. Exercise as a treatment for depression: an update. Clin Psychol Rev.

13. Greist, J.H., Klein, M.H., et al. 1979. Running as treatment for depression. Comp Psychiatry 20:41–53.

14. Doyne, E.J., Bowman, E.D., et al. 1983. A Comparison of Aerobic and Nonaerobic Exercise in the Treatment of Depression. Association for the Advancement of Behavior Therapy, Washington, DC.

15. Greist, J.H. 1984. Exercise in the Treatment of Depression. Coping With Mental Stress: The Potential and Limits of Exercise Intervention. National Institute of Mental Health, Washington, DC.

16. Martinsen, E.W. 1984. Interaction of Exercise and Medication in the Psychiatric Patient. Coping With Mental Stress: The Potential and Limits of Exercise Intervention. National Institute of Mental Health, Washington, DC.

17. McCann, I.L., Holmes, D.S. 1984. Influence of aerobic exercise on depression. J Pers Soc Psychol 46:1142–1147.

18. Powell, R.R. 1974. Psychological effects of exercise therapy upon institutionalized geriatric mental patients. J Gerontol 29:157–161.

19. Dustman, R.E., Ruhling, R.O., et al. 1984. Aerobic exercise training and improved neuropsychological function of older individuals. Neurobiol Aging 5:35–42.

20. Schade, D. 1981. Stress hormone response to exercise. In: Appenzeller, O., Atkinson, R. (eds): Sports Medicine: Fitness, Training, Injuries. Urban & Schwarzenberg, Baltimore, pp 135–143.

21. Carr, D.B., Bullen, B.A., et al. 1981. Physical conditioning facilitates the exercise-induced secretion of beta-endorphin and beta-lipotropin in women. N Engl J Med 305:560–563.

22. Farrell, P.A., Gates, W.K., et al. 1982. Increases in plasma β-endorphin/β-lipotropin immunoreactivity after treadmill running in humans. J Appl Physiol 1245–1249.

23. Carlow, T.J., Appenzeller, O. 1981. Neurology of endurance training. In: Appenzeller, O., Atkinson, R. (eds): Sports Medicine: Fitness, Training, Injuries. Urban & Schwarzenberg, Baltimore, pp 41–49.

24. Appenzeller, O. 1981. What makes us run? Editorial. N Engl J Med 305:578–579.

25. Zeiss, A., Lewinsohn, P., et al. 1979. Nonspecific improvement effects in depression using interpersonal skills training, pleasant activities schedules or cognitive training. J Consult Clin Psychol 47:427–439.

26. Little, J.C. 1969. The athlete's neurosis: a deprivation crisis. Acta Psychiatr Scand 45:187–197.

27. Blumenthal, J.A., O'Toole, L.C., et al. 1984. Is running an analogue of anorexia nervosa? JAMA 252:520–523.

28. Gondola, J.C., Tuckman, B.W. 1983. Diet, exercise, and physical discomfort in college students. Percept Mot Skills 57:559–565.

29. Kellner, R., Sheffield, B.F. 1971. The relief of distress following attendance at a clinic. Br J Psychiatry 118:195–198.

30. Thomas, K.B. 1978. The consultation and the therapeutic illusion. Br Med J 1:1327–1328.

31. Kellner, R. 1967. The evidence in favour of psychotherapy. Br J Med Psychol 40:341–358.

32. Meehl, P.E. 1966. Discussion, in Eysenck, H.G. (ed): The Effects of Psychotherapy International Science Press, New York.

SECTION 2
Nutritional and Gastrointestinal Aspects of Sports

.5.

Nutrition for
Physical Performance

Otto Appenzeller

Courses on nutrition are not usually taught in medical schools. This has led to criticism from a variety of activists who claim that physicians know nothing about nutrition, do not consider nutritional deficiencies in the diagnosis and treatment of disease, and rarely recommend nutritional remedies for the maintenance of health and personal well-being. Much of this criticism is unfounded.

Though food preparation is not taught in medical school, biochemistry and physiology are major courses in the first 2 years, and proteins, fats, carbohydrates, minerals, vitamins, and water are topics of primary importance.

Nutrition is especially important during periods of rapid prenatal and postnatal growth, following certain surgical procedures on the gastrointestinal tract, sometimes in cardiology, as part of preventive medicine, and in Third World countries.

Most textbook information on common sense about foods is based on studies of so-called normal people in the Western world. Comparisons between these populations and those in countries where food is sparse suggest that a large part of the world is starving. With the advent of physical activity as a legitimate part of one's daily life, a new view on nutrition is necessary because present opinions of adequate nutrition are based, in part at least, on evaluation of sedentary individuals. Certain principles of nutrition remain valid and need little modification. These include:

1. No single food can guarantee adequate nutrition. The corollary of this is that to be well-nourished, one must eat a variety of foods. This variety should include protein that supplies the essential amino acids in adequate amounts (meat, poultry, fish, eggs, or nuts, and vegetables), milk or milk products (cheese, ice cream, or yogurt), fruits and cereals, some of which should be lightly milled or whole grain.
2. Caloric intake must be balanced with output. The amount of physical activity is important in determining proper caloric intake.
3. Alcohol has a high caloric content; it may predispose to some forms of cancer, but in moderate amounts may retard atherosclerosis.
4. Calories are the same, irrespective of their source; it is important to ingest only as many as are expended, to maintain proper weight.
5. Consumption of one meal a day rather than several tends to increase the total number of

calories over a 24-hr period. It is better, therefore, to have several small meals, rather than one large one.

6. Fluoride is essential for maintaining bones, and it retards or prevents tooth decay. Adequate fluoride is best provided, with few exceptions, by adding it to the water supply. Fluoridation is safe for any age or state of health.

7. Other nutritional supplements are not necessary for most people who consume a balanced diet. Exceptions are pregnancy, when iron and folic acid may be deficient, and certain disease states.

8. Increased blood cholesterol may be a risk factor for cardiovascular disease. Cholesterol levels are influenced not only by cholesterol intake or by the type of fat ingested but also by total caloric intake and expenditure. Cholesterol is made by the body in the absence of exogenous sources, and this is not appreciably influenced by dietary cholesterol. Although it is prudent to reduce dietary cholesterol, such as egg yolks, total fat intake can remain unchanged by partially replacing saturated with unsaturated fats from sunflower, corn, soy, or cottonseed oils, or by using soft margarines with minimum hydrogenation (necessary for solidification of the product made from these oils). Elevated blood cholesterol is only one of many factors favoring atherogenesis, and this subject is controversial. Genetics, hypertension, smoking, etc., also have a role.

9. Salt intake in the United States is much too high and may have something to do with the prevalence of hypertension. Minimizing dietary salt can be helpful in reducing hypertension in those afflicted. The salt used should be iodized.

Prospective studies on how healthy people cope with stress in later life and how they maintain mental and physical health indicate that nutrition, contrary to some beliefs, has little effect. The important factor is the means by which these people mastered their stresses.

MYTHS AND FACTS ABOUT NUTRITION

Nutritional nonsense is bantered about, and patients or athletes have a remarkable repertoire of unfounded beliefs. For example, the notion that healthful foods are found only in health food stores or appropriate health food sections of supermarkets is false. Many of these foods are claimed to have been produced without the use of pesticides and with manures or compost rather than chemical fertilizers.

Plants absorb only inorganic nutrients, and whether these are obtained from the bacterial action on soil, organic compounds in manure, or manufactured fertilizers makes no difference. All foods, if properly used, are healthful.

It is often claimed that processed foods are without nutrients and are inferior in quality to natural foods. Clearly, use of processed foods can contribute to a proper diet and can save time in preparation. If nutrients are missing from processed food, missing agents can be replaced. It is not necessary to know the caloric content of nutritional components, vitamins, and minerals in each food in order to achieve proper nutrition. People do not eat a single food at a meal, but eat groups of foods. The components must be considered in relation to the rest of the intake. An example is the avocado, which provides 260–280 cal, large quantities of vitamin A, and potassium. It also contains about 16% fat, but this is no reason to shun this excellent source of nutrition. Reducing-diets need only eliminate calories and not particular types of foods. Exercise is also helpful in body weight reduction.

Some proponents of health diets claim that sugar is a granular poison. Ordinary sugar makes up only about 15% of the total calories consumed by adults and perhaps up to 25% of those consumed by children. Most sugar is eaten as a constituent of other foods, as in ice cream or cakes. Sugar is completely utilized nutritionally. Carbohydrates in the diet, including honey, promote tooth decay when teeth are not cleaned after eating. It is the frequent consumption of sugar and the consistency of the sugar used, not its quantity, that cause tooth decay. Milk might be anticariogenic because of its phosphate content. If fluoridated water is consumed by children from birth or infancy, however, there will be, irrespective of the sugar consumption, a 70% reduction in tooth decay in comparison to those who do not drink fluoridated water.

Megavitamin therapy in excess of 10 times the recommended daily requirement is advocated by some for prevention of a variety of diseases. Large amounts of certain vitamins, particularly A and D, are toxic and cause, rather than prevent, disease. Moreover, there is no good evidence that megavitamin therapy can prevent cancer, cure colds, or achieve other similar claims.

It has been claimed by some that bananas and avocados have high cholesterol and fat content and should be avoided, particularly by those attempting weight reduction. This is false. Bananas, avocados, and other fruits and vegetables do not contain cholesterol, which is found only in animal products. Fat is present in trace amounts in bananas, which contain more carbohydrate than other fruits. Fat content in avocados is higher than in other fruits, but avocados are an excellent source of vitamins and minerals, and both bananas and avocados are good sources of potassium. Because of their high caloric content they should be used in moderation by people attempting to lose weight.

Physicians often err in assessing the nutritional status of their patients. Most patients suffer from problems related to excessive food intake or from the problems associated with food fads, leading to dietary deficiencies. Questions concerning eating between meals, what constitutes the usual breakfast, lunch, and dinner, how much alcohol is consumed, and how much salt is used are important in evaluating the nutritional status of patients and athletes. It should be emphasized that the help of professional dietitians and nutritionists should be sought, for they are an integral part of health care personnel. Certain athletes may require guidance to eat the right foods for a particular sport.

ENERGY EXPENDITURE

During optimal health, function of individual body parts depends upon total body function and vice versa. For this to continue, evolution has provided for a relatively constant cellular environment, and body fluid composition is kept constant. Muscle metabolism varies greatly from rest to maximal exercise. Muscles use about 100 times as much energy during peak activity as is used in rest, and they are similar to neurons during maximum metabolic activity. Nerve cells are always highly active metabolically, regardless of whether a person is asleep or is engaged in demanding mental gymnastics. The widely varying demands of muscles during rest and effort must be accommodated. The "machinery" must, from time to time, be turned on if the muscles and the mechanisms that service them are to be kept in proper working order. The only way to achieve this is by muscular work.

The resting metabolic rate for a 75-kg person is about 7 MJ (1700 kcal) per 24 hr, or equivalent to the energy expended in walking 35–40 km. Walking that distance, of course, requires an additional 7 MJ above that expended at rest. Carbohydrate and fat are the main substrates for muscle metabolism, but protein breakdown also occurs during extended or strenuous physical activity. Increasing work rates during certain athletic performances leads to greater carbohydrate utilization.

Effects of Physical Training

A peculiar and important effect of physical training is the capacity of the body to oxidize fat for energy and decrease the use of glycogen for this purpose. The glycogen-conserving mechanism improves physical performance in many situations, but this is particularly seen in long-distance events. Training improves physical performances in several ways: The number and size of skeletal muscle mitochondria are increased, and mitochondrial enzymes are favorably modified. There is also increased capillary density per unit of muscle tissue, which reduces the distance nutrients have to travel between capillaries and muscle cells. With continuous and regular training, other benefits include increased tendon, muscle, and bone strength; better coordination; and perhaps delay in onset of fatigue.

Maintenance of constant body weight depends upon balanced energy intake and expenditure, even though energy expenditure may vary widely. If daily exercise is prolonged and intensive, calorie intake is often less than energy output, and reduction in body weight occurs (Tables 5-1, 5-2).

Effects of Lack of Activity

On the other hand—and more commonly—if energy expenditure is less than calorie intake, and particularly if the energy expenditure is below a certain level, the surplus intake leads to obesity. In this condition, satiety is reached only after larger amounts of energy have been taken in than have been utilized. Much of the obesity widespread in the Western world is the result of too little physical activity in the face of excessive food intake, and the hypothalamic satiety center is set well above the energy expenditure. This state occurs in children who are reduced to little physical activity by modern conveniences and in adults who, because of the nature of their work, often lead a sedentary life.

It is important that the energy intake and satiety be regulated by the energy output, which can be achieved only if young people are encouraged to exercise regularly and if obese adults consciously regulate their diets to match energy output. If obesity occurs in infancy, the number of fat cells is increased and may predispose to obesity later in life. Treatment of obesity in such people is often difficult.

Appetite, which may have been a reliable guide to energy requirements and to the intake of appropriate nutrients in the past, is no longer a reliable indicator because it is manipulated by food manufacturers and the preparation of food. Therefore, under modern Western conditions, food intake dictated by appetite even over short periods cannot be used to judge energy requirements. Two important changes that have occurred in modern society are social and cultural influences favoring large energy intake and reduction in the demand for physical work. The need for most nutrients, as opposed to the need for energy, is, to a large extent, independent of the individual activity level. Therefore, a subject who is less active runs the risk of nutritional inadequacies because the overall food intake is small if the subject is in energy balance (Wretlind [1]).

Table 5-1 Weight Maintenance Based on Ordinary Activities 22 Hr/Day

Activity	Length of Time* (h)	Energy Expenditure (MJ)†	
		M	F
Sleeping (rest in bed)	8	2.3	2
Sitting	6	2.3	1.75
Standing	6	3.75	2.25
Walking	2	1.5	1.25
Maintenance energy intake (total)		9.85 (2364 kcal)	7.25 (1740 kcal)

*Suggested 2 hr of exercise daily not included
†One MJ ≃ 240 kcal

Table 5-2 Energy Expenditure in Ordinary Activities and Some Sports*

Type of Activity	Expended Energy (MJ)†	Type of Activity	Expended Energy (MJ)†
Housework	0.5	Waterskiing	2
Cycling 6 mph	1	Tennis singles	2
Tennis doubles	1.5	Paddleball	2.3
Cycling 8 mph	1.5	Cycling 12 mph	2.3
Volleyball	1.5	Alpine skiing	2.3
Badminton	1.5	Jogging 5 mph	2.3
Walking 4 mph	1.7	Swimming (continuous)	2.75
Cycling 10 mph	1.7	Running 8 mph	2.75
Cycling 11 mph	2	Cycling 13 mph	2.75
Walking 5 mph	2		

*For remaining 2 hr or 24-hr cycle (male and female)
†1MJ ≈ 240 kcal

Thus, a linear relationship exists between the energy supply per 24 hr and the supply of certain nutrients such as protein, calcium, thiamine, iron, and vitamin A. In general, a diet of about 12.5 MJ (3000 kcal) per day supplies the necessary nutrients to normal people, but it has been shown that the energy intake must exceed 10.5 MJ (2500 kcal) for an adequate supply of many nutrients. The Western diet seems to be geared to an energy requirement of at least 10.5 MJ (2500–3000 kcal), an intake that is totally unsuitable for the majority of consumers. This, of course, accounts for obesity and malnutrition in areas where food is plentiful. The so-called "diseases of modern society," including iron deficiency, diabetes mellitus, and constipation, may at least in part be ascribed to chronic malnutrition or to inappropriate energy expenditure. One may speculate that low energy consumption and its associated malnutrition may be improved by providing more essential nutrients per unit of energy than are presently available; therefore, a change in dietary constituents is necessary for those who require only 6–8.6 MJ (1500–2000 kcal per day), or those people should become high energy consumers by participating in physical activity in different forms. By increasing energy output they can, without risking obesity, eat more and get adequate amounts of essential nutrients (Åstrand [2]).

BODY WEIGHT

The ease of weighing a person and assessing nutritional state has obscured the complexity of the processes that underlie weight change. A number of athletes are anxious to decrease their weight, either to qualify for weight limits or to improve performance in long-distance events in which additional weight may be a disadvantage. Weight loss reflects a decrease in one or more body constituents sufficent to produce decreased body mass. Practically, the constituents usually contributing to weight loss over a short period are water, fat, protein, and glycogen. Over a longer term, deficits in mineral from bones and other areas may make a small contribution to weight loss.

Components of Weight Loss

To assess the components of weight loss, one must remember that protein and glycogen are constituents of tissues and part of complex hydrated organic materials. Therefore, when glycogen or protein is lost, "obligatory water" that reflects the hydration ratio (grams of water per gram of body constituent) is also lost. The ratio for glycogen and protein is about 3–4:1 and for nitrogen alone is 19–25:1. These ratios are approximate because of individual variations; also, the range of hydration coefficients given in the literature is wide. Whether adipose tissue loses water in association with the mobilization of triglycerides is not known. In addition to the obligatory water losses with protein and glycogen, deficits, and sometimes retention of water during weight loss that are unexplained by hydration coefficients, occur. In these situations, the water seems to be drawn from the extracellular compartment or from a disproportionate loss of intracellular water, or a combination of both processes. During early weight loss, the composition of the loss is varied, depending on the diet and, what is more important for athletes, on the preexisting nutritional state of the subject. The variability of weight loss during the early stages is due to a varying water loss that, under some circumstances, may account for 100% of the weight reduction—for example during diuretic therapy or during excessive heat loads and physical activity.

With prolonged caloric restriction, however, water can be retained on occasion to the point that it may cause weight gain even though fat and protein losses continue. It is well known that on a weight-reducing regimen, all subjects tend to lose weight rapidly during the first week or two. Much of this rapid loss of weight is water, which reflects the natriuresis and reduction in renal-concentrating capacity that accompanies early starvation. The mechanism of the water and sodium losses in these situations is not fully understood. This may, perhaps, be related to increased glucagon secretion, and the increased anion load placed on the nephron by nutritional ketosis may explain the additional sodium excretion.

In addition, the obligatory water loss of 600–800 ml accompanies the depletion of body glycogen that occurs during fasting or carbohydrate deprivation. Attempts must be made to assess the meaning of weight loss, because it is essential to know the type of tissue that is being lost. One can estimate this from the energy value of the loss per unit weight. For example, the energy value is largest if a given kilogram of weight is entirely composed of body fat. On the other hand, if a given unit of weight loss is largely protein and water, less energy has been lost.

Quality of Weight Loss

Empirically it has been found that the energy deficit or the quality of weight loss is likely to be highest when the rate of decrease in weight is slowest. To make an adequate judgment about the quality of the weight loss, however, the proportion of water per unit of weight lost needs to be assessed. Then, a better idea of the quality of weight loss can be based on the relative contribution made by fat and body protein to the energy deficit. It is customary to assume that an average weight loss of 0.45 kg (1 lb) corresponds to an energy deficit of approximately 14.5 MJ (3500 kcal). This, however, implies that 98% of the energy burned is derived from depot fat, the remainder being body protein. This very favorable composition of energy loss is, however, rarely achieved in weight control or reducing attempts. It is likely to occur only in obese subjects who fast for long periods, and the relative water loss is low. It is not likely to occur in nonobese subjects or athletes who are attempting to lose weight.

Rate of Weight Loss   Attempts to interpret the rate of weight loss with different diets can now be made by considering the differences between obese and nonobese subjects, both with respect to short- and long-term adherence to weight-reducing diets. Physically active adult male volunteers maintained for several weeks on approximately 5 MJ (1000 kcal) carbohydrate diets lost approximately 0.8 kg per day during the first 3 days, but the loss decreased to about 0.23 kg/day at the end of the second week. This difference was almost entirely due to increased water loss in the early phase of the diet and to some degree of water retention later on (Brozek et al. [3]).

Thirty-two male volunteers ate only salmon for 24 weeks. This diet supplied approximately 6.5 MJ (1570 kcal) per day, and was composed of 50 g protein, 30 g fat, and 275 g carbohydrates. The weight loss during the first 11 weeks was approximately 40% fat, 12% protein, and 48% water. During the remainder of the time, the mean composition of weight loss was 54% fat, 9% protein, and 37% water, and weight loss was only about 49 g/day during the second half of the experiment, compared to 150 g/day during the first half. The decreased weight loss was attributed to an adaptation of these nonobese subjects to the low-calorie diet. At the end of 24 weeks, the basal metabolic rate of the participants had dropped by an average of 31%, and their voluntary physical activity had decreased by 55%. More-over, fat breakdown increased from a mean of 88% during the first half of the semi-starvation to a mean of 93% during the second half. In contrast to the energy equivalent of 14.5 MJ (3500 kcal) per 0.45 kg (1 lb) weight loss previously cited, the average energy equivalent in these nonobese subjects was only about 8 MJ/0.45 kg during the first 11 weeks of the experiment and about 10 MJ/0.45 kg during the second part of the experiment. This finding underscores the fact that in nonobese subjects during adaptation to undernutrition, the energy value of 0.45-kg weight loss is far below that usually cited.

In obese subjects, the rate of weight loss during the first 5 days of adherence to a diet comprised of 5 MJ (1200 kcal) was 0.45 kg (1lb) per day (Yang and Van Itallie [4]). There is, therefore, no difference in the rapidity of weight loss in the early phases of energy restriction in obese and nonobese subjects. In this situation, 66% of the weight loss was water, and the rest was very similar to that found in nonobese subjects.

Ratio of Carbohydrates to Fat When the proportion of carbohydrates to fat was changed drastically and obese subjects were given a diet containing 90 g carbohydrate or a ketogenic diet containing only 10 g carbohydrate, but each yielding an energy of only 3.3 MJ (800 kcal), an absolute weight loss of 0.34 kg/day occurred, compared to 0.31 kg/day on the nonketogenic diet. The difference between the two rates of weight loss was due to increased water loss on the ketogenic diet.

Starvation Diet In the same subjects studied during 10 days of complete starvation, the daily weight loss was 50% higher than the loss during the ketogenic diet, and the increase in loss was due to the greater energy deficit. Surprisingly, however, during the total fast, the energy lost was the same as that lost during the ketogenic diet, and the increased weight loss during complete starvation was entirely due to water loss.

During prolonged dietary restriction, obese subjects increase the energy contributed to maintaining metabolic activity by adding more of their fat stores to the fuel mixture. After 6 weeks on a very-low-energy diet, obese subjects oxidized a fuel mixture that was much higher in fat and lower in protein than that utilized by nonobese volunteers during similar stringent dietary restriction. Obese subjects, therefore, during prolonged severe intake curtailment, use the fuel reserves (fat) more efficiently than do lean persons. They also do not have the substantially decreased basal metabolic rate that occurs in nonobese volunteers, and they do not voluntarily decrease their physical activity, as occurs in their nonobese counterparts. Thus, obesity predisposes to a continued and better quality weight loss after prolonged periods of semistarvation, whereas nonobese subjects, left to their own devices, decrease physical activity and, thus, energy expenditure, considerably. Similarly, in exercising individuals who are physically well trained, those whose skin-fold thickness is above the median tend to lose fat as determined by skin-fold measurements during prolonged exertion, whereas those who are below the median, eating the same diet and participating in the same daily exertions, show no loss of subcutaneous fat (Fig. 5-1).

From these studies, it is clear that the rate of body-fat loss correlates best with the energy deficit during food restriction. At a given energy deficit, the rate of loss in body weight depends upon the composition of the loss, and particularly on the proportion of

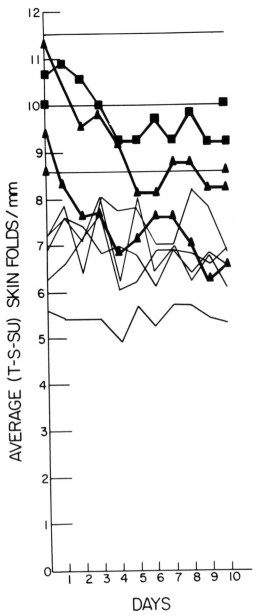

5-1 Change in skin fold thickness (subcutaneous fat) in 8 runners in the Himalayas over 10 days. No decrease in subcutaneous fat if initial measurements were below normal for sedentary subjects of comparable age. Average daily mileage 26 km (range 9–37 km). Horizontal lines range of normal for sedentary subjects. T = triceps fold; S = subscapular fold, SU = suprailiac fold.

water. During early calorie restriction, diuresis often occurs, and this can be increased and continued beyond its natural duration by a low-calorie ketogenic diet or by fasting. During prolonged restricted calorie intake, adaptation develops, and energy from fat stores is used to make up the deficit and conserve protein and water. Obese subjects adapt more successfully and can continue physical activities much longer than nonobese persons under similar dietary restriction (Van Itallie and Yang [5]). It cannot be determined from these studies, however, whether further adaptation occurs in athletes who continue physical activity during starvation. Athletes would undoubtedly hope that a continuous high-energy weight loss composed largely of fats with relative sparing of protein could occur.

FOOD SELECTION

Selection of food is determined by a number of factors, the most important of which is the satisfaction of hunger. During famine, habits and preferences are forgotten and sometimes products not normally regarded as fit for human consumption are eaten. Unfortunately, when ample food is available, the food choice is often largely influenced by habit. These habits are complicated and stem from a number of influences, especially the food available locally. For example, fish are a common part of the diet in coastal areas or near lakes or rivers. Where climate is appropriate, grain, complex carbohydrates, yams, tapioca, or similar plants are consumed.

In the Western world the wide variety of foods available makes the choice abundant and often leads the consumer astray. When common foods become scarce, as they did during World War II, they may be regarded as luxury items and eaten only rarely, together with those that are not considered appetizing. An example of this is the present shortage of herring in Europe, which a few years ago was a part of the daily diet of the poorer population but now is considered a delicacy because of its high price. The converse, of course, is also true when so-called luxury foods drop in price and become plentiful.

In addition to habits formed in early childhood, which are, of course, subject to familial traditions, religious and cultural influences play a large part in determining customary food intake. In many cultures, for example, the Indian culture, food is not only nourishment but is also an integral part of religious and other ceremonies. Of course, even today restrictions of certain foods, based on religious beliefs, are found in almost all countries.

Clearly, the dietary rules given in the Bible, the Koran, and the Talmud play an important part in the food selection of various ethnic groups. Moreover, the prescribed fasting during religious ceremonies and abstinence from certain foods play an important part in physical condition and food habits. Because of the very early adherence to a group of foods and habitual consumption of, or abstinence from, other foods, changes in dietary customs are hard for these people to accept and to follow.

However, in those who engage in various sports, food customs can easily be changed because of the athletes' desire for better performance and the promise often implied that consumption of certain foods will lead to improved athletic achievement. Nevertheless, in general, to achieve basic changes in food habits—whether to improve nutrition, prevent disease, or increase athletic achievement—requires strategies and technologies that, at least in the beginning, are integrated as much as possible with previous local habits and religious customs. Giving the impression that the products, timing, or changes proposed are in any way superior to those habitually used by the consumers must be strictly avoided.

NEUROTRANSMITTERS AND FOOD

The brain regulates eating and must receive signals about what has been eaten. This information is different from that received from the sensory input associated with food (taste, smell, or appearance) since many foods have very different energy values and nutrient contents but may be equally bulky and tasty. The brain derives its information, and thus to some extent regulates the contents of the next meal, from the metabolic consequences of food just consumed. One of many possible mechanisms of information flow to the brain about dietary habits is the food-induced change in plasma amino acid patterns, mostly the plasma *tryptophan ratio*. This, in turn, either increases or decreases brain synthesis of an important neurotransmitter, serotonin, of which tryptophan is a precursor. When a carbohydrate-rich and protein-poor meal is consumed, insulin secretion is stimulated. In turn, this diminishes the plasma levels of amino acids, which are able to compete with trytophan for transport mechanisms into the brain. The amino acids involved are leucine, isoleucine, and valine. The tryptophan flux across the blood–brain barrier is thus increased, and subsequently serotonin levels (synthesized from the available tryptophan) are also increased. On the other hand, high-protein meals contribute large quantities of leucine, isoleucine, and valine, which are now actively transported in large quantities into the brain in preference to the relatively scarce tryptophan, thus decreasing the synthesis of the neurotransmitter serotonin. There is some evidence that the brain uses the food-induced changes in its serotonin content to make choices about the content of the next meal (Wurtman and Wurtman [6]).

Disturbances in the mechanisms of food precursor neurotransmitters may induce the carbohydrate craving often associated with obesity and if this is correct, exercise-induced changes in mood may be important in the control of obesity and of carbohydrate craving because serotonin-releasing neurons are involved in the modulation of mood and there is a considerable overlap between appetitive and affective symptoms, particularly in carbohydrate cravers. Since exercise affects both appetite and mood, it is possible that its beneficial effects on obesity and depression are related to an increasing brain serotonin synthesis that could modify depressive symptoms also.

STARVATION

Dietary manipulation to improve athletic performance includes starvation, carbohydrate restriction, protein ingestion, and excessive fat intake. The metabolic events of starvation need, therefore, to be delineated before such manipulations are recommended to athletes for improved physical performance. Human beings live for many months without food and maintain a nearly normal metabolic rate and physical activity (not athletic performance). Survival during starvation depends upon closely integrated adaptive changes.

Interest in starvation is an ancient one, but metabolic studies during starvation in normal people have been performed only recently. In a classic work entitled *A Study of Prolonged Fasting* (Benedict [7]), one subject was sealed in a calorimeter during the night, but was free to write his autobiography during the day. This subject, on the 31st day of fasting, claimed to be feeling very well, was "uplifted," and wished to prolong the fast further because he did not feel a trace of hunger or discomfort. He may of course, have had an easy time, being a professional.

Most other persons fasting for even shorter periods of time would not find it as uplifting. Nevertheless, the study showed that normal subjects can fast for a month without impairing either mental or usual physical capacity.

Available Energy

The available energy during fasting comes mainly from fat (85%). The adipose tissue has little intracellular water and thus contains the most energy per unit of weight. Protein provides about 14% of the available energy, but because of its great importance in enzymatic, structural, and mechanical roles, it is usually preserved until very late, and the body engages in a number of strategems to prevent the breakdown of protein.

Carbohydrates   The carbohydrate store is relatively small, providing only 1% of available energy during fasting, but on the whole, the total energy available to the ordinary human body is enough to last for more than 80 days of total abstinence from food.

Even though carbohydrates are available in such short supply, they are essential for survival, and the clinical manifestations of hypoglycemia, particularly those due to central and peripheral nervous system dysfunction, suggest the importance of glucose. The central nervous system requires 115 g glucose in 24 hr, and more is needed for muscle activity. Other tissues that require glucose for anaerobic glycolysis are, of course, bone marrow, the renal medulla, peripheral nerves, and erythrocytes (about 36 g/day). Total daily body utilization of glucose during fasting is about 150 g, and the small glycogen stores in the liver cannot supply enough for a 1-day fast.

Of the many adaptive changes that occur during fasting, an important one is gluconeogenesis, or production of glucose from proteins. Lactate, a product of glycolysis, can be resynthesized to glucose in the liver and kidney. This does not provide a net energy gain, since lactate was derived from glucose originally, i.e., the energy required for glucose resynthesis is offset by that derived from glycolysis. The advantage of this cycle (the Cori cycle) is twofold: 1) Energy for hepatic glucose synthesis comes from oxidation of fatty acids, which are available in large quantities; 2) the requirements for protein-derived glucose are minimized by the recycling of lactate, the glycolytic product.

Fat   Fat has a direct role as a source of glucose, in addition to providing the energy for glucose resynthesis in the Cori cycle. The glycerol skeleton of triglycerides is readily converted to glucose, yielding about 80 g/24 hr at rest. When lipolysis increases during fasting, the released glycerol becomes an important, though minor, substrate for glucose synthesis.

Amino Acids   Finally, protein-derived amino acids can be used as a major source of glucose through gluconeogenesis, at great expense to the body, as illustrated by an old observation: When dogs are starved to the limit of survival, nitrogen excretion increases just before death, an indication that when all other stores are exhausted, the body turns to its protein. When this happens, death is near.

Fasting humans depend upon glucose production from many sources, but fat is the predominant substrate.

Kidney's Role

The kidney plays an important role in the metabolic adaptation to starvation. It not only contributes to the temporary diuresis at the beginning of starvation but also to gluconeogenesis, which increases to the point of providing almost half the total glucose production. The substrate for renal gluconeogenesis is glutamine, whereas the substrate for hepatic gluconeogenesis is alanine. The nitrogenous by-product of renal gluconeogenesis is ammonia, and the hepatic gluconeogenetic by-product is urea. The ammonia provides additional adaptive advantages because its excretion is in the cationic form, ammonium, which titrates the excess organic acid produced in fasting. Moreover, the ammonia may be resorbed, thus reducing the obligatory nitrogen loss that accompanies the hepatic urea formation. In addition, decreased urea excretion spares the major urinary solute and thus decreases the obligatory water loss and the need for water intake.

Sequence of Events

During the early phase of starvation, blood glucose declines as a result of continuing glucose utilization, particularly by the central nervous system. The lowered blood glucose level signals insulin to fall and glucagon to rise, which in turn facilitate release of fatty acids and amino acids. Fatty acid oxidation, however, provides most of the body's energy requirements and gluconeogenesis supplies glucose to the central nervous system and glycolytic tissues. Insulin is the major regulator of peripheral lipolysis and proteolysis, and glucagon stimulates hepatic glycogen release and liver uptake of alanine for gluconeogenesis.

In early starvation, gluconeogenesis is achieved predominantly by rapid proteolysis. Death from starvation is not caused by hypoglycemia but occurs when one-third to one-half of body protein is lost. Therefore, survival in prolonged starvation necessitates reduction in the rate of protein catabolism. It was observed many years ago that nitrogen loss in starvation decreases with time. When fasting continues beyond 1 week, nitrogen loss measured as urea declines to 3–4 g/day after 4–6 weeks (Owen et al. [8]).

Blood glucose is unchanged after 3 days of starvation without additional physical activity. Therefore, the adaptation to prolonged fasting also includes reduced glycose utilization. Brain requirements for glucose (normally 100–125 g/day), in the face of a daily glucose production of only 80 g, are met by the use of ketone acids, which may provide up to 50–60% of brain fuel needs. The increased use of ketones is, in part, due to a progressive hyperketonemia and, therefore, increased availability of ketones for the brain (Garber et al. [9]).

Ketones   Investigations of prolonged fasting suggest that ketones have a dual role, particularly in the late phase of starvation—that of energy substrate and a signal for change in the type of substrate consumed. The energy to the brain provided by ketones reduces the demand for glucose, and the ketonemia signals to the muscles to reduce protein catabolism and output (Saudek and Felig [10]). The decrease in alanine availability, in turn, causes a reduction in hepatic gluconeogenesis. Ketones coordinate the reduction of glucose utilization and production during prolonged fasts. Thus, metabolic adaptations during starvation maintain glucose homeostasis and conserve body protein. These adaptations are accomplished early by the release of alanine from muscles for hepatic gluconeogenesis. The signals for the initial responses are reduced plasma insulin and increased plasma glucagon. The negative nitrogen balance and depletion of protein stores threaten survival during prolonged fasts, and the organism's metabolism, therefore, shifts toward protein conservation. Hyperketonemia is then the main adaptive mechanism for the late phase.

A number of factors influence the normal human metabolic rate during fasting and refeeding. Normally, metabolic rate increases after a meal, and this increase is even greater when subjects exercise or when they have been overfeeding for several weeks. On the other hand, diminished metabolic rates after a meal were reported in underfed or starved subjects, in obese individuals, and in normal individuals at high altitude (Stock et al. [11]).

Body Changes   The efficiency of the human body changes in response to the nutritional status, and this may provide long-term control of energy balance over and above that provided by food intake. Acute changes in energy intake, such as those often practiced prior to competition by athletes, may also affect diet-induced thermogenesis, and, indeed, the magnitude of the thermic response to a meal during light exercise depends on the previous day's energy intake. Contradictory claims concerning this effect have been reported. More recent investigations of this important dietary manipulation (Stock [12]) showed that acute changes in energy intake do not affect the overall efficiency of the body's energy utilization, either at rest or during exercise. However, the normal changes in blood glucose and free fatty acids in response to food intake are considerably altered by the previous day's diet. The thermic effect of a meal during exercise is enhanced considerably by the subject's having overeaten on the previous day. Thus, carbohydrate loading or starvation prior to competition may profoundly affect the metabolic response to eating on the day of competition. Whether such dietary manipulation and thermic response alter performance has not been established.

DIET AND LIFE SPAN

In laboratory animals, dietary restrictions increase life span. A nutritionally adequate diet was fed every second or third day intermittently with a nutritionally inadequate diet, or animals were fed *ad libitum* a diet with sufficient protein to support maximal growth. The increased life span in animals with dietary manipulation was thought to result from caloric restriction alone. Nutritional manipulation was imposed during early growth and the concept arose that senescence follows growth cessation and is delayed by caloric restriction during early growth.

More recent studies, however, have shown similar beneficial effects of dietary restrictions upon the life span of adult animals. This type of dietary manipulation has not been scrutinized scientifically in human beings. Nevertheless, the increase in life span with a restricted caloric intake has been found in a variety of species and may represent a basic biologic process that is also active in man. The mechanism for this is not known. Physiological and biochemical variables were examined in animals in which dietary manipulation delayed senescence and increased life span. The incidence of various diseases was also studied in these animals. For example, animals with an increaesd life span due to low protein feeding have lower rectal temperatures than controls.

Conversely, little is known about the effect of body temperature on life span in homeothermic animals. The life span of poikilothermic animals increases with decreased environmental temperature. This has been attributed to a lower metabolic rate resulting from a slowing of biochemical reactions by reduced temperature. However, low body temperatures of mice fed a low protein diet are, in fact, associated with increased oxygen consumption. Results are conflicting concerning the relationship of longevity to basal metabolic rate and increased oxygen consumption due to dietary restrictions, and at present the two factors cannot be definitively related.

Several diseases increase with age in animals and humans, but the relationship between the diseases and aging is not known. Dietary restriction and increased life span in mice and rats are associated with delayed onset of a number of diseases, but this is not a consistent occurrence, and the relationship between diet and disease is not clear. Mice fed two dietary regimens, either of which increased life span—namely, a low-protein diet and intermittent feeding—had small cells (judged from the DNA content of hepatic and renal cells) that increased in size with refeeding. The small cells contained less protein and had reduced activities of succinoxidase, cholinesterase, and malic dehydrogenase. No common biochemical alteration was found that could explain the increased life span due to dietary protein restriction or intermittent feeding, nor was there support for the hypothesis that dietary restriction increases life span by reducing protein synthesis and, consequently, reducing use of the genetic code.

Athletes manipulate their diets in many ways. This may include intermittent or continuous insufficient protein intake to sustain cellular activities. However, no studies have been able to relate dietary manipulations or athletic activities during caloric or specific nutrient restriction to longevity.

RECOMMENDED DIETARY ALLOWANCES

It is difficult to establish guidelines for nutrient and energy needs in humans. The standards are estimates based on judgments of expert committees. In the United States, the recommended dietary allowances (RDAs) are only aims to achieve. The RDAs are not minimum requirements but are amounts of nutrients and calories thought to nourish most people adequately in this country. There are no RDAs designed to provide adequate calories and nutrients for athletes in a variety of different sports, though human beings can maintain health within a wide range of nutrient and caloric intake. This includes short-term deficits in both caloric and dietary essentials. Most short-term deficits can be made up, but the effects of prolonged dietary inadequacies for those actively engaged in physical work have not been sufficiently studied. Nevertheless, for sedentary individuals, the most common nutritional deficit in this country is iron.

Achieving a Suitable Balance

Excessive intake of nutrients and calories, on the other hand, is not always associated with deleterious effects. What is excess for a sedentary individual might not be excessive for an athlete. Moreover, the efficiency of liver and kidney function and the presence of compensatory and detoxification mechanisms are important in determining whether caloric and nutrient excess will be associated with symptoms. There are no recognized advantages to the ingestion of nutrients, and certainly not of calories, that are vastly greater than those needed for either correction or deficiency or replenishment caused by exaggerated requirements or by metabolic or absorptive diseases. Because of this, a widely varied diet makes the probability of excessive exposure to a noxious component, either natural or environmental, less likely. Moreover, it also assures that adequate essential nutrients are taken.

Differences in Dietary Needs   The balance of energy intake and output and of nutritional sufficiency is most acutely disturbed in the mature members of our society. The only-too-common weight gain is related to overeating and, even more importantly, to lack of exercise. Metabolic rate and energy expenditure usually decrease with age in our present society, but total caloric and nutrient intake does not. Therefore, in those who are not habitually physically active, caloric restriction is essential. Nutrient and caloric intake prone to restrictions, particularly in young people who are conscious of weight and figure control, may lead to disease or injury, and, during pregnancy, may compromise the offspring nutritionally.

Nutritional anemias common in women and older men in this country are related to inadequate dietary iron and folic acid. Osteoporosis, also common in elderly women and some men, is related not only to deficient dietary calcium but also to inactivity. Poor nutrition of the elderly in conjunction with their decreased physical activity is a growing public health problem.

Dietary Trends   Surveys of dietary trends in the United States indicate that protein-derived calories are about the same as in 1910. However, in the early part of the century, 50% of the protein came from grains and vegetables, and now 70% of the protein consumed is of animal origin. The increased dietary use of animal protein—meat, poultry, fish, and dairy products—is associated with decreased physical activity.

Carbohydrate consumption has declined, and the carbohydrates used are of different types. Starch consumption has dropped off much more rapidly than that of carbohydrates as a whole during the last six or seven decades, and refined sugar intake has increased, even though it was scarce during World War II. The use of flour and other grain products has also decreased considerably. The reduced use of complex carbohydrates in the diet, accompanied by decreased fiber intake, is a matter of concern for those engaged in dietary advice.

In this country, dietary fat has steadily increased, and has been accompanied by a shift in the type of fat used. Saturated fatty acid content in foods has changed little during the past decades. Polyunsaturated fatty acids have increased only modestly, but noticeably during the last 20 years, mainly as a result of the increased consumption of edible oils. Moreover, cholesterol intake at present is only 10% above that consumed a century ago. Over the past

20 years the consumption of eggs, lard, butter, and various diary products has decreased while meat consumption has increased. These are all trends that are applauded by those advocating dietary manipulation to prevent certain diseases.

Vitamin and mineral intake has not changed much during this century, but calcium, vitamin D, and vitamin A are used slightly more than they were 65 years ago. Since the 1940s, iron, riboflavin, niacin, and thiamine have been added to flour, considerably increasing the per capita availability of these nutrients. The enrichment of certain cereals with the same nutrients has contributed to a slight increase in their consumption.

It should be reemphasized that since the early part of this century, dietary calories in this country have remained essentially the same, but there has also been a concomitant decrease in energy expenditure, related to transportation modes and changes in life-style. This trend has led to major health problems not usually evident in those who are physically active but predominant in the obese sedentary person. It has also contributed, though the mechanism is not understood, to increased vascular disease and other conditions that are probably related to dietary habits. In this setting, the reduced consumption of complex carbohydrates associated with decreased fiber intake has also been blamed for a number of degenerative diseases, but final proof that this aspect of dietary change is, in fact, influencing the occurrence of gastrointestinal disorders such as diverticulosis and certain types of cancer is not available.

MARINE LIPIDS

A long-standing puzzle seems to have recently been explained. It was known that coronary heart disease in Eskimos is very rare, in spite of a very large consumption of fat. It was not, however, realized that their important fat consumption was entirely derived from fish. Thereafter it has been postulated that fish oil is protective against the development of atherosclerosis.

In spite of their high fat intake, compared with that of Western populations, the Eskimos have low plasma lipid levels and a lower incidence of hypertension, but a prolonged bleeding time. All these characteristics were at first thought to be genetically determined but are now felt to be related to the characteristic diet, which consists of cold-water fish, seal, and whale meat. All three dietary sources have large amounts of the marine omega-3 series of polyunsaturated fats. The marine omega-3 series eicosapentaenoic (EPA) and docosahexaenoic (DHA) fatty acides were originally classed together with the structurally similar vegetable oil omega-6 series of polyunsaturated fats, but the differences between these two types of oils in their hypolipidemic activity and antithrombotic effects only recently have been recognized.

A number of hypotheses have been proposed to explain the occurrence of atherosclerosis. Presently, it is thought to be a response to injury. Under this scenario, platelets contribute to lesion formation by their release of important growth factors that cause a proliferation of arterial smooth muscle cells; those cells subsequently accumulate lipid and become the foam cells of atherosclerotic plaques. One of the earliest signs of atherosclerosis is the formation of "fatty streaks" from monocytes, from which foam cells can also be derived. Both platelets and monocytes appear in the arterial endothelium and release growth factors that stimulate smooth muscle proliferation. It is thought that marine lipids reduce the adherence of monocytes to the arterial wall and that this may be one way in which they beneficially retard the development of atherosclerosis. Of course, they inhibit platelet aggregation as well, which is another important initial step in atherosclerosis.

Prolongation of bleeding time in Eskimos and in subjects receiving supplements of dietary omega-3 fatty acids is thought to result from changes in prostaglandin synthesis, and these fatty acids, together with the omega-6 series, serve as substrates for formation of prostaglandins that modulate platelet aggregation. These are thromboxane A_2 and prostaglandin I_2 (prostacyclin). Thromboxane A_2 is produced, among other sites, in platelets, and promotes platelet aggregation and vasoconstriction. Prostacyclin, on the other hand, is synthesized predominantly in vascular endothelial cells and inhibits platelet aggregation and is also a vasodilator. The omega-3 fatty acids compete with omega-6 fatty acids and produce prostaglandins that retard platelet aggregation and promote vasodilatation. The consumption of these marine fatty acids rather than fatty acids derived from plant oil produces diminished amounts of the aggregatory thomboxane A_2. It does not alter, and may even increase, prostacyclin effects. The resultant influence of marine fatty acid supplementation is a reduction in platelet aggregation and a prolongation of bleeding time, similar to that found in Eskimos.

Experimental studies in which non-Eskimo persons were given a diet consisting mainly of mackerel and salmon for a total of 2–3 g of EPA daily showed that after 6 weeks there was a reduction in platelet aggregation and a prolongation of bleeding time. Additional experimental studies with mainly fish diets showed an increase in platelet survival time and a lowering of plasma thromboglobulin. All these and other effects contribute to the prolongation of the bleeding time. Similar results have also been found in patients with established ischemic cardiovascular disease.

Additional studies in human healthy subjects given EPA and DHA daily showed that inhibition of chemotactic responses of neutrophils to endothelial cells could be achieved. This supports the idea that EPA and DHA may have anti-inflammatory effects as well. Anecdotal evidence suggests that dietary supplement of marine fatty acids improves the joint symptoms of degenerative osteoarthritis in some runners.

There are three classes of fatty acids: saturated fatty acids (stearic palmitic), which are hypercholesterolemic in their effects; monosaturated fatty acids, which either are neutral or have a mild cholesterol lowering effect; and polyunsaturated fatty acids, which have a moderate hypocholesterolemic effect. Of the two types of polyunsaturated fatty acids, the omega-6 vegetable oils (containing linoleic and arachidonic acids) are widespread, and the omega-3 marine oils, which contain mainly EPA and DHA acids, are more restricted in their distribution. Omega-3 fatty acids and omega-6 fatty acids can compete with each other for cyclo-oxygenase, the enzyme necessary for conversion of these fatty acids to the various types of prostaglandin.

Though dietary polyunsaturated fatty acids have a cholesterol lowering effect, they may have potentially harmful side effects as well. Omega-6 series of fatty acids can enhance cholesterol gallstone formation and decrease immune function. They reduce low-density lipoprotein (LDL) cholesterol levels but also lower the beneficial high-density lipoprotein (HDL). Omega-3 fatty acids do not have these unwanted side effects, but their safety has not yet been fully assessed, except in an epidemiologic sense where evidence of harm to populations such as the Eskimos has not been found. In healthy volunteers, a comparison of salmon oil with vegetable oil supplement showed significant falls in serum cholesterol levels in both groups, but the salmon oil recipients experienced also a reduction in triglyceride concentrations. In addition, a significant lowering of omega-3 fatty acids on triglyceride-rich lipoproteins, very-low-density lipoproteins, and chylomicrons has also been demonstrated; all of these substances have significant atherosclerogenic effects. Triglyceride-lowering effects are present not only in healthy volunteers but also in patients with type 4 and type 5 hyperlipoproteinemias, conditions associated with marked and early atherosclerosis formation and cardiovascular and cerebrovascular incidents.

Marine omega-3 fatty acids also have an antihypertensive effect that is attributed to changes in prostaglandin production, with a shift from the vasoconstrictor thromboxane A_2 to the less active thromboxane A_3. But, in addition, there is a reduction in norepinephrine levels in treated normal volunteers. In healthy subjects, the isocaloric substitution of either a high-EPA or low-EPA diet was found to cause a significant reduction in systolic and diastolic blood pressures in the high-EPA-treated groups.

The prevention of atherosclerosis is an active endeavor in the aging population, and exercise is thought to promote this or retard the onset of clinical vascular disease. While it has not been conclusively shown that marine lipids prevent coronary artery disease, retrospective evidence suggests that dietary fish consumption is associated with a reduced risk of myocardial infarction. An example of this is a study carried out in the Netherlands, in which information, including a careful dietary history, on a group of 852 middle-aged men was collected in 1960. These subjects were followed for 20 years, and 78 died of coronary heart disease during the follow-up period. An inverse dose-response was found between fish consumption in 1960 and death during the follow-up from coronary heart disease. Mortality from cardiovascular events was more than 50% lower among those individuals who ate at least 30 g of fish per day when compared with those who did not eat fish at all. Therefore, only 2 fish dishes per week may help prevent coronary heart disease in individuals at risk.

Clearly, it seems useful to supplement the protective effects of exercise with marine lipid concentrate, which is now available from health food stores. It remains to be seen whether the prolongation of bleeding time might cause serious tissue extravasation of blood, particularly in the feet of runners or in other parts of the body in other athletes, or whether the change in bleeding time has any effects on exercise performance or can lead to complications from prologed exertion.

The potential of marine omega-3 fatty acids to retard atherosclerosis (particularly in those who already have coronary or cerebrovascular disease) by lowering elevated serum cholesterol and triglyceride levels (by reducing blood pressure and inhibiting platelet aggregation) is of great interest in patients with vascular disorders. Whether such supplements in athletes without clinical evidence of vascular disease might offer further and additional protection over and above the exertion itself, which tends to increase high-density lipoprotein, has not been established (Davidson and Liebson [13]).

Dietary Protein

Dietary protein provides amino acids for growth and tissue maintenance, for enzyme production, and for gluconeogenesis. Amino acids that the body is unable to manufacture, or essential amino acids, are tryptophan, phenylalanine, methionine, lysine, threonine, leucine, isoleucine, valine, and histidine (mainly for infants and possibly for healthy adults). About another 15 amino acids can be made in quantities sufficient to provide the necessary building blocks for body tissues, provided enough nitrogen is available. The biologic value of protein is determined by the dietary composition of essential amino acids, the need for which is related to body requirements.

The need for protein and essential amino acids normally varies with age and is determined by their rate of turnover. In the average sedentary adult, this is about 2.5 g/kg/day or about 175 g of protein. The obligatory losses of nitrogen are only about 30 g protein; there is therefore about an 80% reutilization. The essential amino acids form about 40% of the amino acid content of tissue protein. Essential amino acids need only provide half (20%) of dietary protein in the adult, so they must be even more highly conserved in total turnover of amino acid nitrogen. The essential amino acid requirement for new-tissue formation in growing children is increased to 43% of dietary protein. Standards proposed for a "safe level of protein intake" are 0.55 g/kg/day of excellent quality protein as an average value for adults, and 2 g/kg/day for infants from birth to 6 months of age.

The actual dietary intake of protein in the United States is much higher, and the possible deleterious effects of this on longevity have already been touched upon. Moreover, long-lived people in other parts of the world (Ecuador, Pakistan, and the Caucasus) subsist on low-energy and low-protein diets. These low-protein requirements may help eliminate much of the so-called world "protein gap" but, nevertheless, a number of activists clamor for closure of the protein gap and are reluctant to accept the practical implications of the lastest thinking on protein requirements.

The human body is capable of infinite adaptive changes. When the energy intake falls below the requirement, the living organism burns its own tissue to help bridge the gap between intake and requirement. In the young this is sometimes evidenced by reduction or total cessation of growth. The adaptive changes to low-protein intake, known for years, include reduced urinary nitrogen excretion, especially in the form of urea. In prolonged or even short-lived protein restriction, the hepatic urea cycle is depressed, the amino acid synthesis is increased. The opposite occurs with protein feeding. In severe malnutrition (energy-protein reduction), the most significant deficit is caloric and not protein (McLaren [14]).

Glycogen and free fatty acids are the major energy sources for short-duration physical activity, and protein utilization probably occurs in exercise of long duration. For example, alanine output from skeletal muscle increases in proportion to work intensity (Felig [15]). It may be that amino acids are transaminated in skeletal muscles, thus permitting de novo synthesis of alanine from glucose-derived pyruvate.

An intramuscular enzyme efflux after exercise is another explanation for increased protein involvement in exercise. The enzyme efflux, at least in isolated preparations, occurs only after the muscle work capacity is considerably reduced by fatigue, a finding suggesting that when the muscle's ability to synthesize ATP decreases as a result of glycogen depletion, the cell membrane breaks down and enzymes are released. The enzymes are then degraded into their component amino acids and are subsequently deaminated.

Another possibility is that protein involvement is directly related to the available substrate. Thus, serum urea increases linearly with exercise duration, beginning after about 70 min. At this time, liver glycogen is decreased and muscle glycogen is severely depleted. It is, therefore, possible that protein catabolism occurs with prolonged exercise, similar to that seen in short-term starvation (Saudek and Felig [10]). Therefore, the protein catabolism that occurs during or after prolonged exercise may be related to glycogen depletion and the consequent decreased ATP, and is not directly related to exercise.

The relationship between initial muscle glycogen content and protein catabolism has been examined (Lemon and Mullin [16]). When subjects exercised after carbohydrate depletion, serum and sweat levels of urea nitrogen were significantly higher than those seen with exercise after carbohydrate loading, and serum urea continued to be high into the recovery period. Protein breakdown during carbohydrate depletion was 13.7 g/hr and protein provided 10.4% of the caloric cost of the exercise. The possible mechanisms contributing to increased protein utilization with prolonged exercise have been discussed. In the studies of prolonged exercise in human subjects, the excretion of urea nitrogen in sweat was the most important mechanism in preventing an exercise-induced rise in serum urea nitrogen in both carbohydrate-loaded and -depleted subjects. The importance of urea nitrogen excretion in sweat was emphasized when the highest serum urea values were seen during the recovery period after sweating had ceased. Therefore, serum urea nitrogen probably is not a reliable index of protein catabolism but depends upon the exercising individual's capacity to sweat and on his or her thermoregulatory responses and heat acclimation (see Chapter 2, Temperature Regulation and Sports).

Changes in plasma and urinary amino acids were studied in participants in a 70-km cross-country ski race that lasted $4\frac{1}{2}$–6 hr and was associated with slight dehydration (Refsum et al. [17]). An average of 8 μmol/min/kg body weight of urea were produced during the race. This is more than twice the average urea production for normally active similar persons with ordinary protein intake. A marked change also occurred in plasma amino acids during the race, a finding supporting the suggestion that protein and amino acid metabolism is an integral part of the metabolic response to prolonged heavy exercise. The changes in the amino acid pattern were not influenced by the amino acid composition of serum albumin or muscle, materials probably metabolized during heavy exertion. The explanation was that heavy exercise causes muscle glycogen depletion, reduced pyruvate, and decreased alanine release. The amino acid changes in this study, as in previous studies, were similar to those found during prolonged starvation. Thus, it is clear from many well-conducted studies in humans that prolonged heavy exercise places demands on protein and amino acid stores that should be replenished by appropriate diet.

Excessive Protein Intake   Athletes engaged in heavy short-duration physical activity such as weightlifting, throwing, wrestling, and body building commonly eat excessive amounts of protein. This practice is based upon a tradition that goes back to the ancient Greek athletes who ate large quantities of meat to replace muscles spent during exercise, and is supported by the theory first propounded by J. Von Liebig in 1851 (Consolazio and Johnson [18]) that protein is the principal source of energy for muscle contraction. Though this is clearly not the case, recent reinvestigation of the theory has shed light upon the beneficial effects of increased protein intake, particularly in athletes engaged in muscle building. During such exercise, lean body mass and nitrogen retention increase, and this increase is augmented by higher protein intake. On the other hand, short-term exercise at both high- and low-caloric or nitrogen intake is usually accompanied by increased nitrogen excretion. Thus, athletes engaged in weightlifting, throwing, and other lean-body-mass building exercises over long periods of time and accompanied by increased muscle mass would benefit from increased protein intake on the order of 2.4 g/kg body weight per day. In endurance events, when excessive weight is undesirable, minimal protein intake, as recommended by the World Health Organization, is adequate to replace the muscle breakdown (Marable and Hickson [19]).

Fad Diets   Because increased physical activity is growing in popularity, the desire to lose excessive weight rapidly has tempted many to embark upon severe dietary restrictions and to use some diets that have been recommended for rapid weight loss. In 1976, a book entitled *The Last Chance Diet* was published (Linn and Stuart [20]). Within a short time, several liquid-protein-modified-fast diets became popular and were used for rapid weight reduction by large numbers of people. Though these dietary modifications were intended for the grotesquely obese and were to be the sole source of calories for those attempting this method of weight reduction, it soon became clear that a number of people who wanted to reach ideal weight rapidly to improve athletic performance were also using the diet.

By August 1977, sudden death in several young diet users was reported, and between July 1977 and January 1978, 60 deaths occurred among avid users of the liquid-protein-modified-fast diet. Detailed clinical and necropsy information was available for 17 of these patients who had been healthy except for obesity before embarking on the diet. Electrocardiographic abnormalities, particularly prolongation of the QT interval, were ominous of and may have presaged sudden death in these patients. All those who died suddenly while on the liquid-protein diet were extremely obese, and it was unlikely that they had engaged in physical activity of any sort either before or during the diet. Nevertheless, the temptation to engage in extreme dietary manipulation of this or other types in order to, as it were, lighten the burden, particularly in endurance events, is often great enough that any method might seem minor if it leads to the desired effect. It should be emphasized that the use of various liquid-protein-modified-fast diets is dangerous. Their value in improving athletic performance is certainly questionable, and for those who are more than moderately obese, the chance of serious complications is great (Isner et al. [21]).

Fear of Obesity

Obesity is seen as a serious threat to continued health because of its ill-defined relationships to morbidity and mortality from cardiovascular disease, and a number of other conditions, and those who are obese are often subject to derogatory assessments by themselves and their social contacts. It has been said that "whenever fat people have existed and whenever a literature has reflected aspects of the lives and values of the period, a record has been left of the low regard usually held for the obese by the thinner and clearly more virtuous observer" (Mayer [22]). Because in this country at the moment the obese are classed as immature, passive-dependent, and of low self-esteem, and are given the responsibility for their fatness, they not only face the hazards of their adiposity but also must contend with serious psychologic and social difficulties. It is, therefore, not surprising that some obese individuals embrace exercise and dietary manipulation of the type discussed in the foregoing sections as a panacea for their adiposity. Although both approaches are useful in weight reduction, one should be cognizant of the possible risks of exercise and dietary manipulation in those who are obese and not accustomed to energy expenditure. Moreover, physicians often have negative attitudes toward obese patients, and failure of weight reduction in many individuals may be due to feelings of shame, self-derogation, and the embarrassment that they experience when facing physicians (Maiman and Wang [23]).

Anorexia nervosa is a dramatic disorder characterized by fear of fatness and refusal to maintain a minimally healthy body weight. On the other hand, bulimia, another disorder of eating, is characterized by recurrent episodes of binge eating with a severely restricted diet and often self-induced vomiting and purging. Anorexia nervosa and bulimia, either in isolation or combined, are the most common eating disorders in the United States and are occasionally found among athletes also. The persuasive evidence of the increasing prevalence of eating disorders implies that sports medicine personnel should be prepared for such diagnoses and appropriate treatment in athletes. Anorexia nervosa and bulimia are estimated to affect 10–15% of adolescent girls and young women, and the prevalence of bulimia among college women is said to be as high as 19% (Balaa and Drossman [24]).

Persons wtih anorexia nervosa or bulimia often undertake compulsive ritualistic acts to lose weight. These include not only starvation but also vomiting, the ingestion of cathartics and diuretics, and exercise, often vigorously and to complete exhaustion.

The American College of Physicians Health and Public Policy Committee of 1986 has issued a position paper [25] in which it affirms the necessity for practicing physicians (including those engaged in sports medicine) to be cognizant of the growing problem of eating disorders and their pathogenesis. It is stressed that there is no single psychiatric, physiologic, or pathologic characteristic of anorexia nervosa and that the diagnosis must depend largely upon awareness of the possibility of the condition and the behavioral features of the disorder, which are mostly related to attitudes about body image and eating, two most important aspects of behavior in athletes and dancers.

The diagnosis of anorexia nervosa is based on criteria from the *Diagnostic and Statistical Manual of Mental Disorders (Third Edition)* issued by the American Psychiatric Association (APA), and depends on 1) intense fear of becoming obese that does not diminish as weight loss progresses; 2) disturbance of body image, namely, claiming to "feel fat" even when emaciated; 3) weight loss of at least 25% of original body weight or, if under 18 years of age, weight loss from original body weight plus projected weight gain based on growth charts (to make together 25%); 4) refusal to maintain body weight above a minimum normal weight for age and height; and 5) no known physical illness that would account for the weight loss.

The DSM-III criteria for bulimia are: 1) the presence of recurring episodes of binge eating and 2) at least 3 of the following characteristics: consumption of high-caloric, easily ingested food during binges; inconspicuous eating during a binge, cessation of eating episodes by abdominal pain, sleep, social interuption, or self-induced vomiting; repeated attempts to lose weight through restrictive diets, self-induced vomiting or the use of purging or diuretics; and fluctuation in weight of more than 4.5 kg due to alternate binges and fasts. Excessive exercise (until exhaustion) is also frequently practiced.

Because patients with eating disorders are particularly difficult to identify if they appear healthy, suspicion should be aroused in persons of particular risk, that is, elite women athletes and men who, for no apparent reason, often show increasing deterioration in athletic performance and widely fluctuating body weight.

The following questions have been suggested by the American College of Physicians [25] as important to giving a hint of the presence of eating disorders during history taking in susceptible athletes:

Do you feel helpless in the presence of food?
Are you a binge eater?
Do you try every new diet and always end up gaining back the weight you lose?
Do you try to control your weight by vomiting, using laxatives or diuretics, overexercise, or episodes of starvation?
Do you eat when you are not hungry?
Do you eat when you are anxious?
Do you eat when you are depressed?
Do you feel guilty after an eating binge?
Do you eat sensibly around other people and then "pig out" when you are alone?

OPIOIDS AND FEEDING

Evidence that endogenous opioids are involved in the control of feeding in experimental animals has accumulated, and it is natural to propose that opioids might also be involved in the production of eating disorders in humans. There are a number of experimental obesity settings that are associated with increased opioid production, and an increased number and sensitivity of opiate receptors has been found. Moreover, under experimental conditions, sugar has an effect on feeding behavior that is mediated by opiates. It can be shown, for example, that the obesity-inducing effect of a palatable diet in rodents is blocked by opiate antagonists. Moreover, stress-induced feeding in animals often leads to preferential sucrose ingestion, and this is blocked by opiate antagonists and enhanced by β-endorphin. Whether these effects of nutrients on the endogenous opioid system can occur in humans has not been established. Clinical experience, however, supports the idea that carbohydrates, particularly sugar, are important in binge eating and in obesity, and of course they are of crucial importance in proper nutrition for physical performance. Many binge eaters, not necessarily athletes, preferentially eat sweets during binges, and many obese individuals, of necessity nonathletic, often consume more than half of their total calories in carbohydrates, which is common in healthy athletes. Moreover, sweet snacking is a behavior frequently found during stressful periods. In obese nonathletic individuals sugar can lead to increased β-endorphin production (Fullerton et al. [26]); similar increases can be found in exercising individuals (see Chapter 3, Neurology of Endurance Training). It is tempting, therefore, to speculate that excessive sugar intake resulting in obesity and prolonged exertion sometimes resulting in injury are merely manifestations of addiction to endogenous opioids.

The crucial importance of identifying eating disorders in athletes cannot be overstated. Sudden death in both athletes and in nonathletic patients with anorexia nervosa has repeatedly been reported. In most individuals, this is unexpected, and a cardiac etiology either primary or due to metabolic derangements has often been suggested. Patients with bulimia are also known to be prone to sudden cardiac death. In a study of 43 patients with eating disorders (anorexia nervosa and/or bulimia) it was found that 37% had mitral valve prolapse [25]. Moreover, many of these had cardiac arrhythmias characterized by isolated premature extrasystoles. Since mitral valve prolapse presents an additional risk factor for arrhythmia, the primary association that might exist between mitral valve prolapse syndrome and eating disorders needs to be explored. It has been suggested that anatomic prolapse of the mitral valve is part of a generalized neuroendocrine disorder, and increased vasoconstrictor activity in association with supine bradycardia in such patients has suggested that an increased sympathetic and vagal tone may be present in mitral valve prolapse. A parasympathetic (vagal) increase in tone has repeatedly been documented in athletes and increased plasma catecholamine level is frequently induced with competition in athletics and has also been found in patients with mitral valve prolapse. A hyperresponsiveness to adrenergic stimulation in many patients and perhaps also in some athletes with or without mitral valve prolapse and eating disorders might complicate responses to stress and perhaps account for an occasional sudden death in an otherwise healthy athlete with an unrecognized eating disorder.

LIPID METABOLISM

The main substrate for energy production in human skeletal muscle after prolonged exertion is lipid. Studies were performed, therefore, to assess the effects of training, particularly of the endurance variety, on lipid metabolism. After endurance training, muscle glycogen utilization is reduced and the carbon source of energy for muscular activity is shifted to lipids. This is a major advantage in delaying fatigue in events limited by muscle glycogen content (Gollnick [27]).

Subsequent studies confirmed these findings and showed that equally trained males and females with similar aerobic capacity and muscle fiber composition derive a comparable portion of their energy requirements from lipids. In such persons, however, in vitro measurement of a selected muscle mitochondrial enzyme suggests that female muscle adapts less well than male muscle under similar conditions of training. This finding was attributed to a lesser mitochondrial density in the trained female muscle than in the male muscle. However, even though these in vitro measurements suggest a difference in female muscle fibers, there was no functional effect on lipid utilization during prolonged exertion.

Although the capacity for muscles to metabolize fat is markedly enhanced by endurance training, the actual regulation of lipid use during prolonged physical activity is not limited by the ability of muscle fibers to oxidize fatty acids. Moreover, even untrained muscle can increase lipid oxidation markedly when plasma free fatty acids are increased (Costill and Coyle [28]), a finding that is theoretically explained by the known catecholamine increase with exercise and consequent release of free fatty acids from fat (Appenzeller and Schade [29]). It may be that changes in cyclic AMP are responsible for α- and β-adrenergic stimulation. Catecholamine activity on beta receptors stimulates adenyl cyclase and increases intracellular cyclic AMP, which in turn changes cell function appropriately.

On the other hand, similar interactions with alpha receptors cause decreased cyclic AMP and opposite changes in cell activity. This hypothesis may not apply to all adrenergic responsive cells, but it has been tested in isolated human fat cells, and agrees closely with theoretic considerations (Robison et al. [30]). Epinephrine stimulated cyclic AMP in fat cells from obese subjects in the fed state, and glycerol was released into the incubation medium. Phentolamine (an α-adrenergic receptor blocker) enhanced this action and propranolol (a β-receptor blocker) reduced it to below basal levels.

However, epinephrine suppressed cyclic AMP lipolysis when incubated with fat cells from fasted individuals. The reversal of epinephrine effect on fat cells by fasting appears to be due to decreased β-receptor activity rather than increased α-receptor activity. This change in α- and β-adrenergic receptor action occurred after 1 day of fasting and remained the same for an 8-day observation period.

These findings suggest that during fasting the sympathetic nervous system and circulating catecholamines act to conserve adipose tissue triglycerides (Burns et al. [31]). It should, at this point, be emphasized that some athletes fast prior to competition. If the competition extends beyond 60 min, then clearly the availability of free fatty acids for fuel is crucial to performance. The epinephrine effect of reversal upon lipolysis of human adipocytes from fasting subjects suggests that fasting is not indicated prior to endurance events but may, of course, be of some use during shorter athletic feats.

Exercise Intensity

Under ordinary dietary conditions, the extent to which energy is supplied from carbohydrates or fat is determined by the relative exercise intensity. Increasingly more energy is derived from fat at exercise intensities of 65% maximum oxygen consumption ($\dot{V}O_{2\,max}$) during prolonged activity, but if the intensity rises to 75% $\dot{V}O_{2\,max}$, fat is not used and the muscle needs carbohydrate for fuel. Fat utilization during prolonged exercise is higher after a fat-rich diet than after a carbohydrate-rich or a normal diet.

Thus the implications are clear concerning dietary manipulation prior to sports that require prolonged activity of relatively low intensity, which would benefit, presumably, from a fat-rich rather than a carbohydrate-rich diet. This is not to say, however, that carbohydate "loading" (to be discussed later) is not indicated for athletes who will engage in high-energy activities, even for 2 or more hours. Free fatty acid uptake from plasma into the muscle during exercise is related to plasma concentration of the free fatty acids, but the increased combustion of fat during prolonged exercise—clearly a useful adaptive mechanism—can only in part be explained by increased uptake of plasma free fatty acids. The plasma fatty acids might be supplied in part from hydrolysis of triglycerides by an enzyme (lipoprotein lipase) present at the endothelial surface of muscle capillaries. It is possible, therefore, that a training-induced increase in this enzyme might make more fatty acids available during muscular activity in trained individuals.

Lipid Stores

Increased utilization of intramuscular triglyceride occurs in animals and man during prolonged activity, and has been attributed to an intracellular muscle enzyme called hormone-sensitive lipase. In recent studies of lipoprotein lipase activity and lipid stores in human skeletal muscles during prolonged exercise (Lithell et al. [32]), the enzyme increased in skeletal muscle during an 85-km cross-country ski race. Moreover, this increase was most striking in those athletes who had the best training and the fastest times in this competition. The training and $\dot{V}O_{2\,max}$, as well as the finishing times, were closely correlated so that it is not possible to be certain which of these factors was, in fact, the determinant for the increased lipoprotein lipase activity. In the best-trained athletes, the largest triglyceride stores occurred during competition. The lipoprotein lipase activity increased only minimally in the best competitors. The least-trained participants in this study, on the other hand, had a sixfold increase in lipoprotein lipase during the race so that in these subjects there was greater capacity for free fatty-acid uptake from serum triglycerides in comparison to highly trained participants in the same race. Thus, these studies confirm numerous previous reports that muscular energy during prolonged heavy physical work is, in part, and probably most efficaciously, derived from intracellularly stored lipids, and in highly trained subjects the stores are both larger and more easily used than in less-well-trained competitors. It seems, therefore, advantageous to increase fat consumption during training in order to make free fatty acids more available and, perhaps, induce lipoprotein lipase formation in muscle capillary endothelium.

DIETARY FIBER

It has been suggested that the increasing prevalence of obesity in Western countries may, in part, be due to increased refined carbohydrate, and, therefore, reduced fiber in the diet. Several physiologic activities of dietary fiber tend to reduce the chances of obesity. Fiber displaces nutrients from the diet and requires more chewing, thus reducing the rate of food ingestion. It also promotes secretion of saliva and gastric juice, which contributes to gastric distention and satiety, and decreased small bowel absorption of some foods, particularly fat and protein. Moreover, consumption of refined products such as white flour and sugar are more likely to cause excess calories because they can be eaten rapidly and absorbed efficiently.

In countries where obesity is rare, the population usually ingests a diet rich in complex carbohydrates with their high fiber complement. *Ad libitum* intake of high-fiber diets provides greater satiety than does that of low-fiber diets of comparable energy content. This finding is attributed to a larger undigested residue in the intestine with corresponding increase in the feeling of bulk and distention.

The Egyptian sand rat, which normally eats a high-fiber diet, becomes obese on reduced-fiber diets, and rats given snack foods become obese and then revert to normal weight when the ordinary rat-pellet diet is reinstituted. Snack foods are high in energy and sugar and are practically devoid of fiber. The overall role of food fiber in obesity is far from clear. It is, however, believed that consumption of fiber-rich food may help prevent obesity and promote weight loss in obese people if calories are simultaneously restricted.

Vegetarian Diet

The dietary practices of athletes vary widely according to their sport. Many endurance athletes are vegetarians. Most, fortunately, are "lacto-ovo" vegetarians or are, at least lacto-vegetarians. It is rare to find "pure" vegetarians or those who refuse eggs, dairy products, and all flesh foods. The true or pure vegetarian (vegan) whose philosophy prohibits exploitation or "cruelty" toward animals is at risk of serious malnutrition, particularly when engaging in high-energy output for a prolonged time.

Many athletes, and particularly vegetarians, also prefer organic or natural foods in the belief that vegetables grown with the addition of pesticides, herbicides, or inorganic fertilizers are, somehow, contaminated and have lost their nutritive values. This idea, of course, is not supported by scientific evidence, and belongs to the cultists espousing counter-culture philosophies, which have, until recently, also included the so-called Zen macrobiotic diet.

Athletes using vegetarian diets, however, have a large fiber intake, which affects gastrointestinal motility and nutrient absorption, both important considerations before competition. For example, if food energy content is reduced because of fiber, then adequate energy may not be available during competition, particularly in endurance events. The bulky residue and decreased speed of absorption of high-fiber foods may seriously affect performance by causing increased bowel motility and gastrointestinal discomfort.

The role of high-fiber foods in the maintenance of desired weight in some athletic disciplines is not clear. Nevertheless, vegetarianism is now widespread among certain athletes and merits consideration of its effect on performance during both competition and training (Calkins [33]). Claims have been made that increased dietary fiber prevents or treats diabetes, atherosclerosis, cancer of the large bowel, and many other disorders. Most of these claims are based on epidemiologic data comparing very different populations and important factors other than dietary fiber that may have been instrumental in changing the disease incidence.

Dietary fiber is the skeletal remnant of plant cells, which resists human gastrointestinal enzymatic digestion. Phytic acid (inositol hexaphosphate), closely associated with dietary fiber and an important component of bran and whole-grain flour, may combine with calcium, magnesium, iron, and zinc and cause deficiency of these ions when dietary sources are marginal or when the body requires larger amounts of them. Other constituents of the plant skeleton may have profound effects. These include silica and lipids found in fruit leaves and seeds, and nonmetabolizable sugars, such as raffinose, which may promote production of bowel gas in humans. Whether these effects of dietary fibers are detrimental to athletic performance has not been determined.

Effects of Fiber on Carbohydrates and Lipids

Well-documented clinical studies suggest that some types of food fiber have a beneficial effect on carbohydrate metabolism in diabetes. All studies agree on the glucose-lowering effect of guar and pectin often found in fruits. The glucose-lowering effects of dietary fibers, particularly cellulose, are less certain. In some diabetic patients, food fiber may significantly decrease or totally eliminate the need for insulin, an advantage that may be particularly valuable in those diabetics who are athletes.

Dietary fiber is also important in serum lipid regulation. For example, Seventh Day Adventists who are lacto-ovo vegetarians have a greatly reduced risk of coronary artery disease in comparison to others, but the specific dietary component responsible for the reduced risk in this group has not been identified. Neither cellulose nor bran has a definable effect upon serum cholesterol, whereas dietary guar and pectin lower it.

The role of high-fiber diets in the treatment of hypercholesterolemia is not established. Attempts have also been made to assess the value of dietary fiber in changing triglyceride levels in the management of atherosclerosis, but at present, information is insufficient to reach a conclusion. The value of athletic pursuits in the prevention or treatment of certain so-called degenerative diseases, including atherosclerosis, is also not clear because most athletes manipulate their diets, a factor that may affect the target disease in addition to increasing energy output.

Unquestionably, dietary fiber decreases transit time through the colon and also increases the average daily weight of stools. Small bowel transit time is relatively constant. A high-fiber diet also alters gastrointestinal bacterial flora. The lack of dietary fiber has been implicated on epidemiologic grounds as, perhaps, responsible for widespread diverticulosis in North America. Bran, which is not widely used by most people, shortens bowel transit time in normal subjects and in those with diverticular disease. Whether dietary fiber is at least partly responsible for builky and frequent stools often occurring in endurance athletes is not clear.

Dietary fiber may also influence certain so-called degenerative diseases of Western society. The typical "Western diet," high in fat and protein and low in fiber, has been blamed for a number of ills, and the thrust is increasing for dietary modification to prevent disease, particularly among athletes. The effect of increasing dietary fiber upon athletic performance, in preventing diabetes, atherosclerosis, diverticulitis, and perhaps colonic cancer is poorly understood, and one may not conclude, on the basis of present studies, that high dietary fiber benefits athletic performance or prevents disease (Levin and Horwitz [34]).

NUTRITIONAL SUPPLEMENTS AND VITAMINS

Certain conditions must be met to evaluate claims for nutritional supplements and vitamins. These include answers to the following questions: Is the information based on personal observation, or can it stand the scrutiny of other scientists? Is it anecdote or science? Can the results be reproduced by those not involved in promoting the product, or does the recommended dietary change work just in the hands of its promoters, as suggested in a Harvard Medical School Health Letter [35]? Did control studies show that treatments are superior to placebos or "doing nothing"? What happens in the absence of supplementation or therapy? Are the results pure coincidence, the result of the natural history of the disorder, or the effect of other not-controlled-for conditions? Has the recommended manipulation, dietary or otherwise, been proven to be safe when compared with doing nothing or with other therapy? Is the risk of taking the supplement justified? In other words, what is the risk:benefit ratio? Lastly, the burden of proof that a certain dietary manipulation or therapy is effective is upon those who propose it, particularly if it involves methods or procedures that are not generally accepted medically.

Megavitamins

Megavitamin therapy is the use of one or several vitamins in amounts that are 10 or more times greater than those recommended by the Committee on Dietary Allowances of Food and Nutrition, National Research Council of the United States. The recommended daily allowance (RDA) for each vitamin is substantially above the range that is commonly found in proper nutrition, to allow for a safety factor. Over the years, the RDA for most vitamins has decreased as knowledge about nutritional requirements has improved. Megavitamin therapy, as advocated by various cultists, is chemical and not nutrient therapy.

In general, vitamins function as coenzymes or hormones, or when combined with body protein to form holoenzymes, usually referred to as enzymes. A vitamin is useful only when combined with its apoenzyme, and the apoenzyme that is manufactured per unit of time is limited. Saturation of apoenzyme occurs at vitamin levels that are roughly those recommended in the dietary allowances, and excess vitamins become pharmacologic agents. Therefore, they are no longer nutrients, but are then medication.

A vitamin is an organic compound that the body cannot make in adequate amounts— that is, not protein, fat, or carbohydrate—and that is necessary for normal human metabolism. Vitamin deficiency produces a specific disease such as beriberi, rickets, or scurvy, which is corrected by administration of the deficient vitamin.

The 13 human vitamins need not be enumerated here. Four of them are fat soluble and nine are water soluble. The last vitamin to be discovered was B_{12} in 1948, and further intensive research has not added new ones. Several growth factors, para-aminobenzoic acid, bioflavonoids, choline, inositol, lipoic acid, and ubiquinone, are necessary for other organisms such as bacteria. Some of these are also used by humans but can be produced in the body as needed.

Megavitamin therapy is rational and efficacious in certain genetic diseases associated with an inborn error of metabolism, in which the defect in vitamin utilization may be overcome by large doses of the vitamin. Occasionally, disorders occur that are associated with defective transport of vitamins across membranes. Megadose vitamins may be useful for treatment of toxic states produced by antivitamins—such as methotrexate, used in the treatment of malignancy; the antibacterial agent, trimethoprim; or the diuretic, triamterene. Megadoses of vitamin A have resulted in death, and death occurred in one person who had received 80 g of vitamin C intravenously (Herbert [36]).

There are no scientifically acceptable published data indicating that healthy, usually active individuals need vitamin supplementation, provided they eat a diet that includes grain, fruits, vegetables, meat, and milk products. It is not clear whether increased physical activity, including athletic performance, raises the demand for certain vitamins. Acceptable studies, for example, have not shown that vitamin C supplementation in excess of 200 mg/day is safe. In spite of these caveats, many athletes take megadoses of a variety of vitamins and, in particular, vitamin C. In this population, vitamin C ingestion of 15–20 g/day for many years has not, however, produced adverse effects, and the influence of such doses on athletic performance is purely anecdotal. Benefits from megadoses of vitamin E, also widely ingested by athletes, are anecdotally reported.

Vitamin C Usage

The effects of large doses of ascorbic acid (vitamin C) on a variety of functions of human and animal cells have been assessed. Enhanced neutrophil motility to endotoxin-activated autologous serum, a chemotactic stimulus, occurred in normal adults after the ingestion of 2 and 3 g of ascorbate daily, whereas lower doses had no effect. Other functions of neutrophils were unaltered by vitamin C. Serum immunoglobulins and mitogen-induced protein synthesis were totally unaltered by ascorbic acid. Thus, vitamin C stimulates some cellular but not humoral immune function in humans. This effect should be considered when assessing the value of supplementary vitamin C in the protection from certain infections (Anderson et al. [37]).

Physical stress may require additional vitamin C. In studies of black mine workers in South Africa, subclinical vitamin C deficiency was common despite adequate daily intake from dietary sources. To prevent this, the addition of approximately 250 mg per person per day was recommended by the National Research Institute for Nutritional Diseases (Visagie et al. [38]).

Recent reports indicate that vitamin C stimulates prostaglandin E_1 formation in human platelets. This occurs at physiologic concentrations of vitamin C. Prostaglandin E_1 is important in lymphocyte function and, therefore, plays an important role in immune responses. Moreover, prostaglandin E_1 is also important in collagen and ground substance, in the metabolism of cholesterol, in the regulation of insulin, and in the responsiveness of the human body to insulin. It may be that defective prostaglandin E_1 formation accounts for many features of scurvy or partial vitamin C deficiency and additionally explains many of the reputed therapeutic effects of vitamin C. These hypotheses are unproven, but if correct, vitamin C is of value only if adequate dihomogammalinolenic acid, the precursor of prostaglandin E_1, is available. The adequate precursor, in turn, depends upon the presence of enough essential fatty acids, pyridoxine and zinc (Horrobin et al. [39]).

Because metals are involved in the function of various vitamins, studies were done to assess the bio-availability of dietary iron, copper, and zinc, and how this might be affected by vitamin C megadoses. It is known, for example, that such megadoses enhance absorption of iron and inhibit dietary copper absorption. Since zinc is particularly important in the reputed therapeutic effects of megadoses of vitamin C, its bio-availability after ascorbic acid supplementation was also examined in humans, and no effect was found over a dose range of up to 2 g ascorbic acid per day (Solomons et al. [40]). Because many athletes consume a relatively high fiber diet, it was also suggested that this might interfere with absorption of trace metals. Lacto-ovo-vegetarian nonathlete adolescents were compared to omnivores with regard to zinc in hair and dietary fiber. A significant positive correlation between zinc and fiber intake in the omnivores was noted. No significant correlation was found in the vegetarians, but a slight inverse relationship between zinc in hair and dietary fiber was present. This was attributed to the chelation effect by dietary fiber of, perhaps, phytic acid on zinc in the vegetarians (Treuherz [41]).

NUTRITION AND NERVOUS SYSTEM FUNCTION

Numerous studies have shown that inadequate nutrition during development can cause permanent structural and chemical changes in the nervous system, which correlate with long-term alterations in intellectual and sensorimotor activities. It is also agreed that the effect of such malnutrition is not as easily reversed when it occurs early in development as during later growth. In spite of the necessity still to prove that early malnutrition results in later behavioral alterations, overwhelming evidence exists for the great vulnerability of the nervous system to dietary manipulations or malnutrition during the time when glial cell hyperplasia and neuronal migration are most active. On the other hand, during adolescence and adulthood, the effects of malnutrition on nervous system function are easily reversed by improved nutrition.

More recent findings, however, suggest that brain composition, neurotransmitters, interneuronal communication, and therefore, nervous system function are sensitive to quantity and quality of food throughout the organism's life span, irrespective of whether growth is occurring. All central and peripheral neurotransmitters are dietary components or are relatively simple metabolites of dietary constituents. Minor changes in nutrient quality and quantity can, not surprisingly, produce changes in brain neurotransmitters and in the physiologic and behavioral responses of the organism, which depend, to a large extent, on the levels of these neurochemicals. In laboratory animals, for example, changes in the available tyrosine, tryptophan, or choline effect the synthesis of dopamine, norepinephrine, serotonin, and acetylcholine in the central nervous system (Wurtman et al. [42]).

It has not been established whether nutritional manipulation during maturity or senescence alters brain function by either structural alterations or change in neurotransmitter storage, release, or inactivation comparable to that in immature animals. Nevertheless, elderly people are particularly prone to nutritional deficiency as a result of social factors, advancing chronic disease, or mental dysfunction. Even in those who have access to complete diets, nutritional deficiencies may develop because of medical or dental dysfunction, gastrointestinal diseases, or other causes, thus limiting nutrients to the brain for appropriate neurotransmitter synthesis and maintenance of neurons and glia.

Whether morphologic abnormalities found in human and animal brains with advancing years are the result of insidious malnutrition has not been established. It is possible that the decreasing functional capacity of the aged nervous might, in fact, be related to dietary abnormalities in some way still to be defined. The need exists to understand the relationships between aging, nutrition, nervous system structure, and the effect of physical activity on all three. Physical activity, however, has been shown to slow certain aging-associated processes of the human nervous system. Moreover, it is not known to what extent age-induced changes in brain structure, chemistry, and function directly alter nutritional status by influencing dietary habits and food utilization. Clearly, then, answers to these questions may provide understanding of the effects of nutrition on physical performance and, in turn, knowledge of how these interrelate with nervous-system aging and perhaps change its rate of progression. It should be remembered, however, that "no man can have a peaceful life who thinks too much about lengthening it" (Lucius Annaeus Seneca).

An accepted practice and one often suggested to those engaging in athletic activities is to indulge in the craving for certain foods if these develop. Recent evidence from animal studies suggests that such cravings may indicate nutritional requirements and may, in fact, result from changes in neuronal systems due to dietary-induced alterations in neurotransmitters.

Thus, although it has been recognized for years that extremes in dietary protein content and composition result in distortion of plasma amino acid patterns and depressed food consumption, it is now borne out in laboratory rats that shifts in plasma amino acids caused by normal food intake signal messages to the brain that control feeding behavior. These signals arise from amino acids that function as neurotransmitters or their precursors. Since it is known that at least two neuronal systems, one depending on 5-hydroxytryptamine and the other on catecholamines for neurotransmitters, are involved in the control of food intake, it is postulated that the neurotransmitters are influenced by the availability of their dietary amino acid precursors. The synthesis, for example, of 5-hydroxytryptamine and of the catecholamines is directly related to the level of precursors, tryptophan and tyrosine, respectively, in the brain. The brain uptake of these amino acids is exquisitely regulated by their plasma level. Therefore, changes in plasma amino acid patterns and availability influence serotonergic and catecholaminergic neurons to signal behavioral responses to food.

For example, if an animal selects among dietary options, it can change either the quantity or the quality of food consumed. Thus, evidence indicates that the quantity of food intake is influenced by shifts in plasma tyrosine in relation to other large neutral amino acids with a consequent alteration in brain tyrosine and catecholamine activity. On the other hand, changes in plasma tryptophan in relation to other large neutral amino acids alter brain tryptophan and 5-hydroxytryptamine, alter food preference, and regulate protein consumption. It is easy, therefore, to suggest (without scientific evidence) that the often reported cravings for certain foods during athletic activities or during changes in athletic performance and, perhaps, at other periods of life (pregnancy) are the result of changing levels of amino acids at least and possibly of other nutrients, and that they are best followed, in order to ensure adequate nutrition and energy balance for the task at hand (Anderson [43]).

Endogenous opiate-like substances have tentatively been linked with symptoms in some schizophrenic patients, and other anecdotal reports suggest that such patients may improve on gluten-free diet. Investigators at the National Institute of Mental Health looked at the possibility that peptic digestion of a variety of proteins, including wheat gluten, might produce opiate-like activity, and to their surprise, this was the case. These compounds are called exorphins, analogous to endorphins and the endogenously produced opiate-like materials. Isolation and sequencing of the peptides in hydrolysates of β-casein (a constituent of milk) with opioid properties show them to be slightly different from the endogenously produced enkephalins, including β-endorphin, and they have been called β-casomorphins. These substances, like the endogenously produced β-endorphin, produce a pain-free state (analgesia) after intracerebroventricular injections in animals, which is reversible by the opium antagonist, naloxone. It is not clear whether exorphins produce central nervous system effects after oral ingestion.

The instillation of digested gluten into the stomach of animals produces a rapid rise in postprandial peripheral insulin and glucagon, and simultaneous administration of naloxone intragastrically prevents increase in these blood hormones. This supports the view that the digested gluten test meal activates opiate receptors.

Other peptide-like substances have been isolated from foods. For example, a peptide with thyrotropin-releasing hormone (TRH) activity has been found in alfalfa; it differs from endogenous TRH, a prolactin releaser, by inhibiting prolactin release. TRH, distributed throughout the gastrointestinal tract, affects gastric acid and pancreatic secretions and gut mobility. Oat leaves contain a substance with activity similar to luteinizing hormone-releasing hormone. The biologic significance of the neuropeptides has not been determined.

While some evidence exists that these food hormones are absorbed unaltered and produce systematic effects, the present feeling is that they have a significant role locally. Clearly, their local effects on gut motility, absorption of energy-producing foods, and other gastrointestinal functions also influence mood and performance (Morley [44]).

DIETARY CONSTITUENTS AND DISEASE

The eating habits of athletes include vegetarianism, and the effect of this on dietary lipids is of great interest, particularly in view of the reputed effects of exercise upon atherosclerosis (reviewed in another chapter). In acute clinical studies in human volunteers, it was shown that onion and garlic supplementation prevents alimentary hyperlipemia and increases fibrinolytic activity, effects that would presumably decrease lipid deposition in vessel walls and reduce atherosclerosis. Moreover, evidence also indicates that garlic and onion have hypocholesterolemic activity. In experimental animals, garlic inhibits atherogenesis.

In a recent study from India, the effects of dietary use of onion and garlic upon serum cholesterol, triglycerides, lipoprotein, and phospholipids in members of the Jain community were investigated (Sainani and Desai [45]). These people, if strictly adhering to their religious tenets, abstain from garlic and onions. However, many members of Jain families consume either small or large quantities of onion and garlic and these, along with the abstainers, formed the three study groups whose serum lipid profiles were compared. All study participants were vegetarians and consumed fat and refined sugar approximately equally. It was clear, in this long-term epidemiologic review, that total abstention from garlic and onions throughout life was associated with significantly higher levels of serum cholesterol, triglycerides, β-lipoprotein, and phospholipids. Small intake of these vegetables reduced these substances in the blood, and inclusion of large quantities of onion and garlic in the diet reduced serum lipids even more. These findings, combined with vegetarianism, complicate the assessment of the value of exercise in preventing atherosclerosis and its influence on morbidity and mortality due to vascular disease (Sainani and Desai [45]).

Trace Elements

Dietary trace elements also probably influence cardiovascular disease. Geologic, geochemical, and soil maps were compared with epidemiologic maps to assess influence of "geochemistry on the incidence of cardiovascular disease" (Masironi [46]). Changes in the content or in the availability of trace elements in rocks or water may contribute to certain chronic diseases including atherosclerosis.

The geographic distribution of cardiovascular disease is associated with geochemical differences, a trend particularly evident in the United States and Europe, where mortality from cardiovascular disease is high. High mortality rates from cardiovascular disease correlate well with areas where the underlying soil is poor in essential trace elements.

This finding has been further confirmed by observing a relationship between the incidence of cardiovascular disease and the degree of mineralization of water supplies. Thus, in parts of the world served by soft water, there is usually a high rate of cardiovascular death compared to parts of the world served by hard water. This negative association between mineralization of water with cardiovascular death is not confined to highly industrialized countries but is also present in the developing world.

Thus, evaluation of the reputed beneficial effects of exercise upon cardiovascular disease are further complicated by dietary factors such as the ingestion of hard water, clearly beyond control or manipulative capacity but nevertheless important and, speculatively, even more so to those who ingest large quantities of dietary fiber that may chelate trace elements otherwise available from the water.

The "known" effects of biologic trace elements are a mixture of improbable fact and plausible nonsense. More than 99.9% of animal matter, which includes the human body, is made up of just 11 elements—hydrogen, oxygen, nitrogen, sodium, potassium, chlorine, sulphur, phosphorus, magnesium, calcium, and carbon. The remaining 0.01% of body mass is made up of a variety of elements encompassing about half of the periodic table. Of all these elements, only 10 have been accepted as more or less essential. They include zinc, iron, copper, iodine, cobalt, chromium, selenium, manganese, molybdenum, and fluorine. The function of these elements is very different. For example, zinc, iron, and copper are part of enzymes; cobalt is found in only one molecule; and iodine has only one function. Inessential elements, on the other hand, include many environmental hazards (cadmium, lead, and mercury), others are given in drug form (gold, aluminum, and bromine), and yet others are often used as poisons (antimony and arsenic). The rest of the many elements are thought to be contaminants (Dormandy [47]).

All trace elements have a capacity to excite scientists and laypersons. Even the Greeks, more than 2000 years ago, burned sea sponges as prophylaxis against goiter. They rightly believed the sponges might release a magic element in the smoke. More recently, in central China, a cardiomyopathy was traced to selenium deficiency. Against this background of ancient and modern searches for function of trace elements, the analysis of hair for its elemental components, often present only in the most minute amounts, has gained momentum. Many athletes, when their performance declines, often seek the help of numerous laboratories and, on the basis of the results, supplement their diets with a number of trace elements, some of them essential, others nonessential, and yet others that might be toxic. The many laboratories that offer a "trace element profile" based on hair analyses do not provide, as they say, a guide to the cure of ills that orthodox analytical methods have failed to diagnose. Moreover, the diagnoses reported by such laboratories, which range from lead poisoning to rubidium deficiency, may lead to anxiety and further specialist investigations that are mostly unwarranted. Most such victims of alleged deficiencies or intoxications do not realize, for example, that most trace elements, with the exception of zinc, are present in higher concentration in the hair of women than in that of men. Moreover, there are wide fluctuations depending on age—especially around puberty, pregnancy, and the menopause—and there are wide variations in long-term trends in elemental contents of the hair. Age variations in chromium content of the hair as well as cadmium and the concentration of zinc have been found, the latter being higher in black than in blonde hair, and other variables depending on hair color have also been found. To make matters even more complicated, hair from different regions of the scalp varies in trace element content, and scalp hair is also different from pubic and axillary hair. Some of these variations may be racial, others environmental, but they are difficult to separate. Many other complicating factors remain, but the question of whether hair analysis is ever worthwhile remains unanswered. While most of the time it is not justified, it cannot be dismissed entirely. During the devastating mercury poisoning epidemics in Iraq and Japan, it became clear that hair analysis was a simple and quick, practical and accurate method of measuring the body content of mercury. Hair analysis for the elucidation of frequently declining athletic performance, however, does not seem warranted.

Just like the feasibility of cardiac transplantation is no indication for its performance in the majority of patients with cardiac disease, so the availability of atomic emmission spectroscopy for hair analysis to laboratories is no justification for using the instruments in all athletes.

Environmental Effects

The environmental effects upon nutritional requirements are, of course, multiple and include the effects of altitude upon energy expenditure and intake. For example, it has been shown that body composition changes among sea-level residents when they are abruptly exposed to altitudes of 4000 m or so. It has been suggested that the observed loss in body weight at altitude is due to decreased body fat and reduced blood and plasma volumes, changes, however, that were mostly due to the redistribution of body water.

Body composition does change with acute altitude exposure, and not only fat but protein, water, and minerals are lost. However, when the body fat of natives of high altitude, approximately 4000 m, was compared with that of sea-level natives, no significant differences were observed. The effect of a 10-month sojourn at high altitude on body fat, measured by anthropometric techniques, showed that a significant decline occurred after exposure to 4000 m, but there was an increase in lean body weight, and the total change in body weight was very much smaller than that observed after acute exposure to altitude. Moreover, fluctuations in body fat at high altitudes during a prolonged sojourn might be influenced by the seasons of the year as well (Bharadwaj [48]). During abrupt altitude exposure, increased energy is required to perform standard amounts of work when compared to sea-level requirements. Thus, increased energy is necessary during acute high altitude exposure of about 4000 m, which might, perhaps, be due to the greater metabolic requirements for cardiac and respiratory function at altitude or perhaps to decreased efficiency of performance (Johnson et al. [49]).

Tissue hypoxia in exercising humans leads to increased free fatty-acid mobilization and utilization in spite of ongoing anaerobic metabolism. This has been tentatively ascribed to increased circulating catecholamines (Jones and Robertson [50]).

All these studies attributed the changes in body fat and metabolic alterations during exercise to altitude alone. However, in the field, altitude is almost always accompanied by cold, and the effects of cold have mostly been ignored in these studies. Moderately obese nonathletes fully clothed in arctic clothing exercised for $2\frac{1}{2}$ hr/day for a week in a climatic chamber where the ambient temperature was $-40°C$ and the air was still. Their total daily energy expenditure was about 13 MJ. Only a small energy deficit occurred when energy expenditure was compared to daily caloric intake, but cold exposure led to a significant reduction in skin-fold thickness and increased body density, measured by underwater weighing. The body fat loss during that week was estimated to be from 0.8 kg to 2.3 kg, and lean body mass increased approximately 1.5 kg. These observations were attributed to protein synthesis under cold conditions, ketosis associated with exercise, and a small energy deficit (O'Hara et al. [51]).

Athletes have not been studied under comparable conditions. Their low body fat could affect work in the cold considerably and change the magnitude of body fat loss, energy intake, and lean body mass from that seen in moderately obese, middle-aged nonathletic males. High-density lipoproteins reached 148 ± 29 mg/dl in whole blood in male mountaineers during a strenuous 8-week climb. This rise was attributed not only to the physical exertion and improvement in athletic fitness, but also to cold exposure, the hypoxia itself, and perhaps to mental stress. Other factors that affect high-density lipoproteins such as body weight, alcohol consumption, or cigarette smoking did not change significantly during the climb, though dietary changes were significant in that the caloric intake increased considerably and consisted mainly of carbohydrates, which tend to decrease high-density lipoproteins. The rapidity with which high-density lipoproteins rose under these conditions is extraordinary. Similar studies should be undertaken to see what the actual rate of change might be. During high altitude exertion, changes in blood constituents of even greater magnitude have been observed within several hours (Nestel et al. [52]) (see Chapter 18, Oxygen Transport During Exercise at Sea Level and High Altitude).

DIETARY PRINCIPLES

For optimum support of athletic performance, appropriate timing of food intake is essential. Clearly, large, infrequent meals cause discomfort during athletic performance and provide excessive calories. Meals before training or competition should be varied. The training diet should be the standard one for a particular sport and should not precede physical effort too closely.

Ideally, 4–6 hr should elapse between the last meal and the beginning of competition. A time lapse of several days exists between carbohydrate ingestion and muscle glycogen storage. The food mix is important. Free carbohydrates should be avoided before prolonged competition, since insulin release often leads to reactive hypoglycemia if physical activity is continued during the metabolism of sugar. The importance of fats in preparation for endurance competition has already been mentioned, and the value of vitamin supplements is not established. Most endurance athletes use megavitamin supplementation, but the effect upon their performance has not been documented.

The *Oxford English Dictionary* defines *brawn* as "pickled or potted boar's flesh." This is an apt description of the large, lean body mass that is attained by a diet that is predominantly proteins and fats and few carbohydrates.

Endurance events, on the other hand, require high caloric intake in the form of carbohydrates and fats and relatively little protein in proportion to the total calories consumed. The quantity of fiber in the diet is important when preparing for competition. For events lasting more than a few minutes, dietary fiber should not be taken, if possible, for a day or two to avoid gastrointestinal motility problems and defecation at inappropriate times.

CARBOHYDRATE LOADING

Muscle glycogen supercompensation by athletes in endurance events is traceable to a report claiming that this improved marathon running significantly. Not all world-class endurance athletes find carbohydrate loading useful. Proper carbohydrate loading requires that the muscles be receptive to glycogen storage, which is the case only during the first 10 hr after exhaustive exercise, and that muscles can sustain carbohydrate abstention, or total depletion of muscle glycogen. Moreover, the mean time to achieve maximum glycogen storage is approximately 3 days, with considerable individual variation.

The high carbohydrate intake, best ingested in the form of complex carbohydrates, must be preceded by an exhaustive workout, and followed by little or no exercise of the muscles to be used during competition. Moreover, the considerable changes in body weight—first the decrease associated with body water loss, and then the inordinate increase in body weight occasioned by water utilization in glycogen synthesis—make athletic performance sometimes difficult, particularly at the beginning of a long-distance race.

Investigations of substrate utilization during prolonged exercise preceded by the ingestion of glucose in glycogen-depleted and control subjects has shown that the principal substrate for energy in controls is carbohydrate, whereas in those who are glycogen depleted it is lipid (Ravussin et al. [53]). Clearly, therefore, for prolonged exertion, the glycogen depletion without repletion is preferable, since lipids are a better source of energy during long-distance races than carbohydrates. Moreover, in spite of glycogen depletion, these subjects did not utilize ingested glucose to a greater extent than did control subjects. This was probably due to their high free fatty-acid plasma levels, a factor that again suggests that the glucose intake during prolonged energy expenditure is not advantageous. Muscle glycogen use was not improved, and glucose ingestion may cause decreased water resorption from the gastrointestinal tract.

Thus, while it is well-established that during exercise the endogenous glycogen stores of muscles are an important source of energy, they are also the limiting factors in prolonged exertion. The alternate energy source from lipids is preferable if athletic performance is to continue beyond 1 hr. The assumption that the exogenously administered glucose during exercise improves its utilization in those who are glycogen depleted has not been proved, and the experience of many suggests that such glucose intake may, in fact, lead to hypo-glycemia during continued athletic performance and thus decrease the quality of and ability to prolong physical activity (Ravussin et al. [53]).

The views expressed by Mark Twain, that the only way to keep your health is to eat what you don't want, drink what you don't like, and do what you'd rather not, have no scientific foundation except that they point to an important principle that, taking into account the foregoing cautions, is still the leading nutritional doctrine to be advocated: Indulge moderately in what you like, partake of a great variety of foods, and keep your energy expenditure high.

REFERENCES

1. Wretlind, A. 1967. Nutrition problems in healthy adults with low activity and low caloric consumption. In: Blix, G. (ed): Nutrition and Physical Activity, Almquist and Wiksell, Uppsala.

2. Åstrand, P.O. 1979. Diet and exercise—How to secure an adequate intake of essential nutrients. Intern Med 1:23–26.

3. Brozek, J., Grande, F., et al. 1957. Changes in body weight and body dimensions in men performing work on a low calorie carbohydrate diet. J Appl Physiol 10:412–420.

4. Yang, M.-U., Van Itallie, T.B. 1976. Composition of weight lost during short term weight reduction: metabolic responses of obese subjects to starvation and low-calorie ketogenic and non-ketogenic diets. J Clin Invest 58:722–730.

5. Van Itallie, T.B., Yang, M.-U. 1977. Diet and weight loss. N Engl J Med 297:1158–1161.

6. Wurtman, R.J., Wurtman, J.J. 1986. Carbohydrate craving, obesity and brain serotonin. Appetite 7 (Suppl 99): 103.

7. Benedict, F.G. 1915. A study of prolonged fasting, Pub. 203. Carnegie Institute, Washington, D.C.

8. Owen, O.E., Felig, P., et al. 1969. Liver and kidney metabolism during prolonged starvation. J Clin Invest 48:574–576.

9. Garber, A.J., Menzel, P.H., et al. 1974. Hepatic ketogenesis and gluconeogenesis in humans. J Clin Invest 54:981–984.

10. Saudek, C.D., Felig, P. 1976. The metabolic events of starvation. Am J Med 60:117–126.

11. Stock, M.J., Morgan, N.G., et al. 1978. Effect of high altitude on dietary-induced thermogenesis at rest and during light exercise in man. J Appl Physiol 45:345–349.

12. Stock, M.J. 1980. Effects of fasting and refeeding on the metabolic response to a standard meal in man. Eur J Appl Physiol 43:35–40.

13. Davidson, M.H., Liebson, P.R. 1986. Marine lipids and atherosclerosis: a review. Cardiovasc Rev Rep 7:461–471.

14. McLaren, D.S. 1974. Dietary protein in medical practice. Practitioner 212:441–447.

15. Felig, P. 1975. Amino acid metabolism in man. Annu Rev Biochem 44:933–956.

16. Lemon, P.W.R., Mullin, F.P. 1980. Effect of initial muscle glycogen levels on protein catabolism during exercise. J Appl Physiol 48:624–629.

17. Refsum, H.E., Gjessing, L.R., et al. 1979. Changes in plasma amino acid distribution and urine amino acids excretion during prolonged heavy exercise. Scand J Clin Lab Invest 39:407–413.

18. Consolazio, C.F., Johnson, H.L. 1972. Dietary carbohydrate and work capacity. Am J Clin Nutr 25:85–87.

19. Marable, N.L., Hickson, J.F., Jr. 1979. Urinary nitrogen excretion as influenced by a muscle-building exercise program and protein intake variation. Nutr Rep Int 19:795–805.

20. Linn, R., Stuart, S.L. 1976. The Last Chance Diet. Lyle Stuart Inc, Secaucus, N.J.

21. Isner, J.J., Sours, H.E., et al. 1979. Sudden, unexpected death in avid dieters using the liquid-protein-modified-fast diet. Observations in 17 patients and the role of the prolonged QT interval. Circulation 60:1401–1412.

22. Mayer, J.R. 1968. Overweight: Causes, Cost and Control. Prentice-Hall Inc, Englewood Cliffs, N.J.

23. Maiman, L.A., Wang, V.L. 1979. Attitudes toward obesity and the obese among professionals. J Am Diet Assoc 47:331–335.

24. Balaa, M.A., Drossman, D.A. 1985. Anorexia nervosa and bulimia: the eating

disorders DM 31:1–52.

25. American College of Physicians Health and Public Policy Committee 1986. Eating disorders: anorexia nervosa and bulimia. Ann Int Med 105:790–794.

26. Fullerton, B.T., Getto, C.J., et al. 1985. Sugar opioids and binge eating. Brain Res Bull 14:673–680.

27. Gollnick, P.D. 1977. Free fatty acid turnover and the availability of substrates as a limiting factor in prolonged exercise. In: The Marathon, Physiological, Medical, Epidemiological and Psychological Studies. Ann NY Acad Sci 301:64–71.

28. Costill, D.L., Coyle, E. 1977. Effects of elevated plasma FFA and insulin on muscle glycogen usage during exercise. J Appl Physiol 43:695–699.

29. Appenzeller, O., Schade, D.S. 1979. Neurology of endurance training. III. Sympathetic activity during a marathon race. Neurology 29:540.

30. Robison, G.A., Butcher, R.W., et al. 1967. Adenyl cyclase as an adrenergic receptor. Ann NY Acad Sci 139:703–707.

31. Burns, T.W., Boyer, P.A., et al. 1979. The effect of fasting on the adrenergic receptor activity of human adipocytes. J Lab Clin Med 94:387–394.

32. Lithell, H., Orlander, J., et al. 1979. Changes in lipoprotein-lipase activity and lipid stores in human skeletal muscle with prolonged heavy exercise. Acta Physiol Scand 107:257–261.

33. Calkins, A. 1979. Observations on vegetarian dietary practice and social factors: the need for further research. J Am Diet Assoc 74:353–355.

34. Levin, B., Horwitz, D. 1979. Dietary fiber. Med Clin North Am 63:1043–1055.

35. How to evaluate medical information. 1978. Harvard Medical School Health Letters 3:6.

36. Herbert, V. 1979. Facts and fictions about megavitamin therapy. J Fla Med Assoc 66:475–481.

37. Anderson, R., Oosthuizen, R., et al. 1980. The effects of increasing weekly doses of ascorbate on certain cellular and humoral immune functions in normal volunteers. Am J Clin Nutr 33:71–76.

38. Visagie, M.E., DuPlessis, J.P., et al. 1975. Effect of vitamin C supplementation on black mineworkers. S Afr Med J 49:889–892.

39. Horrobin, D.F., Oka, M., et al. 1979. The regulation of prostaglandin E₁ formation: a candidate for one of the funda-mental mechanisms involved in the actions of vitamin C. Med Hypoth 5:849–858.

40. Solomons, N.W., Jacob, R.A., et al. 1979. Studies on the bioavailability of zinc in man. III. Effects of ascorbic acid on zinc absorption. Am J Clin Nutr 32:2495–2499.

41. Treuherz, J. 1980. Zinc and dietary fibre: observations on a group of vegetarian adolescents. J Hum Nutr 29:10A.

42. Wurtman, R.J., Cohen, E.L., et al. 1977. Control of brain neurotransmitter synthesis by precursor availability and food consumption. In: Usdin E., Hambur, D.A., Barchas J.D. (eds): Neuroregulators and Psychiatric Disorders. Oxford University Press, New York, pp. 103–121.

43. Anderson, G.H. 1979. Control of protein and energy intake. Role of plasma amino acids and brain neurotransmitters. Can J Physiol Pharmacol 57:1043–1057.

44. Morley, J.E. 1982. Food peptides. JAMA 247:2379–2380.

45. Sainani, G.S., Desai, D.B. 1979. Effect of dietary garlic and onion on serum lipid profile in Jain community. Indian J Med Res 69:776–780.

46. Masironi, R. 1979. Geochemistry and cardiovascular diseases. Philos Trans R Soc Lond [Biol] 288:193–203.

47. Dormandy, T.L. 1986. Trace element analysis of hair. Br Med J 293:975–976.

48. Bharadwaj, H. 1972. Effect of prolonged stay at high altitude on body fat content—an anthropometric evaluation. Human Biol 44:303–316.

49. Johnson, H.L., Consolazio, C.F., et al. 1971. Increased energy requirements of man after abrupt altitude exposure. Nutr Rep Int 4:77–82.

50. Jones, N.L., Robertson, D.G. 1971. Effects of hypoxia on fat metabolism in exercising humans. J Physiol [Lond] 222:30.

51. O'Hara, W.J., Allen, C., et al. 1979. Fat loss in the cold—a controlled study. J Appl Physiol 46:872–877.

52. Nestel, P.J., Podkolinski, M., et al. 1979. Marked increase in high density lipoproteins in mountaineers. Atherosclerosis 34:193–196.

53. Ravussin, E., Pahud, P., et al. 1979. Substrate utilization during prolonged exercise preceded by ingestion of ¹³C-glucose in glycogen depleted and control subjects. Pflügers Arch 382:197–202.

.6.

Sports and the Gastrointestinal Tract and Liver

Nicholas A. Volpicelli and Monroe H. Spector

Disorders of gastrointestinal and hepatic function may either adversely affect athletic performance or be precipitated by athletic activity and associated factors, such as diet and nutritional supplements. Moderate physical activity probably aids digestive function and prevents or treats certain digestive disturbances, such as peptic ulcer and constipation. On the other hand, excessive training and effort or attempts to increase strength and endurance with fad diets and hormones may lead to serious and life-threatening medical illnesses.

ABDOMINAL PAIN

Abdominal pain that occurs during strenuous physical activity, especially running, is referred to as a "stitch." This pain is transient and probably results from muscular spasm or trapped intestinal gas. Abdominal pain that persists after rest or that is chronic warrants medical investigation. It is particularly important to keep this in mind when evaluating athletes who participate in contact sports, since these individuals may have a ruptured spleen, liver, or pancreas and require immediate diagnosis and treatment. Chronic abdominal pain unrelated to trauma usually indicates an underlying disorder such as peptic ulcer and should be diagnosed and treated as in the nonathlete. Further considerations, especially in runners, include cecal trauma (Porter [1]) and cecal volvulus (Pruett et al. [2]) due to excessive motion of the cecum.

NAUSEA AND VOMITING

Nausea and vomiting in athletes may result from nervous tension. Strenuous exercise inhibits gastric emptying (Ramsbottom and Hunt [3]); Fordtran and Saltin [4]; Costill and Saltin [5]); food and liquids ingested shortly before and during an athletic event may therefore remain in the stomach and lead to nausea and vomiting. Nevertheless, it is often necessary to replace some of the fluids, electrolytes, and energy lost during long events. Dilute solutions of glucose or sodium chloride may be used for this, since these substances are depleted and absorbed during submaximal exercise (Fordtran and Saltin [4]; Costill and Saltin [5]). Glucose concentrations greater than 139 mM retard gastric emptying (Costill and Saltin [5]), as do amino acids or fats (Cooke [6]), and should therefore be avoided. Other factors that may contribute to decreased gastric motility during exercise include changes in intestinal blood supply, and the circulating levels of adrenal hormones, gastrointestinal hormones, prostaglandins, and endogenous opioids. Toxic metabolites acting on the vomiting center may cause nausea and vomiting. Finally, head trauma is a cause of nausea and vomiting and can be a sign of increased intracranial pressure, a potential medical and surgical emergency. The occurrence of migraine headache (with nausea and vomiting) in relation to competition is unusual. Forceful vomiting and retching can cause lacerations at the esophagogastric junction (Mallory-Weiss syndrome) and produce hematemesis and shock.

DIARRHEA

Acute or chronic diarrhea is not uncommon in athletes. Acute diarrhea is usually of bacterial or viral origin. In most instances, the illness is self-limited and therapy is not indicated except to replace fluid and electrolytes. Nevertheless, acute diarrhea should be avoided if possible since it decreases or prevents maximal physical performance. Special advice should be given to athletes travelling to countries where risk of exposure to diarrheal illness is high. The most common cause of acute infectious diarrheal illness contracted in foreign countries is enterotoxigenic E. coli (Gorbach et al. [7]), though shigella, samonella, amebiasis, and giardiasis are still prevalent. Hygiene is the mainstay of prevention; athletes travelling to underdeveloped countries should avoid ingesting local water in any form, including ice cubes and uncooked vegetables and fruits. Daily doxycycline prevents most toxigenic E. coli diarrheas and should be considered in those athletes at risk (Sack et al. [8]). This antibiotic does not prevent diarrhea in all travelers and, if overused, may lead to emergence of resistant organisms or untoward drug reactions (Merson [9]). Acute diarrhea in the "traveler" athlete may be relieved with bismuthsubsalicylate (Pepto-Bismol®), 30–60 ml every 30 min for eight doses (total 240–480 ml) (Du Pont et al. [10]). If this brings no relief, then fluids and electrolytes should be replaced. If gastrointestinal bleeding occurs or symptoms persist more than 24–48 hr, the stool should be cultured for enteric pathogens and examined for parasites so that appropriate drug therapy can be instituted. The urge to defecate and diarrhea are the most frequent gastrointestinal symptoms of long-distance runners (Fogoros [11]; Volpicelli et al. [12]; Keeffe et al. [13]), especially during increased or more severe training and strenuous races. This usually subsides as training levels off or decreases. The cause of diarrhea in long-distance runners is unknown, but contributing factors may include: 1) relative intestinal ischemia due to shunting of blood away from the intestine to the heart and skeletal muscle; 2) changes in gut motility; 3) changes in gastric and intestinal secretion and absorption; 4) mechanical jiggling of the colonic contents in the upright position (Sullivan [14]); and 5) increased calories and dietary fiber (Sullivan [14]). Modifications in gut motility, secretion, and absorption are at least in part hormonally mediated. Hypothetical candidates include prostaglandins (Demers et al. [15]) and motilin (Rennie et al. [16]), which accelerate gastrointestinal motility and also increase with marathon running. Endorphins are elevated in long-distance runners (Appenzeller et al. [17]), and increasing evidence indicates that these and related opioid compounds affect gastrointestinal motility, absorption, and secretion (Ambinder and Schuster [18]; McKay et al. [19]). Most long-distance runners with loose bowel movements take vitamin and iron supplements, which also may contribute to changes in bowel habits (Volpicelli et al. [12]). Though most diarrheas in athletes are acute and self-limited, chronic diarrhea may also occur. When it does, one should search for an underlying disorder such as ulcerative colitis, Crohn's disease, sprue, giardiasis, etc. A common but frequently unrecognized cause of bloating, chronic diarrhea, and abdominal pain is lactase deficiency. This hereditary abnormality is especially common in blacks, orientals, Jews, and those of southern Mediterranean origin. Avoidance of milk and milk products leads to cessation of symptoms. Likewise, caffeine, which has been recommended as an aid to athletic performance and endurance (Ivy et al. [20]), can cause diarrhea in some persons (Wald et al. [21]).

GASTROINTESTINAL BLEEDING

Gastrointestinal bleeding in the athlete may be due to hemorrhoids, peptic ulcer, inflammatory bowel disease, polyps, cancer, etc. The diagnosis and management is the same as in the nonathlete. Gastrointestinal bleeding in long-distance runners occurs during strenuous training or maximal effort and disappears when training declines or reaches a plateau (Fogoros [11]; Volpicelli et al. [12]). The authors have seen two long-distance runners with recurrent gastrointestinal bleeding presenting with melena. Neither was taking aspirin or other medications. In both instances, clotting parameters and radiologic and endoscopic studies of the upper and lower gastrointestinal tracts were normal. Bleeding ceased in each when training was reduced but recurred when effort was increased to maximal levels. In one patient, bleeding did not recur when the total distance run was increased more gradually. In addition to these two cases, of 20 long-distance runners (15 men, 5 women) participating in races of marathon or greater distances who were instructed to avoid all medications at least one week prior to the race, 4 (3 women, 1 man) had gastrointestinal blood loss (guaiac-positive stools) prior to and/or immediately after the race. Two of these (1 man, 1 woman) had a history of recurrent gastrointestinal hemorrhage that had been investigated medically with no source found. Further support for occult gastrointestinal bleeding has been reported from two independent studies showing that competitive long-distance running induces blood loss (McMahon et al. [22]; Stewart et al. [23]) measured by the Hemoccult® guaiac card and the newer and quantitative HemoQuant® methods.

The cause of gastrointestinal bleeding in long-distance runners is unknown. It may be related to intestinal ischemia or jarring of the bowel during long runs. Whether this occurs in other athletes is unknown. Gastrointestinal blood loss should not be attributed to strenuous exercise until appropriate studies are done to exclude the usual medical causes. Hemoglobin concentration may decline after strenuous conditioning, such as long-distance running (Bunch [24]) due to hemodilution from increased plasma volume, not from loss of red blood cells or iron. Therefore, a fall in hemoglobin concentration in the well-conditioned athlete should not be interpreted as evidence of gastrointestinal blood loss, unless there is blood in the stool or low serum iron.

HEPATITIS

Both hepatitis A (infectious) and hepatitis B may occur as a result of a close association with a "community" of athletes.

Hepatitis A

Hepatitis A is transmitted primarily by the fecal–oral route. Therefore, close personal contact with infected individuals or ingestion of contaminated water or food can lead to illness.

For example, an outbreak occurred in 1969 among members of the Holy Cross football team when they drank contaminated water (Morse et al. [25]); Chang and O'Brien [26]). Of 97 players, coaches, and trainers, 90 were thought to have evidence of acute hepatitis. Of these, 32 were icteric and 58 anicteric based on clinical grounds. Recently, the stored serum samples from this team were tested for IgM antibody to hepatitis A. It was found that only 32 icteric team members were positive (Friedman et al. [27]), indicating a much lower attack rate than previously assumed.

A more usual circumstance confronting athletes, trainers, and doctors is when one or more members of a team develops acute hepatitis A. In this instance, one must care for affected individual(s) and for the potentially exposed team members. Medical management of the athlete with acute hepatitis A is no different from that of other individuals. Since there is no specific treatment, care is supportive and should include a balanced diet and observation for increasing jaundice, encephalopathy, prolongation of the prothrombin time, and hypoglycemia, signs of hepatic failure. If the patient cannot eat or if hepatic failure develops, hospitalization is necessary. There is no evidence that bed rest enhances healing, and if the patient is able, moderate exercise has been recommended (Chalmers et al. [28]; Repsher and Freehorn [29]), though this recommendation is still controversial (Krikler and Zilberg [30]; Krikler [31]). Strenuous activity should be avoided during the acute stages. When liver function is normal again, the patient may return to full activity. Hepatitis A does not lead to chronic hepatitis, and infection appears to confer lifelong immunity. Individuals in close personal contact (roommates, household contacts, etc.) with hepatitis A patients should be passively immunized with immune globulin to prevent or decrease the severity of the acute illness. Passive immunization is not necessary unless all team members are in close personal contact. Furthermore, if a team has been exposed to a common source of infection, such as contaminated water, attempts to immunize after an index case is recognized would probably be too late. Stool viral concentrations in affected individuals are highest during the incubation period and begin to fall with the onset of clinical hepatitis (Rakela and Mosly [32]). Therefore, the risk of transmitting infection is less if close personal contact occurs after the onset of jaundice, and it is negligible once the patient recovers. Since most hepatitis A infections are subclinical (Szmuness et al. [33]), it is necessary to measure liver function in each member of a team to determine who is already afflicted. In those with abnormal liver function, the presence of IgM antibody to hepatitis A confirms acute infection (Decker et al. [34]). The presence of IgG antibody without IgM antibody indicates remote infection and immunity.

Hepatitis B

Hepatitis B is primarily transmitted by direct inoculation of infected blood or blood products into a susceptible host. In athletes, this is most likely to occur in contact sports in which open wounds are common. However, one of the largest reported outbreaks of hepatitis B occurred in Sweden among cross-country track-finders (Ringertz and Zetterberg [35]). In this noncontact sport, runners traverse a course along check points in the shortest possible time. Frequently, they sustain open leg wounds from contact with surrounding obstacles and plants. After much investigation, it was concluded that hepatitis B was probably transmitted after the race by runners using common bathing sites where infected blood from one individual came in contact with open wounds of others who were susceptible. Runners were subsequently required to wear protective clothing, including leg shields, and arrangements were made for more sanitary conditions. Following these measures, the outbreak, which lasted from 1958 to 1962, disappeared. Although similar outbreaks of hepatitis B associated with athletics have not been reported, it should be kept in mind that transmission from an open sore of one athlete to another should be avoided. Documentation of hepatitis B has been simplified by serologic tests sensitive and specific for hepatitis B surface antigen (HbsAg). Transmission of blood containing HbsAg into the blood stream of a previously uninfected individual, by whatever means, including cuts and abrasions, can lead to infection. In these instances, the recipient of infected blood should be passively immunized with hepatitis-specific immunoglobulin, since ordinary immunoglobulin may not contain enough hepatitis B antibodies to be protective. The treatment of acute hepatitis B is the same as that for hepatitis A. However, unlike hepatitis A, hepatitis B infection may occasionally become chronic and lead to cirrhosis. There is no effective treatment for chronic hepatitis B. In addition, a small proportion of infected individuals may become chronic carriers of the hepatitis B virus, without evidence of active liver disease. Therefore, those with acute hepatitis B should be followed medically until liver function is normal and HbsAg disappears from the serum to document full recovery. Further evidence for complete recovery is the demonstration of antibody to HbsAg in the serum of those previously infected. Whether to allow chronic carriers of hepatitis B to participate in sports where they might transmit infection to others remains an ethical problem. With the exception of the Swedish track-finders, major outbreaks of hepatitis B have not been reported in association with sports. Moreover, athletes might be infected with hepatitis B by close contact with nonathletes, sexual contacts, dental procedures, etc. It would be difficult to trace isolated cases to another "carrier" athlete. Until specific guidelines are established, the decision regarding athletic participation by a chronic carrier of hepatitis B virus must be individualized. For those athletes at high risk of exposure, an effective vaccine is now available.

Non-A, Non-B Hepatitis

Non-A, non-B hepatitis, presumably due to another virus or viruses, is now well described (Feinstone et al. [36]) and accounts for most cases of posttransfusion hepatitis. The clinical illness and potential for chronic hepatitis (Knodell et al. [37]) are similar to that of hepatitis B, though the incubation period is shorter. There are no reports as yet to link this infection to athletics, but the potential exists.

Liver Function Tests

Occasionally, the physician is confronted with a well-trained, otherwise healthy athlete who has "abnormal liver functions" including elevations in the bilirubin, serum glumatic-oxaloacetic transaminase (SGOT), and alkaline phosphatase. These abnormalities are particularly common in long-distance runners (Bunch [24]), but can occur in other athletes. Liver disease can be excluded if creatine phosphokinase (CPK) is also elevated and the serum gammaglutamlyl transpeptidase (GGPT), glutamic-pyruvate transaminase (SGPT), albumin, and total protein are normal (Bunch [24]). the use of androgenic–anabolic steroids to increase strength and endurance is another potentially serious cause of abnormal liver function in athletes and has been associated with peliosis hepatis (dilated blood-filled cystic spaces within the liver) and hepatocellular carcinoma (Johnson [38]). The use of steroids is therefore undesirable. For the many other causes of abnormal liver function, athlete cases should be evaluated and treated like nonathlete cases.

Chronic Hepatitis and Cirrhosis

There is no evidence that strenuous exercise aggravates chronic liver disease or cirrhosis. Patients usually avoid physical exertion, depending upon the severity and activity of the liver disease. Cirrhosis may be associated with pulmonary arteriovenous shunts (Bashour and Cochran [39]), leading to decreased arterial oxygen saturation. A decrease in available oxygen not only adversely affects athletic performance, but also may result in anoxia to vital organs during strenuous exercise.

EXERCISE AND GASTROINTESTINAL HEALTH

It has been shown epidemiologically that physical exercise reduces the risk of subsequent peptic ulcer (Paffenbarger et al. [40]). Though this might be explained by decreased alcohol and nicotine consumption in athletes, it is noteworthy that submaximal exercise reduces gastric acid secretion in normals (Ramsbottom and Hunt [3]) but not in those with established duodenal ulcers (Markiewiczk et al. [41]). This effect of exercise on peptic ulcer may be mediated humorally, since experimental ulcers in rats are inhibited by administration of sera from well-trained athletes (Frankl et al. [42]; Frankl [43]). Gastric carcinoma, on the other hand, may be increased in individuals engaging in greater amounts of physical activity, because they eat more and are consequently exposed to more potential gastric carcinogens (Stukonis and Doll [44]). Constipation is common in bedridden and hospitalized patients and disappears when they resume normal activity. As noted previously, many long-distance runners have loose and more frequent bowel movements during strenuous training. Therefore, chronic constipation in otherwise healthy individuals might respond to treatment with exercise such as jogging, eliminating the need for cathartics. There is experimental evidence that regular exercise decreases the lithogenicity of bile in humans and animals (Simko [45]) and thus possibly decreases the incidence of cholesterol gallstones.

CONCLUSION

Much needs to be learned regarding the effects of exercise and physical conditioning on gastrointestinal and hepatic function. Although gastrointestinal illness adversely affects athletic performance, it is unknown whether certain inborn or acquired characteristics of gastrointestinal and hepatic function actually enhance athletic performance. It is commonly assumed that regular exercise improves gastrointestinal and hepatic function and eventually will be utilized to prevent and treat some functional disorders in these areas.

REFERENCES

1. Porter, A.M.W. 1982. Marathon running and the caecal slap syndrome. Br J Sports Med 16:178.
2. Pruett, T.L., Wilkins, M.E., et al. 1985. Cecal volvulus: a different twist for the serious runner. N Engl J Med 312:1262.
3. Ramsbottom, N., Hunt, J.N. 1974. Effect of exercise on gastric emptying. Digestion 10:1–8.
4. Fordtran, J.S., Saltin, B. 1967. Gastric emptying and intestinal absorption during prolonged severe exercise. J Appl Physiol 23:331–335.
5. Costill, D.L., Saltin, B. 1974. Factors limiting gastric emptying during rest and exercise. J Appl Physiol 37:679–683.
6. Cooke, A.R. 1975. Control of gastric emptying and motility. Gastroenterology 68:804–816.
7. Gorbach, S.K., Kean, B.H., et al. 1975. Travelers' diarrhea and toxigenic Escherichia coli. N Engl J Med 292:933–936.
8. Sack, R.B., Froehlich, J.L., et al. 1979. Prophylactic doxycycline for travelers' diarrhea. Gastroenterology 76:1368–1373.
9. Merson, M.H. 1979. Doxycycline and the traveler. Gastroenterology 76:1485–1488.
10. Du Pont, H.L., Sullivan, P., et al. 1977. Symptomatic treatment of diarrhea with

bismuth subsalicylate among students attending a Mexican university. Gastroenterology 73:715–718.

11. Fogoros, R.N. 1980. "Runners' trots." Gastrointestinal disturbances in runners. JAMA 243:1743–1744.

12. Volpicelli, N.A., Levin, A., et al. Unpublished data.

13. Keeffe, E.B., Lowe, D.K., et al. 1984. Gastrointestinal symptoms of marathon runners. West J Med 141:481–484.

14. Sullivan, S.N. 1984. The effect of running on the gastrointestinal tract. J Clin Gastroenterol 6:461–465.

15. Demers, L.M., Harrison, T.S., et al. 1981. Effect of prolonged exercise on plasma prostaglandin levels. Prostagland Med 6:413–418.

16. Rennie, J.A., Christofides, N.D., et al. 1979. Stimulation of human colonic activity by motilin. Gut 20:A912.

17. Appenzeller, O., Standefer, J., et al. 1980. Neurology of endurance training. V. Endorphins. Neurology 30:418–419.

18. Ambinder, R.F., Schuster, M.M. 1979. Endorphins: new gut peptides with a familiar face. Gastroenterology 77:1132–1140.

19. McKay, J.A., Linaker, B.D., et al. 1981. Influence of opiates on ion transport across rabbit ileal mucosa. Gastroenterology 80:279–284.

20. Ivy, J.L., Costil, D.L., et al. 1979. Influence of caffeine and carbohydrate feedings on endurance performance. Med Sci Sports 11:6–11.

21. Wald, A., Back, C., et al. 1976. Effect of caffeine on the human small intestine. Gastroenterology 71:738–742.

22. McMahon, L.F., Ryan, M.J., et al. 1984. Occult gastrointestinal blood loss in marathon runners. Ann Intern Med 100:846–847.

23. Stewart, J.G., Ahlquist, D.A., et al. 1984. Gastrointestinal blood loss and anemia in runners. Ann Intern Ned 100:843–845.

24. Bunch, T.W., 1980. Blood test abnormalities in runners. Mayo Clin Proc 55:113–117.

25. Morse, L.J., Bryan, J.A., et al. 1970. Holy Cross football team hepatitis outbreak. Antimicrob Agents Chemother 10:30–32.

26. Chang, L.W., O'Brien, T.F. 1970. Australian antigen serology in the Holy Cross football team hepatitis outbreak. Lancet 2:59–61.

27. Friedman, L.S., O'Brien, T.F., et al. 1985. Revisiting the Holy Cross football team hepatitis outbreak (1969) by serological analysis. JAMA 254:774–776.

28. Chalmers, T.C., Eckardt, R.K., et al. 1955. The treatment of acute infectious hepatitis: controlled studies of the effects of diet, rest, and physical reconditioning on the acute course of the disease and on the incidence of relapses and residual abnormalities. J Clin Invest 34:1163–1235.

29. Repsher, L.H., Freehorn, R.K. 1969. Effects of early and vigorous exercise on recovery from infectious hepatitis. N Engl J Med 281:1393–1396.

30. Krikler, D.M., Zilberg, B. 1966. Activity and hepatitis. Lancet 2:1046–1047.

31. Krikler, D.M. 1971. Hepatitis and activity. Postgrad Med J 47:490–492.

32. Rakela, J., Mosly, W.J. 1977. Fecal excretion of hepatitis A virus in humans. J Infect Dis 135:933–938.

33. Szmuness, W., Dienstag, J.L., et al. 1976. Distribution of antibody to hepatitis A in urban adults. N Engl J Med 295:755–759.

34. Decker, R.H., Overby, L.R., et al. 1979. Serologic studies of transmission of hepatitis A in humans. J Infect Dis 139:74–82.

35. Ringertz, O., Zetterberg, B. 1967. Serum hepatitis among Swedish track finders. N Engl J Med 276:540–546.

36. Feinstone, S.M., Kapikian, A.Z., et al. 1975. Transfusion-associated hepatitis not due to viral hepatitis type A or B. N Engl J Med 292:767–770.

37. Knodell, R.G., Conrad, M.E., et al. 1977. Development of chronic liver disease after acute non-A, non-B post-transfusion hepatitis: role of gamma globulin prophylaxis in its prevention. Gastroenterology 72:902–909.

38. Johnson, F.L. 1975. The association of oral androgenic–anabolic steroids and life-threatening disease. Med Sci Sports 7:284–286.

39. Bashour, F.A., Cochran, P. 1966. Alveolar-arterial oxygen tension gradients in cirrhosis of the liver. Am Heart J 71(6):734–740.

40. Paffenbarger, R.S., Wing, A.L., et al. 1974. Chronic disease in former college students. XIII. Early precursors of peptic ulcer. Am J Epidemiol 100:307–315.

41. Markiewiczk, M., Cholwea, M., et al. 1975. Gastric basal secretion during exercise and restitution in patients with chronic duodenal ulcer. Acta Hepato-Gastroenterol 26:160–165.

42. Frankl, R., Csalay, L., et al. 1969. Antiulcerogenic effect of blood sera from hu-

man subjects and from albino rats adapted to physical exercise and from inactive controls. Acta Med Acad Sci Hung 26(1):41–46.

43. Frankl, R. 1971. Humoral mechanism of ulcer-resistance of the organism adapted to physical exercise. Acta Med Acad Sci Hung 28(1):69–73.

44. Stukonis, M., Doll, R., 1969. Gastric cancer in man and physical activity at work. Int J Cancer 4:248–254.

45. Simko, V. 1978. Physical exercise and the prevention of atherosclerosis and cholesterol gall stones. Postgrad Med J 54:270–277.

.7.

Fuel Metabolism in the Long-Distance Runner

Neil Kaminsky

The principles of fuel metabolism in the marathoner are poorly understood by laypersons and blatantly oversimplified by self-styled "experts" who lack knowledge of intermediary metabolism. Such "experts" have substituted hearsay and anecdotal information for reason and scientific evidence in approaching the subject, often giving absurd nutritional recommendations. Unfortunately, many runners unquestioningly follow such recommendations without first ensuring their validity.

There has been a great deal of investigation into fuel metabolism, many studies comparing normal with diabetic individuals, and a number of reliable laboratories have conducted scientific studies on energy utilization in the long-distance runner. Many of these are assembled in a "marathon issue" published by the New York Academy of Science (Milvy [1]). Other comprehensive summaries have been completed by Newsholme [2], Essen [3], Ahlborg et al. [4], Scheele et al. [5], Locksley [6], and Sherman and Costill [7].

In this chapter substrate metabolism in the long-distance runner is examined and a basis given for individuals to assess their nutritional needs. Nutritional recommendations, based on what is scientifically known, are also included.

FUEL UTILIZATION AND STORAGE

To begin, one must compare substrate utilization and hormone fluxes in the fasting versus the fed state (Cahill [8]; Randel et al. [9]). It soon becomes clear that running a marathon is a telescopic representation of a prolonged fast.

Fed and Fasted States

Several processes are at work in the fed and fasted states (see Fig. 7-1). As a meal is ingested, gut hormones are liberated that, in effect, tell the pancreas a meal is coming. As glucose begins to rise in the blood, the storage hormone insulin is released from the pancreatic beta cell. Glucose is absorbed by the liver, muscle, brain, and other organs, and any excess glucose not needed for immediate energy is stored in the liver and muscle as glycogen. Once glycogen stores in the muscle and liver have been saturated, further excess

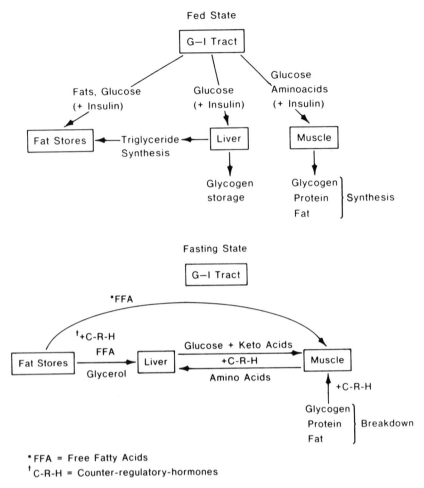

7-1 The fed and fasting states.

glucose is converted to fat in the liver. This fat is transported through the blood to fat depots, where it is stored as triglycerides. Fats that are ingested are likewise deposited in fat storage depots under the influence of insulin. Amino acids—breakdown products of protein formed in the gastrointestinal tract—are stored in muscle as protein, an action also enhanced by insulin. As with glycogen, muscle stores of protein also become saturated, and any protein taken in above the amount that muscle can accommodate loses "amino groups" and is stored as fat. (So much, then, for the "training table" and the high-protein diet to put on more muscle mass.)

Insulin, therefore, is the storage hormone that in response to an ingested meal facilitates the storage of 1) carbohydrates as glycogen and fat, 2) fat in fatty depots, and 3) amino acids as proteins in muscle and other tissue. Some of the ingested glucose, also affected by the action of insulin, is used for immediate energy needs. On the other hand, the counter-regulatory hormones—glucagon from the pancreas, epinephrine, growth hormone, and corticotrophin-cortisol—are suppressed with the balanced meal or high-carbohydrate meal.

Fuel Mobilization

After fasting, the reverse of the fed state occurs as the body demands to be supplied with energy sources for metabolism (Fig. 7-1). Since fuel stores must be broken down, the storage hormone, insulin, falls to low levels; the counterregulatory hormones rise and (with the decrease in insulin) the following sequence occurs: 1) glycogenolysis (breakdown of stored glycogen) initially, 2) gluconeogenesis (the making of new glucose), and 3) lipolysis (breakdown of stored fat). Fat, stored as triglycerides, yields fatty acids and glycerol. Thus, basic fuels for metabolism are provided in the fasted state. Specifically, glycogen breaks down in muscle and the liver to form glucose. Glucose from the liver is liberated into the blood stream, where it is taken up by other tissues and oxidized to CO_2 and water. During oxidation, high-energy phosphate bonds (e.g., adenosine triphosphate [ATP]) for metabolism are formed (e.g., brain function, muscle contraction, etc.) (Fig. 7-2). The glucose derived from muscle glycogen acts locally in the muscle and does not enter the blood stream because of the absence of a certain enzyme (glucose 6-phosphatase) in muscle. However, lactate derived from muscle and other tissues together with special amino acids from muscle stores enter the liver and are transformed into new glucose.

Fat is the largest potential source of energy. It breaks down into glycerol and free fatty acids. Glycerol is then converted to glucose, and fatty acids have several possible metabolic pathways. They can be taken up and metabolized directly by muscle, or they can travel to the liver where they are broken down and excreted back into the blood as ketoacids. These ketoacids can be directly used by muscle and brain as energy sources.

Therefore, going from the fed to the fasted state is a hormonal shift that allows for fuel storage in times of plenty and fuel mobilization in times of fasting. This metabolic shift is a finely tuned automatic continuum.

The hormonal profile and the metabolic events that occur in fasting are generally the same as those in a marathon run. However, in a marathon, the events in fasting are "telescoped" into 2–4 hr of maximum effort. There is no mystery to the fuel shifts, but considerable mystique surrounds attempts to improve the stores and the efficiency of their utilization.

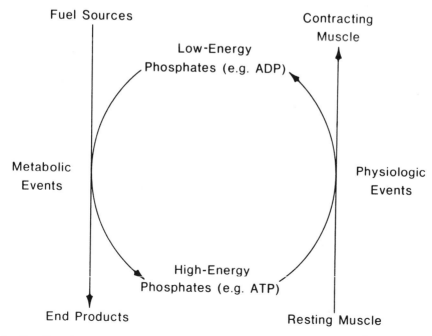

7-2 Coupling of energy production with utilization. High-energy phosphates are produced from fuel sources. Physiologic events, such as muscle contraction, use high-energy phosphates.

FUEL METABOLISM IN EXERCISE

Use of Glycogen and Fat

In aerobic exercise, the production of high-energy phosphate bonds is able to keep pace with the utilization of these bonds by exercising the muscle (Fig. 7-2). Anaerobic metabolism occurs at the point where high-energy phosphates are used in excess of those produced (this is in excess of 100% $\dot{V}_{O_2 \, max}$) (Newsholme [2]).

Carbohydrate is the preferred fuel source (Essen [3]). The simple explanation is that carbohydrate is totally combustible—there is an oxygen atom for every carbon atom. Regrettably, total body carbohydrate store is only about 200 g, two-thirds of which is in muscle. Muscle glycogen depletion occurs at about 20–25 miles and has been proposed as one of the causes of what is euphemistically called "hitting the wall" (Locksley [6]).

Why doesn't the body just switch to fat metabolism? Part (or maybe all) of the answer is that carbohydrate is a more combustible fuel, even though fat gives more energy per unit weight than does carbohydrate. Fatty acids are also metabolized at a slower rate, by oxidation to 2 carbon fragments followed by oxidation of these fragments to CO_2 and water, an energy-producing process. In contrast, glucose produces energy as it is broken down to 2 carbon fragments. It is known that resting muscle in the fasting state uses principally fat. But let that muscle work at 70–80% $\dot{V}_{O_2 \, max}$, and carbohydrate becomes the obligate fuel source until it runs out. Presumably, when the carbohydrate stores are depleted, fat cannot maintain the previous fast pace (Fig. 7-3).

Some excellent studies have been done by Newsholme [2], Essen [3], and Essen et al. [10] that map fuel utilization at different levels of effort. Returning to the starvation analogy, nonexercising muscle uses principally fat (Randel et al. [9]). Even at levels of intensity up to 60 $\dot{V}_{O_2 \, max}$, lipids are the most important substrate for exercising muscle. The analogy doesn't apply at higher levels of effort, as glycogen becomes the preferred substrate; the reason, in all likelihood, is the combustible nature of carbohydrate, but the exact mechanism for the shift to carbohydrate is unclear.

Carbohydrate Loading

A great deal of effort has been expended to try to increase carbohydrate stores in muscle. J. Bergstrom and E. Hultman devised experiments correlating increased muscle glycogen stores and improved performance, thus providing the rationale for carbohydrate loading (Bergstrom et al. [11]; Karlsson and Saltin [12]; Bergstrom and Hultman [13]). Using a bicycle ergometer on one leg and using the other nonexercising leg as the control, subjects rode the bicycle until the glycogen was depleted in the experimental leg muscle. After the subjects were refed carbohydrate-rich, carbohydrate-poor, or mixed diets, both muscles were rebiopsied and the experimental leg was reexercised. The experimenters were able to show that the carbohydrate-rich diet both increased the muscle glycogen stores and improved physical performance (Fig. 7-4). In applying the carbohydrate loading concept to distance running, Karlsson and Saltin [12] studied 10 athletes who ran two 30-km races separated by 3 weeks. Before each race they ate a mixed diet or followed a carbohydrate-loading protocol consisting of a glycogen-depleting run, then 2 days of carbohydrate-poor feeding followed by a high-carbohydrate diet for 3 days. The runners' leg muscles were biopsied before and after each run. The runners were found to have a higher muscle glycogen content and a better performance on the carbohydrate-loading protocol than on a simple mixed diet without carbohydrate loading. Thus, there is experimental evidence suggesting that carbohydrate loading improves performance, that is, the duration of high performance, but not the speed.

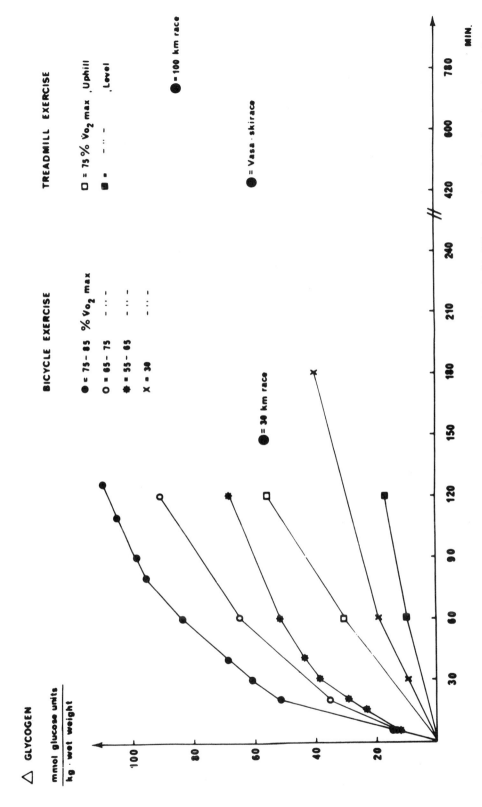

7-3 Glycogen utilization in the quadriceps femoris (vastus lateralis) at different work intensities and with different modes and duration of exercises. Values taken from References 3, 4, 5, 6, 8, 9, 11, 18, and 26. (From Essen, B. 1977. Intramuscular substrate utilization during prolonged exercise. Ann NY Acad Sci 301:30–44. Reprinted with permission.)

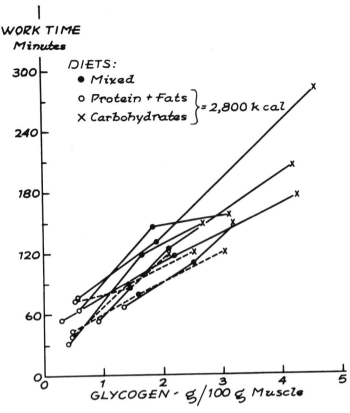

7-4 Effect of carbohydrate meals and duration of exercise—the carbohydrate loading effect. (From Bergstrom, J., Hermansen, et al. 1967. Diet, muscle glycogen and physical performance. Acta Physiol Scand 71:140–150. Reprinted with permission.)

The "Glycogen Burst"

The biggest drain on glycogen stores occurs at the beginning of a marathon run (Essen et al. [10]), when approximately 20% of the available glycogen is used in the first 5 min. Energy requirements are, obviously, instantaneous. Since glucose uptake early on is limited, the energy needs are supplied by glycogen breakdown. To utilize fat early and preserve glycogen, some investigators have recommended increasing triglycerides and fatty acids before a marathon. Since blocking fatty acid mobilization with nicotinic acid has been shown to accelerate glycogen utilization, it is assumed that the converse may be true, that increasing fatty acid availability will spare glycogen. In fact, Newsholme [2] has shown that fatty acids slow glycolysis at several points in the breakdown of glycogen. Further, Costill et al. [14] have demonstrated a significant decrease in glycogen utilization during a 70% $\dot{V}O_{2\ max}$ 30-min treadmill run when subjects were given heparin immediately after a fatty meal. The heparin activates lipoprotein lipase and thereby increases fatty acids. Elevating free fatty acids may well be a reasonable suggestion for runners who begin their race relatively slowly with a $\dot{V}O_{2\ max}$ below 70–80%, but is questionable at higher levels of effort.

The body's requirement for high-energy phosphates is the final determinant of the fuel source, which is a function of the race's pace. The contractile process using ATP is coupled to the generation of ATP (Fig. 7-2). Given a continuum of preferred substrates (fatty acids to glycogen), if fatty acids are elevated at the beginning of effort, more fat will be utilized at the lower level of effort (where less ATP is needed), and perhaps less glycogen will be used at a higher level of effort. The elite marathoner would be using glycogen early since he or she has a greater demand for high-energy phosphates.

Lipolysis

In any event, fats break down either from fat depots or from fat stores in muscle itself (visually, "marbled" beef). Jones et al. [15] investigated fat utilization in light (35% $\dot{V}O_{2\ max}$) versus heavy (70% $\dot{V}O_{2\ max}$) exercise by having subjects pedal for 40 min on a bicycle ergometer. Using plasma turnover rates of several fatty acids, it was found that light exercise was accompanied by mobilization of fat from peripheral adipose tissue stores. In heavy work, triglycerides within muscle broke down and the fatty acids were used directly by muscle. Glycerol, the other component of stored fat, was not used directly by muscle during heavy work and escaped into the blood stream to be taken up by the liver for gluconeogenesis.

In both muscle and liver, fatty acids are broken down to acetate, which is used directly for energy production. Much of the liver acetate is converted to ketoacids, which are then liberated into the blood stream and taken up by muscle, brain, and other tissues. Ketoacids function as a substrate for ATP synthesis. Fatty acids, therefore, whether liberated from perhipheral stores, from muscle itself, or from a combination of both, contribute to ATP synthesis in two ways: either directly through the metabolism of acetate or indirectly through the oxidation of ketoacids (Hagenfeldt [16]).

Gluconeogenesis

So far, the discussion of metabolism has centered on fuel stored as glycogen and fat. The third major fuel source comes through the provision of new glucose from protein and from breakdown products of glycogen and glucose metabolism itself. The reader is referred to a recent outstanding review of amino acid metabolism in exercise by Lemon and Nagle [17].

With the onset of effort, glucose uptake by exercising muscle begins along with the other hormonally induced metabolic events mentioned previously. Maximum gluconeogenesis rose many times above basal levels and provided roughly one-third of the fuel for ATP synthesis in Wahren's experimental model (Wahren [18]). More reliance is placed upon improved fat metabolism in conditioned runners, so glucose use is less (Fig. 7-5). The beginning substances for new glucose formation are lactate and pyruvate from muscle glycogen breakdown, the amino acid alanine from muscle, and glycerol from fat breakdown. The most important of these substrates for new glucose is lactate through the Cori cycle. By a reversal of the anaerobic glycolytic pathway, lactate and pyruvate are converted to glucose through an energy-using process (Ahlborg and Felig [19]).

It is interesting to find that lactate levels do not fall despite muscle glycogen depletion in the legs. The continued source of lactate for gluconeogenesis are the "nonexercising" muscles, such as those in the arms (Ahlborg and Felig [19]). In fact, the highest lactate levels are recorded during the recovery phase as the body immediately begins to replace leg muscle glycogen through gluconeogenesis. At variance, Koivisto et al. were not able to demonstrate arm muscle glycogen depletion during endurance exercise to explain the high lactate levels [20].

The glucose-alanine cycle is represented in Fig. 7-6. Certain amino acids, probably coming from muscle, provide an amino group that combines with pyruvate in muscle to form alanine. Alanine travels through the blood to the liver where the amino group is shaved off, forming pyruvate again. Pyruvate is then converted to glucose, which enters the circulation for muscle, brain, and other tissue uptake.

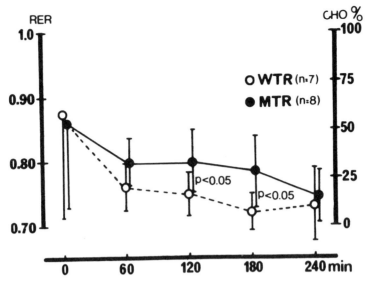

7-5   Respiratory exchange ratio (RER) and relative contribution of carbohydrates (CHO %) to the total energy production in well-trained (WTR) and moderately trained (MTR) groups of healthy men during a 4-hr bicycle ergometry exercise. (From Rahkila, P., Soimajarvia, J., et al. 1980. Lipid metabolism during exercise II—ratio and muscle glycogen content during four hour bicycle ergometry in two groups of healthy men. Eur J Appl Physiol 44:245–254. Reprinted with permission.)

Gluconeogenesis, therefore, provides a significant amount of carbohydrate as fuel for exercising muscle. Since training increases fat usage, less reliance is placed on gluconeogenesis.

Summary

The stages of fuel utilization in endurance exercise are summarized schematically in Fig. 7-7. Muscle glycogen is used as the preferred early fuel (Stage 1). With fat breakdown and gluconeogenesis from glycerol, alanine, and lactate, there is increased fatty acid and

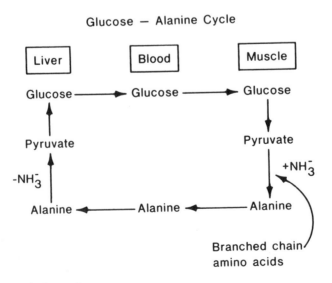

7-6   Glucose-alanine cycle.

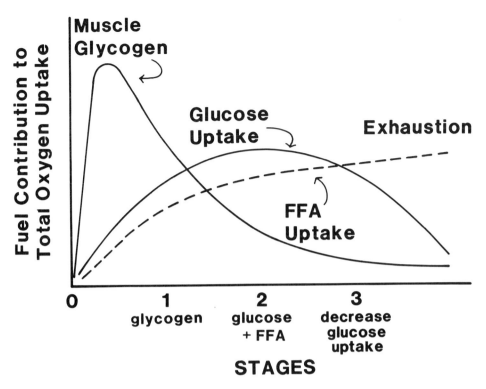

7-7 Stages of fuel utilization during endurance exercise.

glucose uptake, respectively, by exercising muscle (Stage 2). Then, gluconeogenesis falls off, and unless exogenous carbohydrate is provided, glucose uptake declines, leaving fat as the principal energy source (Stage 3). Exhaustion occurs, as fats alone cannot sustain high performance.

EFFECTS OF TRAINING

The preceding section outlines the fuel sources that allow the marathoner to couple high-energy phosphate production to the ultimate goal of muscular contraction. Stored glycogen, lipids, and protein are converted to fuel substrates under hormonal influence. The following brief discussion of the effects of training on substrate metabolism is designed to show that training works—but then, anyone who has put on running shoes and kept them on knows this.

Holloszy et al. [21], Holloszy and Coyle [22], and Costill et al. [23] have investigated training effects in detail. In addition to the salutory changes in heart function and the efficiency of skeletal muscular cellular respiration, training improves glycogen utilization and efficiency of fat use, thereby, in turn, sparing glycogen. Exactly which enzymes are involved in this adaptive and presumably inductive process is largely unknown, but there has been progress in their identification. For example, lipoprotein lipase activity has been known to be significantly higher in both male and female runners than in controls (Nikkila et al. [24]). Furthermore, insulin secretion is less in conditioned athletes than in age- and weight-matched controls (Lohman et al. [25]; Seals et al. [26]), presumably because of enhanced insulin binding to receptors (Heath et al. [27]) as well as postreceptor effects.

Rahkila et al. [28] studied carbohydrate utilization in well-trained versus moderately trained subjects at the same level of effort. The well-trained group used approximately 11% less carbohydrate over the study period (Fig. 7-5).

The inference is that this efficiency is due to improved metabolism of fats and is in accord with previous suggestions that training induces certain lipid-related enzymes to higher efficiency. Training is carbohydrate sparing. Because of this, as well as other metabolic alterations, training does improve performance. Hagen et al. [29] have found that marathon performance improves with low body mass, daily workouts, and training runs of long duration and distance.

One of the most exciting adaptations to training has been suggested by Newsholme [30, 31]. This is the concept of substrate cycles, and it gives some rationale for interval training. By way of analogy, substrate cycling is like racing an engine with the clutch depressed followed by a forward flux through a metabolic pathway as soon as the clutch is released. Newsholme predicts that interval training particularly will "improve the response to hormones of the metabolic systems involved in the control of fuel mobilization" [30, p. 194] and therefore enhance performance.

NUTRITIONAL RECOMMENDATIONS

There is no substitute for training in regard to ultimate performance. All the vitamins, carbohydrates, minerals, lack of red meat, and so on will not matter if the mileage has not been logged. The question therefore is: If the training has been optimal, can nutrition influence performance?

Ideal Body Weight and Maintenance of Glycogen Stores

The first objective of the athlete in training is to project and strive for an ideal body weight. Determining ideal body weight cannot be done by weight–height charts, since they are approximations. The individual runner can look in a mirror and decide if he or she needs to lose weight and generally how much. If one wishes to be more scientific, body fat measurements can be obtained through a physiology laboratory. Generally, female runners should have a body fat composition of 15% or slightly lower, while males should have no more than 10% fat, perhaps ideally 5–8%. If a woman loses fat below a critical amount, she will become amenorrheic, lose bone calcium, and have difficulty with thermoregulation.

Another caution: A balanced diet is important. As an example, after giving a lecture on fuel metabolism some time ago, the author was approached by a fine runner who had just completed the Western States 100-Mile Endurance Run in the United States. During his training, he had serial body fat measurements performed and found that his percentage of body fat was rising while his weight remained stable. There is only one possible answer: He was in negative nitrogen balance and was losing protein mass while replacing it with fat. On further questioning, it was found he had a lactose intolerance and could not drink milk. He was simply not ingesting enough protein from other food sources to replace his muscle protein catabolism. Thus, if one keeps the body supplied with a balanced diet (roughly 55% carbohydrate, 25% protein, and 20% fat) and a liberal enough caloric intake, the body will deposit the fuel stores appropriately. If one wishes to lose weight, then simply decrease the fats in the diet, particularly saturated fats. Do not decrease carbohydrate intake!

Muscle glycogen in trained long-distance runners is roughly 130 mmol/kg/L and falls to 40–60 mmol/kg/L after daily workouts [7]. Failure to take in 2000–2500 carbohydrate cal per day will unfortunately result in glycogen depletion of the muscles and deterioration of performance.

To Carbohydrate-Load or Not?

With regard to carbohydrate loading, there is sufficient evidence that one can supersaturate muscle with glycogen and therefore improve performance (Bergstrom et al. [11]; Karlsson and Saltin [12]; Bergstrom and Hultman [13]; Sherman and Costill [7]). Sherman and Costill have suggested a "modified" regimen that avoids the uncomfortable and potentially dangerous effects of a ketogenic diet while still successfully supercompensating muscle with glycogen (Fig. 7-8).

Elevating Triglycerides

It has been suggested that elevating triglycerides and thereby fatty acids prior to an endurance run minimizes muscle glycogen loss during the glycogen burst at the beginning. This does seem to be the case in experimental animals (Costill et al. [14]) and perhaps in some models (LeBlanc et al. [32]). However, considering the adrenalin-induced increased substrate cycling before a race (vide supra) and a 75% $\dot{V}O_{2\,max}$ effort at the beginning, it is unlikely that any fuel source but carbohydrate will be used. In addition to its questionable role as an ergogenic aide, caffeine, which can elevate triglycerides, has the down-side effect of being a diuretic and therefore the potential for interrupting a run with a forced "pit stop."

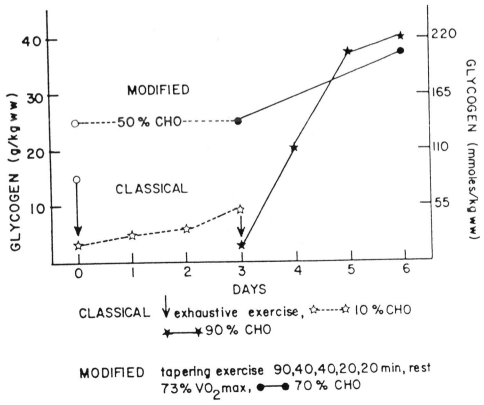

7-8 "Classical" versus "modified" methods for muscle glycogen supercompensation (Sherman and Costill [7]).

Running in the Postabsorptive State

It has been shown that work capacity is impaired if one eats carbohydrate just prior to the onset of exercise (Sherman and Costill [7]; Koivisto and Karonen [33]). Presumably, the elevated insulin will not turn off quickly enough after the beginning of exercise while ingested carbohydrate is rapidly utilized. In the presence of increased insulin levels, glycogen cannot break down, and the resulting hypoglycemia would then impair performance. However, an on-line carbohydrate source begun soon after a race may actually spare muscle glycogen (Koezentowski et al. [34]). Modifying carbohydrate with fat—i.e., a candy bar —may be a satisfactory prerace meal since the addition of fat alters carbohydrate absorption in such a way that hypoglycemia can be prevented (Horton [35]).

Be that as it may, carbohydrate intake during a marathon can only help. As muscle glycogen becomes depleted and gluconeogenesis becomes the carbohydrate source, ingested glucose can help maintain the glucose pool and serve as a fuel source. Sherman and Costill, in fact, recommend a 50–60% glucose solution 20–30 min after beginning a marathon and slightly less concentrated solutions at 20- to 40-min intervals thereafter [7].

In summary, for the successful marathoner, achieving and maintaining ideal body weight is fundamental. There is no evidence to suggest that adding a battery of vitamins, minerals, or exotic concoctions improves performance. The case for carbohydrate loading is valid, but the modified approach should be used [7]. Elevating fats with black coffee prior to a run is of dubious value. The race should be run no sooner than 3 hr after ingesting a meal, and glucose should be taken in during the race. Last, but most important, there is no substitute for training.

THE DIABETIC DISTANCE RUNNER

The diabetic distance runner is special, but there is no reason why a diabetic cannot run a marathon. Muscles of diabetic individuals adapt to training the same way muscles of nondiabetic individuals do (Costill et al. [36]). Diabetic patients, unless there are specific contraindications, should exercise aerobically. Richter et al. [37], Vranic et al. [38], Vranic and Berger [39], and Wahren [40] offer good reviews of diabetes and exercise.

The ideal is to have diabetics begin a run with the same metabolic profile as their nondiabetic counterparts. The blood sugar should be between 80 and 120 mg/dL. The difference between diabetic and nondiabetic runners is that the former may need a dose of insulin, albeit much smaller than usual and in the arm for slower absorption, and they will need to supply much of their fuel needs with ingested glucose during the race. There are no formulas for doing this without knowing the blood sugar level, and the latter should be part of the diabetic runner's training process, requiring an occasional fingerstick blood-sugar test. Appropriate paraphernalia and fluids can be carried during training and competition in a LiquiPac® or the like. Diabetic runners can balance fuel utilization with endogenous stores and exogenous sources, and thus participate in endurance events.

There are successful diabetic cyclists, marathoners, and triathletes. A particular problem area for the endurance-trained diabetic is the replenishing of skeletal muscle with glycogen. Since it takes some 24 hr for muscle stores to be reconstituted, blood sugar is "drained off" at the expense of other tissues during this time. The potential for severe hypoglycemia is there. Decreasing insulin dose and increasing carbohydrate feeding can minimize this potential problem.

REFERENCES

1. Milvy, P. (ed). 1977. The Marathon: Physiological, Medical, Epidemiological and Psychological Studies. Ann NY Acad Sci 301.
2. Newsholme, E.A. 1977. The regulation of intracellular and extracellular fuel supplied during sustained exercise. Ann NY Acad Sci 301:81–91.
3. Essen, B. 1977. Intramuscular substrate utilization during prolonged exercise. Ann NY Acad Sci 301:30–44.
4. Ahlborg, G., Felig, P., et al. 1974. Substrate turnover during prolonged exercise in man. J Clin Invest 53:1090.
5. Scheele, K., Herzog, G., et al. 1979. Metabolic adaptation to prolonged exercise. Eur J Appl Physiol 41:101–108.
6. Locksley, R. 1980. Fuel utilization in marathons: implications for performance (Medical Staff Conference, University of California, San Francisco). West J Med 133:493–502.
7. Sherman, W.M., Costill, D.L. 1984. The marathon: dietary manipulation to optimize performance. Am J Sports Med 12:44–51.
8. Cahill, G. 1981. Metabolism VI-1 to VI-14. In: Rubenstein, E., Federman, D. (eds): Medicine. Scientific American, New York.
9. Randel, P.J., Garland, T.B., et al. 1966. Interaction of metabolism and the physiological role of insulin. Recent Prog Horm Res 22:1–48.
10. Essen, B., Hagenfeldt, L., et al. 1977. Utilization of blood-borne and intramuscular substrates during continuous and intermittent exercise in man. J Physiol 265:489–506.
11. Bergstrom, J., Hermansen, L., et al. 1967. Diet, muscle glycogen and physical performance. Acta Physiol Scand 71:140–150.
12. Karlsson, J., Saltin, B. 1971. Diet, muscle glycogen and endurance performance. J Appl Physiol 31:203–206.
13. Bergstrom, J., Hultman, E. 1972. Nutrition for maximal sports performance. JAMA 22:999–1006.
14. Costill, D.L., Coyle, E., et al. 1977. Effects of elevated plasma FFA and insulin on muscle glycogen usage during exercise. J Appl Physiol 43:695–699.
15. Jones, N.L., Heigenhauser, C.J.F., et al. 1980. Fat metabolism in heavy exercise. Clin Sci 59:469–478.
16. Hagenfeldt, L. 1979. Metabolism of free fatty acids and ketone bodies during exercise in normal and diabetic man. Diabetes 28 (Suppl. I):66–70.
17. Lemon, P.W.R., Nagle, F. J. 1981. Effects of exercise on protein and amino acid metabolism. Med Sci Sports Exerc 13:141–149.
18. Wahren, J. 1977. Glucose turnover during exercise in man. Ann NY Acad Sci 301:45–55.
19. Ahlborg, G., Felig, P. 1982. Lactate and glucose exchange across the forearm, legs, and splenchnic bed during and after prolonged leg exercise. J Clin Invest 69:45–54.
20. Koivisto, V.A., Harkonen, J., et al. 1985. Glycogen depletion during prolonged exercise: influence of glucose, fructose, or placebo. J Appl Physiol 58:731–737.
21. Holloszy, J.L., Tennie, M.J., et al. 1977. Physiological consequences of the biochemical adaptations to endurance exercise. Ann NY Acad Sci 301:440–454.
22. Holloszy, J.O., Coyle E.F. 1984. Adaptations of skeletal muscle to endurance exercise and their metabolic consequences. J Appl Physiol 56:831–838.
23. Costill, D.L., Fink, W.J., et al. 1979. Lipid metabolism in skeletal muscle of endurance-trained males and females. J Appl Physiol 47:787–791.
24. Nikkila, E.A, Taskinen, M.R., et al. 1978. Lipoprotein lipase activity in adipose tissue and skeletal muscle of runners in relation to serum lipoproteins. Metabolism 27:1661–1671.
25. Lohman, D., Liebold, F., et al. 1978. Diminished insulin response in highly trained athletes. Metabolism 27:521–524.
26. Seals, D.R., Hagberg, J.M., et al. 1984. Glucose tolerance in young and older athletes and sedentary men. J Appl Physiol 56:1521–1525.
27. Heath, G.W., Gavin J.R. III, et al. 1983. Effects of exercise and lack of exercise on glucose tolerance and insulin sensitivity. J Appl Physiol 55:512–517.
28. Rahkila, P., Soimajarvia, J., et al. 1980. Lipid metabolism during exercise: II. Respiratory exchange ratio and muscle glycogen content during four-hour bicycle ergometry in two groups of healthy men. Eur J Appl Physiol 44:245–254.
29. Hagan, R.D., Smith, M.G., et al. 1981. Marathon performance in relation to maximal aerobic power and training indices. Med Sci Sports Exerc 13:185–189.
30. Newsholme, E.A. 1978. Substrate cy-

cles: their metabolic, energetic, and thermic consequences in man. Biochem Soc Symp 43:183–205.

31. Newsholme, E.A., Arch, J.R.S. 1983. The role of substrate cycles in metabolic regulation. Biochem Soc Trans 11:52–56.

32. LeBlanc, M., Jobin, J., et al. 1985. Enhanced metabolic response to caffeine in exercise-trained human subjects. J Appl Physiol 59:832–837.

33. Koivisto, V.A., Karonen, S. 1981. Carbohydrate ingestion before exercise: comparison of glucose, fructose and sweet placebo. J Appl Physiol 51:783–787.

34. Koezentowski, G., Jandrain, B., et al. 1984. Availability of glucose given orally during exercise. J Appl Physiol 56:315–320.

35. Horton, E. Personal communication, 1986.

36. Costill, D.L., Cleary, T., et al. 1979. Training adaptations in skeletal muscle of juvenile diabetics. Diabetes 28:818–822.

37. Richter, E.A., Ruderman, M.B., et al. 1981. Diabetes and exercise. Am J Med 70:201–209.

38. Vranic, M., Horvath, S., et al. 1979. Proceedings of a Conference on Diabetes and Exercise 28. Diabetes (Suppl I):1–113.

39. Vranic, M., Berger, M. 1979. Exercise and diabetes mellitus. Diabetes 28:147–163.

40. Wahren, J. 1979. Glucose turnover during exercise in healthy man in patients with diabetes mellitus. Diabetes 28 (Suppl I):1–113.

SECTION 3
Sports and Hormones, Fluids, and Electrolytes

•8•

Hormonal Regulation
of Fluid and Electrolytes
During Exercise

Maire T. Buckman and Glenn T. Peake

There are numerous studies examining the effects of exercise on fluid and electrolyte balance in humans, and substantial information exists regarding the role of various hormones in these processes. This chapter discusses exercise-induced shifts in fluid compartments and changes in electrolyte balance in relation to the hormones that play an important regulatory role in these events. Also, the effects of exercise-induced shifts in fluid compartments and electrolytes on secretion and metabolic effects of these same hormone systems are detailed. Clearly, results of a single study have limited generalized application since each exercise protocol is unique. Exercise has different effects, depending on the specific circumstances at the time of the exercise. For example, exercise acclimation at 39.8°C is associated with an increase in sweat rate, whereas acclimation at 23.8°C is associated with a decrease in sweat rate (Shvartz et al. [1]). Thus, sweating and the associated water and electrolyte losses depend on environmental conditions and acclimation of the individual. Because variable exercise conditions have different effects on salt and water balance and potentially also on hormone secretion, the exercise milieu is precisely defined for each study discussed here.

The variables that characterize each exercise protocol can be divided into: 1) environmental conditions, 2) exercise conditions, and 3) individual conditioning. Environmental conditions include temperature, humidity, wind factors, and altitude. Exercise conditions include position (supine, sitting, standing, upright), type of exercise (weight-lifting, running, climbing, cycling, swimming, etc.), and duration (5 min vs 8 hr, for example). Individual conditioning is the level of exercise training of the participants. Thus, a person who lives a semisedentary life without regular exercise beyond light walking may have a very different response to a given exercise protocol under defined environmental conditions than would a highly trained person who, for example, jogs 10 miles each day. Likewise, sex and age may influence physiologic processes associated with exercise (Plowman et al. [2]). Unfortunately, many exercise studies only partially define these variables, rendering integration of data difficult.

Serum or plasma hormone concentrations are frequently measured to determine hormonal secretory responses. However, other factors influence hormone concentrations independent of stimulus responsiveness. These include the size of the stored hormonal pool available for secretion; the volume for distribution of a hormone, which may change under various conditions; and the clearance of the hormone from the extracellular space. Since exercise in the heat, for example, is associated with a profound decrease in effective arterial blood volume, resulting in diminished renal blood flow, glomerular filtration rate, and splanchic blood flow, the effects on serum hormone concentration may be anticipated to be partially independent of hormone secretion. These effects may result from hemoconcentration, altered hormone distribution, decreased renal excretion, or altered metabolism (Knochel [3]). Thus, an increase in serum or plasma hormone concentration with exercise may not simply reflect enhanced release from its production or storage site. Furthermore, serum hormone concentration may not be the sole determinant of the hormone's biological activity. Tissue or end-organ responsiveness also determines hormonal effects. For example, an increase in the number of aldosterone receptors at the distal renal tubule may enhance aldosterone activity without increased plasma hormone concentrations. Conversely, decreased receptor numbers may diminish the activity at the same hormone concentration. Little is known about the effect of exercise on target-tissue responsiveness, i.e., receptor number and affinity or postreceptor events. However, the variables determining tissue sensitivity to a hormonal stimulus are clearly important. The well-known phenomenon of decreased insulin requirement in exercising diabetics is an example of exercise-induced alteration in tissue responsiveness (Ruderman et al. [4]; Pederson et al. [5]).

Two extensively investigated hormonal systems have a major impact on body fluid and electrolyte homeostasis: the renin–angiotensin–aldosterone system and the neurohypophyseal hormone vasopressin. The anterior pituitary hormones (growth hormone [GH], prolactin [PRL], and adrenocorticotropic hormone [ACTH] through regulation of adrenal steroid secretion) may also affect water and electrolyte balance during exercise, but their effects are less clearly delineated. The recently described cardiac hormone, atrial natriuretic factor or atriopeptin (Cody et al. [6]), may also have an important role; however, studies of its plasma concentration or effects during exercise are in early stages of investigation (Solomon et al. [7]).

RENIN–ANGIOTENSIN–ALDOSTERONE SYSTEM

The renin–angiotensin–aldosterone system is primarily regulated by the renal juxtaglomerular apparatus, which includes the renin-producing segment of the afferent arteriole and the proximal segment of the distal convoluted tubule, the macula densa. Renin secretion is inhibited by increased pressure on stretch receptors within the afferent arteriole, and it is increased by decreased pressure or stretch (Tobian et al. [8]). In addition, renin secretion is modulated by changes in tubular fluid composition at the macula densa (David and Freeman [9]). Volume expansion with sodium chloride has a profound inhibitory effect on renin secretion—more so than comparable expansion with dextran—presumably because of a specific effect of sodium chloride at the macula densa. In addition to these renal mechanisms, renin secretion is influenced by the sympathetic nervous system. Sympathetic tone may be modulated directly via nerve terminals at the juxtaglomerular apparatus (Assaykeen and Ganong [10]) or by circulating catecholamines (Johnson et al. [11]). The neural component of renin secretion appears to be mediated by β-adrenergic receptors (Reid and Morris [12]) with stimulation of β-receptors promoting renin secretion. Once renin is released from the juxtaglomerular cell into the systemic circulation, it cleaves an α-globulin substrate to form the decapeptide angiotensin I, which in turn is enzymatically converted to angiotensin II.

Angiotensin II is a potent vasoconstrictor that stimulates aldosterone biosynthesis and secretion. Aldosterone, in turn, stimulates sodium transport across a number of epithelial membranes, including kidney, sweat glands, salivary glands, and gastrointestinal tract (Knochel [13]; Sharp and Leaf [14]). Aldosterone mediates its effects, primarily via the distal renal tubule, promoting resorption of sodium and excretion of potassium and hydrogen. Thus, the renin–angiotensin–aldosterone system is important in maintaining vascular tone and extracellular fluid volume by enhancing sodium retention and expansion of plasma volume.

Strenuous exercise stimulates the renin–angiotensin–aldosterone cascade in humans. The initiating event in activating this cascade may be, in part, related to pronounced shifts in body fluids that occur with exercise (Fig. 8-1) (Costill [15]). These shifts are characterized by up to a 13% decrease in plasma and effective arterial blood volume occurring during the initial phase of strenuous exercise (Convertino et al. [16]; Geyssant et al. [17]; Melin et al. [18]). Activation of the renin–angiotensin–aldosterone system occurs after each acute bout of exercise, and heat acclimatization does not alter this effect of exercise (Davies et al. [19]). Fluid replacement with physiologic saline blunted, but did not block, renin release.

Several mechanisms account for the decreased blood volume during exercise. Muscular work, independent of environmental conditions, results in massive shunting of blood to skeletal muscle, so-called exercise hyperemia. Quantitatively, muscle blood flow varies almost directly with the degree of work and may increase 20–40 times above resting levels during intense exercise (Barcroft [20]). In addition to shunting blood to skeletal muscle, a substantial shift of plasma water into muscle cells occurs during muscular contraction. This is due to increased osmolality within exercising muscle cells resulting from glycogen

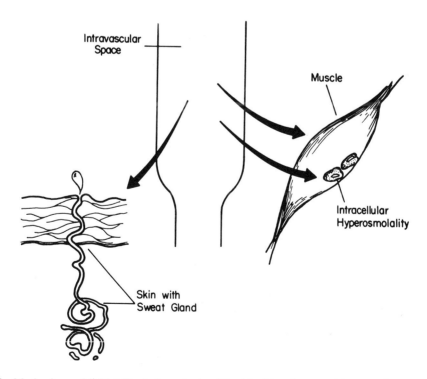

8-1 Mechanisms of fluid shifts during exercise. Blood is shunted to exercising muscle and skin. In muscle, intracellular hyperosmolality induces a shift of plasma water into the cells. Sweat production results in a hypotonic fluid loss. These fluid shifts result in contraction of plasma volume.

breakdown. Glycogen, a major fuel for muscular contraction, is metabolized into smaller intermediary products; since the cell membrane is relatively less permeable to these substances than to water, water moves into the cells. During the early phases of exercise, 10% or more of the inflowing arterial blood may move from plasma into the cell (Schlein et al. [21]). Muscle water increases roughly 8% in active tissue during the early minutes of exercise, and this is associated with an equivalent decline in plasma water (Costill [15]). After the initial shifts, plasma and muscle water tend to be stable over 120 min of strenuous exercise, and only minor changes are observed with continued exertion. However, during the adaptation to continued bouts of exercise, plasma volume increases without a change in red blood cell mass (Convertino et al. [22]). Accompanying the increase in plasma volume is a fall in hemoglobin concentration and hematocrit. Since plasma concentrations of Na^+, K^+, and albumin are maintained despite the increased plasma volume, the total blood content of these substances rises. Thus, acute changes in effective blood volume during acute bouts of exercise promote activation of the renin–angiotensin–aldosterone system; repeated activation of this system promotes expansion of total plasma volume.

Another important factor activating the renin–angiotensin–aldosterone system relates to exercise-induced sweating (Fig. 8-1). Heat generated by muscle contraction and from the environment induces increased peripheral blood flow and sweating (Benzinger [23]), which are important in maintaining thermal equilibrium (Costill [15]). Sweating may further compromise effective arterial blood volume. Fluid and electrolyte losses in sweat depend on environmental conditions (temperature, humidity, wind speed) and on the degree and duration of physical exertion. Furthermore, acclimation modulates sweat losses (Shvartz et al. [1]). Maximum sweat rate in an untrained man may attain 1.5 L/hr (Fasola et al. [24]), whereas marathon runners may lose sweat in excess of 6 L/hr during the race (Costill [15]). Sweat is hypotonic to plasma. The principal ions in sweat are those derived from the extracellular fluid compartment, i.e., sodium and chloride. Sodium in sweat ranges between 10 and 60 mEq/L (Shvartz et al. [1]). Thus, significant fluid and electrolytes can be lost by sweating, and the resultant decrease in extracellular fluid volume may contribute to renin secretion.

An exercise-associated decrease in blood volume, due to fluid shifts and sweat losses, results in reduced renal blood flow and glomerular filtration rate, thereby providing a potent stimulus for renin secretion. In addition, catecholamines increase with exercise (Fasola et al. [24]), and they too are potent stimulators for renin release. Concomitant catecholamine and renin responses during graded exercise suggest that renin secretion is related to enhanced sympathetic activity (Kotchen et al. [25]).

Activation of adrenal aldosterone secretion results principally from the angiotensin II produced as a result of increased renin release during exercise (Fig. 8-2). Although angiotensin II is a potent vasoconstrictor, it has a minor role in blood pressure elevation during exercise (Fagard et al. [26]). In addition to angiotensin II, ACTH and potassium also stimulate aldosterone secretion. Their respective role in exercise-induced aldosterone secretion has not been fully evaluated.

Aldosterone helps to maintain extracellular fluid volume by promoting sodium resorption in the kidney, the gastrointestinal tract, and sweat and salivary glands. The direct renal effect on distal tubular resorption of sodium and excretion of potassium begins 0.5–2 hr after aldosterone administration and lasts 4–8 hr (Barger et al. [27]; Ganong and Mulrow [28]; Ross et al. [29]; Sonnenblick et al. [30]). The delay in onset of aldosterone action on sweat, saliva, and gastrointestinal electrolytes is even longer (August et al. [31]), a fact implying that aldosterone secreted during short bouts of exercise may not become physiologically effective until after exercise is completed. In one study of acute exercise in which plasma aldosterone was measured, a single 60-min exercise bout increased plasma renin and aldosterone nearly sevenfold above baseline (Follenius et al. [32]). Despite *ad libitum*

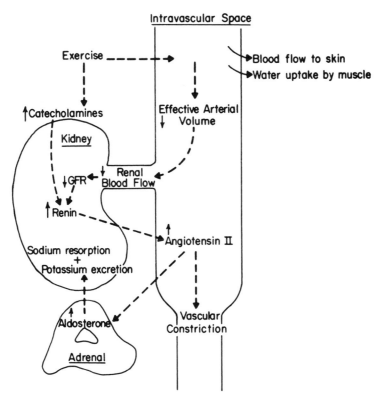

8-2 Proposed sequence of events leading to activation of the renin–angiotensin–aldosterone system during exercise. Significant sodium resorption and potassium excretion may occur at the sweat glands and in the kidney tubule.

water intake, aldosterone remained elevated for 11 hr after exercise completion. The acute plasma aldosterone elevation, therefore, outlasts the exercise to influence the long-term maintenance and expansion of plasma volume.

A variety of environmental factors influence exercise-induced stimulation of the renin–angiotensin–aldosterone system. Aldosterone dynamics during graded exercise at sea level and high altitude have been studied (Maher et al. [33]). Exposure of either low- (400 m) or moderate- (about 2000 m) altitude natives to a high-altitude environment (4200 m) decreased 24-hr urinary aldosterone secretion compared with values observed in these same subjects at low or moderate altitude. Thus, overall production of the hormone was reduced by high altitude. The effects of acute repeated bouts of exercise given in rapid sequence to exhaustion on plasma aldosterone revealed a diminished plasma hormonal response at high altitude in both low-altitude and moderate-altitude natives compared with the responses observed at low altitude in these same individuals. However, the blunting of the exercise-induced hormone rises were more pronounced in the low-altitude natives. Since urinary K^+ fell slightly, whereas urinary Na^+ was unchanged in subjects exposed to high-altitude conditions, the effects of the changes in aldosterone do not appear to have a major effect on renal electrolyte regulation. In another study, healthy males exercised rigorously for 6 weeks on a mechanically braked bicycle ergometer for 20 min at 45% maximum oxygen consumption ($\dot{V}O_{2\,max}$), and after a 1-hr rest period, again for 20 min at 75% $\dot{V}O_{2\,max}$. Plasma renin, angiotensin II, and aldosterone increased in a graded fashion at sea level, and after 11 days at 4300 m. In contrast, on the first day of altitude exposure, levels of all three hormones were significantly lower than those at sea level and after adaptation to altitude. It was proposed that the acute hypoxemia of high altitude, known to increase renal blood flow, may signal a decrease in renin release and, secondarily, a decrease in aldosterone secretion (Hogan et al. [34]). This hypothesis is consistent with evidence suggesting that renal blood flow changes are the primary activators of the renin–angiotensin–aldosterone system during exercise (Fig. 8-2). In some studies, renin secretion was affected less severely by altitude or hypoxia than was aldosterone secretion (Keynes et al. [35]), and in some situations renin secretion rose with hypoxia as aldosterone fell (Milledge and Catley [36]). This led to the suggestion that hypoxia may decrease the activity of the enzyme responsible for conversion of angiotensin I to angiotensin II, since the latter is responsible for regulation of aldosterone secretion (Milledge and Catley [36]). However, direct measurements of angiotensin-converting enzyme activity during an hypoxic challenge, in which plasma aldosterone fell substantially, failed to reveal any decrease in the activity of this enzyme (Colice and Ramirez [37]). In a separate study, plasma angiotensin II levels rose with the induction of hypoxia while aldosterone was falling (Raff and Levy [38]). In another recent investigation (Shigeoka et al. [39]), hypoxemia was shown to blunt exercise-induced renin secretion and to totally obliterate the expected rise in aldosterone to treadmill exercise. From their studies and those of others they reviewed, Sigeoka et al. concluded that hypoxemic exercise results in the release of a substance that blocks the effects of angiotensin II on adrenal aldosterone release. Alternately, hypoxia may have a direct effect on adrenal zona glomerulosa steroidogenesis. From the available contradictory studies, it appears that the mechanism(s) by which high altitude or hypoxemia blunts the renin–angiotensin–aldosterone response to exercise have not been fully elucidated.

Another environmental factor influencing activation of the renin–angiotensin–aldosterone system is heat. Prolonged exercise in heat results in large water and salt losses from sweating. This may further compromise intravascular volume and result in counter-regulatory sodium conservation by enhanced renal sodium resorption and by decreased sodium concentration in sweat. Moderately conditioned normal men (average $\dot{V}O_2$ max 42 ml O_2/kg/min) exercised in a room maintained at 32°C and 45–50% relative humidity to promote large salt and water losses from sweating. Activity consisted of cycling at 50% $\dot{V}O_2$ max for eight 15-min intervals spaced by 5-min rest periods. During rest periods, subjects ingested water equal to sweat volume losses. The change in plasma aldosterone paralleled that of plasma renin. Both hormones were significantly lower if water was replaced by electrolyte solution containing 20 mEq/L sodium, 20 mEq/L potassium and 23 g/L glucose (Francis and MacGregor [40]). This study suggests that sodium losses from sweating are an additional stimulus to aldosterone secretion, which can be partially reversed by sodium intake.

Under extreme conditions, e.g., during basic military training in hot climates, more than 12 L of fluid can be lost per day in sweat (Robinson and Robinson [41]). Sodium in sweat averaged about 40–60 mEq/L, and potassium 4–9 mEq/L. Such training can therefore result in sodium losses in excess of 500 mEq and potassium losses of more than 100 mEq per day. These volume and electrolyte losses are potent stimuli for aldosterone secretion. Both aldosterone excretion and secretion are high in those engaging in intense physical conditioning in a hot climate (Knochel et al. [42]). Serial estimations of exchangeable ^{42}K showed a marked potassium deficit due to sweat and urinary losses. Inappropriately high urinary potassium losses for the potassium-depleted state occurred in those training in hot climates, an indication of an aldosterone effect on the kidney. Similar experiments in cooler climates did not show potassium depletion. Potassium deficits may be associated with rhabdomyolysis. Therefore, overproduction of aldosterone with exercise in the heat may be dangerous (Knochel et al. [42]).

In another study, performed over a period of 5 days during intense military training, during which subjects were deprived of sleep and food, basal renin and aldosterone levels were markedly elevated. Acute exercise at 60% $\dot{V}O_2$ max on the third day of training resulted in further elevations of both renin and aldosterone. In subjects calorically replenished to the level of caloric expenditure, the changes in renin and aldosterone were less pronounced but still were present. Catecholamines were noted to rise throughout the training period, and this rise was blunted in the calorically augmented group. Allowing sleep in calorically deprived trainees minimally blunted the hormonal changes (Opstad et al. [43]).

In one study, subjects were exposed to heat without exercise. This resulted in fluid shifts similar to those seen during exercise, i.e., increased blood flow to the skin and marked elevation in plasma aldosterone (Costill [15]). This study implied that during acute heat exposure, decreased plasma volume from sweating and shifting of blood to skin from the central circulation may stimulate aldosterone secretion.

Other factors that potentially affect renin secretion have been investigated. Since plasma β-endorphin rises with exercise (Faioli et al. [44]; Carr et al. [45]; Gambert et al. [46]), an effect of this opioid peptide on renin and aldosterone plasma concentrations was investigated. In one study, moderate doses of maloxone, a drug that blocks several classes of opiate receptors, had no effect on exercise-induced elevations of either renin or aldosterone (Brammert and Hokfelt [47]). However, larger doses of naloxone were observed to enhance the renin and aldosterone responses to exercise (Grossman et al. [48]). These studies indicate minor effects of opioids on suppressing the renin–angiotensin–aldosterone system.

Potential effects of prostanoids and their related bioactive fatty acid derivatives on exercise-induced renin and aldosterone secretion have been sought by blocking production of these compounds with a drug that blocks the cyclo-oxygenase enzyme system responsible for formation of all of these related compounds (Staessen et al. [49]). When indomethacin was given to normal volunteers, recumbent and upright renin levels were reduced and the rise in renin following exercise to 100% $\dot{V}O_{2\ max}$ was reduced in treated subjects. Although recumbent aldosterone levels were not different in control and treated subjects, upright aldosterone levels were reduced, and the exercise-induced rise also was diminished in treated subjects. In contrast, plasma catecholamine responses were not altered by indomethacin treatment. Thus, the net effect of endogenous prostanoids may be to facilitate renin and aldosterone secretion both in the resting state and during exercise, but the exercise-induced rise in renin and aldosterone does not appear to be solely dependent on the prostanoids and their related fatty acid derivatives.

The effects of activation of the renin–angiotensin–aldosterone system on renal electrolyte handling would be expected to enhance sodium reabsorption by decreasing urinary sodium losses and to promote potassium excretion, thereby enhancing urinary potassium losses. In most studies, the urinary sodium does indeed decrease as predicted, but the effects on potassium excretion are variable (reviewed in Lijnen et al. [50]). However, severe prolonged exercise resulting in sustained elevations of aldosterone secretion does promote renal potassium wastage (Castenfors [51]; Dobrev et al. [52]; Carraz et al. [53]). Less severe exercise programs have been reported to produce variable effects on urinary potassium, including a decrease in its excretion (Lijnen et al. [50]).

VASOPRESSIN (ANTIDIURETIC HORMONE)

Vasopressin is produced in the supraoptic and paraventricular nuclei of the anterior hypothalamus, and its granules are stored in the posterior pituitary gland (neurohypophysis). The primary function of vasopressin is to preserve tonicity of body fluids, and its secretion is regulated primarily by changes in plasma osmolality (Robertson et al. [54]). This system is exquisitely sensitive; minute changes in plasma osmolality of 1–2% result in significant changes in plasma vasopressin (Robertson et al. [54]). Increased plasma osmolality, as with hypotonic dehydration, results in increased vasopressin secretion and subsequent enhanced free-water resorption by the kidney. Decreased plasma osmolality after free-water intake, in contrast, causes suppression of vasopressin release and increased water excretion. Thus, small changes in extracellular fluid tonicity regulate vasopressin secretion, which in turn modulates renal handling of water in a way that restores extracellular fluid osmolality to normal.

The function of vasopressin to preserve body fluid tonicity is compromised only when hemodynamic factors reach threatening proportions. Blood volume must be decreased by 10–15% before vasopressin release is significantly stimulated (Robertson and Athar [55]). At this level, tonicity may be increasingly compromised to conserve blood volume. When a normal adult was depleted of sodium by sweating in a heat chamber, body water tonicity did not decline until extracellular fluid volume was reduced by approximately 12% (McCance [56]). Major shifts in extracellular fluids may also be associated with alterations in vasopressin secretion. Increased ambient temperature from 25°C to 50°C was associated with increased plasma antidiuretic hormone; the hot environment dilates peripheral vascular beds and decreases central blood volume (Moore [57]). Volume receptors regulate hypovolemia-induced vasopressin secretion. Conversely, decreased ambient temperature from 26°C to 13°C was associated with decreased plasma vasopressin. Cooling caused peripheral vasoconstriction and increased central blood volume, which in turn decreases vasopressin secretion (Moore [57]). Thus, major changes in central blood volume, whether secondary to extracellular fluid loss or to redistribution, regulate vasopressin secretion.

Prolonged strenuous exercise is associated with decreased urine formation (Castenfors [58]; Refsum and Stromme [59]). Increased shunting of blood to exercising muscle results in decreased splanchnic and renal circulation (Castenfors [58]). Decreased renal blood flow is proportional to the severity of exercise (Castenfors [58]). This causes decreased creatinine clearance (C_{cr}), which is quantitatively related to decreased urine formation (Castenfors [58]). The significant correlation between decreased C_{cr} and urine flow suggests that the diminished urine flow occurs, at least in part, secondary to decreased glomerular filtration. Maximum concentrating ability is decreased during exercise because of presumed reduction of interstitial sodium and urea secondary to decreased glomerular filtration. Nevertheless, the antidiuretic action of vasopressin may also be operative, and this possibility has recently been examined by several groups of investigators.

Vasopressin Secretion

Plasma vasopressin increases with exercise in men and women (Reid and Morris [12]; Convertino et al. [16, 22, 63]; Geyssant et al. [17]; Williams et al. [60]; Wade and Claybaugh [61]; Nielsen et al. [62]; Vallotton et al. [64]; Dessypris et al. [65]). Several variables have been identified that might modulate vasopressin secretion, including exercise intensity, duration, and mode; training; and hydration status.

Exercise Intensity A threshold of exercise intensity for vasopressin secretion has been described in several studies:

Plasma vasopressin in untrained men working on a cycle ergometer for 6 min at a time at work loads ranging from 100 W (40% $\dot{V}_{O_2\,max}$) to 225 W (90% $\dot{V}_{O_2\,max}$) did not increase at a work load performed at 40% $\dot{V}_{O_2\,max}$; however, at higher work loads, vasopressin increased in a curvilinear fashion (Convertino et al. [16]). In a subsequent study by the same group (Convertino et al. [63]), vasopressin rose only when work intensity exceeded 50% $\dot{V}_{O_2\,max}$. The same threshold was observed in untrained men both before and after an 8-day training period. Thus, a work intensity threshold above 50% $\dot{V}_{O_2\,max}$ is necessary to stimulate vasopressin secretion.

To evaluate the mechanism of exercise-induced vasopressin secretion, volume and os-molar variables were examined. Plasma volume decreased at each exercise level, with the maximum change of -12.4% to -13.7% occurring at the highest work load (Convertino et al. [16]). Plasma osmolality increased in a curvilinear fashion from a mean resting level of 287 mOsm/kg to a mean maximum level of 302 mOsm/kg at the maximum work load. Changes in plasma osmolality were significantly correlated with changes in vasopressin concentrations. Thus, the investigators concluded that hyperosmolality is important in the regulation of vasopressin release during acute bouts of exercise. Decreased plasma volume may also contribute to vasopressin secretion.

Exercise Duration The increase in plasma vasopressin with exercise may be dependent on exercise duration. Wade and Claybaugh [61] noted no change in vasopressin after a 20-min period of treadmill exercise at 70% of max heart rate. However, 60 min of exercise at the same intensity elicited a vasopressin response.

Exercise Mode Paired studies in 5 healthy men exercising at approximately 60% $\dot{V}O_{2\ max}$ suggest that positional and perhaps other factors may influence vasopressin secretion (Nielsen et al. [62]). Exercise on a bicycle ergometer resulted in a significant increase in vasopressin concentration, whereas swimming at approximately the same work intensity failed to induce vasopressin secretion. Plasma volume changes were similar in both groups and thus could not account for the differential vasopressin responses observed. Plasma osmolality, however, was not measured in this study and thus its contribution, if any, cannot be evaluated.

Exercise Training Effects of exercise training on basal and stimulated vasopressin secretion have been studied by several groups of investigators.

Pre-exercise vasopressin levels have been reported to be unaffected by training in male subjects (Geyssant et al. [17]; Convertino et al. [22, 63]). However, Maresh et al. [66] observed an increase in basal vasopressin concentrations in women basketball players after a 5-month training season. Since time of menstrual cycle was not controlled in this study, and cyclic estrogen secretion may alter the vasopressin response to exercise (Maresh et al. [66]), further studies are necessary to clarify whether training is an independent variable in enhancing basal vasopressin secretion in women.

Exercise-induced vasopressin secretion in relation to training has been studied. Convertino et al. [22] examined plasma vasopressin responses in men working on a bicycle ergometer at 160 W (65% $\dot{V}O_{2\ max}$) for 2 hr/day over a period of 8 days. Increased plasma volume, to 112% above baseline, occurred during the 8-day study period and was associated with maintenance of the resting plasma osmolality; this observation suggests that the exercise-associated volume expansion consisted of a corresponding isotonic increase in total solutes. Mean plasma vasopressin concentrations increased eight- to ninefold over resting levels at completion of each exercise period; the magnitude of the increase was similar on the first and last days of the exercise program, indicating that the increased total plasma volume failed to exert an inhibitory influence on vasopressin secretion. The increase in vasopressin correlated significantly with the acute increase in plasma osmolality and plasma sodium during exercise. Thus, vasopressin response to acute exercise bouts correlated with hyperosmolality and was unaffected by an 8-day training period, during which an expansion of plasma volume occurred.

Longer training periods, likewise, do not affect the vasopressin response to acute exercise bouts in men and women. Geyssant et al. [17] examined the effect on plasma vasopressin concentrations in four untrained men of a 5-month endurance program consisting of working on a bicycle ergometer at 87% $\dot{V}O_{2\ max}$ 4 times per week to exhaustion. A significant increase in plasma vasopressin was observed after each training session. The magnitude of the increase was similar at the beginning and the end of the 5-month program. Likewise, a study in women college basketball players indicated a similar vasopressin response to maximal exercise before and after the training season (Maresh et al. [66]). Similar findings were reported in a population study (Melin et al. [18]). Subjects were divided into well-trained, trained, and untrained groups on the basis of $\dot{V}O_{2\ max}$. The three groups then exercised on a bicycle ergometer at 80% $\dot{V}O_{2\ max}$ to exhaustion. Plasma vasopressin measured by bioassay increased significantly after exercise in all three groups to a comparable level. Thus, all of the studies demonstrated that vasopressin responses to acute exercise bouts did not depend on the level of training or physical fitness.

Hydration Status Since vasopressin secretion is regulated by both osmolar and volume mechanisms, hydration status would be expected to modulate vasopressin secretion.

Wade and Claybaugh [61] studied the effect of hydration on vasopressin response in young men after 1 hr of treadmill running at a heart rate approximately 35%, 70%, and 100% of predicted maximum rate. Subjects exercised following 10 hr of water deprivation and after ingesting 30 ml of water. As in the previous studies, vasopressin changes correlated significantly with work intensity. In addition, the increase in vasopressin after maximum exercise was greater following 10 hr of water deprivation than after water supplementation. Plasma vasopressin returned to resting values 1 hr after completion of exercise. Pre-exercise, resting vasopressin levels, however, were similar in the two groups. In contrast to previous studies, plasma vasopressin concentration did not correlate with plasma osmolality changes or plasma volume changes during exercise. However, a positive correlation was observed between plasma renin activity (PRA) and vasopressin, suggesting that angiotensin II may have influenced vasopressin secretion. Other investigators have reported conflicting results regarding the role of angiotensin II on vasopressin release (Schrier et al. [67]).

In summary, several factors are involved in the regulation of exercise-induced vasopressin secretion. Plasma vasopressin increases acutely with exercise; quantitatively, the increase depends on work intensity, work duration, and hydration status. Mode of exercise, including positional variants, may affect vasopressin secretion. Repetitive exercise does not alter the vasopressin response to acute exercise, and long-term training has no modulatory effect on this response. The mechanism of vasopressin secretion is related principally to the hyperosmolality that accompanies vigorous physical work and, to a lesser extent, to the hypovolemia associated with exercise. It has also been suggested that angiotensin II plays a role in exercise-associated vasopressin release. In addition, since vasopressin is primarily metabolized by the liver and the kidneys, decreased blood flow to these organs during exercise may contribute to increased plasma levels of the hormone (Wade and Claybaugh [61]).

Physiologic Effects of Increased Plasma Vasopressin During Exercise

Physiologic consequences of increased plasma vasopressin during exercise have not been studied extensively. Exercise has been associated with an increase in free-water clearance during exercise (Wade and Claybaugh [61]) and immediately after exercise (Melin et al. [18]). The decreased urine volume associated with exercise appears to be primarily due to a decrease in osmolar clearance. Since vasopressin decreases free-water clearance, Melin et al.'s observations suggest absence of a substantial role for vasopressin in the exercise-associated antidiuresis. However, since preexercise free-water clearance was already negative in these studies, antidiuretic hormone biologic effect could have already been maximal at the onset of exercise, and the decreased negative free-water clearance could represent exercise-associated changes in renal solute handling. Nielsen et al. [62] further suggested that the relative diuresis observed during swimming compared with bicycling was associated with stable vasopressin levels with swimming in contrast to the rise observed when exercise was performed in the vertical position.

Other factors may modulate vasopressin activity at the renal tubule. Exercise increases renal prostaglandins, which may interfere with vasopressin action at the kidney (Oliw [68]; Share and Claybaugh [69]; Zambraski and Dunn [70]). Furthermore, norepinephrine released during exercise may play a role in the antidiuresis observed with exercise (Schrier et al. [67]). Norepinephrine administered by intravenous infusion increases renal water excretion in humans. This diuretic effect appears to be associated with α-adrenergic stimulating properties of norepinephrine. In vitro studies show that norepinephrine interferes with the cellular action of vasopressin. Serum cortisol increases with vigorous exercise and enhances free-water excretion. Although the precise respective roles of renal prostaglandins, norepinephrine, and cortisol in modulating the vasopressin effect on the renal tubule during exercise have not been studied, experimental data suggest that such interactions may be important in explaining the apparent contradictory findings of increased plasma vasopressin and enhanced free-water clearance with exercise.

ANTERIOR PITUITARY HORMONES

Adrenocorticotropic hormone is the major determinant of adrenal cortisol secretion. Exercise is associated with increased ACTH and cortisol secretion (Few [71]). The function of the elevated cortisol is not clear, but it may help maintain or re-establish normal glomerular filtration and enhance water diuresis.

Growth hormone rises during exercise, but the effect is markedly blunted when exercise is performed in a cold environment (Frewin et al. [72]) and is potentiated in persons adapted to high altitude (Raynaud et al. [73]). In diabetic subjects, when blood glucose is increased, GH response to exercise is more marked, and this effect is no longer evident when blood glucose is chronically normal (Tamborlane et al. [74]). Since atropine will block the exercise-induced rise in plasma GH, a cholinergic mechanism may mediate GH release during exercise (Few and Davies [75]).

A potential role for opioid peptide neuroregulation of GH secretion has been sought. In one study, administration of the opiate receptor blocker naloxone failed to alter the exercise-induced rise in GH (Mayer et al. [76]), while Spiler and Molitch [77] found that naloxone blunted the rise in GH induced by a similar bicycle ergometer work load. Further investigations are warranted to delineate a role for the opioids in the exercise-induced secretion of GH.

Growth hormone has a variety of metabolic effects that might be involved in adaptation to exercise. It increases glomerular filtration and enhances renal resorption of sodium chloride, thus potentially contributing to an expanded plasma volume. Growth hormone also increases renal resorption of magnesium and potassium; increases plasma volume, erythrocyte mass, and interstitial fluid volume; increases feee fatty acid release from fat cells; and increases blood glucose and muscle glycogen stores (Daughaday [78]). Whether GH is primarily responsible for these effects is not clear, since it may also modulate potent metabolic actions of other hormones.

Serum prolactin concentrations rise with strenuous exercise in men and in women (Smallridge et al. [79]; Hale et al. [80]; Baker et al. [81]). The prolactin rise may be enhanced by athletic training and improved physical conditioning compared with the untrained state (Roland et al. [82]; Brisson et al. [83]). Increased core temperature without exercise is a potent stimulus to prolactin secretion (Mills and Robertshaw [84]). Therefore, ambient and/or core temperature changes during exercise may modulate the observed prolactin responses (Frewin et al. [72]). The precise role of changes in core temperature during exercise under various environmental and internal physiologic conditions remains to be elucidated. In addition to temperature, several neuroendocrine mediators facilitating prolactin release have been proposed, including the dopaminergic system (Moretti et al. [85]) and opiate peptides (Faretti et al. [86]). The opiate peptide hypothesis seems especially attractive in view of the observation that opiate receptor blockade with naloxone infusion significantly decreases serum prolactin concentration in trained athletes.

The possible role of physiologic hyperprolactinemia during exercise has not been studied. Breast milk production is an established metabolic effect of prolactin. Numerous other metabolic actions have been suggested but remain controversial. Further study of exercise-induced prolactin secretion may provide a novel model by which to study extramammary prolactin effects. We have proposed a role for prolactin in renal water and salt retention by observing that chronically hyperprolactinemic women conserve iso-osmolar fluid during an acute water load (Buckman et al. [87]). This effect may occur directly at the kidney or via prolactin modulation of other hormonally mediated renal events as suggested from studies in animals (Mills et al. [88]). Prolactin's role in extracellular volume maintenance during acute exercise and volume expansion during chronic training remains to be clarified.

SUMMARY

Major secretory changes of anterior and posterior pituitary and adrenal hormones occur during exercise. These result from alterations in fluid distribution, catecholamine secretion, and other poorly understood mechanisms. The altered plasma hormones tend to restore effective intravascular volume by preventing salt and water loss through the kidneys and sweat glands. The renin–angiotensin–aldosterone and vasopressin systems, according to extensive studies, have a primary influence on fluid and electrolyte balance during exercise. Other hormones have been investigated, but their roles are not clearly defined. Growth hormone and possibly adrenocorticotropic hormone, through regulation of cortisol secretion, may influence metabolic changes that occur during exercise, other than those associated with salt and water balance. Although still controversial, a role for prolactin directly or indirectly in renal handling of solutes and water has been suggested.

REFERENCES

1. Shvartz, R., Bhattacharya, A., et al. 1979. Deconditioning-induced exercise responses as influenced by heat acclimation. Aviat Space Environ Med 50:893–897.
2. Plowman, S.A., Drinkwater, B.L., et al. 1979. Age and aerobic power in women: a longitudinal study. J Gerontol 34:512–520.
3. Knochel, J.P. 1974. Environmental heat illness. Arch Intern Med 133:841–864.
4. Ruderman, N.B., Ganda, O.P., et al. 1979. The effect of physical training on glucose tolerance and plasma lipids in maturity-onset diabetes. Diabetes 28 (Suppl. 1):89–101.
5. Pederson, O., Beck-Nielsen, H., et al. 1980. Increased insulin receptors after exercise in patients with insulin-dependent diabetes mellitus. N Engl J Med 302:886–890.
6. Cody, R.J., Atlas, S.A., et al. 1986. Atrial naturetic factor in normal subjects and heart failure patients. Plasma levels and renal, hormonal and hemodynamic responses to peptide infusion. J Clin Invest 78:1362–1374.
7. Solomon, S., Corwin, S., et al. In press. Atrial natriuretic factor and prolonged exertion in endurance trained subjects. Ann Sports Med.
8. Tobian, L., Tomboulian, A., et al. 1959.

The effect of high perfusion pressures on the granulation of juxtaglomerular cells in an isolated kidney. J Clin Invest 38: 605–610.

9. David, J.O., Freeman, R.H. 1976. Mechanisms regulating renin release. Physiol Rev 56:2–56.

10. Assaykeen, T.A., Ganong, W.R. 1971. The sympathetic nervous system and renin secretion. In: Martini, L., Ganong, W.F. (eds): Frontiers in Neuroendocrinology. Oxford University Press, London, pp 67–102.

11. Johnson, M.D., Fahri, E.R., et al. 1979. Plasma epinephrine and control of plasma renin activity: possible extrarenal mechanisms. Am J Physiol 236:854–859.

12. Reid, I.A., Morris, B.J. 1978. The renin-angiotensin system. Annu Rev Physiol 40:377–410.

13. Knochel, J.P. 1977. Aldosterone. In: Kurtzman, N.A., Martinez-Maldonado, M. (eds): Pathophysiology of the Kidney. Charles C Thomas, Springfield, IL, pp 446–472.

14. Sharp, G.W.G., Leaf, A. 1973. Effects of aldosterone and its mechanism of action on sodium transport. In: Orloff, J., Berliner, R.W. (eds): Handbook of Physiology-Renal Physiology. American Physiological Society, Washington, DC, pp 815–830.

15. Costill, D.L. 1977. Sweating: its composition and effects on body fluid. Ann NY Acad Sci 301:160–170.

16. Convertino, V.A., Keil, L.C., et al. 1981. Plasma volume, osmolality, vasopressin, and renin activity during graded exercise in man. J Appl Physiol 50:123–128.

17. Geyssant, A., Geelen, G., et al. 1981. Plasma vasopressin, renin activity, and aldosterone: effect of exercise and training. Eur J Appl Physiol 46:21–30.

18. Melin, B., Echache, J.P., et al. 1980. Plasma AVP, neurophysin, renin activity, and aldosterone during submaximal exercise performed until exhaustion in trained and untrained men. Eur J Appl Physiol 44:141–151.

19. Davies, J.A., Harrison, M.H., et al. 1981. Effect of saline loading during heat acclimatization on adrenocortical hormone levels. J Appl Physiol 150:605–612.

20. Barcroft, H. 1963. Circulation in skeletal muscle. In: Handbook of Physiology: A Critical Comprehensive Presentation of Physiologic Knowledge and Concepts (Vol. 3). Williams & Wilkins, Baltimore, MD, pp 1353–1386.

21. Schlein, E.M., Jensen, D., et al. 1973. The effect of plasma water loss on assessment of muscle metabolism during exercise. J Appl Physiol 34:568–572.

22. Convertino, V.A., Brock, P.J., et al. 1980. Exercise training-induced hypervolemia: role of plasma albumin, renin, and vasopressin. J Appl Physiol 48:665–669.

23. Benzinger, T.H. 1959. On physical heat regulation and the sense of temperature in man. Proc Natl Acad Sci USA 45:645–659.

24. Fasola, A.F., Martz, B.K., et al. 1966. Renin activity during supine exercise in normotensives and hypertensives. J Appl Physiol 21:1709–1712.

25. Kotchen, T.A., Hartley, L.H., et al. 1971. Renin, norepinephrine and epinephrine responses to graded exercise. J Appl Physiol 31:178–184.

26. Fagard, R.A., Reybrock, T., et al. 1978. Effect of angiotensin antagonism at rest and during exercise in sodium-depleted man. J Appl Physiol 45:403–407.

27. Barger, A.C., Berlin, R.D., et al. 1958. Infusion of aldosterone, 9-alpha-fluorohydocortisone and antidiuretic hormone into the renal artery of normal and adrenalectomized, unanesthetized dogs: effect on electrolyte and water excretion. Endocrinology 62:804–815.

28. Ganong, W.F., Mulrow, P.J. 1958. Rate of change in sodium and potassium excretion after injection of aldosterone into the aorta and renal artery of the dog. Am J Physiol 195:337–342.

29. Ross, E.J., Redy, W.J., et al. 1959. Effects of intravenous infusions of d,l-aldosterone acetate on sodium and potassium excretion in man. J Clin Endocrinol Metab 19:289–296.

30. Sonnenblick, E.H., Cannon, P.J., et al. 1961. The nature of the action of intravenous aldosterone: evidence for a role of the hormone in urinary dilution. J Clin Invest 40:903–913.

31. August, J.T., Nelson, D.H., et al. 1958. Response of normal subjects to large amounts of aldosterone. J Clin Invest 37:1549–1555.

32. Follenius, M., Brandburger, G., et al. 1979. Plasma aldosterone, prolactin and ACTH: relationships in man during heat exposure. Horm Metab Res 11:180–181.

33. Maher, J.T., Jones, L.G., et al. 1975. Aldosterone dynamics during graded exercise at sea level and high altitude. J Appl Physiol 39:18–22.

34. Hogan, R.P., Kotchen, T.A., et al. 1973. Effect of altitude on renin-aldosterone

system and metabolism of water and electrolytes. J Appl Physiol 35:385–390.

35. Keynes, R.J., Smith, G.W., et al. 1982. Renin and aldosterone at high altitude in man. J Endocrinol 92:131–140.

36. Milledge, J.S., Catley, D.M. 1982. Renin, aldosterone, and converting enzyme during exercise and acute hypoxia in humans. J Appl Physiol 52:320–323.

37. Colice, G.L., Ramirez, G. 1985. Effect of hypoxemia on the renin-angiotensin-aldosterone system in humans. J Appl Physiol 58:724–730.

38. Raff, H., Levy, S. 1986. Renin-angiotensin II-aldosterone and ACTH-cortisol control during acute hypoxemia and exercise in patients with chronic obstructive pulmonary disease. Am Rev Respir Dis 133:396–399.

39. Shigeoka, J.W., Colice, G.L., et al. 1985. Effect of normoxemic and hypooxemic exercise on renin and aldosterone. J Appl Physiol 59:142–148.

40. Francis, K.T., MacGregor, R. III. 1978. Effect of exercise in the heat on plasma renin and aldosterone with either water or a potassium-rich electrolyte solution. Aviat Space Environ Med 49:461–465.

41. Robinson, S., Robinson, A.H. 1954. Chemical composition of sweat. Physiol Rev 34:202–220.

42. Knochel, J.P., Dotin, L.N., et al. 1972. Pathophysiology of intense physical conditioning in a hot climate. J Clin Invest 51:242–255.

43. Opstad, P.K., Oktedalen, O., et al. 1985. Plasma renin activity and serum aldosterone during prolonged physical strain. Eur J Appl Physiol 54:1–6.

44. Faioli, F., Morett, C. 1980. Physical exercise stimulates marked concomitant release of β-endorphin and adrenocorticotropic hormone (ACTH) in peripheral blood in man. Experimentia 36:987–988.

45. Carr, D.B., Bullen, B.A., et al. 1981. Physical conditioning facilitates the exercise-induced secretion of beta-endorphin and beta-lipotropin in women. N Engl J Med 305:560–563.

46. Gambert, S.R., Garthwaite, T.L., et al. 1981. Running elevated plasma β-endorphin immunoreactivity and ACTH in untrained human subjects. Proc Soc Exp Biol Med 168:1–4.

47. Brammert, J., Hokfelt, B. 1985. Lack of effect of naloxone in moderate dosage on the exercise-induced increase in blood pressure, heart rate, plasma catecholamines, plasma renin activity and plasma aldosterone in healthy males. Clin Sci 68:185–191.

48. Grossman, A.P. Boulous, P., et al. 1984. The role of opioid peptides in the hormonal responses to acute exercise in man. Clin Sci 67:483–491.

49. Staessen, J., Cattaert, A., et al. 1984. Hemodynamic and humoral effect of prostaglandin inhibition in exercising humans. J Appl Physiol 56:39–45.

50. Lijnen, P., Hespel, P., et al. 1985. Urinary excretion of electrolytes during prolonged physical activity in normal man. Eur J Appl Physiol 53:317–321.

51. Castenfors, J. 1967. Renal clearances and urinary sodium and potassium excretion during supine exercise in normal subjects. Acta Physiol Scand 70:207–214.

52. Dobrev, D., Stefanova, D., et al. 1969. Veranderungen des Gasaustausches und der biochemis chenBlut and Herzzusammensetzung von Teilnehmern und Marathonschwimmen. Med Sport 9:276–279.

53. Carraz, G., Pin, G., et al. 1960. Fatigue, potassium et corticoides [Fatigue, potassium, and corticoids]. Med Educ Phys Sport 34:299–305.

54. Robertson, G.L., Athar, S., et al. 1977. Osmotic control of vasopressin function. In: Andreoli, T.E., Grantham, J.J., et al. (eds): Disturbances in Body Fluid Osmolality. American Physiological Society, Bethesda, MD, pp 125–148.

55. Robertson, G.L., Athar, S. 1971. The interaction of blood osmolality and blood volume in regulating plasma vasopressin in man. J Clin Endocrinol Metab 42:613–620.

56. McCance, R.A. 1936. Experimental sodium chloride deficiency in man. Proc R Soc Lond (Biol) 119:245–268.

57. Moore, W.A. 1971. Antidiuretic hormone levels in normal subjects. Fed Proc 30:1387–1394.

58. Castenfors, J. 1977. Renal function during prolonged exercise. Ann NY Acad Sci 301:151–159.

59. Refsum, H.E., Stromme, S.B. 1978. Renal osmol clearance during prolonged heavy exercise. Scand J Clin Lab Invest 38:19–22.

60. Williams, E.S., Ward, M.P., et al. 1979. Effect of the exercise of seven consecutive days' hill-walking on fluid homeostasis. Clin Sci Mol Med 56:305–316.

61. Wade, C.E., Claybaugh, J.R. 1980. Plasma renin activity, vasopressin concentration, and urinary excretory responses to exercise in men. J Appl Physiol 49:930–936.

62. Nielsen, B., Sjogaard G., et al. 1984. Cardiovascular, hormonal and body fluid

changes during prolonged exercise. Eur J Appl Physiol 53:63–70.

63. Convertino, V.A., Keil, L.C., et al. 1983. Plasma volume, renin, and vasopressin responses to graded exercise after training. J Appl Physiol 54:508–14.

64. Vallotton, M., Merkelbach, U., et al. 1983. Studies of the factors modulating antidiuretic hormone excretion in man in response to the osmolar stimulus: effects of oestrogen and angiotensin II. Acta Endocrinol (Copenh) 104:295–302.

65. Dessypris, A., Wager, G., et al. 1983. Marathon run: effects on blood cortisol—ACTH, iodothyronines—TSH and vasopressin. Acta Endocrinol (Copenh) 95(2):151–157.

66. Maresh, C.M., Wang, B.C., et al. 1985. Plasma vasopressin, renin activity, and aldosterone responses to maximal exercise in active college females. Eur J Appl Physiol 54:398–403.

67. Schrier, R.W., Berl, T., et al. 1977. Nonosmolar control of renal water excretion. In: Andreoli, T.E., Grantham, J.J., et al. (eds): Disturbances in Body Fluid Osmolality. Williams & Wilkins, Baltimore, MD, pp 149–178.

68. Oliw, E. 1979. Prostaglandins and kidney function. Acta Physiol Scand (Suppl) 461:1–55.

69. Share, L., Claybaugh, R.J. 1972. Regulation of body fluids. Annu Rev Physiol 34:235–260.

70. Zambraski, E., Dunn, M. 1979. Renal prostaglandin (PG) secretion in exercising dogs. Fed Proc 38:893.

71. Few, J.D. 1974. Effect of exercise on the secretion and metabolism of cortisol in man. J Endocrinol 62:341–353.

72. Frewin, D.B., Frantz, A.G., et al. 1976. The effect of ambient temperature on the growth hormone and prolactin response to exercise. Aust J Exp Biol Med Sci 54:97–101.

73. Raynaud, J., Drouet, L., et al. 1981. Time course of plasma growth hormone during exercise in humans at altitude. J Appl Physiol 50:229–233.

74. Tamborlane, W.V., Sherwin, R.S., et al. 1979. Normalization of the growth hormone and catecholamine response to exercise in juvenile-onset diabetic subjects treated with a portable insulin infusion pump. Diabetes 28:785–788.

75. Few, J.D., Davies, C.T.M. 1980. The inhibiting effect of atropine on growth hormone release during exercise. Eur J Appl Physiol 43:221–228.

76. Mayer, G., Wessel, J., et al. 1980. Failure of naloxone to alter exercise-induced growth hormone and prolactin release in normal men. Clin Endocrinol 13:413–416.

77. Spiler, I.J., Molitch, M.E. 1980. Lack of modulation of pituitary hormones stress response by neural pathways involving opiate receptors. J Clin Endocrinol Metab 50:516–520.

78. Daughaday, W.H. 1981. The adenohypophysis. In: Williams R. (ed): Textbook of Endocrinology. W.B. Saunders, Philadelphia, pp 87–92.

79. Smallridge, R., Whorton, N., et al. 1985. Effects of exercise and physical fitness on the pituitary-thyroid axis and on prolactin secretion in male runners. Metabolism 34:949–954.

80. Hale, R., Kosasa, T., et al. 1983. A marathon: the immediate effect on female runners' luteinizing hormone, follicle-stimulating hormone, prolactin, testosterone, and cortisol levels. Obstet Gynecol 146:550.

81. Baker, E., Mathur, R., et al. 1982. Plasma gonadotropins, prolactin, and steroid hormone concentrations in female runners immediately after a long-distance run. Fertil Steril 38:38–41.

82. Roland, E., Reggani, E., et al. 1985. Comparison of pituitary responses to physical exercise in athletes and sedentary subjects. Horm Res 21:209–213.

83. Brisson, G., Volle, A., et al. 1980. Exercise-induced dissociation of the blood prolactin response in young women according to their sports habits. Horm Metab Res 12:201–205.

84. Mills, D., Robertshaw, D. 1981. Response of plasma prolactin to changes in ambient temperature and humidity in man. J Clin Endocrinol Metab 52:279–283.

85. Moretti, C., Fabbri, A., et al. 1982. Pyridoxine (B6) suppresses the rise in prolactin and increases the rise in growth hormone induced exercise. N Engl J Med 8:444.

86. Faretti, A., Fabbri, L., et al. 1983. Naloxone inhibits exercise-induced release of PRL and GH in athletes. Endocrinology 18:135–138.

87. Buckman, M.T., Peake, G.T., et al. 1976. Hyperprolactinemia influences renal function in man. Metabolism 25:509–516.

88. Mills, D.E., Buckman, M.T., et al. 1983. Mineralocorticoid modulation of prolactin in effect on renal solute excretion in the rat. Endocrinology 112:823–828.

.9.

Exercise and the Menstrual Cycle

Karen Carlberg, Glenn T. Peake,
and Maire T. Buckman

As women become more active in recreational and competitive athletics, scientific interest in the female's response to exercise continues to grow. An aspect of exercise physiology unique to women concerns the relation of the menstrual cycle to exercise. This chapter summarizes current knowledge about the effects of the menstrual cycle on exercise performance and the effects of regular physical exercise on menstrual function. Physiologic responses to exercise throughout the normal menstrual cycle are described and the effects of regular physical exercise on premenstrual and menstrual symptoms are discussed. Finally, the chapter examines a topic that has attracted considerable research interest in the last few years: The disruption or cessation of the menstrual cycle that sometimes accompanies athletic training.

EFFECTS OF THE MENSTRUAL CYCLE ON EXERCISE PERFORMANCE

It might be expected that fluctuations in sex hormone levels during the normal menstrual cycle would influence exercise performance, since estrogens and progesterone are known to affect a variety of physiologic variables. In addition, the symptoms of premenstrual syndrome, on the days just prior to menstruation, and dysmenorrhea, during menstruation itself, might affect exercise performance in the women who experience these symptoms. Many researchers have studied the effects of menstrual cycle phase on many different parameters of exercise performance. In general, results of these studies have been contradictory and inconclusive.

In several questionnaire studies athletes have been asked to assess their performance during different phases of the menstrual cycle. Erdelyi [1] reviewed several such studies, which revealed that during the menstrual flow 31–48% of the athletes believed that their performance was worse, 42–48% reported no change, and 13–15% claimed to have a better performance. Erdelyi concluded that in most women performance is best in the "postmenstrual" phase and poorest during the "premenstrual" phase and first 2 days of menstruation. Similarly, among 66 participants in the Tokyo Olympics surveyed by

Zaharieva [2], 17% stated that their performance was worse during menstruation, 37% said it made no difference, and 28% reported variable effects.

Evaluation of "perceived exertion" with a questionnaire administered during or immediately after an exercise bout provides a standard technique for measuring the subjective perception of difficulty for a given work load. Perceived exertion is sometimes but not always affected by menstrual phase. Women tested by Higgs and Robertson [3] had a higher perceived exertion during maximal treadmill running (100% maximal oxygen consumption [$\dot{V}O_{2\ max}$]) 2 days prior to and on the day of menstruation onset compared to mid-cycle. However, at 90% $\dot{V}O_{2\ max}$ there were no differences in perceived exertion at different cycle phases. Stephenson et al. [4] found no menstrual cycle effect on perceived exertion at five work loads ranging from 25–100% $\dot{V}O_{2\ max}$ on a bicycle ergometer. Similarly Eston [5] reported no differences in perceived exertion over four menstrual cycle phases in women exercising at 70% and 90% $\dot{V}O_{2\ max}$ on a bicycle ergometer. Thus, perceived exertion may be highest around the onset of menstruation for maximal work loads, but for submaximal work loads menstrual phase appears to have little effect.

The maximal capacity for aerobic exercise can be evaluated by measuring $\dot{V}O_{2\ max}$ or time to exhaustion at a given high work load. These values have been affected by menstrual phase in some but not all studies. Jurkowski et al. [6] reported a longer time to exhaustion during the luteal phase compared with the follicular phase for women exercising on a bicycle ergometer. Conversely, Schoene et al. [7] found a lower $\dot{V}O_{2\ max}$ and shorter time to exhaustion during the luteal phase compared with the follicular phase in women performing cycle ergometry. Higgs and Robertson [3] found that time to exhaustion was lowest 2 days prior to and on the day of menstruation onset during treadmill running. On the other hand, Stephenson et al. [8] reported no menstrual cycle effects on peak oxygen uptake or time to exhaustion in women exercising on a bicycle ergometer. Thus, the evidence for an effect of menstrual phase on maximal aerobic capacity is quite contradictory.

In a study on the effect of menstrual phase on swimming performance (Brooks-Gunn et al. [9]), 4 adolescent competitive swimmers consistently swam their fastest times during menstruation and their slowest times during the 4 days prior to menstruation onset.

Heart rate responses to maximal or submaximal exercise are usually unaffected by menstrual cycle phase (Higgs and Robertson [3]; Jurkowski et al. [6]; Eston [5]). Cardiac output is also unaffected (Jurkowski et al. [6]).

Respiration during exercise may or may not be affected by menstrual cycle phase. Schoene et al. [7] studied ventilatory responses to ergometer exercise. Ventilatory drive, as shown by resting minute ventilation, ventilatory equivalent ($VE/\dot{V}O_2$) during exercise, and ventilatory responses to hypoxia and hypercapnia, was increased in the luteal phase compared with the follicular phase. On the other hand, no menstrual cycle effects were found by Jurkowski et al. [6, 10] on exercise minute ventilation or by Stephenson et al. [4] on exercise minute ventilation, respiratory frequency, or tidal volume.

Some metabolic responses to exercise may be affected by menstrual cycle phase. Jurkowski et al. [6] reported a higher blood lactic acid concentration after heavy and exhaustive exercise in the follicular phase compared with the luteal phase. The rate of lactate disappearance was unaffected, so apparently lactate production was higher in the follicular phase. Bonen et al. [11] studied responses to treadmill walking during the follicular and luteal phases; women were studied in fasted, glucose-loaded, and control states. In the glucose-loaded state, the free fatty acid response to exercise was lower during the luteal phase. In the fasted state, the insulin and growth hormone responses were exaggerated in the luteal phase. Other factors, including blood glucose, lactate, glycerol, and cortisol, were unaffected by menstrual cycle phase. The authors concluded that nutritional status of the subjects is an important consideration in studying menstrual cycle effects on metabolic responses to exercise.

The high progesterone levels of the luteal phase cause a well-known elevation in basal body temperature. Thus, it might be expected that body temperature during exercise would be affected as well. This seems to be true when exercise is performed at normal room temperature, but the menstrual phase effects usually disappear when women exercise in a hot environment. When Stephenson and Kolka [8] exercised women with bicycle ergometry at 23° C, rectal temperatures were slightly higher at mid-cycle and during the luteal phase than they were during menstruation or at mid-follicular phase. However, in hot enviroments ranging from 28° C to 48° C temperature regulatory responses to exercise were unaffected by menstrual phase (Wells and Horvath [12]; Frye et al. [13]; Horvath and Drinkwater [14]). On the other hand, Stephenson and Kolka [15] reported higher body temperatures and higher thresholds for cutaneous vasodilation and sweating in women exercising at 35° C during the luteal phase compared with the follicular phase.

Menstrual phase differences were reported for vascular volume dynamics during exercise in the heat by Gaebelein and Senay [16]. Women were tested during the follicular and luteal phases of the menstrual cycle in hyperhydrated and hypohydrated states. During the follicular phase, particularly following hypohydration, there were more rapid increases in hemoglobin concentration and osmoconcentration, as well as decreases in plasma volume. The authors speculated that higher aldosterone levels associated with the high progesterone levels of the luteal phase may have been responsible for the menstrual phase differences.

In summary, most physiological responses to exercise do not appear to be significantly affected by the hormonal fluctuations or discomforts associated with the menstrual cycle. Exceptions may include some aspects of metabolism and fluid dynamics. The subjects' states of nutrition, hydration, and training may influence experimental results. Intersubject variability is probably considerable and may mask cyclic variations that may be present in some women but not others. For additional reviews, see Jurkowski [17], Eston [5], and Brooks-Gunn et al. [18].

EFFECTS OF EXERCISE ON
PREMENSTRUAL AND MENSTRUAL SYMPTOMS

Premenstrual syndrome (PMS) includes a variety of physiologic and psychologic symptoms occurring during the mid- to late luteal phase of the menstrual cycle. Although PMS is experienced by a large percentage of women, its etiology is not understood (Reid and Yen [19]). Primary dysmenorrhea refers to the pain associated with uterine contractions or ischemia during menstruation. It is believed to be caused by prostaglandins released by the endometrium (Beacham and Beacham [20]). While clinicians sometimes recommend exercise to alleviate these symptoms (Shangold [21]; Havens [22]), there is only a small amount of evidence to support these recommendations.

Several questionnaire studies have been conducted in an attempt to evaluate the effects of exercise training on premenstrual or menstrual symptoms. In a study of 107 Finnish athletes (Ingman [23]), 13% of the women reported a reduction in menstrual pain during training, and 3% reported an increase in menstrual pain during training. Erdelyi [1] studied menstrual cycles in 729 Hungarian athletes, using questionnaires, interviews, and menstrual charts. During training, "unfavorable changes," mostly dysmenorrhea, were found in 18% of athletes under age 18 and in 7% of athletes age 18 and older. Timonen and Procope [24] compared premenstrual and menstrual symptoms in 136 physical education students and 612 university students. The athletic women reported less frequent menstrual pelvic pain, low back pain, headache, anxiety, depression, fatigue, and use of analgesics. There were no differences between the groups in premenstrual pain or edema. Ronkainen et al. [25] mailed questionnaires to 121 Finnish national-level distance runners, 103 skiers, and 83 volleyball players; response rate was 50%. The runners and skiers reported less frequent dysmenorrhea than did the control group (43% vs 64%), while the volleyball players did not differ significantly from the control group in frequency of dysmenorrhea (61% vs 76%). When asked whether physical training affected symptoms of dysmenorrhea, 32% of the runners and skiers and 36% of the volleyball players said that their symptoms were alleviated, 18% and 23% said that their symptoms were aggravated, and 27% and 18% said that exercise did not affect their symptoms.

Golub et al. [26] prescribed a program of calisthenic exercises for 302 junior high school students and questioned them twice yearly for 3 years about premenstrual and menstrual symptoms and regularity in performing the exercises. By the end of the third year, dysmenorrhea had developed in 61% of the girls who did not perform the exercises regularly and in 39% of the girls who continued to exercise. In a controlled prospective study, Prior et al. [27] demonstrated a decrease in premenstrual symptoms during a running exercise training program. The conditioned subjects had fewer breast and fluid symptoms and a decrease in overall molimina. No change in menstrual cycles or reproductive hormones occurred with the training schedule.

In summary, regular physical exercise may improve premenstrual or menstrual symptoms in some women, but other women report a worsening of symptoms or no effects. Shangold [21] suggested that exercise-induced secretion of endorphins or vasodilating prostaglandins may explain the beneficial effects of exercise. However, no studies have attempted to define a mechanism. Further research is needed to provide a better understanding of the effects of exercise on premenstrual and menstrual symptoms. For a more comprehensive review, see Brooks-Gunn et al. [18].

EFFECTS OF ATHLETIC TRAINING ON MENSTRUAL FUNCTION

In the last few years it has become evident that athletic women have a higher incidence of menstrual abnormalities than do nonathletic women. Dancers frequently have menstrual disturbances as well. Common abnormalities include amenorrhea, oligomenorrhea, short luteal phase, and delayed menarche. Despite considerable research activity in this area, the reason for exercise-associated menstrual disturbances is still unknown. Scientific recognition of this phenomenon is too recent for there to be much knowledge about the long-term consequences of exercise-related menstrual dysfunction. At present, the only known significant risk is a loss of bone mineral content similar to that seen in other hypoestrogenic states. In this section the types of menstrual abnormalities that have been characterized in athletes and dancers are described, the various findings of studies in this area are compared, and current recommendations for the treatment of exercise-associated menstrual dysfunction are presented.

Menstrual Disturbances Associated with Athletics and Dance

Oligomenorrhea and Secondary Amenorrhea Oligomenorrhea (infrequent menstruation) and secondary amenorrhea (cessation of menstruation after menarche has occurred) are known to be more common in athletes and dancers than in nonathletic women. Among young, healthy, nonathletic women, 2–5% have secondary amenorrhea (Pettersson et al. [28]; Singh [29]; Bachmann and Kemmann [30]). Among athletes and dancers, the reported frequencies of menstrual disturbances depend on the level of physical activity and on the definitions used for oligomenorrhea and amenorrhea (Lutter [31]).

Large groups of athletes have been surveyed for menstrual characteristics by several investigators. Dale et al. [32] studied 90 runners (more than 30 mile/week), 24 joggers (5–30 mile/week), and 54 nonrunners. Amenorrhea (0–5 menses/year) was present in 24% of the runners, 14% of the joggers, and none of the nonrunners. Lutter and Cushman [33] gave questionnaires to 350 participants in a marathon and a 10-km race. Three percent had not menstruated for at least a year, and 14% menstruated sporadically or no more than every 3 months. Carlberg et al. [34] surveyed 252 college varsity athletes competing in 9 sports and 426 nonathletic college students. Oligo/amenorrhea (no menstrual periods in the previous 3 months or 4 or fewer periods in the previous year) was reported by 12.1% of the athletes and 2.6% of the controls. Oian et al. [35] received 179 questionnaire responses from Norwegian national team members in 27 sports. Ten percent of the women had not menstruated in at least 4 months.

Menstrual function in 475 Nigerian athletes was compared with that in 606 nonathletes (Toriola and Mathur [36]). Irregular menses, oligomenorrhea, or secondary amenorrhea was more common in the athletes. Of the groups of athletes studied, long-distance runners (51%) and ball-game players (36%) most commonly experienced oligomenorrhea. Dysmenorrhea and menorrhagia were more common among the swimmers (37%) and sprinters (42%). Menstrual dysfunction in the athletes was associated with low body fat, low body weight, low relative weight for height, and the stress of the sports activity.

Similar surveys of menstrual function have been done for ballet dancers. Of 89 professional ballet students questioned by Frisch et al. [37], 15% reported secondary amenorrhea (no menses during the previous 3 months), and 9 dancers age 16 or older had primary amenorrhea. Cohen et al. [38] reported that 37% of 30 professional ballet dancers had not menstruated in at least 3 months. Thus, for both athletes and ballet dancers, the prevalence of oligomenorrhea and secondary amenorrhea is consistently higher than that measured in control groups or in large populations of nonathletic women.

Short Luteal Phase The luteal phase of the menstrual cycle may be shortened by regular strenuous exercise in some susceptible women. Shangold et al. [39] monitored 18 menstrual cycles by cervical mucus changes and basal body temperatures in one distance runner. Luteal phase lengths were negatively correlated with mileage run during the follicular phase: Luteal phase was 13–14 days when mileage was less than 5 miles/week and 9 days or less when mileage was greater than 35 miles/week. In this same runner, midluteal progesterone levels were nearly 3 times higher in 3 "control cycles," with little or no running, compared with 3 "training cycles," in which 16–32 miles were run per week.

Prior et al. [40] monitored 48 menstrual cycles by basal body temperatures in 14 women training for the marathon. Sixteen cycles had luteal phases shorter than 10 days and 16 cycles were monophasic, despite normal total cycle lengths for all women. Abnormal cycles were associated with longer training runs. In a more extensive study of two runners, Prior et al. [41] documented luteal phase shortening associated with increased running, which progressed to anovulation in one woman.

Bullen et al. [42] conducted a prospective study of 28 initially untrained women. During an exercise training program, hormone measurements revealed abnormal luteal function in half the women, which progressed to loss of the mid-cycle luteinizing hormone surge in the majority.

In summary, inadequate luteal function may be a common, subtle response to exercise training and may exist with normal total menstrual cycle lengths. The short luteal phase may be associated with infertility (Strott et al. [43]). The data of Prior et al. [41] and Bullen et al. [42] suggest that shortened luteal phases may be an early step in a progression toward anovulation and amenorrhea.

Delayed Menarche Several large survey studies have shown mean age at menarche to be later in athletes than in nonathletic women. For example, mean age at menarche was 13.6 years in 66 collegiate track and field athletes, compared with 12.2 years for 30 college students (Malina et al. [44]); 14.2 years in 18 Olympic volleyball players, compared with 12.3 years in 110 nonathletes (Malina et al. [45]); and 13.4 years in 254 athletes, compared with 12.9 years in 426 control subjects (Carlberg et al. [34]).

Frisch et al. [46] demonstrated that athletes who began training prior to menarche began menstruating later than did athletes who began training after menarche and control subjects; mean ages at menarche were 15.1 years, 12.8 years, and 12.7 years, respectively. Ronkainen et al. [25] found that for runners and skiers, starting training before menarche resulted in greater delays in menarche, thelarche, and pubarche than did starting training after menarche.

While it seems likely that strenuous training can delay puberty, Malina et al. [45] suggested that late-maturing girls may be more likely to excel in sports for both anthropomorphic and social reasons. Stager et al. [47] supported this hypothesis with data showing an association between superior athletic performance and late menarche within a large group of swimmers.

Menarche is delayed in ballet dancers as well. Of 89 ballet students studied by Frisch et al. [37], 69 had undergone menarche at a mean age of 13.7 years, and 20 were still premenarcheal. None of the premenarcheal dancers were older than age 16. Warren [48] followed 15 young ballet dancers for 4 years. Mean age at menarche was 15.4 years. In 10 girls menarche occurred during forced rest due to injury, and in most girls amenorrhea returned with a return to normal physical activity.

Frisch and colleagues have noted that athletes and dancers who begin training prior to menarche or who reach menarche at a late age are more likely to experience menstrual disturbances in later years (Frisch et al. [37, 46]).

Brisson and Dulac [49] emphasized that menarche is a late event in pubertal development, and that earlier neuroendocrine events, including adrenarche and gonadarche, should be considered when studying the effects of physical activity on pubertal development. Malina [50] stated that it is difficult to implicate training as a factor that specifically delays menarche and that the biologic and social factors associated with late menarche must be considered as well.

Factors Associated with Exercise-Related Menstrual Disturbances

When active women with menstrual dysfunction are compared with their peers with normal menstruation, several differences can be seen between the two groups. The factors most often associated with menstrual dysfunction are high levels of exercise intensity and duration and low levels of body weight and body fat.

Exercise Intensity and Duration If physical exercise is causally related to menstrual abnormalities, then high levels of exercise intensity and duration should be associated with higher incidences of menstrual dysfunction. This does seem to be true. Among runners, the amenorrheic women often run farther and faster than do runners who continue to menstruate normally. Feicht et al. [51] found that the incidence of secondary amenorrhea rose from 6% in women running about 10 miles/week to 43% in women running about 80 miles/week. Amenorrheic runners had significantly faster times in the 1500-m race than regularly menstruating runners. Oligo/amenorrheic runners studied by Carlberg et al. [34] averaged 79 km/week compared with 60 km/week for regularly menstruating runners. Oligo/amenorrheic runners studied by Gray and Dale [52] trained at a faster pace than menstruating runners, although weekly mileage was similar.

It appears that participation in almost any sport is associated with a high likelihood of menstrual disturbances. Amenorrhea was reported in 26% of runners, 12% of swimmers, and 12% of cyclists studied by Sanborn et al. [53]. The prevalence of amenorrhea increased with training mileage only among the runners, however. Among athletes surveyed by Carlberg et al. [34], oligo/amenorrhea was more common in each of the 9 sports studied (range 6–18%) than in the control population (2.6%), with the highest incidence among the distance runners.

Body Weight and Composition Extremely low body weight and weight loss are well-known causes of menstrual abnormalities (Fries et al. [54]; Warren [55]; Frisch [56]). It is also well known that athletes often have lower body weights and lower body fat ratios than the average for nonathletic women. The percentage of body fat is commonly between 5 and 20 in athletes (Malina et al. [57]; Wilmore et al. [58]; Sinning [59]) compared with 20–29% for young nonathletic women (Young [60]; Sloan et al. [61]; Wilmore and Behnke [62]). Thus, one of the earliest hypotheses about exercise-related menstrual dysfunction was that it might be attributed to the low percentage of body fat common among athletes (Wilmore et al. [58]).

Many investigators have reported lower average body weights or percentages of body fat in athletes with menstrual dysfunction compared with menstruating athletes. For example, amenorrheic marathon runners surveyed by Shangold and Levine [63] were significantly lighter than regularly menstruating runners. Sanborn et al. [53] found the highest prevalence of amenorrhea among athletes with the highest total body water/body weight ratios (i.e., lowest percent body fat). Of oligo/amenorrheic athletes studied by Carlberg et al. [34], those weighing less than 55 kg tended to be totally amenorrheic, whereas those weighing more than 55 kg continued to menstruate sporadically. Hydrostatic weighing studies conducted by Carlberg et al. [64] indicated that compared with regularly menstruating athletes, oligo/amenorrheic athletes were significantly lower in both fat weight and lean body weight, as well as total body weight. Amenorrheic ballet dancers also tend to be lighter than dancers who continue to menstruate (Frisch et al. [37]; Cohen et al. [38]).

On the other hand, among women with relatively low body weights, changes in menstrual patterns sometimes correlate with changes in activity levels that are not accompanied by changes in body weight or body composition. Such observations have been made in runners (Prior et al. [40]), swimmers (Russell et al. [65]), and ballet dancers (Warren [48]; Abraham et al. [66]).

There may be a synergistic interaction between low body weight and physical activity such that thin women are more susceptible to exercise-induced menstrual changes and physically active women are more susceptible to weight-loss-induced menstrual changes (Vandenbroucke et al. [67]; Carlberg et al. [34]). Bullen et al. [68] documented such an interaction in their prospective study of 28 initially untrained women. While exercise training was accompanied by menstrual disruptions in both their groups of subjects, the menstrual disturbances were more severe in the weight-loss group than in the weight-maintenance group.

The mechanism of interaction between low body weight and reproductive function is not clear. Nonathletic women suffering weight loss-related amenorrhea have numerous aberrations in hypothalamic function, including hypothalamic–pituitary regulatory mechanisms and thermoregulation (Vigersky et al. [69]). In addition, steroid hormones are metabolized to a considerable extent in adipose and muscle tissues, and therefore changes in body composition can alter endocrine function (Siiteri and MacDonald [70]; Fishman et al. [71]; Longcope et al. [72, 73]). Whether low body weight in oligo/amenorrheic athletes and dancers exerts its influence on the hypothalamus, on peripheral steroid metabolism, or on both, has not been determined.

Other Factors Associated with Exercise-Related Menstrual Disturbances Many other factors appear to be associated with exercise-related menstrual disturbances. One is age. Menstrual dysfunction is more common in younger athletes (Speroff and Redwine [74]; Baker et al. [75]). Age affects the incidence of menstrual irregularities in nonathletic women as well (Pettersson et al. [28]).

A history of menstrual irregularity prior to initiation of athletic training may predispose women to exercise-associated menstrual disruption. Shangold and Levine [63] stated that most oligo/amenorrheic runners had similar menstrual patterns before and after beginning intensive training. Schwartz et al. [76] reported that significantly more amenorrheic runners had a history of past irregularity than did normally menstruating runners. However, other investigators have described amenorrheic athletes who claimed to have normal menstrual cycles prior to beginning athletic training (Baker et al. [75]; Carlberg et al. [34]).

Prior pregnancy may protect a woman from exercise-related menstrual disruption. Several investigators have found that amenorrhea is more common among nulliparous athletes than among parous athletes (Dale et al. [77]; Baker et al. [75]; Carlberg et al. [34]). This is also true for nonathletic women (Pettersson et al. [28]). It is not known whether pregnancy somehow affects the hypothalamic–pituitary–ovarian axis to make menstrual disruption less likely, or whether women who are more susceptible to menstrual disturbances are less fertile and therefore less likely to become pregnant.

Diet may influence the menstrual response to athletic training. An association between vegetarianism and menstrual dysfunction in athletes has been noted by several investigators (Carlberg et al. [34]; Frisch [78]; Slavin et al. [79]). A prospective 7-day dietary history administered by Schwartz et al. [76] showed that amenorrheic runners consumed a smaller percentage of their total intake as protein. Deuster et al. [80] obtained 3-day diet records on amenorrheic and eumenorrheic athletes, matched for height, weight, body fat (11–12%) and training distance (113 km/week). Fat intake was lower in the amenorrheic athletes (66 g/day) than in eumenorrheic athletes (97 g/day). Also, zinc intake was very low (10.6 g/day), and plasma zinc levels were lower in the amenorrheic athletes. Surprisingly, the amenorrheic athletes consumed large quantities of vitamin A and dietary fiber. Nelson et al. [81] also used a 3-day diet record to assess nutritional status in eumenorrheic and amenorrheic runners and found that amenorrheic runners had a lower daily caloric intake and a decreased protein intake, which was below the United States Recommended Daily Allowance in 82% of these athletes. However, calcium intake was no different in amenorrheic and eumenorrheic athletes in this study.

Psychologic or emotional stress is a plausible factor in exercise-related menstrual disturbances. Stress and amenorrhea or infertility are sometimes associated in nonathletic women (Seibel and Taymor [82]). It might be that athletes, particularly college varsity athletes, are exposed to more stress than are nonathletes from pressures associated with competition and time commitments. Galle et al. [83] administered a standard psychologic test to runners and found that the amenorrheic women scored significantly higher than regularly menstruating women on obsessive–compulsive behavior and psychoticism and only slightly higher on 7 other measures of emotional distress. Schwartz et al. [76] found that amenorrheic runners associated more stress with their running than did menstruating runners, but did not differ in depression, hypochondriasis, anxiety, or obsessive–compulsive tendencies. Loucks and Horvath [84] did not see any differences between amenorrheic and normally menstruating runners in any traits measured by two psychologic tests. Thus, the available data on psychologic characteristics of amenorrheic athletes are contradictory and deserve further study.

There may be a genetic, or at least familial, component to an athlete's susceptibility to exercise-related menstrual disruption. Carlberg et al. [85] observed similar menstrual responses to athletic training in 4 out of 5 pairs of sisters, including 3 sets of identical twins.

The factors associated with the initiation of menstrual disturbances were also nearly the same within each sister group.

Endocrine Function in Athletes with Menstrual Disturbances

There has been considerable research on endocrine function in athletes with menstrual disturbances. The focus has been on the female reproductive hormones and on hormones that are known to be stimulated by exercise and to have inhibitory effects on the reproductive system. In general, gonadotropic and ovarian hormone secretion is low, as is the case in a variety of other forms of menstrual dysfunction. Several hormonal systems have been investigated as possible links between exercise-induced stress responses and gonadal suppression: the hypothalamic–pituitary–adrenal axis, prolactin, androgens, and β-endorphin.

Ovarian Steroids   Secretion of ovarian hormones is consistently low in athletes with menstrual disturbances. The short luteal phase defect has been characterized by subnormal mid-luteal estradiol, and particularly progesterone, levels (Shangold et al. [39]; Bullen et al. [68]). In amenorrheic athletes, plasma levels of estradiol and progesterone tend to remain near normal early follicular phase values with no cyclic increases (Dale et al. [32]; Boyden et al. [86]; Bullen et al. [68]). Most investigators consider the low steroid levels to be a result of inadequate gonadotropin stimulation of the ovaries.

Gonadotropins   Gonadotropin secretion appears to be suppressed in amenorrheic athletes. In particular, the mid-cycle gonadotropin surge is apparently absent, and the pulsatile pattern of gonadotropin secretion is abnormal. These abnormalities are presumed to result from deficient secretion of gonadotropin-releasing hormone (GnRH) by the hypothalamus. Thus, the problem apparently lies with the hypothalamus rather than the pituitary gland. When gonadotropin levels have been measured in single resting blood samples taken from amenorrheic athletes, concentrations of luteinizing hormone (LH) and follicle-stimulating hormone (FSH) have been reported to be slightly below, slightly above, or the same as those in control subjects, but never very far from the normal follicular range (Baker et al. [75]; Schwartz et al. [76]; Loucks and Horvath [84]). Bullen et al. [68] documented a loss of the mid-cycle LH surge in untrained women who underwent an exercise training program and developed menstrual abnormalities. In oligomenorrheic or amenorrheic runners, gonadotropin response to synthetic GnRH was found to be normal (Wakat et al. [87]; Veldhuis et al. [88]), supranormal (Yahiro et al. [89]), or subnormal (Boyden et al. [90]). Detailed studies of spontaneous gonadotropin pulsatile secretory patterns have shown abnormalities in both menstruating and amenorrheic runners. Veldhuis et al. [88] found a reduction in LH pulse frequency without any alteration in 24-hr integrated plasma concentrations of LH or FSH in amenorrheic runners. Cumming et al. [91] reported reductions in LH pulse frequency, LH pulse amplitude, and area under the curve over 6 hr for normally menstruating runners compared with sedentary controls. The same normally menstruating runners were followed for an additional 6 hr after a 60-min run and were found to have a further reduction in LH pulse frequency without further reductions in LH pulse amplitude or 6-hr integrated LH levels (Cumming et al. [92]). Thus, LH pulse frequency appears to be the aspect of gonadotropin function most affected by exercise. Reduced frequency of GnRH secretion is presumed to be a common mechanism in various forms of hypothalamic amenorrhea (Reame et al. [93]), and this would be expected to account for the reduced LH pulse frequency observed in these states.

Prolactin   Four hormone systems are known to be stimulated by exercise and to inhibit reproductive systems; these have been investigated with regard to exercise-related menstrual disturbances. The earliest hypothesis was that exercise-induced prolactin secretion inhibited the hypothalamic–pituitary–ovarian axis. Plasma prolactin levels are known to rise during exercise, as well as during other stressful situations (Noel et al. [94]; Brisson et al. [95]; Shangold et al. [96]). Hyperprolactinemia is a well-known cause for amenorrhea and infertility (Jacobs et al. [97]; Archer [98]; Bergh et al. [99]). At the present time, however, it appears that prolactin is unlikely to be involved in exercise-related menstrual disruption. Resting prolactin levels are normal or low in athletes and dancers with menstrual abnormalities (Warren [48]; Chang et al. [100]; Veldhuis et al. [88]). Prolactin responses to exercise are modest (Horgan and Kerstetter [101]; Loucks and Horvath [84]) and may be similar in eumenorrheic and amenorrheic athletes (Chang et al. [102]); prolactin responses to intravenous dopamine infusion are normal in amenorrheic athletes (Chang et al. [100]).

Androgens   A second hypothesis is that exercise-induced androgen secretion inhibits the hypothalamic–pituitary–ovarian axis. Plasma levels of a variety of androgens, presumably of adrenal origin, rise during exercise in women (Sutton et al. [103]; Brisson et al. [104]; Shangold et al. [96]). Amenorrhea and infertility are often associated with hyperandrogenism (Ferriman and Purdie [105]; Rosenfield [106]; Smith et al. [107]). Resting plasma levels of testosterone, androstenedione, dehydroepiandrosterone, and dehydroepiandrosterone-sulfate appear to be normal in amenorrheic athletes (Baker et al. [75]; Schwartz et al. [76]; Oian et al. [35]). Exercise responses for these steroids are also normal in amenorrheic athletes (Loucks and Horvath [84]). However, the ratio of testosterone/estradiol is high in amenorrheic athletes (Loucks and Horvath [84]). Dihydrotestosterone levels, on the other hand, may be unusually high in amenorrheic athletes both at rest and during exercise (Carlberg et al. [108]; Oian et al. [35]). Thus, while levels of most androgens appear to be normal in amenorrheic athletes, dihydrotestosterone, androgen/estrogen ratios, and the amounts of free vs sex-hormone-binding-globulin bound hormone deserve further study.

Endogenous Opioid Peptides   A third hypothesis is that exercise-induced secretion of β-endorphin inhibits hypothalamic GnRH secretion (McArthur [109]). β-Endorphin secretion is stimulated by exercise as well as by other stressors (Appenzeller et al. [110]; Colt et al. [111]; Farrell et al. [112]), and exercise-induced β-endorphin secretion may be facilitated by exercise training (Carr et al. [113]; Bullen et al. [42]). Administration of exogenous opiate substances can inhibit gonadotropin secretion, probably by an action at the hypothalamus (Muraki et al. [114]; Pang et al. [115]; Cicero et al. [116]). Endogenous opioid peptides have been implicated in the normal regulation of the menstrual cycle (Sylvester et al. [117]; Quigley and Yen [118]; Petraglia et al. [119]). Naloxone, an opiate receptor antagonist, has been shown to reverse stress-induced depression of reproductive function in male monkeys (Gilbeau and Smith [120]).

There is some evidence that endogenous opioid peptides may play a role in exercise-related reproductive dysfunction. McArthur et al. [121] reported that naloxone administration was followed by a pronounced increase in LH pulse amplitude in one amenorrheic runner. Russell et al. [65] found that resting β-endorphin levels in female competitive swimmers were about 7 times higher during a strenuous training period than during a moderate training period. Caldwell and Davis [122] reported that naltrexone, another opiate receptor antagonist, reversed exercise-induced estrous cycle disruptions in rats. In contrast, Dixon et al. [123] found that intravenous naloxone administration had no significant effect on LH or FSH secretion in amenorrheic runners. Thus, there is some support for an involvement of endogenous opioid peptides in exercise-related menstrual disturbances, but further research is needed.

Hypothalamic–Pituitary–Adrenal (Glucocorticoid) Axis A fourth hypothesis is that activation of the hypothalamic–pituitary–adrenal axis during exercise results in suppression of the hypothalamic–pituitary–ovarian axis. During acute bouts of exercise there is a rapid rise in ACTH and cortisol (Fraioli et al. [124]), and this appears to be augmented by training (Carr et al. [113]). More recently, Villanueva et al. [125] observed that women runners have increased cortisol production rates, a normal adrenal response to exogenous ACTH, and a normal metabolic disposal of cortisol. Both eumenorrheic and amenorrheic athletes exhibited this abnormality. There are abundant animal studies (Baldwin and Sawyer [126]; Ringstrom and Schwartz [127]; Dubey and Plant [128]; Rivier and Vale [129]; Rivier et al. [130]; Gambacciani et al. [131]) and a few human studies (Boccuzzi et al. [132]; Sakakura et al. [133]) that demonstrate that the hypothalamic–pituitary–adrenal axis hormones interfere with the hypothalamic–pituitary–ovarian axis. Although the site of this inhibition is not clear, suppression of either pituitary LH secretion or of hypothalamic LHRH secretion appears most likely.

Other Endocrine Factors A variety of other endocrine factors have been evaluated in athletes and dancers with menstrual disturbances. The significance of these factors is unknown.

One consistent finding is an elevated estrone/estradiol (E_1/E_2) ratio in both menstruating and amenorrheic athletes compared with sedentary controls (Carlberg et al. [108]; Schwartz et al. [76]; Loucks and Horvath [84]). Boyden et al. [86] found a gradual, although insignificant, increase in E_1/E_2 ratio in women undergoing an endurance training program. The E_1/E_2 ratio reflects both ovarian function and peripheral steroid metabolism, so these results provide further evidence that one or both of these factors are affected by athletic training.

Sex-hormone-binding globulin (SHBG) binds much of the circulating androgens and estrogens and therefore contributes to the activity and balance between these steroids. Baker et al. [75] reported lower SHBG levels in amenorrheic runners compared with menstruating runners. Oian et al. [35] found that SHBG levels were low or low-normal in amenorrheic athletes. It is possible that a low SHBG level would increase the ratio of androgenic activity to estrogenic activity, regardless of the absolute plasma concentrations of the hormones.

Thyroid function may be normal or low in athletes and dancers with menstrual disturbances. Schwartz et al. [76] found that thyroid-stimulating hormone (TSH) levels were significantly lower in amenorrheic runners than in menstruating runners. Warren [48] found low thyroxine (T_4) in one young ballet dancer but normal T_4 and TSH in all other subjects. Marcus et al. [134] measured lower levels of both T_4 and triiodothyronine (T_3) in amenorrheic runners than in menstruating runners. Levels of TSH, T_4, and T_3 were normal in other studies of amenorrheic or oligomenorrheic athletes (Wakat et al. [87]; Oian et al. [35]; Veldhuis et al. [88]).

Bullen and colleagues have suggested that melatonin, secreted by the pineal gland, may be involved in exercise-related menstrual disturbances. Melatonin inhibits secretion of reproductive hormones, probably via the hypothalamus, and its secretion appears to be stimulated by acute stress. These investigators demonstrated a rise in plasma melatonin levels during exercise in menstruating women, which in one study was facilitated by exercise training (Bullen et al. [42, 135]).

Summary In athletes and dancers with menstrual dysfunction, ovarian hormone secretion is low and noncyclic. Gonadotropin secretion and presumably GnRH secretion are also noncyclic and sometimes suppressed. In particular, LH pulse frequency appears to be reduced. The connection between exercise and suppression of the hypothalamic–pituitary–gonadal axis is not known. Exercise-induced prolactin secretion does not appear to be involved. Exercise-induced secretion of androgens or endogenous opioid peptides may be involved, but further study is needed. Activation of the hypothalamic–pituitary–glucocorticoid axis may interfere with the reproductive hormone axis. Further studies are required to clarify this issue. Other factors such as peripheral hormone metabolism and transport and hormone systems related to stress responses and metabolism also deserve further study.

Consequences of Exercise-Related Menstrual Disturbances

Because exercise-related menstrual dysfunction is a recently recognized phenomenon, and because women's involvement in strenuous athletic training is also relatively recent, little is known about the long-term consequences of these menstrual changes. The only risk for which there is much evidence is loss of bone mineral seen in some athletes with long-term estrogen deficiency associated with amenorrhea. The menstrual changes associated with exercise appear to be reversible with cessation or reduction in training.

Bone Mineral Loss (Osteopenia) Bone mineral loss is a known complication of hypoestrogenic states such as the postmenopausal period. Initial reports of bone mineral loss in amenorrheic athletes were met with skepticism because of the known stimulatory effects of exercise on bone mineral deposition (Lutter [136]; Drinkwater [137]). However, there is now enough evidence to conclude that bone mineral loss poses a real risk for athletes with long-term amenorrhea.

Low bone mass in amenorrheic athletes was first reported by Cann et al. [138]. In 11 women with "hypothalamic amenorrhea," 10 of whom were athletic, lumbar vertebral mineral levels were 77% of those in the control group, radial mineral levels were 98% of control levels, and metacarpal thickness was 89% of the control value. Spinal bone mass was higher in women who had been amenorrheic less than a year than in those with longer term amenorrhea. Discrepancies in these 3 methodologic results reflect at least in part differences in sensitivities of the 3 measurements, with vertebral bone density being more sensitive in reflecting changes in bone turnover rates than radius and metacarpal studies.

Subsequent reports have confirmed these findings. Drinkwater et al. [139] found that lumbar mineral density was lower in amenorrheic athletes than in menstruating athletes, although radial mineral densities were not different. Dietary calcium intakes were not different in the two groups. In amenorrheic runners studied by Lindberg et al. [140], cortical and trabecular bone density and trabecular bone mineral content of the radius were lower than in menstruating runners or sedentary women. Lumbar bone mineral content was below the normal range. Stress fractures were reported during the previous year by 49% of the amenorrheic runners and none of the menstruating runners. Marcus et al. [134] reported that lumbar mineral density in amenorrheic runners was lower than in menstruating runners or normal control subjects, but higher than in amenorrheic nonathletic women. Radial mineral density was normal in both groups of runners. Running-related stress fractures were reported by 1 of 11 menstruating runners and by all 6 amenorrheic runners. Serum levels of calcium, phosphorus, parathyroid hormone, alkaline phosphatase, and calcidiol were normal in both groups of runners, but serum calcitriol was lower in the amenorrheic runners. Both groups of runners had low dietary calcium intakes. Thus, vertebral bone mineral was reduced in amenorrheic athletes in all 4 studies in which it was measured, while radial bone mineral was found to be reduced in only one of these studies. Bone turnover in the radius is slow compared with that in the vertebrae; thus, changes in resorption/formation will be reflected in vertebral bone density measurements earlier than in radial studies.

Two additional studies that measured only radial bone mineral concluded that bone mineral was normal in amenorrheic athletes (Linnell et al. [141]; Jones et al. [142]). However, Linnell et al. reported a significant correlation between bone density and both body fatness and body weight among the amenorrheic runners.

Other Health Risks Because estrogens appear to have a protective effect against cardiovascular disease, it has been speculated that exercise-related amenorrhea might affect cardiovascular risk, despite the known cardiovascular benefits of exercise. Serum lipid profiles in amenorrheic athletes, however, reflect only the beneficial effects of exercise. These athletes consistently have elevated high-density lipoprotein (HDL) levels, decreased low-density lipoprotein (LDL) levels, and high HDL/LDL ratios (Dale et al. [77]; Dale and Goldberg [143]; Shainholtz et al. [144]). Thus, amenorrheic athletes appear to share the favorable serum lipid profiles of other endurance-trained athletes.

There has been some speculation that amenorrheic athletes might be at risk for endometrial or breast cancer due to moderate estrogen levels that are unopposed by progesterone (Prior and Vigna [145]; Shangold [146]). No studies of an increased cancer risk have been reported.

Atrophic vaginitis or urethritis can result from hypoestrogenism (Shangold [146]). While data are meager (Warren [48]), it is likely that these symptoms are common among amenorrheic athletes and dancers.

The incidence of musculoskeletal injury was found to be higher in amenorrheic athletes than those with normal menses in the studies of Lloyd et al. [147]. Since they did not study dietary intakes or bone density, it is not clear whether the women who suffered the injuries were the ones with lower bone mineral contents.

Fertility and Contraception Although the menstrual disturbances delineated in women athletes would generally be expected to decrease fertility, the individual woman with exercise-related menstrual dysfunction cannot assume that she is infertile. Amenorrheic athletes occasionally do become pregnant (Carlberg et al. [34]). Sexually active athletes who want to avoid pregnancy should use appropriate contraception (Prior and Vigna [145]).

Reversibility Exercise-related menstrual disturbances appear to be quickly reversible upon reduction of training (Baker [148]; Stager [149]). Questionnaires distributed to former collegiate distance runners by Stager et al. [150] revealed that normal menstrual periodicity returned within 6 months of cessation of training in all women, with an average of 1.7 months. Other investigators have also noted a quick return of normal menses during periods of rest (Warren [48]; Russell et al. [65]), with weight gain (Cohen et al. [38]), or with cessation of training (Prior et al. [41]; Bullen et al. [68]). However, long-term studies are needed.

Fortunately, with the resumption of normal cyclic menstrual function, the decreased vertebral bone mass will return to normal in these women athletes (Drinkwater et al. [151]). This will occur with a reduction in running sufficient to allow menses to return (Lindberg et al. [152]).

Evaluation of the Athlete with Oligo/Amenorrhea

Athletes with delayed menarche (amenorrhea past age 16) or oligo/amenorrhea should be evaluated by standard medical techniques, independent of considerations regarding their exercise status. Without appropriate clinical studies, there is no guarantee that the menstrual dysfunction is due to physical training. Such a cause and effect assumption could be potentially dangerous by delaying appropriate diagnostic studies and subsequent treatment of potentially serious disease states. Exercise-related oligo/amenorrhea syndromes must be diagnoses of exclusion.

There is one exception to the rule mandating a comprehensive diagnostic evaluation of the menstrually dysfunctional athlete. Say a woman with regular menses significantly increases her training duration/intensity in preparation for a competitive event, such as a marathon. During the course of intensified training she stops menstruating. In this setting, the etiology of menstrual dysfunction may well relate to participation in an intensified training regimen. To test the hypothesis, the woman could be observed for a period of several months following participation in the event to determine whether a diminution in exercise intensity is associated with resumption of regular menstrual cycles. If this is the case, no additional studies need to be pursued. If, however, menstruation does not resume within 6 months, a diagnostic evaluation is mandatory.

Pregnancy is a potential, and probably not uncommon, cause of recent-onset secondary amenorrhea among women of childbearing age and should be ruled out before pursuing a medical evaluation. Other nonphysiologic causes of menstrual dysfunction include disorders of the hypothalamic–pituitary axis, ovarian hypo- or hyperfunction, a variety of endocrine disorders including thyroid and adrenal dysfunction, uterine factors, chronic illnesses, and malnutrition, including the anorexia nervosa syndrome.

Treatment of Exercise-Related Menstrual Disturbances

The etiology of exercise-related menstrual disturbances is not understood, and therefore the long-term consequences have not been fully defined. Controlled clinical experiments of various treatment regimens have not been performed. Therapeutic suggestions are largely based on existing knowledge of the pathophysiologic consequences of other types of oligo/amenorrhea. Specific recommendations have been outlined by Shangold [146] and Prior and Vigna [145, 153].

The primary problem relating to oligo/amenorrhea in athletes derives from a deficiency of ovarian estrogen and/or progesterone production. Individual athletes have the option of exploring lifestyle adjustments that may restore a normal hormonal milieu and regular menstrual function. Included in these lifestyle changes are a decrease in exercise duration and intensity; an increase in caloric intake, with positive caloric balance and ensuing weight gain; and a decrease in competition-associated psychologic stress levels by eliminating or decreasing training intensity and participation in highly competitive athletic events. Changes in one or all of these areas may restore normal hypothalamic–pituitary–ovarian–uterine function and might mitigate the need for pharmacologic hormonal replacement programs. Since such lifestyle adjustments result in correction of the problem by entirely physiologic means, we believe they represent the ideal treatment program for a menstrually dysfunctional athlete. If, however, such changes are unacceptable and the athlete prefers to maintain her current athletic lifestyle, pharmacologic measures are available.

Complications related to ovarian dysfunction associated with oligo/amenorrhea include: a) the development of estrogenic states in which some estrogen production is maintained but is unopposed by cyclic progesterone secretion, thus increasing the risk of developing endometrial precancerous and cancerous conditions; and b) the development of hypoestrogenic states in which women develop an increased risk for osteopenia and atrophic changes in the urogenital tract (vagina and urethra). For all these conditions, a preventive approach has distinct advantages over a therapeutic one. This is especially true of the metabolic bone disease, which responds sluggishly to treatment. For those women who maintain some endogenous estrogen production but have anovulatory oligomenorrhea, cyclic progesterone administration will protect the endometrium from hyperplastic and carcinomatous transformation. Regular progesterone withdrawal bleeding further assures some ovarian estrogen production and, presumably, some protection against estrogen deficiency complications; however, vertebral bone density should be assessed in these women to ensure that their level of endogenous estrogen production is indeed adequate. In the absence of progesterone withdrawal bleeding, the patient is estrogen deficient, which can be confirmed by direct measurement of serum estrogen concentrations. In this setting, bone preservation and urogenital mucous membrane integrity can be maintained by administering cyclic estrogen/progestin combinations. Details of these treatment regimens are beyond the scope of this chapter and in the case of an individual athlete are best handled by a qualified physician.

For additional reviews of exercise-related menstrual dysfunction, see Shangold [21], Loucks and Horvath [154], and Puhl and Brown [155].

REFERENCES

1. Erdelyi, G.J. 1962. Gynecological survey of female athletes. J Sports Med Phys Fitness 2:174–179.
2. Zaharieva, E. 1965. Survey of sportswomen at the Tokyo Olympics. J Sports Med Phys Fitness 5:215–219.
3. Higgs, S.L., Robertson, L.A. 1981. Cyclic variations in perceived exertion and physical work capacity in females. Can J Appl Sport Sci 6:191–196.
4. Stephenson, L.A., Kolka, M.A., et al. 1982. Perceived exertion and anaerobic threshold during the menstrual cycle. Med Sci Sports Exer 14:218–222.
5. Eston, R.G. 1984. The regular menstrual cycle and athletic performance. Sports Med 1:431–445.
6. Jurkowski, J.E.H., Jones, N.L., et al. 1981. Effects of menstrual cycle on blood lactate, O_2 delivery, and performance during exercise. J Appl Physiol 51:1493–1499.
7. Schoene, R.B., Robertson, H.T., et al. 1981. Respiratory drives and exercise in menstrual cycles of athletic and nonathletic women. J Appl Physiol 50:1300–1305.
8. Stephenson, L.A., Kolka, M.A. 1982. Metabolic and thermoregulatory responses to exercise during the human menstrual cycle. Med Sci Sports Exer 14:270–275.
9. Brooks-Gunn, J., Gargiulo, J., et al. In press. The effect of cycle phase upon adolescent swimmers' performance. Phys Sportsmed.
10. Jurkowski, J.E., Jones, N.J., et al. 1978. Ovarian hormonal responses to exercise. J Appl Physiol 44:109–114.
11. Bonen, A., Haynes, F.J., et al. 1983. Effects of menstrual cycle on metabolic responses to exercise. J Appl Physiol 55:1506–1513.
12. Wells, C.L., Horvath, S.M. 1974. Responses to exercise in a hot environment as related to the menstrual cycle. J Appl Physiol 36:299–302.
13. Frye, A.J., Kamon, E., et al. 1982. Responses of menstrual women, amenorrheal women, and men to exercise in a hot, dry environment. Eur J Appl Physiol 48:279–288.
14. Horvath, S.M., Drinkwater, B.L. 1982. Thermoregulation and the menstrual cycle. Aviat Space Environ Med 53:790–794.
15. Stephenson, L.A., Kolka, M.A. 1985. Menstrual cycle phase and time of day alter reference signal controlling arm blood flow and sweating. Am J Physiol 249:R191.
16. Gaebelein, C.J., Senay, L.C., Jr. 1982. Vascular volume dynamics during ergometer exercise at different menstrual phases. Eur J Appl Physiol 50:1–11.
17. Jurkowski, J.E.H. 1982. Hormonal and physiological responses to exercise in relation to the menstrual cycle. Can J Appl Sport Sci 7:85–89.
18. Brooks-Gunn, J., Gargiulo, J., et al. 1986. The menstrual cycle and athletic performance. In: Puhl, J.L., Brown, C.H. (eds): The Menstrual Cycle and Physical Activity. Human Kinetics Publishers, Champaign, IL.
19. Reid, R.L., Yen, S.S.C. 1981. Premenstrual syndrome. Am J Obstet Gynecol 39:85–104.
20. Beacham, D.W., Beacham, W.D. 1982. Synopsis of Gynecology (tenth edition). C.V. Mosby, St. Louis, MO.
21. Shangold, M.M. 1984. Exercise and the adult female: hormonal and endocrine effects. In: Terjung, R.L. (ed): Exercise and Sport Sciences Reviews (Volume 12). Collamore Press, Lexington, MA.
22. Havens, C. 1985. Premenstrual syndrome: tactics for intervention. Postgrad Med 77:32–37.
23. Ingman, O. 1952. Menstruation in Fin-

nish top-class sportswomen. In: Karvonen, M.J. (ed): Proceedings of the International Symposium of the Medicine
and Physiology of Sports and Athletics at
Helsinki. Finnish Association of Sports
Medicine.

24. Timonen, S., Procope, B.J. 1971. Premenstrual syndrome and physical exercise. Acta Obstet Gynecol Scand 50:
331–337.

25. Ronkainen, H., Pakarinen, A., et al.
1984. Pubertal and menstrual disorders
of female runners, skiers and volleyball
players. Gynecol Obstet Invest 18:183–
189.

26. Golub, L.J., Menduke, H., et al. 1968.
Exercise and dysmenorrhea in young
teenagers: a 3-year study. Obstet Gynecol
32:508–511.

27. Prior, J.C., Vigna, Y., et al. 1986. Conditioning exercise decreases premenstrual
symptoms: a prospective controlled three
month trial. Eur J Appl Physiol 55:349–
355.

28. Pettersson, F., Fires, H., et al. 1973. Epi-
demiology of secondary amenorrhea: I.
Incidence and prevalence rates. Am J
Obstet Gynecol 117:80–86.

29. Singh, K.B. 1981. Menstrual disorders
in college students. Am J Obstet Gynecol
140:299–302.

30. Bachmann, G.A., Kemmann, E. 1982.
Prevalence of oligomenorrhea and ame-
norrhea in a college population. Am J
Obstet Gynecol 144:98–102.

31. Lutter, J.M. 1986. Prevalence of menstrual change in athletes and active
women. In: Puhl, J.L., Brown, C.H.
(eds): The Menstrual Cycle and Physical
Activity. Human Kinetics Publishers,
Champaign, IL.

32. Dale, E., Gerlach, D.H., et al. 1979.
Menstrual dysfunction in distance runners. Obstet Gynecol 54:47–53.

33. Lutter, J.M., Cushman, S. 1982. Menstrual patterns in female runners. Phys
Sportsmed 10(9): 60–72.

34. Carlberg, K.A., Buckman, M.T., et al.
1983. Survey of menstrual function in
athletes. Eur J Appl Physiol 51:211–222.

35. Oian, P., Augestad, L.B., et al. 1984.
Menstrual dysfunction in Norwegian top
athletes. Acta Obstet Gynecol Scand
63:693–697.

36. Toriola, A.L., Mathur, D.N. 1986. Menstrual dysfunction in Nigerian athletes.
Br J Obstet Gynaecol 93:979–985.

37. Frisch, R.E., Wyshak, G., et al. 1980.
Delayed menarche and amenorrhea in
ballet dancers. N Eng J Med 303:17–19.

38. Cohen, J.L., Kim, C.S., et al. 1982. Exercise, body weight, and amenorrhea in
professional ballet dancers. Phys Sportsmed 10(4):92–101.

39. Shangold, M., Freeman, R., et al. 1979.
The relationship between long-distance
running, plasma progesterone, and luteal
phase length. Fertil Steril 31:130–133.

40. Prior, J.C., Cameron, K., et al. 1982.
Menstrual cycle changes with marathon
training: anovulation and short luteal
phase. Can J Appl Sport Sci 7:173–177.

41. Prior, J.C., Yuen, B.H., et al. 1982. Reversible luteal phase changes and infertility associated with marathon training
(letter). Lancet 2:269–270.

42. Bullen, B.A., Skrinar, G.S., et al. 1984.
Endurance training effects on plasma
hormonal responsiveness and sex hormone excretion. J Appl Physiol 56:1453–
1463.

43. Strott, C.A., Cargille, C.M., et al. 1970.
The short luteal phase. J Clin Endocrinol
Metab 30:246–251.

44. Malina, R.M., Harper, A.B., et al. 1983.
Age of menarche in athletes and non-athletes. Med Sci Sports Exer 15:11–13.

45. Malina, R.M., Spirduso, W.W., et al.
1978. Age at menarche and selected menstrual characteristics in athletes at different competitive levels and in different
sports. Med Sci Sports Exer 10:218–222.

46. Frisch, R.E., Gotz-Welbergen, A.V., et al.
1981. Delayed menarche and amenorrhea
of college athletes in relation to age of onset of training. JAMA 246:1559–1563.

47. Stager, J.M., Robertshaw, D., et al.
1984. Delayed menarche in swimmers in
relation to age at onset of training and
athletic performance. Med Sci Sports
Exer 16:550–555.

48. Warren, M.P. 1980. The effects of exercise on pubertal progression and reproductive function in girls. J Clin Endocrinol Metab 51:1150–1157.

49. Brisson, G.R., Dulac, S. 1982. The onset of menarche: a late event in pubertal
progression to be affected by physical
training. Can J Appl Sport Sci 7:61–67.

50. Malina, R.M. 1983. Menarch in athletes:
synthesis and hypothesis. Ann Human
Biol 10:1–24.

51. Feicht, C.B., Johnson, T.S., et al. 1978.
Secondary amenorrhoea in athletes. Lancet 2:1145–1146.

52. Gray, D.P., Dale, E. 1983. Variables associated with secondary amenorrhea in
women runners. J Sports Sci 1:55–67.

53. Sanborn, C.F., Martin, B.J., et al. 1982.
Is athletic amenorrhea specific to runners? Am J Obstet Gynecol 143:859–
861.

54. Fries, H., Nillius, S.J., et al. 1974. Epidemiology of secondary amenorrhea: II. A retrospective evaluation of etiology with special regard to psychogenic factors and weight loss. Am J Obstet Gynecol 118:473–479.

55. Warren, M.P. 1983. The effects of undernutrition on reproductive function in the human. Endocr Rev 4:363–377.

56. Frisch, R.E. 1985. Fatness, menarche, and female fertility. Perspect Biol Med 28:611–633.

57. Malina, R.M., Harper, A.B., et al. 1971. Physique of female track and field athletes. Med Sci Sports Exer 3:32–38.

58. Wilmore, J.H., Brown, C.H., et al. 1977. Body physique and composition of the female distance runner. Ann NY Acad Sci 301:764–776.

59. Sinning, W.E. 1978. Anthropometric estimation of body density, fat, and lean body weight in women gymnasts. Med Sci Sports Exer 10:243–249.

60. Young, C.M. 1961. Body fatness in normal young women. NY State J Med 61: 1928–1931.

61. Sloan, A.W., Burt, J.J., et al. 1962. Estimation of body fat in young women. J Appl Physiol 17:967–970.

62. Wilmore, J.H., Behnke, A.R. 1970. An anthropometric estimation of body density and lean body weight in young women. Am J Clin Nutr 23:267–274.

63. Shangold, M.M., Levine, H.S. 1982. The effect of marathon training upon menstrual function. Am Obstet Gynecol 143:862–869.

64. Carlberg, K.A., Buckman, M.T., et al. 1983. Body composition of oligo/amenorrheic athletes. Med Sci Sports Exer 15:215–217.

65. Russell, J.B., Mitchell, D.E., et al. 1984. The role of β-endorphins and catechol estrogens on the hypothalamic-pituitary axis in female athletes. Fertil Steril 42:690–695.

66. Abraham, S.F, Beaumont, F.J.V., et al. 1982. Body weight, exercise and menstrual status among ballet dancers in training. Br J Obstet Gynaecol 89:507–510.

67. Vandenbroucke, J.P., Van Laar, A., et al. 1982. Synergy between thinness and intensive sports activity in delaying menarche. Br Med J 284:1907–1908.

68. Bullen, B.A., Skrinar, G.S., et al. 1985. Induction of menstrual disorders by strenuous exercise in untrained women. N Engl J Med 312:1349–1353.

69. Vigersky, R.A., Andersen, A.E., et al. 1977. Hypothalamic dysfunction in secondary amenorrhea associated with simple weight loss. N Eng J Med 297:1141–1145.

70. Siiteri, P., MacDonald, P.C. 1973. Role of extraglandular estrogen in human reproduction. In: Greep, R.O. (ed): Handbook of Physiology. American Physiological Society, Bethesda, MD, pp 615–629.

71. Fishman, J., Boyar, R.M., et al. 1975. Influence of body weight on estradiol metabolism in young women. J Clin Endocrinol Metab 41:989–991.

72. Longcope, C., Pratt, J.H., et al. 1976. In vivo studies on the metabolism of estrogens by muscle and adipose tissue on normal males. J Clin Endocrinol Metab 43: 1134–1145.

73. Longcope, C., Pratt, J.H., et al. 1976. The in vivo metabolism of androgens by muscle and adipose tissue of normal men. Steroids 28:521–533.

74. Speroff, L., Redwine, D.B. 1980. Exercise and menstrual function. Phys Sportsmed 8(5):41–52.

75. Baker, E.R., Mathur, R.S., et al. 1981. Female runners and secondary amenorrhea: correlation with age, parity, mileage, and plasma hormonal and sex-hormone binding globulin concentrations. Fertil Steril 36:183–187.

76. Schwartz, B., Cummings, D.C., et al. 1981. Exercise-associated amenorrhea: a distinct entity? Am J Obstet Gynecol 141:662–670.

77. Dale, E., Gerlach, D.H., et al. 1979. Physical fitness profiles and reproductive physiology of the female distance runner. Phys Sportsmed 7(1):83–95.

78. Frisch, R.E. 1984. Amenorrhoea, vegetarianism, and/or low fat (letter). Lancet 1:1024.

79. Slavin, J., Lutter, J., et al. 1984. Amenorrhoea in vegetarian athletes (letter). Lancet 1:1474–1475.

80. Deuster, P.A., Kyle, S.B., et al. 1986. Nutritional intakes and status of highly trained amenorrheic and eumenorrheic women runners. Fertil Steril 46:636–643.

81. Nelson, M.E., Fisher, E.C., et al. 1986. Diet and bone status in amenorrheic runners. Am J Clin Nutr 43:910–916.

82. Seibel, M.M., Taymor, M.L. 1982. Emotional aspects of infertility. Fertil Steril 37:137–145.

83. Galle, P.C., Freeman, E.W., et al. 1983. Physiologic and psychologic profiles in a survey of women runners. Fertil Steril 39:633–639.

84. Loucks, A.B., Horvath, S.M. 1984.

Exercise-induced stress responses of amenorrheic and eumenorrheic athletes. J Clin Endocrinol Metab 59:1109–1120.

85. Carlberg, K.A., Peake, G.T., et al. 1983. Familial susceptibility to athletic amenorrhea. Ann Sports Med 1:115–116.

86. Boyden, T.W., Pamenter, R.W., et al. 1983. Sex steroids and endurance running in women. Fertil Steril 39:629–632.

87. Wakat, D.K., Sweeney, K.A., et al. 1982. Reproductive system function in women cross-country runners. Med Sci Sports Exer 14:263–269.

88. Veldhuis, J.D., Evans, W.S., et al. 1985. Altered neuroendocrine regulation of gonadotropin secretion in women distance runners. J Clin Endocrinol Metab 61:557–563.

89. Yahiro, J., Glass, A.R., et al. 1987. Exaggerated gonadotropic response to LHRH in amenorrheic runners. Am J Obstet Gynec 156:586–591.

90. Boyden, T.W., Pamenter, R.W., et al. 1984. Impaired gonadotropin resonses to gonadotropin-releasing hormone stimulation in endurance-trained women. Fertil Steril 41:359–363.

91. Cumming, D.C., Vickovic, M.M., et al. 1985. Defects in pulsatile LH release in normally menstruating runners. J Clin Endocrinol Metab 60:810–812.

92. Cumming, D.C., Vickovic, M.M., et al. 1985. The effect of acute exercise on pulsatile release of luteinizing hormone in women runners. Am J Obstet Gynecol 153:482–485.

93. Reame, N.E., Sauder, S.E., et al. 1985. Pulsatile gonadotropin secretion in women with hypothalamic amenorrhea: evidence that reduced frequency of gonadotropin-releasing hormone secretion is the mechanism of persistent anovulation. J Clin Endocrinol Metab 61:851–858.

94. Noel, G.L., Suh, H.K., et al. 1972. Human prolactin and growth hormone release during surgery and other conditions of stress. J Clin Endocrinol Metab 35:840–851.

95. Brisson, G.R., Volle, M.A., et al. 1980. Exercise-induced dissociation of the blood prolactin response in young women according to their sports habits. Horm Metab Res 12:201–205.

96. Shangold, M.M., Gatz, M.L., et al. 1981. Acute effects of exercise on plasma concentrations of prolactin and testosterone in recreational women runners. Fertil Steril 35:699–702.

97. Jacobs, H.S., Franks, S., et al. 1976. Clinical and endocrine features of hyperprolactinaemic amenorrhoea. Clin Endocrinol 5:439–454.

98. Archer, D.F. 1977. Current concepts of prolactin physiology in normal and abnormal conditions. Fertil Steril 28:125–134.

99. Bergh, T., Nillius, S.J., et al. 1977. Hyperprolactinemia in amenorrhoea-incidence and clinical significance. Acta Endocrinol 86:683–694.

100. Chang, F.E., Richards, S.R., et al. 1984. Twenty-four hour prolactin profiles and prolactin responses to dopamine in long distance running women. J Clin Endocrinol Metab 59:631–635.

101. Horgan, F., Kerstetter, T. 1983. Reduced prolactin responses to exercise in amenorrheic athletes. J Sports Sci 1:227–234.

102. Chang, F.E., Dodds, W.G., et al. 1986. The acute effects of exercise on prolactin and growth hormone secretion: comparison between sedentary women and women runners with normal and abnormal menstrual cycles. J Clin Endocrinol Metab 62:551–556.

103. Sutton, J.R., Coleman, M.J., et al. 1973. Androgen responses during physical exercise. Br Med J 1:520–522.

104. Brisson, G.R., Volle, M.A., et al. 1978. Androstenedionemie a l'effort chez la femme (abstract). Can J Appl Sport Sci 3:183.

105. Ferriman, D., Purdie, A.W. 1965. Association of oligomenorrhoea, hirsuties, and infertility. Br Med J 2:69–72.

106. Rosenfield, R.L. 1973. Relationship of androgens to female hirsutism and infertility. J Reprod Med 11:87–95.

107. Smith, K.D., Rodriguez-Rigau, L.J., et al. 1979. The relationship between plasma testosterone levels and the lengths of phases of the menstrual cycle. Fertil Steril 32:403–407.

108. Carlberg, K.A., Peake, G.T., et al. 1981. Androgen response to exercise in oligo-amenorrheic and menstruating athletes (abstract). Program and Abstracts, 63rd Annual Meeting, Endocrine Society, Cincinnati, OH, p 351.

109. McArthur, J.W. 1985. Endorphins and exercise in females: possible connection with reproductive dysfunction. Med Sci Sports Exer 17:82–88.

110. Appenzeller, O., Standefer, J., et al. 1980. Neurology of endurance training: V. Endorphins (abstract). Neurology 30:418–419.

111. Colt, E.W.D., Wardlaw, S.L., et al. 1981. The effect of running on plasma β-endorphin. Life Sci 28:1637–1640.

112. Farrell, P.A., Gates, W.K., et al. 1982. Increases in plasma β-endorphin/

β-lipotropin immunoreactivity after treadmill running in humans. J Appl Physiol 52:1245–1249.

113. Carr, D.B., Bullen, B.A., et al. 1981. Physical conditioning facilitates the exercise-induced secretion of beta-endorphin and beta-lipotropin in women. N Engl J Med 305:560–563.

114. Muraki, T., Tokunaga, Y., et al. 1977. Effects of morphine and naloxone on serum LH, FSH and prolactin levels and on hypothalamic content of LH-RF in proestrous rats. Endocrinol Jpn 24:313–315.

115. Pang, C.N., Zimmerman, E., et al. 1977. Morphine inhibition of the pre-ovulatory surges of plasma luteinizing hormone and follicle-stimulating hormone in the rat. Endocrinology 101:1726–1732.

116. Cicero, T.J., Badger, T.M., et al. 1977. Morphine decreases luteinizing hormone by an action on the hypothalamic-pituitary axis. J Pharmacol Exp Ther 203:58–555.

117. Sylvester, P.W., Chen, H.T., et al. 1980. Effects of morphine and naloxone on phasic release of luteinizing hormone and follicle-stimulating hormone. Proc Soc Exp Biol Med 164:207–211.

118. Quigley, M.E., Yen, S.S.C. 1980. The role of endogenous opiates of LH secretion during the menstrual cycle. J Clin Endocrinol Metab 51:179–181.

119. Petraglia, F., D'Ambrogio, G., et al. 1985. Impairment of opioid control of luteinizing hormone secretion in menstrual disorders. Fertil Steril 43:534–540.

120. Gilbeau, P.M., Smith, O.G. 1985. Naloxone reversal of stress-induced reproductive effects in the male rhesus monkey. Neuropeptides 5:335–338.

121. McArthur, J.W., Bullen, B.A., et al. 1980. Hypothalamic amenorrhea in runners of normal body composition. Endocr Res Commun 7:13–25.

122. Caldwell, C.A., Davis, J.M. 1985. Exercise-associated disturbances of female reproductive function: possible involvement of endogenous opioid peptides (abstract). Med Sci Sports Exer 17:236.

123. Dixon, G., Eurman, P., et al. 1984. Hypothalamic function in amenorrheic runners. Fertil Steril 42:377–383.

124. Fraioli, F., Moretti, C., et al. 1980. Physical exercise stimulates marked concomitant release of β-endorphin and ACTH in peripheral blood in man. Experimentia 36:987–990.

125. Villanueva, A.L., Schlosser, C., et al. 1986. Increased cortisol production in women runners. J Clin Endocrinol Metab 63:133–136.

126. Baldwin, D.M., Sawyer, C.H. 1974. Effects of dexamethasone on LH release and ovulation in the cyclic rat. Endocrinology 94:1397–1403.

127. Ringstrom, S.J., Schwartz, N.B. Cortisol suppresses the LH, but not the FSH, response to gonadotropin-releasing hormone after orchidectomy. Endocrinology 116:472–474.

128. Dubey, A.K., Plant, T.M. 1985. Biol Reprod 33:423.

129. Rivier, C., Vale, W., 1984. Influence of corticotropin releasing factor on reproductive functions in the rat. Endocrinology 114:914–921.

130. Rivier, C., Rivier, J., et al. 1986. Stress-induced inhibition of reproductive functions: role of endogenous corticotropin-releasing factor. Science 231:607–609.

131. Gambacciani, M., Yen, S.S.C., et al. 1986. GnRH release from the mediobasal hypothalamus: in vitro inhibition by corticotropin releasing factor. Neuroendocrinology 43:533–536.

132. Boccuzzi, G., Angeli, A., et al. 1975. Effect of synthetic LHRH on the release of gonadotropins in Cushing's disease. J Clin Endocrinol Metab 40:892–895.

133. Sakakura, M., Takebe, K., et al. 1975. Inhibition of LH secretion induced by synthetic LRH by long-term treatment with glucocorticoids in human subjects. J Clin Endocrinol Metab 40:774–779.

134. Marcus, R., Cann, C., et al. 1985. Menstrual function and bone mass in elite women distance runners. Ann Intern Med 102:158–163.

135. Bullen, B.A., Skrinar, G.S., et al. 1982. Exercise effect upon plasma melatonin levels in women: possible physiological significance. Can J Appl Sport Sci 7:90–97.

136. Lutter, J.M. 1983. Mixed messages about osteoporosis in female athletes. Phys Sportsmed 11(9):154–165.

137. Drinkwater, B.L. 1986. Relationship between altered reproductive function and osteoporosis. In: Puhl, J.L., Brown, C.H. (ed): The Menstrual Cycle and Physical Activity. Human Kinetics Publishers, Champaign, IL.

138. Cann, C.E., Martin, M.C., et al. 1984. Decreased spinal mineral content in amenorrheic women. JAMA 251:626–629.

139. Drinkwater, B.L., Nilson, K., et al. 1984. Bone mineral content of amenorrheic and eumenorrheic athletes. N Engl J Med 311:277–281.

140. Lindberg, J.S., Fears, W.B., et al. 1984. Exercise-induced amenorrhea and bone

density. Ann Intern Med 101:647–648.

141. Linnell, S.L., Stager, J.M., et al. 1984. Bone mineral content and menstrual regularity in female runners. Med Sci Sports Exer 16:343–348.

142. Jones, K.P., Ravnikar, V.A., et al. 1985. Comparison of bone density in amenorrheic women due to athletics, weight loss, and premature menopause. Obstet Gynecol 66:5–8.

143. Dale, E., Goldberg, D.L. 1982. Implications of nutrition in athletes' menstrual cycle irregularities. Can J Appl Sport Sci 7:74–78.

144. Shainholtz, S., Drinkwater, B., et al. 1985. Lipid profiles of amenorrheic and eumenorrheic athletes (abstract). Med Sci Sports Exer 17:214.

145. Prior, J.C., Vigna, Y. 1985. Gonadal steroids in athletic women: contraception, complications and performance. Sports Med 2:287–295.

146. Shangold, M.M. 1985. Causes, evaluation, and management of athletic oligo-/amenorrhea. Med Clin North Am 69:83–95.

147. Lloyd, T., Triantafyllou, S.J., et al. 1986. Women athletes with menstrual irregularity have increased musculoskeletal injuries. Med Sci Sports Exer 18:374–379.

148. Baker, R. 1981. Menstrual dysfunction and hormonal status in athletic women: a review. Fertil Steril 36:691–696.

149. Stager, J.M. 1984. Reversibility of amenorrhoea in athletes. Sports Med 1:337–340.

150. Stager, J.M., Richie-Flanagan, B., et al. 1984. Reversibility of amenorrhea in athletes. N Engl J Med 310:51–52.

151. Drinkwater, B.C., Nilson, K., et al. 1986. Bone mineral density after resumption of menses in amenorrheic athletes. JAMA 256:380.

152. Lindberg, J.S., Powell, M.R., et al. 1987. Increased vertebral bone mineral in response to reduced exercise in amenorrheic runners. West J Med 146:39–42.

153. Prior, J.C., Vigna, Y. 1986. The therapy of reproduction system changes associated with exercise training. In: Puhl, J.L., Brown, C.H. (eds): The Menstrual Cycle and Physical Activity. Human Kinetics Publishers, Champaign, IL.

154. Loucks, A.B., Horvath, S.M.: Athletic amenorrhea: a review. Med Sci Sports Exer 17:56–72.

155. Puhl, J.L., Brown, C.H. The Menstrual Cycle and Physical Activity. Human Kinetics Publishers, Champaign, IL.

·10·

Stress Hormone Response to Exercise

David S. Schade

Exercise requires major changes in metabolic fuels to maintain increased muscle contraction and to supply adequate glucose for the central nervous system. In the basal state, muscle metabolizes lipid exclusively and the central nervous system uses glucose. During exercise, lipid metabolism by muscle increases, but after 90 min, glucose metabolism accounts for 41% of oxygen uptake by leg muscles (Ahlborg et al. [1]), potentially depriving the nervous system of its metabolic fuel (Felig and Wahren [2]). The physiological adaptation that ensures adequate fuel to muscles and the central nervous system is the subject of this chapter.

Energy expended by muscle during exercise is derived from adenosine triphosphate (ATP), generated from adenosine diphosphate (ADP) and high-energy phosphate bonds from creatine phosphate. Sufficient supplies of ATP and creatine phosphate depend upon oxidative phosphorylation of two- and three-carbon molecules from lipid and carbohydrate precursors in muscle mitochondria. When these precursors are not available, ATP decreases and muscle contraction ultimately ceases. Substrates for muscle metabolism are derived from muscle and extramuscular sources, mainly fat and liver cells. The quantities of carbohydrate and lipid precursors in various tissues in humans (Havel [3]) are presented in Table 10-1, which shows that most energy substrate is lipid, stored outside of muscle. Glycogen and triglycerides are the two major storage forms (Fig. 10-1). These are relatively stable and remain in storage sites unless stimulated for release by hormones secreted during exercise. Enzymes involved in making energy available differ and function in a number of reactions for both carbohydrate and lipid precursors. The amount of energy released must meet, but not greatly exceed, the immediate needs of the organism.

Protein, mostly from muscle, can also be used as energy substrate. It is broken down to amino acids, which are converted to glucose in the liver. Alanine and glutamine from this source are the main amino acids used for gluconeogenesis, hence the designation, glucose-alanine cycle (Felig [4]). Although muscle is a potential substrate for glucose production, conservation of muscle protein during exercise is the rule. In spite of this, muscle breakdown during exercise occurs to some extent (Dill et al. [5]). During prolonged fasting, use of carbohydrate and lipid stores precedes muscle catabolism.

This work was supported by PHS grant 5-ROI-DK-31973-05.

Table 10-1 Fuel Stores in a 70-kg Man in Kilocalories and Percent of Total Stored

Site	Tissue	Glycogen		Triglyceride	
		Kcal	%	Kcal	%
Muscular	Muscle	1600	1.4	2,300	2
	Liver	300	0.2	90	0.1
Extramuscular	Fat	100	0.1	108,000	96
Total		2000	1.7	110,390	98.1

Muscle contains small amounts of carbohydrate and lipid, which provide fuel for rapid exercise of short duration (Table 10-1). Continuous exercise for longer periods requires extramuscular sources of energy. Inadequate energy substrate rarely limits muscle contraction in humans.

The hormones that mobilize energy during exercise (Fig. 10-2) are called "stress" hormones and include catecholamines, glucagon, cortisol, and growth hormone. They are also called "counter-regulatory" hormones because their effects are opposite to the anabolic effects of insulin (Eaton and Schade [6]).

There are four "stress" hormones that elevate blood sugar, but only insulin reduces blood sugar. The reasons for four stress hormones are: 1) a deficiency of any one may result in hypoglycemia; 2) each stress hormone has a characteristic onset and duration of action,

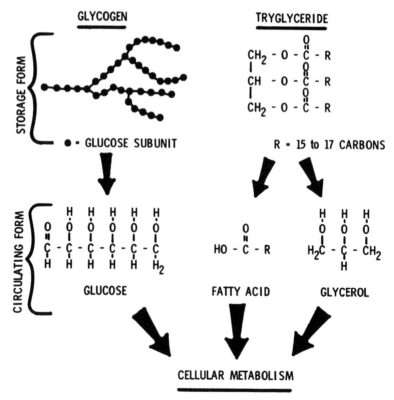

10-1 Storage and circulating forms of metabolic fuels. Carbohydrate is stored as glycogen. Glycogenolysis in liver results in release of glucose into the circulation. Lipid is stored as triglyceride, principally in adipose tissue. Triglyceride is catabolized by a hormone-sensitive lipase, resulting in release of fatty acids and glycerol into blood. Fatty acid is used directly for muscle metabolism, and glycerol is converted to glucose by liver.

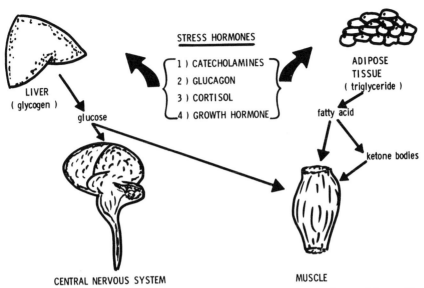

10-2   Metabolic activity of stress hormones. Each mobilizes glucose from liver and fatty acids from adipose tissue. Glucose is used by brain and muscle during exercise. Fatty acids are used by muscle directly or indirectly after their hepatic conversion to ketone bodies. In the absence of stress hormones, circulating energy substrates could not maintain muscle contraction and nervous system function.

and each affects different cells; 3) there is synergism between the stress hormones (Eigler et al. [7]). Thus, this system emphasizes the importance of maintaining adequate blood glucose at all times.

In a runner participating in the 1978 Albuquerque Marathon, all four stress hormones increased acutely (Fig. 10-3a). However, the largest rise in catecholamines occurred between 19 and 26 miles, which might relate to increased fatigue associated with the last 6 miles of the race, or to the excitement of approaching the finish line. In spite of increased uptake of glucose by muscle, plasma glucose rose (Fig. 10-3b) because of increased hepatic glucose production. Plasma nonesterified fatty acids also doubled, and ketone bodies (acetoacetate and 3-hydroxybutyrate) increased ninefold. Although blood flow to muscle may more than triple during strenuous exercise, the lack of energy substrates for muscle metabolism was not limiting this runner. Furthermore, plasma glucose was sufficient for optimal central nervous system function.

INDIVIDUAL STRESS HORMONES

Catecholamines

The catecholamines are structurally related and have potent effects during exercise. Epinephrine originates in the adrenal medulla, and norepinephrine is synthesized in postganglionic sympathetic nerve terminals. These two hormones have similar, but not identical, metabolic functions. They cause vasoconstriction and mobilization of lipids and carbohydrates during exercise. Catecholamines enhance phosphorylation of liver glycogen, which is subsequently hydrolyzed to glucose. Gluconeolysis is particularly important during exercise, when increased muscle use of glucose tends to cause hypoglycemia. Catecholamines may also stimulate gluconeogenesis.

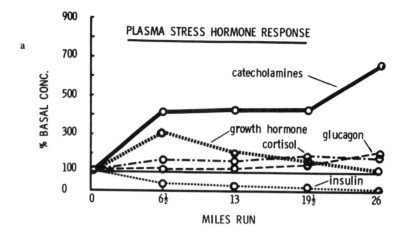

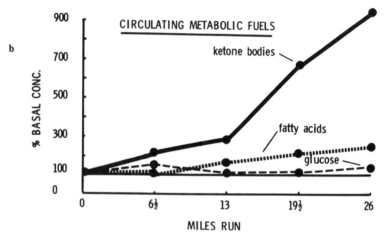

10-3 Elevated plasma stress hormones (a) and energy substrates (b) in a marathon runner. The greatest increase in stress hormones occurred in the catecholamines, which were responsible for the suppression of insulin throughout the 26-mile race. Coincident with the rise in stress hormones, plasma glucose, fatty acids, and ketone bodies also rose in spite of increased use during exercise (b). Plasma levels of these metabolic fuels were never less than basal, suggesting that their availability was not limiting exercise tolerance.

Catecholamines are the most potent lipolytic hormone known. At concentrations of less than 10^{-6} M (one molecule of catecholamine per million molecules of water), these compounds stimulate conversion of fat to fatty acids (Schade and Eaton [8]), which are the main energy source for muscle. Among the other effects of catecholamines (Fig. 10-4) is the suppression of insulin, a potent inhibitor of both glycogenolysis and lipolysis. Suppression occurs during exercise by direct effect of catecholamine on the pancreas in spite of elevated plasma glucose (Iverson [9]). Catecholamines concurrently stimulate pancreatic glucagon, the most potent gluconeogenic hormone in man. Thus, these compounds are probably the most important of the stress hormones.

Glucagon

Glucagon was discovered as a contaminant of insulin. When insulin was injected into an animal, elevation of plasma glucose occurred (glucagon effect) prior to its expected decline

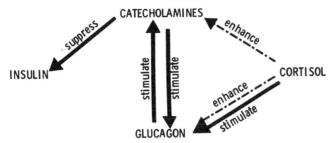

10-4 Hormonal-hormonal interactions during exercise. In addition to its effects on cellular metabolism, each hormone alters concentration or activity of the other stress hormones. Most important of these interactions is suppression of insulin by catecholamines, permitting catabolic activity of all four stress hormones.

(insulin effect). Glucagon is four times more potent in raising plasma glucose than insulin is in decreasing it. Glucagon produces changes in hepatic gluconeogenic hormones in humans within minutes of administration (Greene et al. [10]). It is secreted by pancreatic alpha cells, which adjoin beta cells (insulin-secreting cells) in the islets of Langerhans.

Several studies show that strenuous exercise is a potent stimulus for glucagon secretion in humans, and mild exercise may not induce its release. Glucagon acts mainly on the liver, but when insulin is sufficiently suppressed, it may stimulate lipolysis in adipose tissue. Glucagon enters the portal vein directly after secretion, exposing the liver to elevated plasma concentrations that stimulate gluconeogenesis and glycogenolysis, thus increasing hepatic glucose production. Glucagon stimulates cellular cyclic adenosine monophosphate (AMP), which increases hepatic enzyme activity, rather than promoting synthesis of new enzyme protein.

During the last decade, it was shown that glucagon promotes conversion of fatty acids to ketone bodies in the liver and suppresses their conversion to triglycerides (Schade et al. [11]). This is important during exercise, when fatty acids in plasma exceed the capacity of muscle to use them. Glucagon-mediated conversion of fatty acids to ketone bodies, readily oxidized by muscle cells, ensures additional fuel for muscle. In contrast, triglycerides require hydrolysis before becoming available for muscle oxidation.

Glucagon also exerts hormone-to-hormone interaction. Unlike catecholamines, glucagon stimulates insulin secretion during exercise. However, glucagon also stimulates catecholamine secretion from the adrenal, thereby enhancing glycogenolysis *in vivo* (Gerich et al. [12]). Thus, glucagon, both at hepatic and adrenal levels, helps prevent hypoglycemia during exercise.

Cortisol

Exercise is a potent stimulus for corticotropin secretion which, in turn, stimulates adrenal production of cortisol. Plasma cortisol rises approximately 15 min after initiation of exercise. Increased plasma cortisol, unlike glucagon and the catecholamines, causes metabolic changes in about 90 min, and the effects are prolonged (Schade et al. [13]). This delay reflects the mechanism by which cortisol affects cellular events. Glucagon and catecholamines stimulate cyclic AMP in the cell membrane, and cortisol stimulates new nuclear ribonucleic acid and protein synthesis. Specific proteins in the cytoplasm transport cortisol from the cell surface to the nucleus. The delay in its metabolic effects is due to the time necessary for cortisol transport to the nucleus.

Cortisol affects carbohydrate metabolism by promoting synthesis of hepatic enzymes involved in gluconeogenesis. Recent studies show that cortisol activity is synergistic with that of glucagon and catecholamines. During exercise, when all three hormones are elevated, hepatic glucose production is greatly increased. In addition, cortisol stimulates the release of alanine from muscle, an important gluconeogenic substrate, and inhibits glucose uptake by peripheral tissue, by blocking insulin-dependent and independent pathways.

Corticotropin and cortisol increase plasma nonesterified fatty acids by promoting lipolysis, thus providing additional energy for muscle. Cortisol may also alter hepatic lipid metabolism. Cortisol and other hormones are not known to have synergistic effects on lipid metabolism, but cortisol may affect lipid metabolism indirectly by stimulating glucagon secretion (Marco et al. [14]).

Growth Hormone

Exercise is a major stimulus for growth hormone secretion, and this is used clinically for the hormone's evaluation. Of the four stress hormones, the metabolic activity of growth hormone is least understood. It is both glucogenic and lipolytic, thereby enhancing availability of metabolic fuels during exercise, and it is similar to cortisol in the delay that occurs between elevation in plasma and metabolic effects (Schade et al. [15]). Like cortisol, the delay is related to new protein synthesis.

The lipolytic effect of growth hormone occurs both in vitro and in vivo (Schade et al. [15]). Furthermore, growth hormone causes elevation of plasma ketone bodies and thus increases fuel for muscle during exercise (Schade et al. [15]). Growth hormone also induces hyperglycemia when insulin is suppressed during exercise by catecholamines.

SUMMARY

This chapter reviewed the hormones that provide adequate fuel for muscle and nervous system during exercise. The hormones responsible for raising plasma nonesterified fatty acids, ketone bodies, and glucose are: 1) catecholamines from the adrenal medulla and sympathetic nerve terminals, 2) glucagon from the pancreas, 3) cortisol from the adrenal cortex, and 4) growth hormone from the pituitary gland. These hormones have distinctive actions and temporal profiles of their metabolic effects.

Adequate fuel for muscle contraction is provided by four stress hormones that raise plasma nonesterified fatty acids, and ketone bodies, metabolic fuels that are rapidly used by muscle, sparing muscle glycogen and increasing exercise tolerance. These hormones also raise plasma glucose, which tends to decrease during exercise as muscle blood flow and glucose uptake increases. The avid use of glucose by muscle is partially counteracted by three of the four stress hormones (catecholamines, cortisol, and growth hormone), which inhibit the uptake of glucose by peripheral tissues, thus ensuring an adequate glucose supply for the central nervous system. This intricate hormonal system usually functions well, since exercise-induced hypoglycemia is rare, and limitation of exercise due to inadequate substrate is almost nonexistent.

REFERENCES

1. Ahlborg, G., Felig, P., et al. 1974. Substrate turnover during prolonged exercise in man: splanchnic and leg metabolism of glucose, free fatty acids, and amino acids. J Clin Invest 53:1080–1090.
2. Felig, P., Wahren, J. 1975. Fuel homeostasis in exercise. N Engl J Med 293: 1078–1084.
3. Havel, R.J. 1972. Caloric homeostasis and disorders of fuel transport. N Engl J Med 287:1186–1192.
4. Felig, P. 1973. The glucose-alanine cycle. Metabolism 22:179–207.
5. Dill, D.B., Edwards, H.T., et al. 1935. Effects of adrenalin injection in moderate work. Am J Physiol 3:9–16.

6. Eaton, R.P., Schade, D.S. 1978. Modulation and implications of the counter-regulatory hormones: glucagon, catecholamines, cortisol, and growth hormone. In: Katzen, H.M., Mahler, R.J. (eds): Advances in Modern Nutrition. Diabetes, Obesity, and Vascular Disease (Vol. 2). Hemisphere Publishing Corporation, Washington, DC, pp 341–366.

7. Eigler, N., Sacca, L., et al. 1979. Synergistic interactions of physiologic increments of glucagon, epinephrine, and cortisol in the dog. J Clin Invest 63:114–123.

8. Schade, D.S., Eaton, R.P. 1979. The regulation of plasma ketone body concentration by counter-regulatory hormones in man. III. Effects of norepinephrine in normal man. Diabetes 28:5–10.

9. Iverson, J. 1973. Adrenergic receptors and the secretion of glucagon and insulin from the isolated, perfused canine pancreas. J Clin Invest 52:2102–2116.

10. Greene, H.L., Taunton, O.D., et al. 1974. The rapid changes of hepatic glycolytic enzymes and fructose-1, 6-diphosphatase activities after intravenous glucagon in humans. J Clin Invest 53:44–51.

11. Schade, D.S., Woodside, W., et al. 1979. The role of glucagon in the regulation of plasma lipids. Metabolism 28:874–886.

12. Gerich, J.E., Karam, J.H., et al. 1973. Stimulation of glucagon secretion by epinephrine in man. J Clin Endocrinol Metab 37:479–481.

13. Schade, D.S., Eaton, R.P., et al. 1977. Glucocorticoid regulation of plasma ketone body concentration in insulin deficient man. J Clin Endocrinol Metab 44:1069–1079.

14. Marco, J., Calle, C., et al. 1973. Hyperglucagonism induced by glucocorticoid treatment in man. N Engl J Med 288:128–131.

15. Schade, D.S., Eaton, R.P., et al. 1978. The regulation of plasma ketone body concentration by counter-regulatory hormones in man. II. Effects of growth hormone in diabetic man. Diabetes 27:916–924.

·11·

Exercise and the Kidney

Kenneth D. Gardner, Jr.

Exercise and the kidney interrelate in two important ways: One, physical exertion alters normal renal function. Two, individuals with impaired renal function engage in athletic endeavors. In this chapter each of these issues is addressed, with emphasis on the question of whether and to what extent renal function can be permanently impaired by strenuous activity.

EXERCISE AND THE NORMAL KIDNEY

Background

Collier in 1907 [1] described the postexercise appearance of protein in the urine and deduced that physical exertion, not renal disease, was responsible. A report describing an increase in the rate of cast excretion in the urines of marathon runners followed in 1910 (Barach [2]). These characteristics of the alterations that manifest in urine after exercise were confirmed by numerous subsequent studies. In 1954 Amelar and Solomon [3] added hematuria to the list of urinary changes. They studied urines obtained from boxers before and after matches. Amelar and Solomon attributed hematuria after boxing to renal injury—blows received by the kidneys during the match.

A study was conducted by this author in 1955 in which the urinary sediments of a team of college football players were followed over the course of two weeks in midseason. The severity of proteinuria and cylinduria was found to correlate with the degrees of individual physical exertion (Gardner [4]). Of significance in this study was the observation that exercise induced not only an abnormal degree of proteinuria and an increase in the numbers of hyaline and granular casts, but also the transient appearance of red blood cell casts in some urines. Because the urinary sediments of athletes can resemble those passed by patients with the nephritic syndrome (proteinuria occurring with hyaline, granular, and red blood cell casts) and because of the transient nature of these abnormalities (they disappear with abstinence from exercise, unlike those of acute nephritis), the term "athletic pseudonephritis" was coined.

In 1958 the question of whether trauma to kidneys was responsible for any or all of the urinary abnormalities that are found after exercise was addressed directly. Alyea and Parish [5] recorded proteinuria, hematuria, and cylinduria in athletes after their participation in

Table 11-1   Features of Athletic Pseudonephritis

Proteinuria
  Albuminuria
  Globulinuria
  Myoglobinuria (usually mild and transient)
  Hemoglobinuria (mild; presence parallels hematuria)
Formed elements
  Hyaline casts
  Granular casts
  Red blood cells
  White blood cells
  Red blood cell casts
Clinical setting
  Occurs within 7 days of last exertion
  Abnormalities clear with rest
  Abnormalities occur immediately postexercise with, but later (more than one day)
    without, depression of glomerular filtration rate

the relatively nontraumatic sports of rowing and swimming. Results of this study substantially excluded the possibility that direct trauma to the kidney caused proteinuria and hematuria in athletes. Thus, by the late 1950s, it was generally held that "athletic pseudonephritis" was a confirmed, benign entity and that the passage of protein, blood, and casts after exercise was little more than a clinical curiosity (Table 11-1).

The simplicity and the erroneous nature of this judgment soon became obvious. Reports began to appear of clear-cut renal failure brought on by physical exertion. In 1960, Howenstine [6] reported the renal consequences of excessive performance of "squat jump" calisthenics among Marine Corp recruits. Dark urine, albuminuria, hematuria, pyuria, red blood cell casts, myoglobinuria, hemoglobinuria, and severe swelling of quadriceps muscles appeared in 19 of 60 individuals. One of the 19 experienced an episode of acute renal failure. From this study and subsequent reports over the next decade (Arnett and Gardner [7]; Smith [8]; Hamilton et al. [9]; Ritter et al. [10]), it became evident that strenuous exercise, especially by unconditioned individuals stressed by heat (Schrier et al. [11]), carried risks of myolysis, acute tubular necrosis, and acute renal failure. Thus did malignant "athletic nephritis" (Table 11-2) join benign "athletic pseudonephritis" as the second of two clinical syndromes that might occur following exercise in previously normal individuals (Gardner [12]).

Physiology and Pathophysiology

With exercise, a series of changes occur in renal function, urinary composition, and hormonal activity. Effective renal plasma flow, as measured by p-aminohippurate clearance, declines (Grimby [13]; Castenfors [14]). Blood received by the kidney diminishes with increasing oxygen uptake as the severity of exercise is increased. These changes can be detected within minutes after exertion is initiated. They remit with rest.

The decline in renal plasma flow is paralleled by a drop in glomerular filtration rate (GFR) (Kachadorian [15]). The GFR returns, albeit slowly, toward normal when exercise is ended. Hydration appears to be effective in blunting the reduction in GFR that is induced by exercise (Castenfors [14]).

Urine volume lessens and urine concentration rises, evidently the consequence of increased antidiuretic hormone (ADH) activity (Wade and Claybaugh [16]). As is the case with GFR, hydration tends to blunt the degree of change, in this case the extent of hyperosmolality. During exercise urinary sodium excretion falls as an apparent result of increased reabsorption of sodium by the renal tubules. Urinary potassium excretion varies in less

Table 11-2   Features of Exercise-Induced Renal Failure

Proteinuria
  Albuminuria
  Globulinuria
  Hemoglobinuria (usually marked)
  Myoglobinuria (usually marked)
Formed elements
  Hyaline casts (usually marked)
  Granular casts (usually many; often broad)
  Cellular casts
  Red blood cells
  Red blood cell casts
  Hemoglobin/myoglobin casts (often broad; not inevitable)
  Tubular epithelial cells
Clinical setting
  Worsening azotemia
  Developing oliguria
  Elevated muscle enzymes in serum
  Persisting metabolic acidosis
  History of little previous physical conditioning (usual but not inevitable)
  Elevated body temperature (may persist in spite of hydration and rest)

predictable fashion (Kachadorian [15]), making the routine prediction of replacement needs for this ion unreliable. Relative to other ions and solutes, Poortmans has documented reductions in the urinary excretion of chloride, calcium, phosphorus, and urea (Poortmans [17]).

Accompanying changes in urinary composition, and in all likelihood causing most of them, are increases in plasma aldosterone levels and renin activity (Galbo [18]; Hansson et al. [19]). Despite repeated observations, the pathophysiology of athletic pseudonephritis remains speculative. Intrarenal vasoconstriction as the consequence of activation of the renin–angiotensin axis is suspect (Poortmans [17]). Epinephrine injection is followed by proteinuria in several experimental models and humans.

The pathophysiology of exercise-induced acute tubular necrosis is better understood. The combination of metabolic acidosis and myolysis with myoglobinemia and myoglobinuria is one that is lethal to many if not all renal tubular epithelial cells. Thus, a direct toxic effect of acid myetin on tubular epithelia is held responsible for athletic nephritis (Falk et al. [20]; Kagen [21]; Gabow et al. [22]).

The appearance of myoglobin per se in blood and urine is not the harbinger of inevitable renal failure. Both can occur with exercise, accompanied by rises in serum levels of aldolase and creatine phosphokinase (Schrier et al. [11]). Using radioimmunoassay to detect myoglobin, Ritter et al. documented delayed (6-hr) rises in serum myoglobin levels after severe exercise among 16 U.S. Army recruits (Ritter et al. [10]). These workers showed further that conditioning reduced the degree of myoglobinemia among the same individuals. In the absence of subsequent functional impairment, however, extreme rises in serum muscle components are rarely encountered. Therefore, greater amounts of myoglobinuria and higher serum levels of muscle enzymes can be considered to carry with them the greater likelihood of impending renal shutdown.

Laboratory Evaluation

Studies into the nature of the protein excreted after exercise reveal two types: One is uromucoid known as Tamm-Horsfall mucoprotein, derived from the lower nephrons and collecting ducts of the kidney, the primary matrix component of hyaline casts, and probably of benign significance. The other is serum-derived protein, including albumin and smaller molecular-weight globulins (Poortmans [17]). Presumably, passage of these proteins into urine reflects increased permeability of the glomerulus to them. Diminished tubular reabsorption may contribute.

Routine urine tests are useful in assessing degrees of albuminuria, myoglobinuria, and hemoglobinuria. The popular dipstick method detects primarily albuminuria, while the less specific sulfosalicylic acid (SSA) precipitation test will yield positive results to not only albumin but also to the hemo- and myoglobins. A weaker dipstick reaction in face of a strongly positive SSA precipitation test suggests globulinuria and serves as grounds to pursue a search for hemoglobinuria and myoglobinuria. The dipstick test for blood utilizes orthotolidine and, in fact, demonstrates the presence of organic iron (myo- as well as hemoglobin) in urine. Thus the dipstick test for blood can be used at the bedside (trackside) to strengthen suspicions of significant pigmenturia that are raised by discrepant proteinuria test results. Dipstick results do not distinguish between myoglobin and hemoglobin. In the past, distinction has been advocated on the basis of results from solubility and differential filtration tests. These tests are simple to perform, require little in the way of special equipment, and therefore, have enjoyed a popularity that far outweighs their reliability. They yield both false positives and false negatives with alarming frequency. In their stead results from the more time-consuming, (unfortunately) less accessible, and far more reliable immunofluorescent, immunoradiographic, or electrophoretic techniques should be depended on.

Differential Diagnosis

The task of differential diagnosis in athletic pseudonephritis is simplified immensely by the temporary nature of the abnormal urinary findings. Awareness of the syndrome and appreciation of the fact that urinary abnormalities clear within 7 days, usually less (Gardner [4]), should allow one to distinguish pseudonephritis from post-beta-streptococcal glomerulonephritis, nephritis secondary to collagen vascular disease, etc. Virtually no form of organic nephritis with urinary abnormalities runs its course within a single week. Furthermore, in most of these entities, renal function can be impaired. The confirmation of azotemia, for example, requires that a diagnosis other than pseudonephritis be considered.

Trauma to the kidney typically causes pain localized to the area and may be accompanied by microscopic or gross hematuria. Significant myoglobinuria and proteinuria (4 +) are not found. Their presence, the absence of a history of trauma, and the presence of bilateral renal tenderness should suggest the syndrome of postexercise acute renal failure, not renal trauma.

Therapy

The design of a program to minimize the likelihood of serious renal complications after exercise is based on elements of the just-completed discussion. Recognizing that an ounce of prevention is worth a pound of cure, health professionals may advise their colleagues and clients as follows: A program of graded physical conditioning before strenuous exercise reportedly can protect against myolysis (Ritter et al. [10]). Adequate fluid intake favorably influences the tendencies for dehydration, reduced GFR, and increased ADH activity that accompany or soon follow strenuous exertion (Poortmans [17]; Wade [23]).

Voluntary exertion in a hot environment should be avoided (Schrier et al. [11]). The appearance of pigmenturia after exercise, while not an invariable forerunner of acute renal failure, should be cause for concern. If followed by persistent low urinary volumes in spite of adequate rehydration and a fall in peak exercise pulse rate, medical advice should be obtained. Sustained oliguria and pigmenturia, i.e., for more than 8–12 hr postexercise, are adequate justification for nephrologic consultation. Whether impending oliguria can be reversed by aggressive management, e.g., with osmotic or loop diuretics to promote urinary flow and/or with alkali to reverse acidosis, remains debatable. The same may be said about the ability of these measures to shorten the period of morbidity. Under specialist supervision in the hospital, these measures probably should be employed; their potential benefit appears to outweigh their risks.

PROGNOSIS

The outlook generally is good for those unfortunate enough to suffer acute renal failure. While a period of days (usually less than 21) in the hospital are required, renal function most frequently returns to normal. Studies dealing with the longevity of athletes fail to reflect an increased incidence of deaths, premature or not, from renal causes (Montoye et al. [24]; Schnohr [25]; Polednak [26], [28]; Baskin et al. [27]; Shepard [29]). Thus, it seems likely that exercise, irrespective of its short-term effects, imposes no long-lasting consequences on kidney function or viability. For that rare individual who may experience permanent loss of renal function, dialysis and transplantation are available.

EXERCISE AND THE DISEASED KIDNEY

Exercise and Acute Renal Failure

A significant degree of physical exertion in the presence of acute renal disease is not advised. It matters not from what basis azotemia has occurred. Bed rest and passive exercises are advised for those with post-beta-streptococcal glomerulonephritis until edema, azotemia, and hypertension are controlled. The restrictions on those with azotemia from other forms of nephritis are less severe. Nonetheless, the acutely diseased kidney is unable to regulate adequately the body's fluid and salt contents and acid–base balance and to excrete its nitrogenous wastes. Any added provocation from exercise, with its tendencies to accelerate catabolic activity, increase hydrogen and nitrogen turnover rates, and shunt blood from the kidney, is held to be contraindicated.

Exercise and Chronic Renal Disease

In the setting of chronic renal disease, exercise enjoys increasing notoriety in two ways: 1) as a provocative measure in the early diagnosis of Type 1 diabetic nephropathy and 2) as a therapeutic measure in chronic hemodialysis patients.

Among Type 1 diabetics, as it does among nondiabetic subjects, exercise provokes albuminuria (Feldt-Rasmussen et al. [30]; Mogensen and Christensen [31], [32]; Viberti et al. [33]; Schmitz et al. [34]). There is more to the story, however. Among Type 1 diabetics whose urines are negative to dipstick testing for albumin at rest, the excretion of greater than 15 μg/min of albumin and a GFR in excess of 150 ml/min portend subsequent progression to diabetic nephropathy (Mogensen and Christensen [31]). Elevated systemic blood pressure appears to play a contributory but not causative role in the renal changes (Mogensen and Christensen [32]). Feldt-Rasmussen et al. [30] examined the possibility but were unable to demonstrate any special provocative effect of exercise on microalbumin excretion by the Type 1 diabetic kidney.

Individuals with chronic renal disease exhibit significant departures from normal in their cardiac and metabolic responses to exercise. Overall tolerance to exercise is reduced

(Painter and Zimmerman [35]). Exercise capacity as measured by maximal oxygen consumption is low (Painter et al. [36]). Lactic acidosis develops more rapidly (Parrish et al. [37]). Left ventricular stroke work does not increase normally, and left ventricular end diastolic pressure is abnormally raised (Pehrrson et al. [38]). These results indicate that the chronically azotemic individual, whether or not on hemodialysis, has an abnormality in the muscle handling of lactate (Parrish [39]) and impaired myocardial function. Nonetheless, a program of carefully graded exercise appears to be physically beneficial among patients on maintenance hemodialysis. Shalom and associates recorded a 42% improvement in work capacity during treadmill testing among 7 hemodialysis patients who regularly attended a 12-week exercise testing program (Shalom et al. [40]). Seven additional patients who attended significantly fewer sessions showed no such response. The psychological benefits of exercise to hemodialysis patients, however, remains equivocal. Compliance with the exercise regimen is relatively poor (Painter and Zimmerman [35]). The fact that only 14 of 174 patients chose to participate led Shalom et al. to conclude that few appear willing to participate to an extent sufficient to induce physiologic change (Shalom et al. [40]). At present, therefore, programs of graded exercise appear to offer moderate but definite physiologic but only problematic psychologic benefits to the chronic renal failure (hemodialysis) population.

REFERENCES

1. Collier, W. 1907. Functional albuminuria in athletes. Br Med J 1:4–6.
2. Barach, J.H. 1910. Physiological and pathological effects of severe exercise (the marathon race) on the circulatory and renal system. Arch Intern Med 5:382–405.
3. Amelar, R.D., Solomon, C. 1954. Acute renal trauma in boxers. J Urol 72:145–148.
4. Gardner, K.D. 1956. "Athletic Pseudonephritis"—Alteration of the urine sediment by athletic competition. JAMA 161:1613–1617.
5. Alyea, E.P., Parish, H.H. 1958. Renal response to exercise—urinary findings. JAMA 167:807–813.
6. Howenstine, J.A. 1960. Exertion-induced myoglobinuria and hemoglobinuria. JAMA 173:99–499.
7. Arnett, J.H., Gardner, K.D. 1961. Urinary abnormalities from over-use of muscles. Am J Med Sci 241:55–58.
8. Smith, R.F. 1968. Exertional rhabdomyolysis in naval officer candidates. Arch Intern Med 121:313–319.
9. Hamilton, R.W., Gardner, L.B., et al. 1972. Acute tubular necrosis caused by exercise-induced myoglobinuria. Ann Intern Med 77:77–82.
10. Ritter, W.S., Stone, M.J., et al. 1979. Reduction in exertional myoglobinemia after physical conditioning. Arch Intern Med 139:644–647.

11. Schrier, R.W., Hano, J., et al. 1970. Renal, metabolic, and circulatory responses to heat and exercise. Ann Intern Med 73:213–223.
12. Gardner, K.D. 1971. Athletic nephritis: pseudo and real. Ann Intern Med 75:966.
13. Grimby, G. 1965. Renal clearances during prolonged supine exercise at different loads. J Appl Physiol 20:1294–1298.
14. Castenfors, J. 1967. Renal function during exercise. Acta Physiol Scand 70:1–44.
15. Kachadorian, W.A. 1972. The effects of activity on renal function. In: Alexander, J.F., Serfass, R.C., Tipton, C.M. (eds.): Fitness and Exercise. Athletic Institute, Chicago, pp 97–116.
16. Wade, C.E., Claybaugh, J.R. 1980. Plasma renin activity, vasopressin concentration and excretory responses to exercise in men. J Appl Physiol 49:930–936.
17. Poortmans, J.R. 1984. Exercise and renal function. Sports Med 1:125–153.
18. Galbo, H. 1982. Endocrinology and metabolism in exercise. Curr Probl Clin Biochem 11:26–44.
19. Hansson, B.G., Dymling, J.F., et al. 1977. Long-term treatment of moderate hypertension with beta-receptor blocking agent metaprolol. Eur J Clin Pharm 11:239–245.
20. Falk, K., Rayyes, A.N., et al. 1973. Myoglobinuria with reversible acute re-

nal failure. NY State J Med 73:537–543.

21. Kagen, L.J. 1970. Immunofluorescent demonstration of myoglobin in the kidney: case report and review of forty-three cases of myoglobinemia and myoglobinuria identified immunologically. Am J Med 48:649–652.

22. Gabow, P.A., Kaehny, W.O., et al. 1982. The spectrum of rhabdomyolysis. Medicine 61:141–152.

23. Wade, C.E. 1984. Response, regulation, and actions of vasopressin during exercise: a review. Med Sci Sports Exerc 16:506–511.

24. Montoye, H.J., Van Huss, W.D., et al. 1956. Study of the longevity and morbidity of college athletes. JAMA 162:1132–1134.

25. Schnohr, P. 1971. Longevity and causes of death in male athletic champions. Lancet 2:1364–1366.

26. Polednak, A.P. 1972. Longevity and cause of death among Harvard College athletes and their classmates. Geriatrics 27:53–64.

27. Baskin, A.M., Freedman, L.R., et al. 1972. Proteinuria in Yale students and 30-year mortality experience. J Urol 108:617–618.

28. Polednak, A.P. 1972. Mortality from renal diseases among former college athletes. Ann Intern Med 77:919–922.

29. Shepard, R.J. 1986. Exercise in coronary heart disease. Sports Med 3:26–49.

30. Feldt-Rasmussen, B., Baker, L., et al. 1985. Exercise as a provocative test in early renal disease in type 1 (insulin-dependent) diabetes: albuminuric, systemic, and renal hemodynamic responses. Diabetologia 28:389–396.

31. Mogensen, C.E., Christensen, C.K. 1985. Blood pressure changes and renal function in incipient and overt diabetic nephropathy. Hypertension 7:1164–1173.

32. Mogensen, C.E., Christensen, C.K. 1984. Predicting diabetic nephropathy in insulin-dependent patients. N Engl J Med 311:89–93.

33. Viberti, G.C., Hill, R.D., et al. 1982. Microalbuminuria as predictor of clinical nephrophathy in insulin-dependent diabetes mellitus. Lancet 1:1430–1432.

34. Schmitz, O., Hansen, H.E., et al. 1985. End-stage renal failure in diabetic nephropathy: pathophysiology and treatment. Blood Purif 3:120–139.

35. Painter, P., Zimmerman, S.W. 1986. Exercise in end-stage renal disease. Am J Kid Dis 7:386–394.

36. Painter, P., Messer-Rehak, D., et al. 1986. Exercise capacity in hemodialysis, CAPD, and renal transplant patients. Nephron 42:47–51.

37. Parrish, A.E., Zikria, M., et al. 1985. Oxygen uptake in exercising subjects with minimal renal disease. Nephron 40:455–457.

38. Pehrrson, S.K., Jonasson, R., et al. 1984. Cardiac performance in various stages of renal failure. Br Heart J 52:667–673.

39. Parrish, A.E. 1981. The effect of minimal exercise on the blood lactate in azotemic subjects. Clin Nephrol 16:35–39.

40. Shalom, R., Blumenthal, J.A., et al. 1984. Feasibility and benefits of exercise training in patients on maintenance dialysis. Kidney Int 25:958–963.

Heart, Blood Vessels, Pulmonary and Hematologic Adaptation to Exercise

•12•

Cardiovascular Adaptations to Sustained Aerobic Exercise

Jerome E. Goss and Neal Shadoff

Sustained aerobic exercise requires increased oxygen delivery to muscle cells. Improved aerobic performance comes about mainly through changes in the cardiovascular system, which improves oxygen transport, and through adaptation in skeletal muscles. These changes are modified by coronary artery disease and aging.

This chapter reviews the cardiovascular adaptations that develop with aerobic training and explores the modifications produced by coronary artery disease and aging.

HEART RATE AND STROKE VOLUME

The easiest physiologic function to measure and compare longitudinally in individuals or between groups of subjects is heart rate. Whether a person is an elite marathoner or a quality middle-aged distance runner, his or her resting heart rate is 15–20 beats/min slower than the average heart rate (Kasch [1]; Paolone et al. [2]; Morganroth et al. [3]). This has been attributed to alterations in the autonomic nervous system (Lin and Horvath [4]; Scheuer and Tipton [5]). The sinoatrial node in the right atrium is influenced by the autonomic nervous system, which controls intrinsic heart rate. Controversy exists concerning relative changes in parasympathetic and sympathetic activities to the heart as a result of training, but in the resting state increased parasympathetic activity is operative (Scheuer and Tipton [5]). There does not seem to be any consistently significant changes in myocardial or plasma levels of catecholamines at rest (Christensen et al. [6]; Cousineau and Ferguson [7]; Peronnet et al. [8]). Increased parasympathetic activity or increased vagal tone explains some of the atrioventricular conduction changes seen in the resting electrocardiogram of endurance athletes (Lichtman et al. [9]).

Reduction in maximal heart rate from endurance training (Scheuer and Tipton [5]; Rowell [10]; Ekblom [11]) has been attributed to: 1) changes in autonomic control (Blomqvist and Saltin [12], 2) increased stroke volume, and 3) reduction in circulating catecholamines (Scheuer and Tipton [5]; Hartley et al. [13]; Christensen and Galbo [14]). Endurance training decreases heart rate for a submaximal work load and increases stroke volume (Scheuer and Tipton [5]; Froelicker [15]). Peripheral responses to training are also important in the exercise/heart rate response. It has been shown in bicycle ergometry studies that the reduced heart rate response to a work load occurs only when using trained muscles (Clausen et al. [16]). One group of subjects used arms and one group used legs. After training, the subjects were tested with alternate arm and leg exercises. The lower heart rate response to exercise load was seen only when the trained limb was used.

Stroke volume also increases with endurance training (Morganroth et al. [3]; Hanson et al. [17]; Rowell [10]; Ekblom [11]; Hartley et al. [18]). Echocardiographic techniques were used to compare 15 long-distance runners with a control group of noncompetitive students (Morganroth et al. [3]). A statistically significant increase in stroke volume ($p < .01$) in the endurance-trained athletes was found. Seven elite runners who had a mean stroke volume of 189 ml at maximum oxygen consumption ($\dot{V}O_{2\,max}$) were studied by dye dilution techniques (Ekblom [11]). Less well trained endurance runners at $\dot{V}O_{2\,max}$ had a stroke volume of 149 ml and 8 untrained subjects at $\dot{V}O_{2\,max}$ had a stroke volume of 122 ml. Endurance training, therefore, increased stroke volume by 55% in elite runners compared with untrained subjects.

MAXIMAL OXYGEN CONSUMPTION AND CARDIAC OUTPUT

Endurance training significantly increased the maximal work capacity, commonly expressed as $\dot{V}O_{2\,max}$ (Scheuer and Tipton [5]; Hanson et al. [17]). Sedentary middle-aged men had a $\dot{V}O_{2\,max}$ of 30 ml/kg/min; football defensive linemen trained in strength and not endurance had an average $\dot{V}O_{2\,max}$ of 45 ml/kg/min (Wilmore [19]); soccer stars had a $\dot{V}O_{2\,max}$ of 58 ml/kg/min; and elite distance runners a $\dot{V}O_{2\,max}$ of 79 ml/kg/min (Gettman and Pollock [20]). Values as high as 85 ml/kg/min were reported in endurance runners (Saltin and Astrand [21]).

Increased $\dot{V}O_{2\,max}$ is a function of increased maximal cardiac output and increased arteriovenous difference in oxygen concentration (Ekblom [11]; Froelicker [15]). Stroke volume is greater in trained athletes both at rest and during exercise (Rowell [10]). Since the heart rate in trained athletes at $\dot{V}O_{2\,max}$ is not increased, the increased maximal cardiac output is due to increased stroke volume. In 7 well-trained distance runners, an average cardiac output of 36 L/min was recorded, the highest value being 42.3 L/min. Eight untrained males had maximum cardiac output of 23.9 L/min (Ekblom [11]). Thus, endurance-trained athletes had about 50% greater maximal cardiac output than did untrained controls. Enhanced oxygen extraction (i.e., widening arteriovenous oxygen difference) during maximum exercise accounts for the other 50% of increased oxygen supplied to cells of endurance-trained athletes (Rowell [10]). In those whose cardiac output can be only minimally increased with training, oxygen extraction by the tissues is the major factor in increasing oxygen supply and maximal work capacity. A patient with limited left ventricular function and an artificial pacemaker would be an example. The mechanism for increased extraction is primarily redistribution of blood flow from the areas of low extraction, such as the splanchnic bed, to areas of high extraction, i.e., skeletal muscles (Rowell [10]). Submaximal work loads require the same oxygen consumption after training so that total body efficiency is unchanged (Froelicker [15]). Therefore, cardiac output and arteriovenous oxygen differences are unchanged at submaximal work loads by aerobic training in normal subjects (Scheuer and Tipton [5]; Hartley et al. [13]; Froelicker [15]; Mitchell [22]).

BLOOD PRESSURE

In studies of more than 3,000 men, the resting systolic and diastolic pressures were significantly lower in physically fit persons than in those in poor physical condition (Cooper et al. [23]), and both resting systolic and diastolic pressures in 66 middle-aged men were significantly lower after 1 year of modest aerobic training (Paolone et al. [2]). Similar observations of less magnitude were made in untrained men, ages 52–88 years, after only 6 weeks of aerobic training (de Vries [24]). Others have noted no decrease in blood pressure with endurance training (Hanson et al. [17]; Ekblom et al. [25]; Frick et al. [26]), but significant reduction in blood pressure of hypertensive patients placed in exercise programs was found (Boyer and Kasch [27]; Choquette and Ferguson [28]). Personal observation supports the concept of variation in blood pressure response to endurance training. The importance of initial blood pressures was pointed out by Hellerstein et al. [29]. If a person had low blood pressure before training, the pressure did not change, but if blood pressure was initially elevated, both resting systolic and diastolic pressures decreased significantly after aerobic conditioning, perhaps explaining some of the contradictory observations.

The mean arterial pressure in trained athletes at $\dot{V}O_{2\,max}$ may be increased, unchanged, or slightly decreased (Scheuer and Tipton [5]). Reduction in systolic blood pressure at $\dot{V}O_{2\,max}$ with aerobic training occurred in middle-aged men (Paolone et al. [2]), and significant ($p < .01$) decrease in the diastolic pressure from 86 mm Hg to 76 mm Hg was noted after 1 year of training, with further decline to 66 mm Hg after 2 years of modest aerobic training. With exercise, systolic pressure increases in normal subjects, but usually not above 210 mm Hg, and the diastolic pressure remains the same or is decreased (Hellerstein et al. [29]). If systolic blood pressure exceeds 220 mm Hg and the diastolic pressure is above 95, the response to exercise is considered to be abnormal and suggests underlying hypertension (Hellerstein et al. [29]).

The mechanism for blood pressure change with exercise is based on the relationship of arterial blood pressure (BPa) to cardiac output (CO) and peripheral resistance (PR) (BPa = CO × PR). When exercise commences, skeletal muscle activation increases venous return and cardiac output. At the same time, the arterioles supplying the exercising muscles dilate and peripheral vascular resistance decreases. The net result of these initial changes is decreased blood pressure. Early activation of the sympathetic nervous system and withdrawal of parasympathetic tone increase heart rate, stimulate the myocardium, and constrict splanchnic and renal arterial and venous beds, which raise cardiac output and peripheral vascular resistance. The overall result is increased arterial pressure or no change (Hellerstein et al. [29]; Clausen [30]). During exercise, plasma norepinephrine increases with the intensity of work, but in well-trained athletes the sympathetic response is less than in untrained individuals for the same work load (Hellerstein et al. [29]).

MYOCARDIAL CONTRACTILITY AND PERFUSION

Endurance training improves myocardial contractility, shown by increased mean ventricular ejection rate and maximal first derivative of the pressure pulse by as much as 35% (Hanson et al. [17]). Several studies of aerobically untrained rats showed increased cardiac actomyosin ATPase activity, which provides metabolic support for hemodynamic alterations, thus implying improved myocardial contractility (Penpargkul and Scheuer [31]; Scheuer and Stezoski [32]; Bhan and Scheuer [33]).

Aerobic training appears to improve myocardial perfusion (Cohen [34]; Scheuer [35]). The diameters of main coronary artery lumens were up to three times their usual width in necropsy studies of great endurance athletes (Currens and White [36]). Coronary arterial beds, estimated by the weight of vinyl acetate corrosion casts, were increased in aerobically treated rats (Tepperman and Pearlman [37]), and the ratio of the cross-sectional area of the coronary artery capillary lumen to ventricular muscle fibers was also increased with exercise (Mitchell [22]). The capillary:ventricular fiber ratios in exercise-trained rats from youth to old age were significantly increased for trained animals in another study (Tomanek

[38]). Hypoxia produced by restriction of coronary blood flow in dogs caused increased collateral flow (Eckstein [39]). Mild circumflex coronary artery narrowing produced increased collateral blood flow only in the aerobically untrained animals. In those with moderate to severe narrowing, both the trained and untrained animals showed increased collateral flow, but the effect was enhanced by endurance training. These studies support the concept that aerobic training improves both macro- and microcoronary blood flow.

CARDIAC HYPERTROPHY

In contrast to skeletal muscle, cardiac muscle does not increase its respiratory capacity, but it does hypertrophy in response to endurance training: Trained athletes have larger hearts than sedentary controls of similar body weight (Morganroth et al. [3]; Holloszy [40]; Blair et al. [41]). Echocardiograms on college swimmers, runners, wrestlers, and control subjects showed that swimmers and runners had significantly ($p < .001$) larger left ventricular volumes. The swimmers, runners, and wrestlers had significantly ($p < .001$) larger left ventricular size, but only wrestlers had a significantly ($p < .001$) thicker ventricular wall. This finding indicates that endurance-trained athletes develop increased cardiac volume in contrast to wrestlers, whose exercise is mainly isometric and consequently leads to mural cardiac hypertrophy (Morganroth et al. [3]). When male national and international standard aerobically trained athletes were compared to matched untrained controls, both ventricles were significantly larger in the trained athletes. Left ventricular volume was 43% larger ($p < .002$), and right ventricular volume was 24% larger ($p < .005$) (Blair et al. [41]). Increased left ventricular size increases work capacity since positive correlation exists between heart size and maximal cardiac output (Holloszy [40]; Blair et al. [41]).

MYOCARDIAL OXYGEN CONSUMPTION

Myocardial oxygen consumption is determined by: 1) basal oxygen requirement, 2) electrical activity, 3) internal work (tension × heart rate), 4) external work (load × shortening), and 5) the contractile state (Mitchell [22]; Sonnenblick et al. [42]). The basal oxygen requirement (Mitchell [22]) and oxygen consumed by electrical activity are low (Klocke et al. [43]). Oxygen consumption induced by internal work is about twice that induced by external work (Coleman et al. [44]; Sonnenblick et al. [45]). Tension, heart rate, and contractile state are the principal determinants of myocardial oxygen consumption (Mitchell [22]; Sonnenblick et al. [42]). Measurement of myocardial oxygen consumption is difficult at rest and almost impossible during exercise. For this reason, a number of calculations that approximate myocardial oxygen consumption are used (Froelicker [15]; Mitchell [22]). The double product (peak systolic blood pressure × heart rate), the triple product (peak systolic blood pressure × heart rate × ejection time), and the tension-time index (area under the left ventricular or aortic pressure curve during systole × heart rate) are all used as estimates of myocardial oxygen consumption (Froelicker [15]; Hanson et al. [17]; Mitchell [22]).

Hanson et al. [17] demonstrated a significant reduction in tension-time index (myocardial oxygen consumption) with aerobic training in a group of middle-aged men at rest and at all levels of exercise: The greatest decrease occurred in the mid-range of exercise intensity. After 1 year of modest aerobic training, 45 middle-aged men had an 18% reduction in double product (myocardial oxygen consumption) (Paolone et al. [2]), which is important when the modest intensity of the program is considered. Although myocardial oxygen consumption is difficult to measure, aerobic training in humans appears to reduce myocardial oxygen consumption both at rest and during exercise.

ADAPTATIONS IN CORONARY ARTERY DISEASE

In patients with coronary artery disease (CAD) aerobic training produces many of the same cardiovascular adaptations that occur in normal people (Mitchell [22]; Hartley et al. [46]; Frick and Katila [47]; Ehsani et al. [48]), but the severity of CAD and the amount of functional cardiac muscle that is present may limit adaptation. Viable cardiac muscle and, to some extent, ischemic cardiac muscle (Scheuer and Stezoski [32]) can adapt, but areas of dyskinetic scar cannot. Regeneration of myocardial cells does not occur. Heart rate, at rest and with submaximal work, is decreased in patients with CAD after aerobic training (Frick and Katila [47]; Ehsani et al. [48]; Varnauskas et al. [49]; Clausen and Trap-Jensen [50]; Redwood et al. [51]). Stroke volume has not been consistently improved by aerobic training, a finding that is probably related to the extent of left ventricular scarring (Hartley et al. [46]). Frick and Katila [47] showed significant ($p < .05$) increase in stroke volume at submaximal work loads in 7 patients who had undergone modest aerobic training after suffering myocardial infarction, but the findings of Detry et al. [52] did not support this. Mean systemic blood pressure reduction at submaximal work load in aerobically trained patients with CAD was noted in several studies summarized by Hartley et al. [46]. A significant reduction ($p < .02$) in systolic blood pressure from 153 to 137 mm Hg with modest aerobic training using stationary bicycle ergometers has also been found (Redwood et al. [51]).

Aerobic training almost uniformly improved $\dot{V}O_{2\,max}$ (aerobic power) in patients with CAD (Mitchell [22]; Ehsani et al. [48]; Redwood et al. [51]; Detry et al. [52]). In patients with CAD but without angina, $\dot{V}O_{2\,max}$ increased by 18%, and in those with angina $\dot{V}O_{2\,max}$ increased by 30% after aerobic training (Detry et al. [52]). Patients with ischemic cardiomyopathy and severe depression of the left ventricular ejection fraction may have normal exercise tolerance. (Litchfield et al. [53]; Franciosa et al. [54]; Port et al. [55]; Wilson and Ferraro [56]; Higginbotham et al. [57]). When patients with left ventricular dysfunction and ejection fractions of 30% or less (normal $> 50\%$) were exercised on a treadmill, 50% had normal exercise tolerance in spite of significant left ventricular dysfunction, and some had incredible exercise capacity considering their degree of dysfunction. One such patient had an ejection fraction of only 14%, but was able to exercise on a graded treadmill for 15.5 min (Sheffield protocol: normal > 11 min) (Benge et al. [58]).

Certain patients with CAD can perform high levels of aerobic work. Seven patients with previous myocardial infarctions completed the Boston Marathon after training (Kavanagh et al. [59]). Their average race speed was 5.4 mph, corresponding to 81% of their $\dot{V}O_{2\,max}$. Since most patients with CAD do not perform at maximal work loads, an increased $\dot{V}O_{2\,max}$ allows the aerobically trained patient to work at submaximal loads at a lower percentage of maximal work capacity. Aerobic training improves exercise capacity before appearance of angina pectoris. Seven patients with previous myocardial infarction and angina pectoris increased the average $\dot{V}O_{2\,max}$ at the onset of anginal pain from 9.6 to 15 ml/kg/min ($p < .01$), allowing them to cycle 6.8 min longer with 6 weeks of training (Redwood et al. [51]).

The mechanism by which patients with CAD improve exercise performance with aerobic training is unclear (Froelicker [15]; Mitchell [22]; Frick and Katila [47]; Varnauskas et al. [49]; Clausen and Trap-Jensen [50]; Detry et al. [52]). Patients with CAD showed increased arteriovenous oxygen difference after aerobic training in one study (Detry et al. [52]) and no change during submaximal exercise load in another study (Frick and Katila [47]). No significant change in cardiac output but increased stroke volume was reported by two groups of investigators (Frick and Katila [47]; Clausen and Trap-Jensen [50]), while others (Varnauskas et al. [49]; Detry et al. [52]) reported decreased cardiac output during submaximal exercise after training. Cardiac output and arteriovenous oxygen difference at submaximal work loads are usually unchanged by training in normals. Increased arteriovenous oxygen difference during submaximal work in patients with CAD after training thus supports the concept that improved peripheral extraction is more important than cardiac function in increasing work capacity of the trained CAD patient (Froelicker [15]). The relative importance of cardiac function and peripheral circulatory changes in exercise capacity after aerobic training varies from patient to patient, depending on the extent of left ventricular dysfunction.

Several studies of CAD patients after exercise training suggest that there is reduced myocardial oxygen consumption at submaximal work loads (Frick and Katila [47]; Redwood et al. [51]; Detry et al. [52]). One study used the tension-time index to show this (Frick and Katila [47]). In another study the exercise load required to produce angina pectoris was defined in 7 patients with CAD, and the triple product at that load was calculated (Redwood et al. [51]). The subjects then trained for 6 weeks and were retested at the same work load that had previously produced angina. Only 1 of the 7 experienced angina, and the triple product decreased from 4300 to 3521 ($p < .025$). The same subjects continued training with progressively increasing work loads until angina pectoris reappeared. A significant increase in triple product occurred at the onset of angina (4885 vs 4300; $p < .05$). These findings suggest that training reduces myocardial oxygen requirement at a given exercise load and may enhance myocardial oxygen delivery in patients with coronary artery disease.

ADAPTATIONS IN AGING

Aging is a progressive process that results in decline in work capacity ($\dot{V}O_{2\ max}$), loss of flexibility, and delayed reaction time. Obesity is also an accepted part of aging in many parts of the world. Fig. 12-1, an adaptation of a chart from Cantwell [60], illustrates the progressive decline in $\dot{V}O_{2\ max}$ that occurs at all levels of physical fitness with aging. Fifty percent decline in $\dot{V}O_{2\ max}$ occurs from age 30 to 70 for the average fit person. This decline may be greater if the person is well trained as a youth but not fit when older. The loss of work capacity is primarily due to reduction in maximal heart rate (Kasch [1]; Gertenblith et al. [61]; Kavanagh and Shephard [62]; Pollock [63]; Granath et al. [64]), stroke volume (Granath et al. [64]), and cardiac output (Kasch [1]; Granath et al. [64]). Increased systemic blood pressure (Kavanagh and Shephard [62]; Pollock [63]; Granath et al. [64]) and peripheral resistance (Kasch [1]) also occur, and both require increased left ventricular work.

Right heart catheterization during recumbent exercise showed oxygen consumption of 1.46 L/min in men ages 60 to 83, compared to 2.06 L/min in men of average age 23 (Granath et al. [64]). Cardiac output was also lower (13.1 L/min) in the older group compared to 18.5 L/min in the younger group. Heart rate and stroke volume were reduced in the older group, compared to the younger group. Systolic blood pressure was 39 mm Hg higher in the older group at maximal work load. Average pulmonary artery wedge pressure was 7 mm Hg higher in the older group. Higher pulmonary artery wedge pressures and left ventricular end-diastolic pressures were found in another study of older subjects during exercise (Tartulier et al. [65]). This suggests that the ventricle in the older person is less compliant and has increased resistance to filling at heavy work loads.

Since reduction in physical work capacity ($\dot{V}O_{2\ max}$) is a recognized indicator of physiologic aging, it can be used to assess the effect of aerobic training on the aging process. Sedentary males ages 40 to 50 have $\dot{V}O_{2\ max}$ of 29–35 ml/kg/min (Kasch [1]; Pollock [63]), which places them in the low to average fitness category (Fig. 12-1). Comparison of the data in Table 12-1 indicates that the older endurance runners have a high maximal work capacity for age (Pollock [63]). Even runners over age 70 had a 14% higher maximal work capacity than sedentary 40–50-year-old men. Reduction in maximal work capacity (aerobic power) occurs with age, even in endurance-trained athletes, with the largest decrease appearing

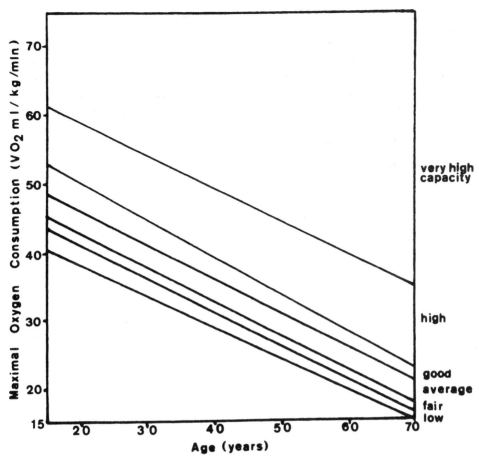

12-1 Decline in cardiopulmonary fitness with aging in untrained individuals. (Adapted from Cantwell, J.D. 1977. Stress testing indicated in a variety of complaints. Physician Sportsmed 5(2):70–74).

after age 70 (Kavanagh and Shephard [62]; Pollock [63]). In older endurance competitors, a decrease of about 8 ml/kg/min of $\dot{V}O_{2\,max}$ (aerobic power) occurred between 35 and 65 years of age, compared to a steady decline in the average person of 4–5 ml/kg/min per decade from age 25 to 65 (Kavanagh and Shephard [62]). The rate of decline of $\dot{V}O_{2\,max}$ is therefore 33–45% slower in endurance-trained competitors compared to the average population.

These studies were of competitive endurance athletes. What about the recreational aerobic runner? Sixteen active men, age 45, ran 24 km/week for 10 years (Kasch [1]). At age 45 their average $\dot{V}O_{2\,max}$ was 43.1 ml/kg/min, placing them in the high maximal work capacity for age (Fig. 12-1). After 10 years of training, their average $\dot{V}O_{2\,max}$ was not significantly changed (44.4 ml/kg/min), but they were now in the very high work capacity range

Table 12-1   Maximal $\dot{V}O_2$ (ml/kg/min) of Older Endurance Runners

Age (yr)	Kavanagh and Shephard (1977)	Pollock (1974)	Asano et al. (1976)	Grimby and Saltin (1966)
40–50	49.9	57.5	49.7	57
50–60	46.0	54.4	45.1	53
60–70	41.6	51.4	42.2	43
>70	29.0	40.0	38.9	—

Adapted from Kavanagh, J., and Shephard, R.J., 1977. The effects of continued training on the aging process. Ann NY Acad Sci 301:656–670.

for age. Basically, these men kept their maximal work capacity stable over a 10-year period while maximal work capacity for the general population was declining.

Whether increased survival of older people or animals occurs as a result of exercise is not clear (Goodrick [66]). Mean longevity of 6-week-old male and female Wistar rats in either standard laboratory cages or in cages with activity wheels was 11.5% longer in female rats allowed voluntary exercise than in female rats that were not allowed to exercise ($p < .01$), and was 19.3% longer in male rats allowed voluntary exercise than in inactive males ($p < .01$) (Goodrick [66]). Although endurance training does not allow the immortality hoped for by some (Scaff [67]), it modifies many aspects of aging.

REFERENCES

1. Kasch, F.W. 1976. The effects of exercise on the aging process. Phys Sportsmed 4(6):64–69.
2. Paolone, A.M., Lewis, R.R., et al. 1976. Results of two years of exercise training in middle-aged men. Phys Sportsmed 4(12):72–77.
3. Morganroth, J., Maron, B.J., et al. 1975. Comparative left ventricular dimensions. Ann Intern Med 82:521–524.
4. Lin, T., Horvath, S.M. 1972. Autonomic nervous control of cardiac frequency in the exercise trained rat. J Appl Physiol 33:796–799.
5. Scheuer, J., Tipton, C.M. 1977. Cardiovascular adaptations to physical training. Annu Rev Physiol 39:221–251.
6. Christensen, N.J., Galbo, H., et al. 1979. Catecholamines and exercise. Diabetes 28:58–69.
7. Couisineau, D., Ferguson, R.H., 1977. Catecholamines in coronary sinus during exercise in man before and after training. J Appl Physiol 43:801–806.
8. Peronnet, F., Cleroux, J., et al. Plasma norepinephine response to exercise before and after training in humans. J Appl Physiol 51:812–818.
9. Lichtman, J., O'Rourke, R.A., et al. 1973. Electrocardiogram of the athlete. Arch Intern Med 132:763–770.
10. Rowell, L.B. 1974. Human cardiovascular adjustments to exercise and thermal stress. Physiol Rev 54:75–159.
11. Ekblom, B. 1969. Effect of physical training on oxygen transport system in man. Acta Physiol Scand (Suppl) 328:5–45.
12. Blomqvist, C.G., Saltin, B. 1983. Cardiovascular adaptation to physical training. Annu Rev Physiol 45:169–197.
13. Hartley, L.H., Mason, J.W., et al. 1972. Multiple hormone responses to prolonged exercise in relation to physical training. J Appl Physiol 33:607–610.
14. Christensen, N.J., Galbo, H. 1983. Sympathetic nervous activity during exercise. Annu Rev Physiol 45:139–168.
15. Froelicker, V.F. 1976. The hemodynamic effects of physical conditioning in healthy young men and middle-aged individuals, and in coronary heart disease. In: Naughton, J.P., Hellerstein, H.K. (eds): Exercise Testing and Exercise Training in Coronary Heart Disease. Academic Press, New York, pp 63–77.
16. Clausen, J.P., Trap-Jensen, J., et al. 1971. Evidence that the relative exercise bradycardia induced by training can be caused by extra cardiac factors. In: Larsen, O.A., Malmborg, R.P. (eds): Coronary Heart Disease and Physical Fitness. University Park Press, Baltimore, MD, pp 27–28.
17. Hanson, J.S., Tabakin, B.S., et al. 1968. Long-term physical training and cardiovascular dynamics in middle-aged men. Circulation 38:783–788.
18. Hartley, L.H., Grimby, G., et al. 1969. Physical training in sedentary middle-aged and older men. III. Cardiac output and gas exchange at submaximal and maximal exercise. Scand J Clin Lab Invest 24:335–344.
19. Wilmore, J.H. 1976. Football pros' strength and CV weakness—charted. Phys Sportsmed 4(10):44–54.
20. Gettman, I.R., Pollock, M.L. 1977. What makes a superstar? A physiological profile. Phys Sportsmed 5(5):64–68.
21. Saltin, B., Astrand, P.O. 1967. Maximal oxygen uptake in athletes. J Appl Physiol 23:353–358.
22. Mitchell, J.H. 1975. Exercise training in the treatment of coronary heart disease. Adv Intern Med 20:249–272.
23. Cooper, K.H., Pollock, M.I., et al. 1976. Physical fitness levels vs. selected coronary risk factors. JAMA 236:166–169.
24. de Vries, H.A. 1970. Physiological effects of an exercise training regimen upon men aged 52 to 88. J Gerontol 25:325–336.
25. Ekblom, B., Astrand, P.O., et al. 1969.

Effect of training on circulatory responses to exercise. J Appl Physiol 24:518–528.

26. Frick, M.H., Konttinen, A., et al. 1963. Effects of physical training on circulation at rest and during exercise. Am J Cardiol 12:142–147.

27. Boyer, J.L., Kasch, F.W. 1970. Exercise therapy in hypertensive men. JAMA 211:1668–1671.

28. Choquette, G., Ferguson, R.J. 1973. Blood pressure reduction in "borderline" hypertensives following physical training. Can Med Assoc J 108:699–703.

29. Hellerstein, H.K., Boyer, J.L., et al. 1976. Exploring the effects of exercise on hypertension. Phys Sportsmed 4(12):36–49.

30. Clausen, J.P. 1977. Effect of physical training on cardiovascular adjustments to exercise in man. Physiol Rev 57:779–803.

31. Penpargkul, S., Scheuer, J. 1970. The effect of physical training upon the mechanical and metabolic performance of the rat heart. J Clin Invest 49:1859–1868.

32. Scheuer, J., Stezoski, S.W. 1972. Effect of physical training on the mechanical and metabolic response of the rat heart of hypoxia. Circ Res 30:418–429.

33. Bhan, A.K., Scheuer, J. 1972. Effects of physical training on cardiac actomyosin adenosine triphosphate activity. Am J Physiol 223:1486–1490.

34. Cohen, M.V. 1983. Coronary and collateral blood flows during exercise and myocardial vascular adaptations to training. Exerc Sport Sci Rev 11:55–59.

35. Scheuer, J. 1982. Effects of physical training on myocardial vascularity and perfusion. Circulation 66:491–495.

36. Currens, J.H., White, P.D. 1961. Half a century of running. N Engl J Med 265:988–993.

37. Tepperman, J., Pearlman, D. 1961. Effects of exercise and anemia on coronary arteries of small animals as revealed by the corrosion-cast technique. Circ Res 9:576–584.

38. Tomanek, R.J. 1969. Effects of age and exercise on the extent of the myocardial capillary bed. Anat Rec 167:55–62.

39. Eckstein, R.W. 1957. Effect of exercise and coronary artery narrowing on coronary collateal circulation. Circ Res 5:230–235.

40. Holloszy, J.O. 1973. Long-term metabolic adaptations in muscle to endurance exercise. In: Naughton, J.P., Heilerstein, H.K. (eds): Exercise Testing and Exercise Training in Coronary Heart Disease. Academic Press, New York, pp 211–222.

41. Blair, N.L., Youker, J.E., et al. 1980. Echocardiographic assessment of cardiac chamber size and left ventricular function in aerobically trained athletes. Aust N Z J Med 10:540–547.

42. Sonnenblick, E.H., Ross, J. Jr, et al. 1968. Oxygen consumption of the heart: newer concepts of its multifactorial determination. Am J Cardiol 22:328–336.

43. Klocke, F.H., Braunwald, E., et al. 1966. Oxygen cost of electrical activation of the heart. Circ Res 18:357–365.

44. Coleman, H.N., Sonnenblick, E.H., et al. 1969. Myocardial oxygen consumption associated with external work: the Fenn effect. Am J Physiol 217:291–296.

45. Sonnenblick, E.H., Ross, J. Jr, et al. 1965. Velocity of contraction as a determinate of myocardial oxygen consumption. Am J Physiol 309:919–927.

46. Hartley, L.H., Jones, L.G., et al. 1973. The usefulness of exercise therapy in the management of coronary heart disease. Adv Cardiol 9:174–202.

47. Frick, M.H., Katila, M. 1968. Hemodynamic consequences of physical training after myocardial infarction. Circulation 37:192–202.

48. Ehsani, A.A., Martin, W.H., et al. 1982. Cardiac effects of prolonged and intense exercise training in patients with coronary artery disease. Am J Cardiol 50:246–254.

49. Varnauskas, E., Bergman, H., et al. 1966. Haemodynamic effect of physical training in coronary patients. Lancet 2:8–12.

50. Clausen, J.P., Trap-Jensen, J. 1970. Effects of training on the distribution of cardiac output in patients with coronary artery disease. Circulation 42:611–624.

51. Redwood, D.R., Rosing, D.R., et al. 1972. Circulation and symptomatic effects of physical training in patients with coronary artery disease and angina pectoris. N Engl J Med 286:959–965.

52. Detry, J.R., Rousseau, M., et al. 1971. Increased arteriovenous oxygen different after physical training in coronary artery disease. Circulation 44:109–118.

53. Litchfield, R.L., Kerber, B.E., et al. 1982. Normal exercise capacity in patients with severe left ventricular dysfunction: compensatory mechanisms. Circ 66:129–134.

54. Franciosa, J.A., Park, M., et al. 1981. Lack of correlation between exercise capacity and indexes of resting left ventricular performance in heart failure. Am

J Cardiol 47:33–39.

55. Port, S., McEwan, P., et al. 1981. Influence of resting left ventricular function on the left ventricular response to exercise in patients with coronary artery disease. Circulation 63:856–863.

56. Wilson, J.R., Ferraro, N. 1983. Exercise tolerance in patients with chronic left heart failure: relation to oxygen transport and ventilatory abnormalities. Am J Cardiol 51:1358–1363.

57. Higginbotham, M.B., Morris, K.G., et al. 1983. Determinants of variable exercise performance among patients with severe left ventricular dysfunction. Am J Cardiol 51:52–60.

58. Benge, W., Litchfield, R.L., et al. 1980. Exercise capacity in patients with severe left ventricular dysfunction. Circulation 61:955–959.

59. Kavanagh, T., Shephard, T.H., et al. 1974. Marathon running after myocardial infarction. JAMA 229:1602–1605.

60. Cantwell, J.D. 1977. Stress testing indicated in a variety of complaints. Phys Sportsmed 5(2):70–74.

61. Gertenblith, G., Lakatta, E.G., et al. 1976. Age changes in myocardial function and exercise response. Prog Cardiovasc Dis 19:1–21.

62. Kavanagh, T., Shephard, R.J. 1977. The effects of continued training on the aging process. Ann NY Acad Sci 301:656–670.

63. Pollock, M.L. 1974. Physiological characteristics of older champion track athletes. Res Q 45:363–373.

64. Granath, A., Jonsson, B., et al. 1964. Circulation in healthy old men, studied by right heart catheterization at rest and during exercise in supine and sitting positions. Acta Med Scand 176:425–446.

65. Tartulier, M., Bourret, M., et al. 1972. Pulmonary arterial pressures in normal subjects: effects of age and exercise. Bull Physiopathol Resp 8:1295–1321.

66. Goodrick, C.L. 1980. Effects of long-term voluntary wheel exercise on male and female Wistar rats. I. Longevity, body weight, and metabolic rate. Gerontology 26:22–23.

67. Scaff, J.H. Jr, 1977. People Weekly 7(9):88.

.13.

Sudden Cardiac Death in Sports

Jerome E. Goss and Neal Shadoff

Sudden death is generally defined as death occurring within 1 to 24 hr after symptoms (Hinkle [1]; World Health Organization [2]; Goldstein [3]). Exercise or sports-related sudden death usually occurs within 30 sec to several minutes and may be more appropriately categorized as instantaneous death (James et al. [4]; Kuller et al. [5]; Luckstead [6]). When instant death occurs, a fatal arrhythmia, such as ventricular fibrillation followed by immediate circulatory collapse, is suggested (Doyle [7]). The clinical setting for this situation in athletics exists during long-distance running, because plasma norepinephrine, potassium, and lactic acid levels are high, and ventricular premature contractions are frequent (Pickering [8]; Palatini et al. [9]). Although uncommon in sports, sudden death is a dramatic event that gains attention. The risk of sudden death appears to be transiently increased during strenuous sports participation. Conversely, regular vigorous exercise probably reduces the overall chances of sudden death occurring (Siscovick et al. [10]; Morris et al. [11]; Garcia-Palmieri et al. [12]). Identification of every person at risk for such a catastrophic event is not possible, but certain cardiovascular abnormalities are known to be associated with sudden death, and these shall be discussed here.

GENERAL SURVEY

Approximately 450,000 people die suddenly each year in the United States (DeSilva and Lown [13]), but relatively few sudden deaths are sports related (DeSilva and Lown [13]; Vuori et al. [14]; Thompson [15]; Waller [16]). Of 2606 sudden deaths in Finland, only 22 were associated with sports—16 with skiing, 2 with jogging, and 4 with other activities— an incidence of 0.8% compared to 2.2% incidence of sudden death among Finnish sauna bathers. Eight sudden deaths occurred among 1,030,000 cross-country skiers during a 16-year period, or approximately one death in 13,000–26,000 man-hours of cross-country skiing (Vuori et al. [14]). The ski hikes were vigorous, covered from 30–90 km and lasted 5–11 hr. In a small number of skiers, ages 32 to 64, mean heart rates during the hikes were between 132 and 165 beats per minute, or 80–90% of maximal rates.

Twenty-one sudden deaths among athletes were reported in South African newspapers over 18 months, and 19 of them were probably cardiac causes. The sports involved were rugby, 7; refereeing, 4: soccer and tennis, 2 each; and golf, mountaineering, jogging, and yachting, 1 each. Ages ranged from 17 to 58 years. One sudden death per 50,000 player-hours of rugby occurred, and the average age of death was 26 years. Sudden death among rugby referees was 1 per 3000 hr of refereeing, and the average age was 56 years.

Seven subjects with pathologic diagnoses showed advanced coronary atherosclerosis. Two others had ischemic heart disease, according to electrocardiographic evidence of acute myocardial infarction in one and a history of myocardial infarction in the other. In 7 athletes, chest pain preceded death; histories of angina and positive findings in exercise tests in the 7 were thought to be strong indications of ischemic heart disease. In 2 remaining athletes, the clinical picture was "suggestive" of ischemic heart disease (Opie [17]). There have been several reports of myocardial infarction with classic electrocardiographic changes in athletes in whom the coronary arteries were found to be normal at autopsy (Green et al. [18]; Kimbiris et al. [19]; Maron et al. [20]). Transient coronary spasm may have been operative, but chest pain may be a feature of other potentially lethal forms of heart disease such as hypertrophic cardiomyopathy, valvular aortic stenosis, congenital coronary artery anomalies, and mitral valve prolapse. Therefore, chest pain alone cannot be the sole criterion for a diagnosis of ischemic heart disease.

Shephard [21] estimated 1 sudden death per 2500 gymnasium hours among middle-aged businessmen who attended unsupervised gymnasium programs. The estimate was based on reports reaching Ontario newspapers. Ventricular fibrillation occurred less often in supervised programs (Shephard [21]; Pyfer [22]). Pyfer [22] reported eight episodes of ventricular fibrillation occurring over a period of 50,000 gymnasium hours in Seattle, and at the Toronto Rehabilitation Center one episode occurred in over 100,000 hours of exercise (Shephard [21]).

Autopsy studies of 29 competitive athletes showed that death occurred during or shortly after strenuous exercise in 22 (Maron et al. [20]). Subjects included 26 men and 3 women, 20 whites and 9 blacks. Ages ranged from 13 to 30 years. Eleven athletes competed in basketball, 10 in football, 4 in track, 3 in wrestling, and 1 each in swimming, boxing, soccer, tennis, baseball, and gymnastics. Pathologic diagnoses included hypertrophic cardiomyopathy in 14, anomalous origin of the left coronary artery from the anterior sinus of Valsalva in 4, and coronary atherosclerosis in 3. Rupture of the aorta, due to Marfan's syndrome, occurred in 2. Five had idiopathic concentric left ventricular hypertrophy; 2 of these athletes also had narrowed atrioventricular node arteries. In 1 subject both leaflets of the mitral valve prolapsed. The only autopsy findings in 1 athlete were smaller than normal branches from the left circumflex and right coronary arteries to the posterior ventricular wall. The remaining subject had no discernible cardiac abnormality, but complete examination of the conduction system was not possible. Seven of these 29 athletes had undergone premortem evaluation for cardiovascular abnormalities. Five had hypertrophic cardiomyopathy diagnosed pathologically that had been clinically suspected to be normal athlete's heart (3), ventricular septal defect (1), or Wolff-Parkinson-White syndrome (1). In Waller's [16] series of young conditioned subjects who died during or shortly after exercise, 60% (9 of 15) had either hypertrophic cardiomyopathy or idiopathic left ventricular hypertrophy.

SUDDEN DEATH ASSOCIATED WITH RUNNING

With the increase in the popularity of running as a recreational and competition sport for all ages, the occurrence of sudden death during or after a run has drawn attention (Pyfer [22]; Thompson et al. [23]; Noakes and Opie [24]; Noakes et al. [25]; Waller and Roberts [26]; Thompson et al. [27]). Autopsy findings in 18 persons who died while jogging or immediately afterward showed that 13 men died of coronary artery disease and 4 men and 1 woman died of other causes (Thompson et al. [23]). One subject had myocardial lymphocytic infiltrate suggesting myocarditis, and another died of heat stroke. Three remaining subjects had no clear diagnosis, although unexplained myocardial fibrosis was present in 2, suggesting that myocardial bridging was present but unnoticed. Morales et al. [28] report 3 cases of sudden death during exercise in which myocardial bridging was found at autopsy. During rapid heart rate, contraction of bridging muscle may constrict coronary arteries and narrow their lumens more than 75%. Bridging usually involves the left anterior descending coronary artery. The combination of arterial narrowing during systole plus short diastolic filling time can compromise blood supply to the septum. In such cases, focal scarring has been seen in septal areas.

Sudden death in marathon runners from advanced coronary atherosclerosis (Noakes and Opie [24]; Noakes et al. [25]; Waller and Roberts [26]) helps lay to rest the myth that marathon running provides complete immunity from this disorder (Bassler and Cardello [29]). One 44-year-old subject had completed eight marathons and two ultramarathons during the 14 months prior to his sudden death. He was a nonsmoker, but serum cholesterol was 298 mg/dl, high-density lipoprotein cholesterol was 43 mg/dl, and triglycerides were 145 mg/dl, unexpected values for a marathon runner. Sudden death occurred at 19 km in a 24-km road race. Autopsy showed healed anteroseptal infarction with severe (75–100%) atherosclerotic narrowing 5 mm from the origin of the left anterior descending artery, and at 15 mm from its origin, it was occluded by an organized thrombus in which recanalization had occurred. The left circumflex coronary artery showed severe atherosclerotic narrowing 3.5 cm from its origin. Special staining and chemical studies were consistent with acute infarction of the posterior wall (Noakes et al. [25]).

The second death was that of a 41-year-old athlete who had run marathons for 2 years prior to acute inferior myocardial infarction. Angiography confirmed inferior infarction and showed complete occlusion of the left circumflex coronary artery and 50% narrowing in the proximal right coronary artery, with minor irregularities of the lumen in the left anterior descending coronary artery. Cholesterol was 265 mg/dl, and triglycerides, 235 mg/dl. He had smoked pipes and up to 3 cigarettes per day for 20 years, but stopped after the infarction. He was advised to continue jogging but not to participate in marathon races. In the 28 months following infarction, he logged 3624 km and completed 5 marathons. Thirty-one months after infarction he was admitted to the hospital with unstable angina. Coronary angiography showed progression of the atherosclerotic narrowings. The left circumflex was unchanged, with total occlusion, but the right coronary had progressed from 50% narrowing to total occlusion, and the left anterior descending had progressed from irregularities of the lumen to 80% narrowing. While in the hospital awaiting coronary bypass surgery, he developed acute anterolateral infarction followed by death within 1.5 hr. Autopsy revealed severe advanced coronary atherosclerosis, which included severe narrowing in the left anterior descending coronary artery and superimposed total occlusion by fresh thrombus. The left circumflex was totally occluded by long-standing organized thrombus, and the right coronary had severe narrowing, with total occlusion by recent organized thrombus (Noakes et al. [25]).

Waller and Roberts [26] described 5 cases of sudden death in conditioned runners over age 40, 2 of whom were marathoners. All 5 had severe three-vessel disease at autopsy. Both marathon runners had systemic hypertension and hypercholesterolemia with total cholesterol values of 310 mg/dl and 305 mg/dl. One year before death the more experienced marathoner had high-density lipoprotein (HDL) cholesterol of 41 mg/dl while running an average of 173 km per week. He had been running for 10 years and had completed 6 Boston marathons and 7 80-km JFK races. He had had angina pectoris with running for 2 years and positive treadmill stress tests without pain on 2 occasions.

In all 4 cases, advanced coronary atherosclerosis developed while the runners were actively engaged in marathoning. These case reports (Noakes and Opie [24]; Noakes et al. [25]; Waller and Roberts [26]) are important, for most runners and physicians believe in the Bassler hypothesis (Bassler and Cardello [29]), and distance runners may ignore important symptoms because of this unproved popular belief that promises immunity from atherosclerotic cardiovascular events. These reports should caution middle-aged distance runners. Serum lipids in the 4 cases were striking: All four men had high serum cholesterol, and HDL was low in the 2 runners in whom it was measured (Hooper and Eaton [30]). The abnormal lipids are the most apparent reason these 4 marathoners developed advanced coronary atherosclerosis, and their demise might have been sooner if they had not been long-distance runners.

When a person dies during or immediately after running, it is assumed that the exercise caused the death. Koplan [31] estimated the number of cardiac deaths that might occur by chance alone during running. If runners live a marathoner's lifestyle, 4 cardiac deaths while running are expected per year in the United States. If the runners' lifestyle is that of the average white American male, then 15 deaths per year are expected. If the running period includes 2 hr after exercise, expected cardiac deaths are increased to 34 and 119, respectively. The average runner's risk of death during running is somewhere between these two extremes. Without an accurate method for recording deaths during running, it is impossible to say whether a given death was a chance occurrence or was directly related to the last run.

Using information from the Office of the Rhode Island State Medical Examiner and a random-digit telephone survey, it was estimated that one death per 7620 joggers per year or one death per 396,000 hours of jogging occurred in Rhode Island from 1975 to 1980 (Thompson et al. [23]). Although this estimated risk of death is higher than that of Koplan [31], both studies indicate that exercise risk is small and suggest that routine pretraining exercise testing of asymptomatic adults, who are without significant risk factors for coronary artery disease, is not justified.

The more common causes of sudden death in sports are considered in the following sections, with special consideration given to detection and prevention.

CAUSES OF SUDDEN DEATH IN SPORTS

Hypertrophic Cardiomyopathy

Hypertrophic cardiomyopathy, a genetically transmitted disease of cardiac muscle characterized by disproportionate thickening of the ventricular septum (Maron et al. [32]), has frequently been associated with sudden death (Shephard [21]; Maron et al. [32]; Lambert et al. [33]; Sturner and Spruill [34]; Evans et al. [35]; Waller [16]). The hearts of 22 patients with this disorder showed multiple abnormalities in all parts of the conducting system that could be responsible for electrical instability and ventricular fibrillation (James and Marshall [36]). Sudden death has been recognized in symptomatic patients, but most symptomatic patients do not compete in sports.

Maron et al. [32] studied 26 patients in whom sudden death was the first symptom of disease, and 13 of these persons died suddenly during or immediately after moderate to heavy physical exertion. Five were competitive athletes. This group had 2 characteristics: 1) an abnormal electrocardiogram, usually showing left ventricular hypertrophy, and 2) a moderately to severely thickened interventricular septum revealed at autopsy. Evans et al. [35] reported sudden death in two 17-year-old brothers while they were playing basketball, with pathologic changes of hypertrophic cardiomyopathy.

Symptoms associated with hypertrophic cardiomyopathy include chest pain, exertional dyspnea, palpitations, and syncope. Physicians frequently are not alert to the importance of these symptoms in young people. Asymptomatic patients with this disorder may have a systolic murmur at the lower left sternal border and apex. When a patient has the symptoms described and/or a murmur, if the echocardiogram shows disproportional hypertrophy of the intraventricular septum and the electrocardiogram indicates left ventricular hypertrophy, one should consider advising the patient to limit physical activity.

Coronary Artery Anomalies

The incidence of aberrant origin of the coronary arteries is about 0.6% (Liberthson et al. [37]; Kimbiris et al. [38]). In most cases this is a benign condition, and yet anomalous origin of a coronary artery is a very frequent pathologic finding in sports-related sudden death, accounting for 17% of 183 reported cases in one series (Waller [16]). Origin of the left coronary artery from the pulmonary artery is often associated with heart failure in early life and, if not discovered and treated, can result in death. This anomaly has rarely been associated with sudden death during sports (Jokl and Melzer [39]; McClellan and Jokl [40]). The coronary artery anomaly most often associated with exertional sudden death is at the origin of the left coronary from the anterior sinus of Valsalva. The vessel then passes obliquely between the aorta and the pulmonary artery (Shephard [21]; Liberthson et al. [37]; Kimbiris et al. [38]; McClellan and Jokl [40]; Tunstall-Pedoe [41]; Cheitlin et al. [42]; Schaumburg and Simonsen [43]).

The most plausible mechanism of exertional sudden death with this anomaly relates to compromise of the lumen of the coronary artery by the angle formed as it arises from the anterior sinus of Valsalva (Cheitlin et al. [42]). The first part of the left main coronary artery may also be encased in the wall of the aorta (Kimbiris et al. [38]). With increased expansion of the aorta during exercise, the already slitlike opening of the left coronary artery may be further occluded (Cheitlin et al. [42]). Clinical recognition of this anomaly depends on careful evaluation of young athletes with symptoms of exertional chest pain or syncope. Treadmill exercise testing and coronary angiography are used to make the diagnosis, and if established, enlargement of the slitlike ostia corrects the exertional ischemia (Cheitlin et al. [42]).

Atherosclerotic Coronary Heart Disease

Atherosclerosis of the coronary arteries is a disease of all age groups (Opie [17]; Green et al. [18]; Shephard [21]; Noakes and Opie [24]; Noakes et al. [25]; Koskenvuo et al. [44]). Its occurrence in young athletes is always a surprise, and risk factors may be lacking. On the other hand, many middle-aged athletes smoke cigarettes, are hypertensive, have abnormal serum lipids, are diabetic, have a strong family history of atherosclerosis, or have stress-filled lives. Although exercise may modify many risk factors of coronary artery disease (CAD) (Wood et al. [45]; Cooper et al. [46]; Paolone et al. [47]), it cannot make an athlete immune to its development. In the United Kingdom, 30 cases of sudden death associated with playing squash occurred predominantly in middle-aged males with prodromal symptoms of coronary heart disease (Northcote et al. [48]).

Many middle-aged athletes have well-developed CAD before starting to exercise, and symptoms develop with increased physical activity. Exercise in the presence of significant CAD can cause ischemia and transient angina pectoris, life-threatening myocardial infarction, or sudden death. Which condition occurs depends on the extent of disease and the clinical setting. Those who might benefit the most from an exercise program also are most often at risk from exercise. In dogs, a daily exercise program for 6 weeks was able to protect against ventricular fibrillation induced by transient coronary occlusion in a population previously proved to be at risk for sudden death (Billman et al. [49]).

No large experience exists for successfully screening individuals before they start on an exercise program, and controversy prevails among those with limited experience (Vuori et al. [14]; Thompson et al. [23]). Persons with significant risk factors for development of CAD should have treadmill testing to identify exercise-induced ischemia or arrhythmia before they start physical fitness programs. Those with known CAD should be supervised in a coronary rehabilitation program to minimize risks (Green et al. [18]).

Prodromal symptoms before exercise-induced cardiac events are common (Opie [17]; Thompson et al. [23]; Waller and Roberts [26]), but denial by the patient is also common, and the exaggerated claims for the benefits of exercise may contribute to this denial (Noakes et al. [50]). Physicians are also vulnerable to the same claims and may underestimate the significance of new symptoms in athletes. Thompson et al. [23] and others (Opie [17]; Noakes et al. [25]) have pointed out great variation in exercise capacity in subjects whose sudden death was associated with physical activity. The veteran superior athlete is at risk for exercise-induced sudden death, as well as the beginning or middle-aged exercise enthusiast.

These points are not made to discourage sports in mid- and later life but to place the risks involved in perspective. Casualties will continue to occur no matter how careful the screening.

Myocarditis

In a cooperative international study (Lambert et al. [33]) involving 20 pediatric cardiac centers in 10 countries, acute myocarditis accounted for 5% of sudden unexpected deaths, but none were associated with exertion. Sudden death associated with exercise and myocarditis has been reported (Thompson et al. [23]; Jokl and Melzer [39]; Jokl [51]), and several anecdotal reports exist of athletes dying during or shortly after a run to "sweat out" influenza or coryza (Tunstall-Pedoe [41]). Cardiac arrhythmias are common in myocarditis, and presumably death occurs from an arrhythmia potentiated by exercise (Tunstall-Pedoe [41]). Myocardial involvement may be detected during or shortly after even mild viral infections (Tunstall-Pedoe [41]; Barlow [52]; Burch [53]). Verel et al. [54] found that 43% of patients seen during an epidemic of A2 influenza had electrocardiographic changes. Other studies have reported electrocardiographic changes in 14–75% of patients with influenza (Gibson et al. [55]; Walsh et al. [56]). Nonspecific ST segment and T-wave changes are the earliest and most common indicators of myocardial involvement and when present should indicate temporary restriction of athletic activities. Severe exertion during or in early convalescence from an acute viral febrile illness is potentially dangerous and should be discouraged.

Valvular Aortic Stenosis

With critical stenosis of the aortic valve, exercise produces marked elevation of left ventricular pressure, and normal cardiac output may not occur. When the stenosis is present, along with a thickened left ventricle, coronary perfusion may be inadequate for the muscle mass. This produces a relatively ischemic myocardium, which in turn may cause progressive electrical instability and ventricular fibrillation. In the international cooperative study reported by Lambert et al. [33], 38 children died suddenly as a result of valvular aortic stenosis, but only 5 of the deaths occurred during sports. To determine which patients with aortic stenosis were at risk for sudden death, Doyle et al. [57] reviewed the literature and found that most cases were associated with symptoms and/or severe electrocardiographic changes. Left ventricular hypertrophy with "strain pattern" was observed in 70% of reported cases of sudden death, and only 9% of electrocardiograms were normal (Doyle et al.

[57]). Most patients with mild to moderately severe aortic stenosis are asymptomatic, but in cases of sudden death one or more of the following symptoms were present: easy fatigability, chest pain, exertional dyspnea, or syncope.

All athletes with valvular aortic stenosis should undergo thorough history taking, physical examination, and electrocardiogram. If these are consistent with mild stenosis, further studies and limitations are not indicated. If more significant stenosis is suspected, cardiac catheterization should be performed, and the transvalvular gradient at rest and exercise should be assessed. The severity of the stenosis can be determined, and the patient can be counseled regarding participation in sports. Aortic stenosis is a progressive disease; therefore, continued observation for appearance of symptoms and electrocardiographic changes is necessary. Cardiac catheterization studies (Cohen et al. [58]; El-Said et al. [59]) may be repeated to identify progression and, it is hoped, prevent sudden death.

Mitral Valve Prolapse

Mitral valve prolapse is characterized by valvular redundancy and myxomatous thickening of the mitral leaflets, with elongation of the chordae tendineae (Marshall and Shappell [60]). It is commonly found in young women who complain of nonspecific chest pain, palpitations, and dizziness. On physical examination, a mid- to late systolic click and/or a mid- to late systolic murmur of mitral regurgitation can be heard. The electrocardiogram may show nonspecifitic ST–T wave changes in the inferior leads and borderline prolongation of the QT interval (Marshall and Shappell [60]). Echocardiogram and cineangiography will show prolapse of the posterior leaflet or of both leaflets of the mitral valve. The deformity is associated with arrhythmias and sudden death (Marshall and Shappell [60]; Swartz et al. [61]). In a literature review, 6.1% of patients had supraventricular tachycardia, 6.3% had ventricular tachycardia and 1.4% (8 patients) died suddenly (Swartz et al. [61]). However, when compared to the general population, subjects with mitral valve prolapse seem to have no greater incidence of arrhythmias (Savage et al. [62]).

Delayed repolarization arrhythmias have a prolonged QT interval with delayed recovery of parts of the myocardium. This is the essential ingredient to the occurrence of re-entrant arrhythmias such as ventricular tachycardia (Han and Goel [63]). In 94 patients with mitral valve prolapse, 44 (47%) had prolonged QT interval during rest (Swartz et al. [61]); prolonged QT interval has also been reported in patients with prolapsed mitral valve disease during exercise (Pocock and Barlow [64].

Mitral valve prolapse has been reported in 6–10% of asymptomatic young women (Brown et al. [65]; Markiewicz et al. [66]), a finding that could present a formidable problem in determining who should participate in sports. Restriction from sports should be advised only if the patient has paroxysmal ventricular tachycardia that is poorly controlled. Many women complain of postexercise palpitations that are not significant when evaluated by Holter and treadmill exercise testing. The threat of sudden death with this deformity, however, has been overemphasized and has caused undue anxiety and limitation for many patients (Jeresaty [67]).

ACTIVITY GUIDELINES FOR PATIENTS WITH HEART DISEASE

It is impossible to classify the energy requirements of sporting or recreational activities, since people pursue them with different degrees of vigor. For example, swimming may require energy expenditure of less than 5 cal/min or may require more than 20 cal/min, depending on the individual intensity of performance (American Heart Association [68]). A person's skill also determines the amount of energy expenditure in a particular sport.

Table 13-1   Hemodynamic Conditions That Require Restriction of Sports Participation in Subjects with Congenital Heart Defects

Defect	Hemodynamic Parameter
Atrial septal defect	Pulmonary artery pressure > 0.5 of the systemic pressure
Ventricular septal defect	Pulmonary artery pressure > 0.5 of the systemic pressure
Coarctation of the aorta	Severe systemic hypertension or con-concomitant aortic valve disease
Pulmonary stenosis	Peak gradient 50 mm Hg
Patent ductus arteriosus	Pulmonary artery pressure > 0.5 of the systemic pressure or > 2 to 1 shunt

Adapted from Driscoll, D.J., 1985. Cardiovascular evaluation of the child and adolescent before participation in sports. Mayo Clin Proc 60:867–873.

Since many variables exist, a sports participation and skills history must be obtained so that more accurate prescriptions of activities can be outlined. Treadmill exercise testing with maximal oxygen consumption can be helpful in verifying the safety of the proposed exercise prescription.

Sports requiring isometric work, such as weight-lifting, wrestling, and gymnastics, demand special consideration because of a disproportionate increase in systemic blood pressure relative to oxygen consumption (American Heart Association [68]). Although specific information is not available regarding the effects of transient systemic blood pressure elevation, it seems wise to discourage patients with left ventricular outflow obstruction, aortic insufficiency, significant coarctation of the aorta (American Heart Association [68]), and moderate or severe hypertension from participating in sports that require primarily isometric work.

Patients who have had repair of congenital defects and are without symptoms may be too casually evaluated. Special attention should be given to patients who have undergone total repair of tetralogy of Fallot. Trifascicular block and right bundle branch block with premature ventricular contractions have been associated with a high incidence of sudden death in this group (Quattlebaum et al. [69]), but none of these deaths were associated with sports. If a patient with repaired tetralogy of Fallot seeks advice regarding sports participation, the presence or absence of right bundle branch block or trifascicular block should be determined. If either is present, the patient should have Holter monitoring and treadmill exercise testing before a decision on sports participation is made. If significant ventricular arrhythmia is present, the patient should receive appropriate antiarrhythmic therapy and should be advised that moderate restriction be observed in choosing sports activities.

Patients with unrepaired congenital heart defects must be counseled on an individual basis depending on the hemodynamic abnormalities present, the potential for arrhythmias, and the specific activities to be performed. A complete fitness evaluation, including measurement of maximal oxygen consumption, may be the most specific approach to an activity or exercise prescription in individuals with congenital heart disease (Driscoll [70]), but Table 13-1 provides general guidelines for the most commonly encountered defects.

REFERENCES

1. Hinkle, L.E., Thaler, H.T. 1982. Clinical classification of cardiac deaths. Circulation 65:457–464.

2. World Health Organization. 1970. Report of the 4th working group with revised operating protocol. Working Group on

Ischemic Heart Disease Registers, June 29–July 1, 1970, Copenhagen. Regional Office for Europe, World Health Organization, EURO 5010(4), Copenhagen.

3. Goldstein, S. 1982. The necessity of a uniform definition of sudden coronary death: witnessed death within 1 hour of the onset of acute symptoms. Am Heart J 103:156–159.

4. James, T.N., Froggatt, P., et al. 1967. Sudden death in young athletes. Ann Intern Med 67:1013–1019.

5. Kuller, L., Lillienfeld, A., et al. 1967. An epidemiological study of sudden and unexpected death in adults. Medicine 46:341–361.

6. Luckstead, E.F. 1982. Sudden death in sports. Pediatr Clin North Am 29:1355–1362.

7. Doyle, J.T. 1975. Profile of risk of sudden death in apparently healthy people. Circulation 52 (suppl 3): 176–179.

8. Pickering, T.G. 1979. Jogging, marathon running, and the heart. Am J Med 66:717–719.

9. Palatini, P., Maraglino, G., et al. 1985. Prevalence and possible mechanisms of ventricular arrhythmias in athletes. Am Heart J 110:560–567.

10. Siscovick, D.S., Weiss, N.S., et al. 1984. The incidence of primary cardiac arrest during vigorous exercise. N Engl J Med 311:874–877.

11. Morris, J.N., Everitt, M.E., et al. 1980. Vigorous exercise in leisure-time: protection against coronary heart disease. Lancet 2:1207–1210.

12. Garcia-Palmieri, M.R., Costas, R. Jr., et al. 1982. Increased physical activity: a protective factor against heart attacks in Puerto Rico. Am J Cardiol 50:749–755.

13. DeSilva, R.A., Lown, B. 1978. Ventricular premature beats, stress, and sudden death. Psychosomatics 19:649–661.

14. Vuori, I., Makarainen, M., et al. 1978. Sudden death and physical activity. Cardiology 63:287–304.

15. Thompson, P.D. 1982. Cardiovascular hazards of physical activity. Exerc Sport Sci Rev 10:208–235.

16. Waller, B.F., 1985. Exercise-related sudden death in young (age ≤ 30 years) and old (age ≥ 30 years) conditioned subjects. In: Wenger, N.K. (ed): Exercise and The Heart. Volume 2. Cardiovascular Clinics. FA Davis Company, Philadelphia, pp 9–73.

17. Opie, L.H. 1975. Sudden death and sport. Lancet 1:263–266.

18. Green, L.H., Cohen, S.I., et al. 1976. Fatal myocardial infarction in marathon racing. Ann Intern Med 85:704–706.

19. Kimbiris, D., Segal, B.L., et al. 1972. Myocardial infarction in patients with normal patient coronary arteries as visualized by cineangiography. Am J Cardiol 29:724–728.

20. Maron, B.J., Roberts, W.C., et al. 1980. Sudden death in young athletes. Circulation 62:218–229.

21. Shephard, R.J. 1974. Sudden death—a significant hazard of exercise. Br J Sports Med 8:101–110.

22. Pyfer, H. 1974. Group exercise rehabilitation for cardiopulmonary patients. A five year study. 20th World Congress of Sports Medicine, Melbourne, Australia.

23. Thompson, P.D., Stern, M.P., et al. 1979. Death during jogging or running. JAMA 242:1265–1267.

24. Noakes, T.D., Opie, L.H. 1979. Marathon running and heart: the South African experience. Am Heart J 98:669–671.

25. Noakes, T.D., Opie, L.H., et al. 1979. Autopsy-proven coronary atherosclerosis in marathon runners. N Engl J Med 301:86–89.

26. Waller, B.F., Roberts, W.C. 1980. Sudden death while running in conditioned runners aged 40 years or over. Am J Cardiol 45:1292–1300.

27. Thompson, P.D., Funk, E.J., et al. 1982. Incidence of death during jogging in Rhode Island from 1975 through 1980. JAMA 247:2535–2538.

28. Morales, A.R., Romanelli, R., et al. 1980. The mural left anterior descending coronary artery, strenous exercising, and sudden death. Circulation 62:230–237.

29. Bassler, T.J., Cardello, F.P. 1976. Fiber feeding and atherosclerosis. JAMA 235:1841–1842.

30. Hooper, P.L., Eaton, R.P. 1978. Exercise, high density lipoprotein and coronary heart disease. In: Appenzeller, O., Atkinson, R. (eds): Health Aspects of Endurance Training (Vol. 12, Medicine and Sports Series). Karger, Basel, Switzerland, pp 72–84.

31. Koplan, J.P. 1979. Cardiovascular deaths while running. JAMA 242:2578–2579.

32. Maron, B.J., Roberts, W.C., et al. 1978. Sudden death in patients with hypertrophic cardiomyopathy: characterization of 26 patients without functional limitation. Am J Cardiol 41:803–810.

33. Lambert, E.C., Menon, V.A., et al. 1974. Sudden expected death from cardiovascular disease in children. Am J Cardiol 34:89–96.

34. Sturner, W.Q., Spruill, F.G. 1974. Asymmetrical hypertrophy of the heart:

two sudden deaths in adolescents. J Forensic Sci 19:565–571.

35. Evans, A.T., Korndorffer, W.E., et al. 1980. Sudden death of two brothers while playing basketball: familiar hypertrophic cardiomyopathy. Texas Med J 76:45–51.

36. James, T.N., Marshall, T.K. 1975. Asymmetrical hypertrophy of the heart. Circulation 51:1149–1166.

37. Liberthson, R.R., Dinsmore, R.E., et al. 1974. Aberrant coronary artery origin from the aorta. Circulation 59:744–779.

38. Kimbiris, D., Iskandrian, A.S., et al. 1978. Anomalous aortic origin of coronary arteries. Circulation 58:606–615.

39. Jokl, E., Melzer, L. 1971. Acute fatal nontraumatic collapse during work and sport. In: Jokl, E., McClellan, J.T. (eds): Exercise and Cardiac Death (Vol. 5, Medicine and Sport Series). Karger, Basel, Switzerland pp 5–18.

40. McClellan, J.T., Jokl, E. 1971. Congenital anomalies of coronary arteries as cause of sudden death associated with physical exertion. In: Jokl, E., McClellan, J.T. (eds): Exercise and Cardiac Death (Vol. 5, Medicine and Sports Series). Karger, Basel, Switzerland, pp 91–98.

41. Tunstall-Pedoe, D. 1979. Exercise and sudden death. Br J Sports Med 12:215–219.

42. Cheitlin, M.D., DeCastro, C.M., et al. 1974. Sudden death as a complication of anomalous left coronary origin from the anterior sinus of Valsalva. Circulation 50:780–787.

43. Schaumburg, H., Simonsen, J. 1978. Sudden death due to congenital malformation of the left coronary artery: a case report. Forensic Sci Int 12:83–85.

44. Koskenvuo, K., Karvonen, M.J., et al. 1978. Death from ischemic heart disease in young Finns aged 15 to 24 years. Am J Cardiol 42:114–118.

45. Wood, P.D., Haskell, L. et al. 1977. Plasma lipoprotein distribution in male and female runners. Ann NY Acad Sci 301:748–763.

46. Cooper, K.H., Pollock, M.L., et al. 1976. Physical fitness levels vs. selected coronary risk factors. JAMA 236:166–169.

47. Paolone, A.M., Lewis, R.R., et al. 1976. Results of two years' training in middle-aged men. Phys Sportsmed 4(12):72–77.

48. Northcote, R.J., Evans, A.D., et al. 1984. Sudden death in squash players. Lancet 1:148–150.

49. Billman, G.E., Schwartz, P.J., et al. 1984. The effects of daily exercise on susceptibility to sudden cardiac death. Circulation 69:1182–1189.

50. Noakes, T., Opie, L., et al. 1977. Coronary heart disease in marathon runners. Ann NY Acad Sci 301:593–619.

51. Jokl, E., 1971. Sudden death after exercise due to myocarditis. In: Jokl, E., McClellan, J.T. (eds): Exercise and Cardiac Death (Vol. 5, Medicine and Sport Series). Karger, Basel, Switzerland, pp 99–101.

52. Barlow, J.B. 1976. Exercise, rugby, football and infection. S Afr Med J 50:1351.

53. Burch, G.E. 1976. Of URI and cardiomyopathy. Am Heart J 91:538.

54. Verel, D., Warrack, A.J.N., et al. 1976. Observations on the A2 England influenza epidemic. Am Heart J 92:290–299.

55. Gibson, T.C., Arnold, J., et al. 1959. Electrocardiographic studies in Asian influenza. Am Heart J 57:661–668.

56. Walsh, J., Burch, G.E., et al. 1958. A study of the effects of type A (Asian strain) influenza on the cardiovascular system. Ann Intern Med 49:502–528.

57. Doyle, E.F., Arumugham, P., et al. 1974. Sudden death in young patients with congenital aortic stenosis. Pediatrics 53:481–489.

58. Cohen, L.S., Friedman, W.F., et al. 1972. Natural history of mild congenital aortic stenosis elucidated by serial hemodynamic studies. Am J Cardiol 30:1–5.

59. El-Said, G., Galioto, F.M., et al. 1972. Natural hemodynamic history of congenital aortic stenosis in childhood. Am J Cardiol 30:6–12.

60. Marshall, C.E., Shappell, S.D. 1974. Sudden death and the ballooning posterior leaflet syndrome. Arch Pahol 98:134–138.

61. Swartz, M.H., Terchholz, L.E., et al. 1977. Mitral valve prolapse. A review of associated arrhythmias. Am J Med 62:377–389.

62. Savage, D.D., Levy, D., et al. 1983. Mitral valve prolapse in the general population. 3. Dysrhythmias: the Framingham study. Am Heart J 106:582–586.

63. Han, J., Goel, B.G. 1972. Electrophysiologic precursors of ventricular tachyarrhythmias. Arch Intern Med 129:749–755.

64. Pocock, W.A., Barlow, J.B. 1980. Post exercise arrhythmias in the billowing posterior mitral leaflet syndrome. Am Heart J 80:740–745.

65. Brown, O.R., Kloster, F.E., et al. 1975. Incidence of mitral valve prolapse in the asymptomatic normal (abstract). Circulation 51 (suppl 2):77.

66. Markiewicz, W., Stoner, J., et al. 1975.

Mitral valve prolapse in one hundred presumably healthy females (abstract). Circulation 51 (suppl 2):77.

67. Jeresaty, R.M. 1976. Sudden death in the mitral valve prolapse-click syndrome. Am J Cardiol 37:317–318.

68. Ad Hoc Committee on Rehabilitation of the Young Cardiac, Council on Cardiovascular Disease in the Young, American Heart Association. 1976. Activity guidelines for young patients with heart disease. Phys Sportsmed 4(8):47–52.

69. Quattlebaum, T.G., Varghese, P.J., et al. 1976. Sudden death among postoperative patients with tetralogy of Fallot. Circulation 54:289–293.

70. Driscoll, D.J. 1985. Cardiovascular evaluation of the child and adolescent before participation in sports. Mayo Clin Proc 867–873.

.14.

Exercise and High-Density Lipoprotein
A Mechanism for Coronary Artery Disease Risk Reduction

Philip L. Hooper and Stephen F. Crouse

On the basis of 1981 estimates regarding the leading causes of death in the United States, cardiovascular diseases accounted for about 990,000 deaths, or nearly 50% of the total annual mortality (American Heart Association [1]). The annual estimated economic cost associated with medical treatment of this disease and lost revenue due to worker disability is a staggering $64.4 billion. The magnitude of personal tragedy associated with these deaths is immeasurable. Coronary artery disease (CAD) is the most prevalent manifestation of cardiovascular disease and, of itself, accounts for 56% of all cardiovascular disease deaths. In spite of many modern scientific advances, CAD still accounts for nearly 1 in 3 deaths and remains the single leading cause of death in the United States. However, recent mortality statistics have shown a modest decline in CAD deaths (Gordon [2]; Gordon and Thom [3]), possibly due at least in part to factors such as increased exercise, better management of heart disease, prudent diets, and less cigarette smoking. It is evident to even the casual observer that a virtual "exercise explosion" has taken place in recent years, exhibited best by the increased number of individuals participating in endurance-type activities such as jogging and swimming. Individuals express various reasons for exercising, such as weight or stress reduction, improvement in a sense of well-being, and heightened enjoyment of life. A significant number of people exercise because they believe that exercise reduces the risk of CAD.

EXERCISE AND CORONARY ARTERY DISEASE

A review of the literature related to the influence of physical exercise on CAD risk demonstrates the difficulty in designing an investigation that establishes exercise as an independent, causative factor in CAD risk reduction. Indeed, the ideal study to unequivocally demonstrate the influence of exercise on CAD would require a random assignment of individuals at birth into high- and low-activity groups and an observational period from birth to death. The obvious impractibility of such a study has necessitated the acceptance of other, less direct methods of inquiry to address this problem. In this regard, epidemiologic methods of research have proved useful to determine the relationship between exercise and CAD incidence and prevalence.

Epidemiologic studies have isolated physical activity as a protective factor against CAD. In the first study to address this question, Morris et al. [4] compared sedentary bus drivers with more active bus conductors in a population of 31,000 London transport employees. They found the sedentary drivers had 1.5 times the number of CAD deaths and twice the incidence of sudden death after the first myocardial infarction as did the conductors. In a subsequent study, Morris [5] examined death certificates and occupations of 2 million middle-aged men in Great Britian. Lower CAD mortality was found in those with higher levels of job-related physical activity. Both studies have been criticized because job selection created a natural bias (Froelicher and Oberman [6]).

Paffenbarger et al. [7] reported on a 22-year follow-up of 3686 longshoremen in San Francisco. Work energy requirements were determined from measurements of oxygen consumption in each job assignment. When CAD risk factors such as cigarette smoking, blood pressure, and cholesterol were taken into account, the study revealed that workers with jobs requiring high energy outputs had one-third the incidence of fatal CAD compared to workers with less active jobs.

In a subsequent study by this same group (Paffenbarger et al. [8]), physical activity as an index of CAD risk was studied in 16,936 Harvard male alumni. Those who had not been particularly athletic as students but who had a high level of physical activity in middle age were at lower risk of heart attack than former athletes whose later exercise levels were low. Furthermore, they found that middle-aged men who exerted less than 2000 kcal in exercise per week had 64% higher risk of CAD than alumni who exerted more than 2000 kcal per week.

Other retrospective epidemiologic studies seem to support the concept that regular, vigorous exercise reduces morbidity and mortality from CAD in middle-aged men. There are few studies showing no benefit from long-term exercise, and none report that exercise aggravates CAD or hastens the development of clinical disease. The interested reader is referred to two excellent reviews on this topic: Blackburn [9] and Paffenbarger and Hyde [10]. The weight of the evidence supports the view that those who exercise have a lower risk of coronary disease, though exercise above a minimum threshold level is probably required (Superko et al. [11]).

The mechanism by which exercise reduces the risk of CAD is probably composed of many factors. Improved cardiovascular function associated with exercise is well established and reviewed elsewhere. The health-conscious life-style of the exercise enthusiast often reduces CAD risk (weight control, prudent dietary habits, abstinence from smoking, etc.). One recently identified benefit of exercise is an increase in the antiatherogenic fat transport substance, high-density lipoprotein (HDL, α-lipoprotein).

HIGH DENSITY LIPOPROTEIN

Though the recent literature has revealed the pathology of CAD to be of multifactorial dimensions, lipids and lipoproteins appear to play a central role. The association between total serum cholesterol and clinical manifestations of this disease has been established for some time, but a causal relationship between cholesterol and CAD-related mortality and morbidity has only recently been demonstrated (Lipid Research Clinics Program [12]). In addition to the amount of circulating cholesterol, several lines of research have demonstrated that the manner in which total cholesterol is distributed among the major lipoprotein carrier molecules is particularly useful in explaining the contribution of this lipid to atheroma formation and to CAD pathogenesis. Through interactions with enzymes and cell surface receptors, the protein constituents (apoproteins) of each lipoprotein species direct the cholesterol-containing molecule to its site of metabolism. Of particular relevance to this discussion is the role of HDL in CAD risk and the influence of exercise on this important cholesterol transport molecule.

High-Density Lipoprotein in Coronary Artery Disease

In 1951, Barr et al. [13] studied atherosclerosis and serum lipoproteins. They stated that "the outstanding fact in our observations is the relative and absolute reduction of α-lipoprotein (HDL) in atherosclerosis" (p. 481). They also observed that human infants and laboratory animals had elevated HDL and were resistant to CAD. Therefore, they proposed that HDL has a protective effect upon the heart. Unfortunately, the majority of lipid research since 1951 has focused on total serum cholesterol and its major lipoprotein carrier, low-density lipoprotein (LDL), rather than HDL. However, recent data from large prospective studies indicate that HDL is a better predictor of CAD risk than either serum cholesterol or LDL.

The highly publicized Framingham Heart Study (Gordon et al. [14]) gave evidence that HDL is an important CAD risk factor and shifted medical attention from serum cholesterol levels to serum HDL levels. The Framingham Study was initiated in 1948 when the United States Public Health Service began a comprehensive study of factors associated with the development of atherosclerotic and hypertensive cardiovascular disease. A sample of the adult population of Framingham, Massachusetts, was observed for 30 years. In 1968, 2815 of these men and women, ages 40–82, had lipids and lipoproteins determined. Four years after the measurements, 142 subjects had developed CAD even though their average cholesterol level was normal (244 mg/100 ml). Interestingly, most people dying from CAD in the United States have normal serum cholesterol levels, which suggests at least two possibilities: 1) So-called normal serum cholesterol levels are in reality dangerously high, or 2) more lipid information than only the total cholesterol level is required to accurately assess the lipid contribution to CAD risk.

This latter hypothesis was addressed in the Framingham Study, in which it was shown that subjects with HDL-cholesterol levels below 35 mg/100 ml had an incidence of CAD 8 times higher than did those with HDL levels greater than 65 mg/100 ml. In addition, a study in Georgia (Castelli et al. [15]), the Tromso Heart Study in Norway (Miller and Miller [16]), the Hiroshima Study (Kajiyama et al. [17]), the Stockholm Prospective Study (Carlson [18]), and the Honolulu Heart Study (Rhoads et al. [19]) have all shown the same inverse relationship between HDL levels and CAD.

Further evidence that HDL protects the heart from atherosclerosis comes from studies of conditions associated with high or low HDL levels. Glueck et al. [20] identified 18 kindred with genetically elevated HDL levels. The average HDL-cholesterol in this group was 81 mg/100 ml compared to 53 mg/100 ml in controls. In kindreds with elevated HDL, life expectancy was longer and incidence of CAD was lower compared to those in the general United States population.

Women have higher HDL levels than men (Gustafson et al. [21]) and they also have one fifth the number of CAD deaths compared to men age 50 (*Statistical Bulletin* [22]). Lower HDL values are seen with obesity (Wilson and Lees [23]), poorly controlled diabetes mellitus (Lopez-Virella et al. [24]), chronic renal failure (Brunzell et al. [25]), and smoking (Garrison et al. [26]). All these conditions significantly increase CAD risk. Therefore, the foregoing epidemiologic findings demonstrate with regards to CAD risk that a high HDL level seems beneficial and that, conversely, a low HDL level is detrimental.

In an attempt to simplify the complex relationships between the relative levels of the major lipoprotein classes and CAD risk, the Framingham group has proposed the use of a total cholesterol/HDL-cholesterol ratio for assessing lipid-related risk of CAD (Castelli et al. [27]). This ratio relates the reputedly anti-atherogenic aspect of HDL-cholesterol to the atherogenic aspect of total cholesterol and was shown to be a strong predictor of CAD. Though this ratio may prove useful for screening purposes because of its simplicity, the authors cautioned that it may not be as informative about the risk of developing CAD as the information contained in the configuration of the specific values of cholesterols. Despite this caution, this risk marker has found its way into widespread clinical use.

Recently, the relationships between apo A-I, the major HDL apoprotein, and CAD have been investigated. Fager et al. [28] compared apo A-I levels in patients suffering an acute myocardial infarction (MI) with those of individuals in a cholesterol-matched and randomly selected control group. The results showed that apo A-I levels were lower in the patients than in the controls even when various other risk factors, i.e., cholesterol and smoking, were taken into account. In addition, Avogaro et al. [29] concluded that apo A-I was a better discriminator between MI survivors and age- and sex-matched controls than were any of the individual lipoprotein-lipids. Maciejko et al. [30] concluded on the basis of stepwise discriminant analysis that apo A-I was a powerful discriminator of angiographically documented CAD superior to that of HDL-cholesterol, though both were significantly lower in patients diagnosed as having CAD. Furthermore, the ratio of apo B (the primary apoprotein in LDL) to apo A-I has been shown to be a powerful discriminator for either the presence or severity of angiographically defined CAD (Noma et al. [31]). This recent work is indeed promising and suggests that apolipoprotein concentrations may be valuable CAD risk markers in the general population. Thus, apolipoprotein assessments could replace or enhance the effectiveness of lipid measurements in screening tests for predicting the future occurrence of CAD.

Other investigators have determined that the knowledge obtained by applying analytical ultracentrifugation to HDL lipoprotein fractions to obtain the HDL subclasses (HDL_2 and HDL_3) adds further precision to serum lipid information and may prove useful in refining the role of HDL in lipid metabolism and atherogensis. Though the biological role of these HDL subclasses is as yet not well understood, it has been reported that HDL_2 was significantly lower in patients with documented CAD and was related to the number of partial and complete coronary artery stenoses (Miller et al. [32]); was higher in females, who have a lower risk of CAD, than in their male counterparts (Wood and Haskell [33]); and was inversely related to the development of CAD (Goffman et al. [34]). High-density lipoprotein-3 (HDL_3) is apparently inert with respect to CAD risk. Though this preliminary information is encouraging, conclusive evidence relating the role of HDL subclasses to the etiology and pathology of CAD awaits further investigation, and at present HDL subfractioning techniques remain primarily a research tool.

Ethanol and High-Density Lipoprotein

Ethanol ingestion is known to increase HDL levels. Belfrage et al. [35] gave nonintoxicating doses of alcohol to 9 healthy males for 5 weeks. Plasma HDL concentration steadily rose to 30% above control values over the experimental period. Levels fell as soon as alcohol was discontinued. Johansson and Medhus [36] found elevated HDL levels in 60 of 69 alcoholic patients admitted to an alcohol withdrawal unit. After 2 weeks of abstinence, the HDL values of the patients returned to normal. Yano et al. [37] studied the relationship of alcohol consumption to CAD in 7705 Japanese men living in Hawaii over a period of 6 years. Those who drank 40 ml of alcohol per day (equivalent to 3 bottles of beer, 3 glasses of wine, or 2½ jiggers of hard liquor) had less than one-half the CAD events experienced by nondrinkers. The HDL levels in the drinkers were found to be higher than in the coronary-prone nondrinkers. Very recently it was demonstrated that ethanol consumption can affect the plasma concentration of apo A-I, the major protein constituent of HDL. Plasma concentrations of apo A-I fell 11% when men who were normally moderate consumers of alcohol (38 ml/day) abstained from alcohol consumption for 5 weeks. Subsequent reversion to normal alcohol intakes for 6 weeks in these same men caused a 14% rise in apo A-I (Camargo et al. [38]). These studies suggest that alcohol consumption may reduce CAD risk—perhaps by increasing HDL-cholesterol or HDL apoproteins.

However, evidence related to the HDL_2 and HDL_3 response to alcohol ingestion has been reported and suggests a note of caution. Though chronic alcohol consumption by alcoholics has been shown to raise the HDL_2:HDL_3 ratio (Taskinen et al. [39]), moderate alcohol consumption by healthy men resulted in an elevation of HDL_3 and not of the reputedly beneficial HDL_2 subclass (Eichner [40]; Haskell et al. [41]). Furthermore, moderate ethanol ingestion appears to have no effect on HDL levels in men who engage in regular running or jogging (Hartung et al. [42]). These studies generally support the view that ethanol ingestion may raise HDL concentrations, but also suggest that the response in men consuming moderate amounts of alcohol may not be associated with an increase in the appropriate HDL subclass. Further research will be required to resolve this issue. Despite the potentially beneficial influence of alcohol on the lipid profile, the known toxicity and abuse potential of ethanol ingestion decreases its usefulness as an antiatherogenic agent and limits its therapeutic value.

Pathogenesis of Coronary Artery Disease

Research in coronary atherosclerosis has focused on cholesterol accumulation within proliferating smooth muscle cells of blood vessels. The accumulation of cholesterol in these cells is the result of three processes: synthesis, deposition, and removal.

In the normal state, synthesis of cholesterol in the cell is thought to contribute little to cholesterol accumulation. Goldstein and Brown [43] have shown that cholesterol synthesis in the cell is blocked when its receptor is occupied by LDL. Since only 25 mg/100 ml of LDL-cholesterol is required to suppress synthesis, the mean level of LDL-cholesterol in individuals from Western societies (120 mg/100 ml) is normally sufficient to inhibit this cellular process.

Cholesterol deposition in smooth muscle cells of blood vessels by circulating lipoproteins has received much attention. The cholesterol within atherosclerotic plaques is thought to come predominantly from LDL (Portman [44]). Low-density lipoprotein is derived from very-low-density lipoproteins (VLDL) by degradation (Fig. 14-1). Very low-density lipoprotein is synthesized in the liver and is the major transport vehicle for endogenous triglycerides. The triglyceride fraction is hydrolyzed by lipoprotein lipase, and in the process, the VLDL particle is degraded to intermediate density lipoprotein (IDL), then further degraded to LDL. Low-density lipoprotein is left with the remaining cholesterol and is the major cholesterol carrier in the body (Eaton et al. [45]). It is slowly cleared from the blood by a number of processes, including deposition into smooth muscle cells of blood vessels. The LDL binds to specific binding sites on cell membranes and is taken up by pinocytosis to form intracellular vacuoles (Fig. 14-2); cellular lysosomes then digest these lipoprotein vacuoles (Peters and DeDuve [46]). Accumulation of cholesterol occurs when LDL blood levels are high (Smith and Slater [47]) and when intracellular degradation is impaired (Peters and DeDuve [46]).

Until recently, emphasis has been placed on LDL influx as the major determinant of

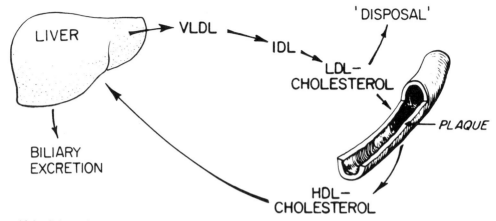

14-1 Schematic representation of the low-density lipoprotein generating system (LDL) and the high-density lipoproteins (HDL) cholesterol removal system. IDL = intermediate-density lipoproteins; VLDL = very-low-density lipoproteins. (From Hooper, P.L., Eaton, R.P. 1978. Exercise, high-density lipoprotein, and coronary artery disease. In: Appenzeller, O., Atkinson, R.A. (eds): Health Aspects of Endurance Training (Vol. 12, Medicine and Sport Series). Karger, Basel, Switzerland. Reprinted with permission.)

cholesterol accumulation within the cell. Evidence now suggests that cholesterol within smooth muscle cells can be removed by HDL. Moreover, a decrease in the removal of cholesterol from smooth muscle cells, due to a reduced plasma HDL concentration, may be of greater importance in the accumulation of cholesterol than is the excess deposition of cholesterol by LDL. High-density lipoprotein has the unique ability to bind to a cellular receptor (Miller et al. [48]), remove free cholesterol from the cell (Stein et al. [49]), esterify it (Glomset [50]), and transport the cholesterol ester to the bile (Sodhi and Kudchodkar [51]) (Fig. 14-2). This mechanism was first proposed by Glomset [50] in a detailed study of three sisters with a deficiency of the enzyme lecithin:cholesterol acyltransferase (LCAT), an enzyme that catalyzes the esterification of cholesterol. Glomset [50] was fascinated by the cholesterol-burdened foam cells found in the bone marrow and kidneys of these patients, and the similarity to the foam cells seen in familial HDL deficiency (Tangier disease). He postulated that HDL and the LCAT enzyme together esterify the cholesterol load removed from tissues by HDL. The nonpolar cholesterol ester could rapidly be internalized into the core of the HDL (preventing reaccumulation in tissues) and carried to the liver for excretion in the bile.

In addition, Stein et al. [49] have shown rapid cholesterol efflux from cells incubated with HDL apoproteins. Others (Miller et al. [52]) have studied the relationship between plasma lipoproteins and the size of the tissue cholesterol pool. Neither VLDL nor LDL concentrations correlated with total cholesterol pool size. However, HDL concentrations were inversely related to both rapidly and slowly exchanging pools of tissue cholesterol. These findings support the concept that the major determinant of net tissue cholesterol accumulation is the removal of cholesterol by HDL rather than deposition by LDL. Therefore, the mechanism by which HDL may confer a lower CAD risk is through a reduction in the cholesterol burden of the body.

Recent research into the pathogenesis of CAD has focused on both cholesterol accumulation within smooth muscle cells and the rate of proliferation of these cells. Ross [53] has reviewed literature that supports the following sequence of events leading to atherosclerotic plaque formation: 1) arterial endothelial injury, 2) platelet degranulation, 3) smooth muscle migration from the arterial media to the intima, and finally 4) smooth muscle cell proliferation in the intima accompanied by lipid deposition that leads to the formation of the

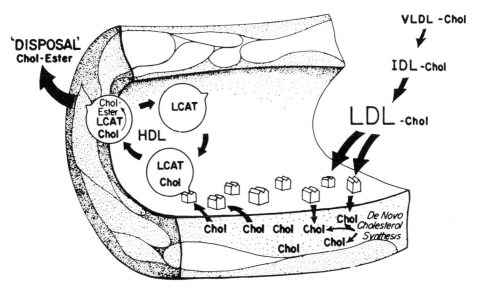

14-2 Cholesterol (Chol) accumulation in arterial smooth muscle cells: a net result of low-density lipoprotein (LDL) cholesterol disposition, de novo synthesis and high-density lipoprotein (HDL) cholesterol removal. IDL = intermediate-density lipoproteins; LCAT = lecithin:cholesterol acyltransferase; VLDL = very-low-density lipoprotein. (From Hooper, P.L., Eaton, R.P. 1978. Exercise, high-density lipoprotein, and coronary artery disease. In: Appenzeller, O., Atkinson, R.A. (eds): Health Aspects of Endurance Training (Vol. 12, Medicine and Sport Series). Karger, Basel, Switzerland. Reprinted with permission.)

characteristic atheroma. Research currently supports the concept that lipoprotein-lipids influence this disease process in a number of ways. In this context, LDL has been shown to have both direct and indirect toxic effects on endothelial cells in culture. In contrast, HDL seems to have a protective effect on endothelial cells, as a consequence of either a) its stimulation of endothelial prostacyclin production, thus preventing platelet adherance; or b) its role in the prevention of membrane cholesterol overloading (Henriksen et al. [54]). In addition, serum factors such as lipoproteins (Fisher-Ozoga et al. [55]), platelet factors (Ross et al. [56]), and hormones (Stout et al. [57]) have been shown to stimulate smooth muscle cell proliferation. Low-density lipoprotein has been found to be a particularly potent stimulus for smooth muscle proliferation (Fisher-Ozoga et al. [55]), whereas HDL appears to inhibit this process. A recent study in Finland (Tammi et al. [58]) revealed that sera from physically active lumberjacks (high in HDL) were more effective than sera from sedentary men in inhibiting the rate of smooth muscle DNA synthesis. Thus, HDL may also protect against CAD through inhibition of arterial smooth muscle proliferation.

What is High-Density Lipoprotein?

High-density lipoprotein consists of spherical micelles, approximately 110 μm in diameter, with a hydrophobic inner core of esterified cholesterol and triglyceride and a hydrophilic outer shell of protein, free cholesterol, and phospholipid (Stoffel et al. [59]). The composition of HDL is approximately 50% protein, 25% phospholipid, 20% cholesterol, and 5% triglyceride. This may be compared with LDL, which is composed of 46% cholesterol and carries 70–80% of the total circulating cholesterol. Very-low-density lipoprotein primarily transports endogenous triglyceride, being composed of 60–70% triglyceride and about 17% cholesterol (Jackson et al. [60]).

Existing evidence suggests that HDL particles (nascent disks) are produced in three ways: synthesized by the liver, synthesized by the intestinal epithelial cells, and generated by triglyceride-rich lipoprotein hydrolysis. High-density lipoprotein is a dynamic particle undergoing constant change in lipid and apoprotein composition; it participates in the generation of cholesterol esters from free cholesterol and lecithin via the enzyme LCAT. In addition, HDL is involved in a number of other lipid-lipoprotein regulatory processes via apoprotein exchange or interaction with other circulating lipoproteins. The major site of HDL degradation appears to be the liver and involves the action of the hepatic lipase enzyme. The half-life of HDL in human plasma is about 5 days, the longest of any lipoprotein.

The protein fraction of the lipoprotein is termed the *apoprotein* and several distinct types have been identified. These include three apo A (apo A-I, -II, and -IV), two apo B, three apo C (apo C-I, -II, and -III), apo D, and several polymorphic forms of apo E. The protein constituents serve to provide structural support and stability for the lipoprotein particles, provide recognition sites for cell membrane receptors, and act as cofactors for enzymes involved in lipoprotein metabolism. The primary apoproteins of HDL are A-I, A-II, and C peptides, though very small amounts of apo B, C, D, and E are also associated with the HDL particle (DuFaux et al. [61]). The exact role played by each of these apoproteins in the lipid transport and metabolism mediated by HDL is not completely understood. However, it does appear that the A-I peptide, the major apoprotein of HDL, initiates binding to cellular surface receptors and may participate in the LCAT reaction (Fielding et al. [62]). The A-II peptide of HDL is present in about one fourth the concentration of A-I and has as yet no recognized metabolic function (Chenny and Albers [63]). At least four peptide units with differing functions have been identified in the C-peptide group. The C-peptides dynamically shuttle between the HDL, VLDL, and IDL circulating in the plasma (Havel et al. [64]). The C-II peptide functions as a major activator of lipoprotein lipase, while C-I and C-III peptides inhibit human tissue lipoprotein lipase (Ekman and Nilsson-Ehle [65]). The activation of lipase activity at the surface of VLDL and IDL accelerates degradation of VLDL into IDL and, subsequently, IDL into LDL in the process of lipid clearance from the blood.

Total HDL levels are determined by sophisticated ultracentrifugation or electrophoretic procedures. With electrophoresis, the HDL migrates as the α-lipoprotein. Measurements of cholesterol within the HDL fractions are easily performed and correlate well with total HDL values (Albers et al. [66]). The determination of HDL-cholesterol is made by first adding phosphotungstate and magnesium, or manganese and heparin, to either plasma or serum, which precipitates all lipoprotein fractions except for HDL. A simple cholesterol analysis of the remaining supernatant solution will result in an HDL-cholesterol determination (Lopez-Virella et al. [67]). The simplicity of the HDL-cholesterol determination has permitted its utilization in large epidemiologic studies of CAD. More complex ultracentrifugal techniques have been used to separate HDL into the subclasses HDL_2, HDL_3, and, more recently, HDL_1. However, these procedures are limited almost exclusively to research settings at this time.

Exercise and High-Density Lipoprotein

Several lines of current research suggest that exercise affects serum levels of lipids and lipoproteins. Though exercise-induced alterations in the levels of these CAD risk factors have not been universally demonstrated, the evidence generally supports the contention that exercise may alter CAD risk via induced changes in lipid-lipoprotein metabolism, particularly as related to HDL.

Cholesterol and Triglyceride   Until recently, studies of exercise and lipid metabolism, like studies of CAD, had focused on total serum cholesterol and triglyceride. It is now generally concluded, when factors such as age, adiposity, and pretraining cholesterol levels are taken into account, that exercise has little or no influence on the plasma total cholesterol but does reduce triglyceride levels (Haskell [68]). This reduction in triglyceride appears to have both acute and chronic components and is not evident when pretraining values are low. The mechanism of this exercise-induced triglyceride reduction may be related to a decrease in VLDL production by the liver (Simonelli and Eaton [69]). This effect can be demonstrated in normal and Zucker rats, the animal model for type IV hyperlipoproteinemia. In humans with type IV hyperlipoproteinemia, only 30 min of treadmill walking a day for 4 days has a similar effect (Gyntelberg et al. [70]). With regard to LDL, the major cholesterol transport lipoprotein, DuFaux et al. [61] have identified 22 studies that document a lower LDL level in endurance-trained versus sedentary individuals and a reduced LDL in response to physical training programs. However, no difference and higher values in endurance-trained individuals have also been reported (Haskell [68]). When differences between trained and sedentary groups have been noted, the magnitude of the difference has been relatively small, usually about 10–12%, and generally occurs in runners who are very lean.

High-Density Lipoprotein Cholesterol In contrast to the variable and sometimes conflicting findings related to total serum cholesterol and LDL-cholesterol, the effects of exercise on HDL-cholesterol documented in both cross-sectioned and longitudinal studies appear quite consistent. The results of several studies comparing HDL-cholesterol in exercising and nonexercising populations are presented in Table 14-1. These studies are representative of the numerous cross-sectional investigations that have been conducted and demonstrate the nearly universal finding that those who are endurance trained possess significantly higher levels of HDL-cholesterol than do their sedentary counterparts. Furthermore, job and leisure time physical activity appears to be conducive to HDL elevation. Those who are more active generally demonstrate higher mean concentrations of HDL compared with less active controls (Haskell et al. [79]), though the differences are of less magnitude (5 mg/dl) than when endurance-trained individuals are contrasted with sedentary individuals (12–20 mg/dl). In addition, Schwane and Cundiff [80] found a significant correlation between HDL-cholesterol and aerobic capacity as assessed by a treadmill test. Berg and Keul [81] have reported similar findings and, in addition, have demonstrated a significant correlation between apo A-I and maximum aerobic capacity. However, patients with restricted activity due to injury or disease have demonstrated lower HDL-cholesterol levels (La Porte et al. [82]).

Such results suggest the existence of a dose–response relationship between exercise and HDL levels. Indeed, it appears that both the amount and type of exercise are important determinants of HDL elevation. Hagan et al. [83] and Hartung et al. [77] have concluded that the distance run during exercise training was the best predictor of HDL-cholesterol levels—superior to dietary factors, body-mass index, age, or percentage body fat. Other research suggests that a threshold of physical activity exists below which beneficial HDL increases do not occur; for runners this appears to be at 8 (Wood et al. [84]) to 10 miles (Williams et al. [85]) run per week. Athletes participating in anaerobic speed and power events such as weight-lifting and sprinting generally demonstrate HDL levels similar to (Farrell et al. [86]; Lehtonen and Vikari [76]; Nikkila et al. [74]) or less than (Berg et al. [87]) those of age- and sex-matched sedentary controls. These results from weight-lifters may be confounded by the failure to control for the use of anabolic steroids, since chronic use of these compounds has been shown to dramatically reduce HDL levels (Alen and Rahkila [88]). In contrast to the previously cited studies, Goldberg et al. [89] reported that strength training promoted a rise in the HDL-cholesterol level and a decrease in the total cholesterol to HDL-cholesterol ratio in previously sedentary, steroid-free men and women. However, these results remain equivocal since a control group was not included in the study

Table 14-1 Cross-Sectional Studies of Exercising and Nonexercising Populations and Their HDL-Cholesterol Levels

Subjects			HDL-cholesterol		
Type of Exercise		Sex and No.	Mg/100 ml ± SD	p	Location and Study

Type of Exercise	Sex	No.	Mg/100 ml ± SD	p	Location and Study
Runners, at least 15 miles/week	M	41	64 ± 13		
				<.05	Stanford, CA (Wood et al. [71])
Controls	M	145	43 ± 10		
Runners	F	43	75 ± 14		
				<.05	
Controls	F	101	56 ± 14		
Lumberjacks		12	67 ± 10		Finland (Lehtonen and Viikari [73]
				<.001	
Electricians		15	49 ± 11		
Runners and skiers	M	23	69 ± 15		Finland (Lehtonen and Viikari [73])
				<.01	
Controls	M	15	54 ± 12		
Sprinters, 12–23 miles/week	M	8	50 ± 6		
				<.01	
Long-distance runners, 62–82 miles/week	M	12	66 ± 7		Finland (Nikkila et al. [74])
				<.01	
Controls	M	10	47 ± 6		
Long-distance runners, 25–58 miles/week	F	6	74 ± 19		
				<.05	
Controls	F	16	61 ± 3		
Boston Marathon runners	M	49	55 ± 14		
	F	1		<.001	Massachusetts (Adner and Castelli [75])
	M	42	45 ± 9		
Controls	F	1			
Ice hockey players (not endurance trained)	M	24	50 ± 7		
				<001	Finland (Lehtonen and Viikari [76])
Soccer team players (endurance trained)	M	21	64 ± 14		
				<.001	
Controls	M	61	53 ± 9		
Marathon runners, 40 miles/week	M	59	65 ± 15		
				<.001	
Joggers, 6 miles/week	M	85	58 ± 18	<.001	Houston, Texas (Hartung et al. [77])
Controls	M	74	43 ± 14		
Long-distance running >40 miles/week	M	21	59 ± 12		
				<.01	Albuquerque, New Mexico (Crouse et al. [78])
Controls	M	23	49 ± 7		

design. Hurley et al. [90] demonstrated that bodybuilders, whose weight-lifting routines typically consisted of high-repetition exercises, had HDL levels similar to runners and significantly higher than power-lifters, who normally use low-repetition exercises. These results suggest that the weight-lifting method that promotes higher caloric expenditure per session and is more aerobic in nature may promote beneficial lipoprotein changes.

Weaknesses in the cross-sectional design used in many studies preclude the control of various confounding variables and selection bias that may influence HDL levels apart from physical activity. For example, the Stanford runners evidenced much higher HDL levels but also smoked less, ate differently, weighed less, and consumed nearly 6 times as much wine compared with their untrained counterparts (Wood et al. [71]). Hartung et al. [77] concluded on the basis of the strength of the associations between measured variables that diet, smoking, and alcohol habits alone could not explain the differences in HDL levels among runners, joggers, and sedentary subjects. However, the use of the longitudinal study design allows for more adequate control of the various extraneous factors, which could invalidate conclusions made on the basis of cross-sectional study results.

In general, results of longitudinal training studies support the contention that exercise elevates HDL-cholesterol concentrations. Altekruse and Wilmore [91] were early investigators to document this. Thirty-nine sedentary males averaging 33 years of age were studied before and after 10 weeks of walking, jogging, or running 3 times a week. Subjects trained an average of 5.2 miles per week at an average pace of 7.5 miles per hour. Mean weight loss was 1 kg. Diet, alcohol consumption, and cigarette smoking were not measured. Levels of HDL increased from 36.9% to 55.5% of total lipoprotein at the expense of VLDL and LDL.

Lopez et al. [92] studied 13 medical students who exercised 4 times a week for 7 weeks. Each exercise period consisted of 10–15 min of jogging, 5–10 min of bicycling, and 5–10 min of calisthenics. No weight loss occurred in response to training, and diet, alcohol consumption, and cigarette smoking were not monitored. Total HDL rose 16% from 57 mg/100 ml to 66.4 mg/100 ml ($p < .01$). Others have documented a rise in HDL in post-myocardial infarction patients who walked/jogged 30–45 min 3 times per week (Erkelens et al. [93]; Streja and Mymin [94]).

DuFaux et al. [61] have reviewed 31 training studies related to HDL-cholesterol. Two thirds of these studies documented an increase in HDL-cholesterol, while one third showed no change or a decrease in the plasma concentration of this lipoprotein. Results from studies conducted by Wood et al. [84] and Williams [85] indicate that failure to control for amount of exercise performed per week may confound the results of training studies. These researchers have shown that the magnitude of HDL-cholesterol change over the course of a training program is highly correlated with the amount of exercise performed. Furthermore, it appears that a minimum of 8–10 miles run per week is required to induce an HDL increase.

Vu Tran et al. [95] have concluded that several factors may contribute to the ambiguity noted in the literature with respect to training-induced changes in lipoprotein levels. The statistical technique meta-analysis was used to aggregate the results of 66 training studies involving the measurement of human blood lipid-lipoprotein changes over time. Age, length and intensity of training, maximal oxygen uptake, body weight, and percentage body fat were shown to interact with exercise and changes in lipid-lipoprotein levels. Of particular interest, initial levels of HDL-cholesterol were strongly correlated ($p < .01$) with their training-induced changes. Thus, failure to account for these potential confounding factors in training studies may lead to spurious results.

These results suggest the exercise-induced changes in HDL levels may not be independent of changes in body weight and/or body fat. Indeed, Brownell et al. [96] have concluded that weight reduction may independently increase HDL-cholesterol concentrations, at least in obese men and women. Sopko et al. [97] have attempted to define the independent and combined effects of exercise conditioning and weight loss in young obese men. Subjects were randomly assigned to 1 of 4 groups: control, exercise training and constant weight, inactive and weight loss through caloric restriction, and a combination of exercise training and weight loss. Their results showed that the inactivity–weight loss modality and the exercise–constant weight modality each significantly increased HDL-cholesterol, and the effect of exercise with weight loss produced an additive effect of HDL elevation above that produced independently by either modality. Thus, it appears that exercise and weight loss separately and independently increase HDL-cholesterol in obese males, and that their effects are additive.

High-Density Lipoprotein Subfractions Relatively little information is available regarding the influence of exercise on the major HDL subclasses HDL_1 and HDL_2. Wood and Haskell [98] reported that the antiatherogenic HDL_2 subclass was elevated in men and women runners compared with sedentary controls, while HDL_3 was not related to exercise status. In addition, male athletes reportedly demonstrate a higher HDL_2:HDL_3 ratio than do untrained controls (DuFaux et al. [61]), and it appears that HDL_2 levels are significantly related to bicycle work performance ($r = .52; p > .05$) (Kuusi et al. [99]). Results of longitudinal training studies have been inconsistent and have shown 1) no change in HDL_2 or HDL_3 levels over a 6-week training period (Lipson et al. [100]), 2) an increase in HDL_2 with a concomitant decrease in HDL_3 following 10 weeks of exercise training (Nye et al. [101]), and 3) changes in HDL_2 levels with training that are correlated with miles run per week (Wood et al. [84]). Thus, conclusive evidence that HDL subfractions are differentially affected by exercise training awaits future research.

High-Density Lipoprotein Apoproteins A change in measured HDL-cholesterol may simply reflect an increase in the ability of the HDL particle to transport cholesterol; i.e., the proportion of the cholesterol transported in relation to the protein and phospholipid may be altered. However, evidence now indicates that HDL protein constituents are also elevated by exercise. Lehtonen et al. [102] found apo A-I to be 32% higher in athletes than in age-matched controls, while no difference was found for apo A-II levels. Others have reported similar results from cross-sectional comparisons of athletes and controls (Thompson et al. [103]; Wood et al. [98]). Evidence from longitudinal training studies is very limited and not conclusive; studies have shown either an increase (Kiens et al. [104]) or no change (Wood et al. [84]) in apo A-I levels in response to 12 weeks to 1 year of physical training. Clearly, definitive evidence is presently lacking concerning the effect of exercise on the apolipoprotein profile, and this problem merits further research.

Postulated Mechanisms by Which Exercise Alters High-Density Lipoprotein

From the foregoing discussion, it is clear that physically active individuals have higher levels of HDL-cholesterol than do the sedentary majority and that the association is in all likelihood a causal one. However, the regulation of the synthesis and catabolism of the lipoproteins in general is poorly understood, and until more is learned about this problem the mechanism by which exercise may induce alterations in HDL metabolism will remain unresolved. Though much remains to be learned, the information that is available at least allows for speculation concerning the role of exercise in the modulation of HDL levels. Recent evidence suggests that exercise, by dramatically increasing energy expenditure and promoting catabolic metabolic processes, may alter the phosphorylation state of regulatory enzymes involved in lipoprotein and/or cholesterol synthesis and degradation. In addition, it has been postulated that exercise may alter the enzymes lipoprotein lipase (LPL), hepatic lipase (HL), or LCAT, which are involved in plasma triglyceride and cholesterol metabolism.

Enzyme Phosphorylation   Though current lipid research offers some insight into the role of HDL in cholesterol metabolism, little is known about de novo synthesis of HDL apoproteins. It is known that at least 35 enzymes are regulated by external, physiologic stimuli acting through phosphorylation/dephosphorylation mechanisms (Cohen [105]). Recently it has been demonstrated that 3-hydroxy-3-methylglutaryl coenzyme A reductase (the major regulatory enzyme for cholesterol biosynthesis) may be inactivated by phosphorylation in response to cholesterol feeding (Arebalo et al. [106]). Furthermore, beta-adrenergic antagonists lower HDL-cholesterol (Loren et al. [107]), while beta-adrenergic agonists appear to raise HDL levels (Hooper et al. [108]). Hooper and Scallen [109] have concluded that factors that increase HDL levels are associated with physiologic states in which catabolic reactions are favored and regulatory proteins are phosphorylated. In contrast, low HDL levels are associated with physiologic states in which anab1olic (biosynthetic) reactions predominate and the involved regulatory proteins are dephosphorylated. They proposed that hormonal or drug stimuli increase cyclic adenosine monophosphate, with subsequent activation of protein kinase(s), which in turn phosphorylates an enzyme (or enzymes) that either increases HDL apoprotein synthesis or decreases its catabolism. The specific enzyme system or systems that may participate in HDL apoprotein synthesis or degradation remain to be identified. Though this hypothesis is attractive and could explain exercise-induced changes in HDL levels, it presently lacks experimental verification.

Lipoprotein Lipase   Research related to the potential role of LPL in exercise-induced HDL increase has been critically reviewed by Haskell [110]. The essentials of this argument involve the fact that exercise appears to increase LPL activity, which could in turn reduce plasma triglyceride concentration. It is postulated that some of the cholesterol, phospholipid, and apoprotein made available from the potentiated VLDL catabolism are transferred to discoidal HDL particles (nascent disks) secreted by the liver resulting in an increased plasma HDL mass. In support of this hypothesis, endurance runners generally demonstrate higher muscle and adipose tissue LPL activity than do untrained controls. In addition, adipose tissue LPL activity is strongly correlated with HDL levels (Nikkila et al. [74]). However, Peltonen et al. [111] were not able to demonstrate a significant correlation between HDL-cholesterol and postheparin or adipose tissue LPL either before or after training. Both LPL and HDL increased in response to the training stimulus, but most of the LPL increase occurred in the first week of training, suggesting that LPL elevation may be an acute response to exercise. Though evidence suggests that LPL may be related to HDL metabolism, a causal relationship between exercise-induced changes in LPL activity and HDL elevation has not been documented.

Hepatic Lipase   Hepatic lipase apparently functions in the removal of HDL_2 by the liver and the generation of the denser HDL_3 subfraction (DuFaux et al. [61]). Haskell [110] reported that exercise may result in decreased HL activity and that a negative correlation has been documented between HDL-cholesterol and HL in runners, active military academy students, and middle-aged men before and after training. In contrast, Sutherland et al. [112] reported a 27% increase in HDL-cholesterol and a 29% increase in postheparin HL activity following 18 weeks of moderate training. Thus, the role of HL in modulating HDL levels in response to exercise requires clarification by additional research.

Lecithin:Cholesterol Acyltransferase   The enzyme LCAT is involved in the esterification of cholesterol and transfer of the cholesterol esters formed to HDL particles. Activation of LCAT probably requires HDL apoproteins. Thus, an increase in LCAT activity could increase the circulating levels of HDL-cholesterol. Haskell [110] noted that an increase in LCAT activity has been demonstrated in physically active rats, in endurance-trained sportsmen, and in response to endurance training in middle-aged men. It appears that short-term (6-week) exercise withdrawal does not affect LCAT activity or HDL_2 and HDL_3 levels (Thompson et al. [113]). Marniemi (114) reported that changes in LCAT activity were correlated with increased HDL-cholesterol and total cholesterol levels following moderate training in men, though this finding is not universal. It is evident that the relationship among exercise, LCAT activity, and HDL-cholesterol is not well understood and that conclusive evidence of a causal link between exercise and increased LCAT activity awaits future research.

CONCLUSION

In spite of recent advances in the diagnosis and treatment of CAD, this malady still remains the number one cause of death in the United States. Several lines of research have provided evidence for the existence of certain biological and behavioral factors that appear to influence an individual's risk for developing this disease. In this regard, elevated levels of circulating HDL-cholesterol appear to confer some measure of protection against CAD development and pathology. Physical activity also has been identified as a major protective factor against CAD; those who are employed in more physically demanding occupations or who habitually engage in exercise during leisure time have a lower incidence and prevalence of CAD. This beneficial modification of CAD risk associated with exercise may be explained at least in part by exercise-induced changes in serum lipid-lipoprotein levels, particularly levels of HDL-cholesterol. Exercise promotes an increase in the HDL-cholesterol concentration, with a concomitant decrease in the total cholesterol:HDL-cholesterol ratio. It seems fairly certain that exercise also induces an increase in the antiatherogenic HDL_2 subclass and in the concentration of circulating apoprotein A-I. The mechanism by which physical exercise promotes these lipoprotein alterations is probably not independent of the caloric expenditure or the training modality used during exercise. The intracellular phosphorylation state and enzymes such as LPL, LCAT, and HL, which are known to influence lipid metabolism, have been shown to be related to the exercise stimulus. Such findings have provided the theoretical basis for several proposed mechanisms through which exercise may act to modify HDL concentrations. An exercise threshold does exist below which no change in HDL occurs. This threshold appears to be relatively low, amounting to 8 to 10 miles run per week (or an equivalent), but greater amounts of activity do result in even greater increases in HDL. The hypothesis that an exercise-induced elevation of HDL-cholesterol results in protection from CAD is attractive and scientifically sound, but as yet unproved. Well-controlled, long-term longitudinal studies of active and sedentary individuals are needed to clarify this issue. In the meantime, the existing evidence clearly supports a principle that has been intuitively evident all along: regular exercise is a heathful practice.

REFERENCES

1. American Heart Association. 1985. Heart Facts. Dallas, TX.
2. Gordon, T. 1982. Recent decline in coronary disease mortality in the United States: part of a general decline in mortality. Am Heart J 103:151–152.
3. Gordon, T., Thom, T. 1975. The recent decrease in coronary heart disease mortality. Prev Med 4:115–125.
4. Morris, J.N., Heady, J.A., et al. 1953. Coronary heart-disease and physical activity of work. Lancet 2:1053–1057, 1111–1120.
5. Morris, J.N. 1960. Epidemiology and cardiovascular disease of middle age: I, II. Mod Concepts Cardiovasc Dis 29: 625–631.
6. Froelicher, V.F., Oberman, A. 1972.

Analysis of epidemiologic studies of physical inactivity as a risk for coronary artery disease. Prog Cardiovasc Dis 15:41–65.

7. Paffenbarger, R.S., Jr, Hale, W.E., et al. 1977. Work-energy level, personal characteristics and fatal heart attack; birth cohort effect. Am J Epidemiol 105:200–213.

8. Paffenbarger, R.S., Jr, Wing, A.L., et al. 1978. Physical activity as an index of heart attack risk in college alumni. Am J Epidemiol 108:161–175.

9. Blackburn, H. 1983. Physical activity and coronary heart disease: a brief update and population view (Part I and II). J Cardiac Rehab 3:101–111, 171–174.

10. Paffenbarger, R.S., Jr., Hyde, R.T. 1984. Exercise in the prevention of coronary heart disease. Prev Med 13:3–22.

11. Superko, R.H., Wood, P.D., et al. 1985. Coronary heart disease and risk factor modification. Is there a threshold? Am J Med 78:826–838.

12. Lipid Research Clinics Program. 1984. The lipid research clinics coronary primary prevention trial results. I. Reduction in incidence of coronary heart disease. II. The relationship of reduction in incidence of coronary heart disease to cholesterol lowering. JAMA 251:351–374.

13. Barr, D.P., Russ, E.M., et al. 1951. Protein–lipid relationships in human plasma. Am J Med 11:480–495.

14. Gordon, T., Castelli, W.P., et al. 1977. High density lipoprotein as a protective factor against coronary heart disease. Am J Med 62:707–714.

15. Castelli, W.P., Doyle, J.T., et al. 1972. HDL-cholesterol and other lipids in coronary heart disease: the cooperative lipoprotein phenotyping study. Circulation 55:767–772.

16. Miller, G.J., Miller, N.E. 1975. Plasma high density lipoprotein concentrations and development of ischaemic heart disease. Lancet 1:16–19.

17. Kajiyama, G., Mizuno, T., et al. 1974. The lowered serum phospholipids in alpha-lipoprotein in patients with atherosclerosis. Hiroshima J Med Sci 23:229–236.

18. Carlson, L.A. 1973. Lipoprotein fractionation. J Clin Pathol 26 (suppl 15):32–37.

19. Rhoads, G.G., Gulbrandsen, C.L., et al. 1976. Serum lipoproteins and coronary heart disease in a population study of Hawaii Japanese men. N Engl J Med 294:293–298.

20. Glueck, C.J., Gartside, P., et al. 1976. Longevity syndromes: familial hypobeta- and familial hyperalpha-lipoproteinemia. J Lab Clin Med 88:941–957.

21. Gustafson, A., Lillienberg, L., et al. 1974. Human plasma high-density lipoprotein composition during the menstrual cycle. Scand J Clin Lab Invest 137 (suppl):63–70.

22. Statistical Bulletin. 1975. 56:1–6, June.

23. Wilson, D.E., Lees, R.S. 1972. Metabolic relationships among the plasma lipoproteins. J Clin Invest 51:1051–1057.

24. Lopes-Virella, M.F.L., Stone, P.G., et al. 1977. Serum high-density lipoprotein in diabetic patients. Diabetologia 13:285–291.

25. Brunzell, J.D., Albers, J.J., et al. 1977. Prevalence of serum lipid abnormalities in chronic hemodialysis. Metabolism 26:903–910.

26. Garrison, R.J., Kannel, W.B., et al. 1977. Cigarette smoking and HDL-cholesterol: the Framingham Study. Circulation 55–56 (suppl III):44.

27. Castelli, W.P., Abbott, R.D., et al. 1983. Summary estimates of cholesterol used to predict coronary heart disease. Circulation 67:730–734.

28. Fager, G., Wiklund, O., et al. 1980. Serum apolipoprotein levels in relation to acute myocardial infarction and its risk factors. Apolipoprotein A-I levels in male survivors of myocardial infarction. Atherosclerosis 36:67–74.

29. Avogaro, P., Don, G.B., et al. 1980. Relationship between apolipoproteins and chemical components of lipoproteins in survivors of myocardial infarction. Atherosclerosis 37:69–76.

30. Maciejko, J.J., Holmes, D.R., et al. 1983. Apolipoprotein A-I as a marker of angiographically assessed coronary-artery disease. N Engl J Med 309:385–389.

31. Noma, A., Yokosuka, T., et al. 1983. Plasma lipids and apolipoproteins as discriminators for presence and severity of angiographically defined coronary artery disease. Atherosclerosis 49:1–7.

32. Miller, N.E., Hammett, F., et al. 1981. Relation of angiographically defined coronary artery disease to plasma lipoprotein subfractions and apolipoproteins. Br Med J 282:1741–1744.

33. Wood, P., Haskell, W. 1979. The effect of exercise on plasma high-density lipoproteins. Lipids 14:417–427.

34. Goffman, J., Young, W., et al. 1966. Ischemic heart disease, atherosclerosis, and longevity. Circulation 34:679–685.

35. Belfrage, P., Berg, B., et al. 1977. Alterations of lipid metabolism during long-term ethanol intake. Eur J Clin Invest 7:127–131.

36. Johansson, B.G., Medhus, A. 1974. Increase in plasma alpha-lipoproteins in chronic alcoholics after acute abuse. Acta Med Scand 195:273–277.

37. Yano, K., Rhoads, G.G., et al. 1977. Coffee, alcohol, and risk of coronary heart disease among Japanese men living in Hawaii. N Engl J Med 297:405–409.

38. Camargo, C.A., Williams, P.T., et al. 1985. The effect of moderate alcohol intake on serum apolipoproteins A-I and A-II. JAMA 253:2854–2857.

39. Taskinen, M.R., Valimaki, M., et al. 1982. High density lipoprotein subfractions and postheparin plasma lipases in alcoholic men before and after ethanol withdrawal. Metabolism 31:1168–1174.

40. Eichner, E.R. 1985. Alcohol versus exercise for coronary protection. Am J Med 79:231–240.

41. Haskell, W.L., Camargo, C., Jr., et al. 1984. The effect of cessation and resumption of moderate alcohol intake on serum high-density-lipoprotein subfractions: a controlled study. N Engl J Med 310:805–810.

42. Hartung, G.H., Foreyt, J.P., et al. 1983. Effect of alcohol intake on high-density lipoprotein cholesterol levels in runners and inactive men. JAMA 249:747–750.

43. Goldstein, J.L., Brown, M.S. 1977. The low-density lipoprotein pathway and its relation to atherosclerosis. Annu Rev Biochem 46:897–930.

44. Portman, O.W. 1970. Arterial composition and metabolism: esterified fatty acids and cholesterol. Adv Lipid Res 8:41–114.

45. Eaton, R.P., Crespin, S., et al. 1976. Incorporation of 75-seleno-methionine into human apoproteins. III. Kinetic behavior of isotopically labeled plasma apoprotein in man. Diabetes 25:679–690.

46. Peters, T.J., DeDuve, C. 1974. Lysosomes of the arterial wall. II. Subcellular fractionation of aortic cells from rabbits with experimental atheroma. Exp Mol Pathol 20:228–256.

47. Smith, E.B., Slater, R.S. 1972. Relationship between low density lipoprotein in aortic intima and serum lipid levels. Lancet 1:463–469.

48. Miller, N.E., Weinstein, D.B. et al. 1977. Interaction between high density and low density lipoproteins during uptake and degradation by cultured human fibroblasts. J Clin Invest 60:78–89.

49. Stein, Y., Glangeaud, M.C., et al. 1975. The removal of cholesterol from aortic smooth muscle cells in culture and landschutz ascites cells by fractions of human high density apolipoproteins. Biochim Biophys Acta 380:106–118.

50. Glomset, A. 1978. The plasma lecithin:cholesterol acyltransferase reaction. J Lipid Res 9:155–167.

51. Sodhi, H.S., Kudchodkar, B.J. 1973. Correlating metabolism of plasma and tissue cholesterol with that of plasma lipoproteins. Lancet 1:513–519.

52. Miller, N.E., Nestel, P.J., et al. 1976. Relationships between plasma lipoprotein cholesterol concentrations and the pool size and metabolism of cholesterol in man. Atherosclerosis 23:535–547.

53. Ross, R. 1980. The genesis of atherosclerosis. In: National Research Council: 1980 Issues and Current Studies. National Academy of Sciences, Washington, DC.

54. Henriksen, T., Mahoney, E.M., et al. 1982. Interactions of plasma lipoproteins with endothelial cells. Ann NY Acad Sci 401:102–116.

55. Fisher-Ozoga, K., Chen, R., et al. 1974. Effects of serum lipoproteins on the morphology, growth, and metabolism of arterial smooth muscle cells. Adv Exp Med Biol 43:299–311.

56. Ross, R., Glomset, J., et al. 1974. A platelet-dependent serum factor that stimulates the proliferation of arterial smooth muscle cells in vitro. Proc Natl Acad Sci USA 71:1207–1210.

57. Stout, R.W., Bierman, E.L., et al. 1975. Effect of insulin on the proliferation of cultured primate arterial smooth muscle cells. Circ Res 36:319–327.

58. Tammi, M., Ronnemaa, T., et al. 1979. High density lipoproteinemia due to vigorous physical work inhibits the incorporation of (^{3}H) thymidine and the synthesis of glycosaminoglycans by human aortic smooth muscle cells in culture. Atherosclerosis 32:23–32.

59. Stoffel, W., Zierenberg, O., et al. 1976. ^{13}C nuclear magnetic resonance spectroscopic evidence for hydrophobic lipid-protein interactions in human high density lipoproteins. Proc Natl Acad Sci USA 71:3696–3700.

60. Jackson, R., Morrisett, J., et al. 1976. Lipoprotein structure and metabolism. Physiol Rev 56:259–316.

61. DuFaux, B., Assman, G., et al. 1982. Plasma lipoproteins and physical activity: a review. Int J Sports Med 3:123–136.

62. Fielding, C.J., Shore, V.G., et al. 1972.

A protein cofactor of lecithin:cholesterol acyltransferase. Biochem Biophys Res Commun 46:1463–1498.

63. Chenny, M.C., Albers, J.J. 1977. The measurement of apolipoprotein A-I and A-II levels in men and women by immunoassay. J Clin Invest 60:43–51.

64. Havel, R.J., Kane, J.P., et al. 1973. Interchange of apoproteins between chylomicrons and high density lipoproteins during alimentary lipemia in man. J Clin Invest 52:32–38.

65. Ekman, R., Nilsson-Ehle, P. 1975. Effect of apolipoproteins on lipoprotein lipase activity of human adipose tissue. Clin Chim Acta 63:29–35.

66. Albers, J.J., Wahl, P.W., et al. 1976. Quantitation of apolipoprotein A-I of human plasma high density lipoprotein. Metabolism 25:633–644.

67. Lopez-Virella, M.F., Stone, P., et al. 1977. Cholesterol determinations in high-density lipoproteins separated by three different methods. Clin Chem 23:882–884.

68. Haskell, W.L. 1984. Exercise-induced changes in plasma lipids and lipoproteins. Prev Med 13:23–36.

69. Simonelli, C., Eaton, R.P. 1978. Reduced triglyceride secretion: a metabolic consequence of chronic exercise. Am J Physiol 234:221–227.

70. Gyntelberg, F., Brennan, R., et al. 1977. Plasma triglyceride lowering by exercise despite increased food intake in patients with type IV hyperlipoproteinemia. Am J Clin Nutr 30:716–720.

71. Wood, P.D., Haskell, W.L., et al. 1977. Plasma lipoprotein distributions in male and female runners. Ann NY Acad Sci 301:748–763.

72. Lehtonen, A., Viikari, J. 1978. The effect of vigorous physical activity at work on serum lipids with a special reference to serum high-density lipoprotein cholesterol. Acta Physiol Scand 104:117–121.

73. Lehtonen, A., Viikari, J. 1978. Serum triglycerides and cholesterol and serum high-density lipoprotein cholesterol in highly physically active men. Acta Med Scand 204:111–114.

74. Nikkila, E.A., Taskinen, M.R., et al. 1978. Lipoprotein lipase activity in adipose tissue and skeletal muscle of runners: relation to serum lipoproteins. Metabolism 27:1661–1667.

75. Adner, M.M., Castelli, W.P. 1980. Elevated high-density lipoprotein levels in marathon runners. JAMA 243:534–536.

76. Lehtonen, A., Viikari, J. 1980. Serum lipids in soccer and ice-hockey players. Metabolism 29:36–39.

77. Hartung, G.H., Foreyt, J.P., et al. 1980. Relation of diet to high-density lipoprotein cholesterol in middle-aged marathon runners, joggers, and inactive men. N Engl J Med 302:357–361.

78. Crouse, S.F., Hooper, P.L., et al. 1984. Zinc ingestion and lipoprotein values in sedentary and endurance-trained men. JAMA 252:785–787.

79. Haskell, W.L., Taylor, H.L., et al. 1980. Strenuous physical activity, treadmill exercise test response and plasma high-density lipoprotein cholesterol: the Lipid Research Clinic Program Prevalence Study. Circulation 62(suppl IV):53–61.

80. Schwane, J.A., Cundiff, D.E. 1979. Relationships among cardiorespiratory fitness, regular physical activity, and plasma lipids in young adults. Metabolism 28:771–776.

81. Berg, A., Keul, J. 1985. Influence of maximal aerobic capacity and relative body weight on the lipoprotein profile in athletes. Atherosclerosis 55:225–231.

82. La Porte, R.E., Brenes, G., et al. 1983. HDL-cholesterol across a spectrum of physical activity from quadriplegia to marathon running. Lancet 1:1212–1213.

83. Hagan, R.D., Smith, M.G., et al. 1983. High density lipoprotein cholesterol in relation to food consumption and running distance. Prev Med 12:287–295.

84. Wood, P.D., Haskell, W.L., et al. 1983. Increased exercise level and plasma lipoprotein concentrations: a one-year, randomized, controlled study in sedentary, middle-aged men. Metabolism 32:31–38.

85. Williams, P., Wood, P.D., et al. 1982. The effects of running mileage and duration on plasma lipoprotein levels. JAMA 247:2674–2679.

86. Farrell, P.A., Maksud, M.G., et al. 1982. A comparison of plasma cholesterol, triglycerides, and high-density lipoprotein-cholesterol in speed skaters, weightlifters, and non-athletes. Eur J Appl Physiol 48:77–82.

87. Berg, A., Ringwald, G., et al. 1980. Lipoprotein-cholesterol in well-trained athletes. Int J Sports Med 1:137–138.

88. Alen, M., Rahkila, P. 1984. Reduced high-density lipoprotein-cholesterol in power athletes: use of male sex hormone derivatives, an atherogenic factor. Int J Sports Med 5:341–342.

89. Goldberg, L., Elliot, D.L., et al. 1984. Changes in lipid and lipoprotein levels after weight training. JAMA 252:502–506.

90. Hurley, B.F., Seals, D.R., et al. 1984.

High-density lipoprotein cholesterol in body builders v. powerlifters. JAMA 252:507–513.

91. Altekruse, E.B., Wilmore, J.H. 1973. Changes in blood chemistries following a controlled exercise program. J Occup Med 15:110–113.

92. Lopez, A., Vial, R., et al. 1974. Effect of exercise and physical fitness on serum lipids and lipoproteins. Atherosclerosis 20:1–9.

93. Erkelens, W.D., Albers, J.J., et al. 1979. High density lipoprotein-cholesterol in survivors of myocardial infarction. JAMA 242:2185–2189.

94. Streja, D., Mymin, D. 1979. Moderate exercise and high density lipoprotein-cholesterol. JAMA 242:2190–2192.

95. Vu Tran, Z., Weltman, A., et al. 1983. The effects of exercise on blood lipids and lipoproteins: a meta-analysis of studies. Med Sci Sports Exerc 15:393–402.

96. Brownell, K.D., Stunkard, A.J. 1981. Differential changes in plasma high-density lipoprotein cholesterol in obese men and women during weight reduction. Arch Intern Med 141:1142–1148.

97. Sopko, G., Leon, A.S., et al. 1985. The effects of exercise and weight loss on plasma lipids in young men. Metabolism 34:227–236.

98. Wood, P., Haskell, W. 1979. The effect of exercise on plasma high-density lipoproteins. Lipids 14:417–427.

99. Kuusi, T., Nikkila, E.A., et al. 1982. Plasma high-density lipoproteins HDL_2, HDL_3, and postheparin plasma lipases in relation to parameters of physical fitness. Atherosclerosis 41:209–219.

100. Lipson, L.C., Bonow, R.O., et al. 1980. Effect of exercise conditioning on plasma high-density lipoproteins and other lipoproteins. Atherosclerosis 37:529–538.

101. Nye, E., Carlson, K., et al. 1981. Changes in high-density lipoprotein subfractions and other lipoproteins induced by exercise. Clin Chim Acta 113:51–57.

102. Lehtonen, A., Viikari, J., et al. 1979. The effect of exercise on high density (HDL) lipoprotein apoproteins. Acta Physiol Scand 106:487–488.

103. Thompson, P.D., Lazarus, B., et al. 1983. Exercise, diet, or physical charac-teristics as determinants of HDL levels in endurance athletes. Atherosclerosis 46:333–339.

104. Kiens, B., Jorgensen, I., et al. 1980. Increased plasma HDL-cholesterol and apo A-1 in sedentary middle-aged men after physical conditioning. Eur J Clin Invest 10:203–209.

105. Cohen, P. 1982. The role of protein phosphorylation in neural and hormonal control of cellular activity. Nature 296:613–617.

106. Arebalo, R.E., Hardgrave, J.E., et al. 1981. The in vivo regulation of rat liver 3-hydroxy-3-methylglutaryl coenzyme A reductase. J Biol Chem 256:571–574.

107. Loren, P., Foss, P.O., et al. 1980. Effect of propranolol and prazosin on blood lipids: the Oslo study. Lancet 2:4–6.

108. Hooper, P.L., Woo, W., et al. 1981. Terbutaline raises high-density-lipoprotein-cholesterol levels. N Engl J Med 305:1455–1457.

109. Hooper, P.L., Scallen, T.J. 1984. Modulation of high-density lipoprotein: the importance of protein phosphorylation/dephosphorylation. Am Heart J 108:1393–1398.

110. Haskell, W.L. 1984. The influence of exercise on the concentrations of triglyceride and cholesterol in human plasma. In: Terjung, R.L. (ed): Exeriçse and Sports Science Reviews (American College of Sports Medicine Series). Collamore Press, Toronto, Canada, pp. 205–244.

111. Peltonen, P., Marniemi, J., et al. 1981. Changes in serum lipids, lipoproteins, and heparin releasable lipolytic enzymes during moderate physical training in man: a longitudinal study. Metabolism 30:518–526.

112. Sutherland, W.H.F., Woodhouse, S.P., et al. 1984. Post-heparin hepatic lipase activity and plasma high-density-lipoprotein levels in men during physical training. Biochem Med 31:31–35.

113. Thompson, C.E., Thomas, T.R., et al. 1985. Response of HDL cholesterol, apoprotein A-I, and LCAT to exercise withdrawal. Atherosclerosis 54:65–73.

114. Marniemi, J., Dahlstrom, S., et al. 1982. Dependence of serum lipid and lecithin:cholesterol acyltransferase levels on physical training of young men. Eur J Appl Physiol 49:25–35.

•15•

Exercise
and the Lung

Thomas W. Chick and Jonathan M. Samet

The exercising athlete is merely performing work. Thus, his or her activities are appropriately described in terms borrowed from Newtonian physics (Table 15-1). The endurance athlete—the runner, swimmer, or cross-country skier—must work to accelerate and then maintain his or her pace. The isometric athlete—the weight-lifter or football player—also performs work even if no motion occurs. Power, the rate at which work is performed, is the usual measure of work capacity. The mechanical efficiency of work is the portion of energy that is transformed to external work.

Power demands in athletics vary with the type of activity and the rate at which it is performed; for example, an increase in running speed from 8 to 16 km/hr increases oxygen consumption ($\dot{V}O_2$) from 30 to 50 ml/min/kg (Maughan and Leiper [1]). This energy expenditure comprises not only the external work performed but the internal energy costs that accompany exercise, such as cardiac and respiratory work. The hyperpnea of exercise is paralleled by increased oxygen demand by the respiratory muscles themselves. In normal people, even with extreme exertion, the energy required by the respiratory system is never greater than approximately 10% of the total energy expended.

FUEL UTILIZATION DURING EXERCISE

Human work, including athletics, is always accomplished by muscle contraction, which is powered by the high-energy phosphate bonds of adenosine triphosphate (ATP). The ATP stored within muscle can meet energy requirements only transiently, for less than 1 sec (Wasserman and Whipp [2]; Jones [3]). Regeneration of ATP by creatine phosphate is another short-term, limited source of ATP (Astrand and Rodahl [4]; Jones [3]). Sustained exercise with continued demand for ATP ultimately requires the utilization of body energy stores. Fuels available for exercise include fat and carbohydrate; protein utilization requires muscle and parenchymal tissue breakdown and does not occur with ordinary endurance exercise (Felig and Wahren [5]). Body stores are primarily in the form of fat. An untrained 70-kg man has approximately 140,000 kcal of fat and only 2000 kcal of carbohydrate. The carbohydrate is stored in the form of muscle glycogen, 350 g, and hepatic glycogen, 40–90 g (Felig and Wahren [5]). The amount of these fuel supplies varies with diet and exercise patterns.

Table 15-1   Work Performed by the Exercising Athlete

Term	Definition*	Measurement
Force	Accelerates a mass	1 newton = 1 kg $\times$ m $\times$ S^{-2}
Work	Force acting through a distance	1 joule = 1 newton $\times$ 1m
Efficiency	Work output per energy input	percent
Work load	Work demand of a task	watts

*These units are in the International Standard (SI) system. In the previous system, work was measured in kilopond-meters (kpm). For conversion, 1 watt = 6.12 kpm $\times$ min^{-1}

Muscle cells utilize fats and carbohydrates to regenerate ATP through both aerobic and anaerobic processes. The aerobic pathways require adequate numbers of mitochondria, adequate tricarboxylic acid (Krebs) cycle enzymes, and an adequate oxygen (O_2) supply at the mitochondria (Wasserman and Whipp [2]). When these conditions are not met and aerobic metabolism becomes inadequate, ATP regeneration must occur by anaerobic processes.

Exercising muscles use glycogen and blood-borne glucose as carbohydrate fuel. Under both aerobic and anaerobic conditions the initial sequence of glucose metabolism is the same; the glycolytic enzymes convert glucose to pyruvate. When the oxygen supply and mitochondrial numbers are adequate (Idstrom et al. [6]), pyruvate then enters the mitochondria and undergoes oxidative decarboxylation by the tricarboxylic acid cycle enzymes to carbon dioxide (CO_2) and water. Hence aerobic exercise is limited by the availability of muscle glycogen (Costill [7]). Under anaerobic conditions pyruvate is reduced to lactate. During anaerobic exercise, exhaustion can occur when lactic acid accumulation interferes with muscle contractile function (Sahlin et al. [8, 9]; Hogan and Welch [10]; Mainwood and Renaud [11]; Idstrom et al. [6]). Fat is supplied to the muscle as blood-borne free fatty acids. These fatty acids are converted to acetyl coenzyme A, two carbon units, which are metabolized by the tricarboxylic acid cycle (Felig and Wahren [5]); this pathway serves as a glycogen-sparing mechanism and prolongs endurance time (Hickson et al. [12]; Hargreaves et al. [13]).

The ATP yield of aerobic metabolism markedly exceeds that of anaerobic metabolism. Aerobic metabolism yields 37 molecules of ATP for each molecule of glucose, whereas anaerobic metabolism yields 2 ATP molecules for each glucose molecule. Although the energy yield of aerobic metabolism is clearly greater than that of anaerobic metabolism, the external work efficiency of the two processes is remarkably similar, approximately 18% (Gladden and Welch [14]). Fatty acids of composition similar to human adipose tissue are estimated to supply 138 molecules of ATP per molecule of fatty acid; however, the O_2 utilization per molecule of ATP generated from fat metabolism is 12% greater than for carbohydrate metabolism. Therefore, in order to maintain constant power output when fat metabolism predominates, O_2 consumption must increase 12% (Heigenhauser et al. [15]). Aerobic metabolism during prolonged events (such as the marathon) will be sustained after glycogen depletion by fatty acid metabolism, which will require greater O_2 uptake in order to maintain pace. The result is usually a slowing of running pace.

Skeletal muscles are mixtures of two fiber types, which vary in their capacity to sustain aerobic metabolism (Holloszy [16]). Type 1, or slow-twitch fibers, have low myosin ATPase activity, high mitochrondial enzyme activity, and high myoglobin concentration. Type 2, or fast-twitch fibers, have high myosin ATPase activity, low mitochondrial enzyme activity, and low myoglobin content. These contrasting metabolic capacities imply different roles for the two fiber types. The higher aerobic capacity of the Type 1 fibers suggests their suitability for endurance activities. Type 2 fibers, with high ATPase activities, are appropriate for the brief, high-power demands of isometric exercise.

The fuels expended during exercise vary with the intensity and duration of the activity.

Initially, before circulatory compensation occurs, stored ATP and ATP derived from creatine phosphate drive muscle contraction. The contribution of anaerobic glycolysis, also important initially, declines unless the work load is high. In the early phase of sustained exercise, muscle glycogen is the principal energy source. Subsequently, uptake of blood-borne glucose and free fatty acids increases. As muscle glycogen supplies are depleted during the first hour of aerobic exercise, blood-borne glucose becomes the major source of carbohydrate. With continued exercise, glucose utilization may decline while free fatty acid utilization increases and becomes the predominant energy source. Heavy exercise increases the demand for muscle glycogen (Wasserman and Whipp [2]; Felig and Wahren [5]). In fact, heavy and sustained exercise may result in hypoglycemia in some persons (Felig et al. [17]).

The performance of work requires a continuous supply of ATP to sustain muscle contraction. The ATP can be derived from either aerobic or anaerobic metabolism, but the latter yields less energy, more quickly depletes glycogen, and results in lactic acid accumulation. Endurance exercise requires prolonged muscle use and must be accomplished primarily with aerobic metabolism.

MAXIMAL OXYGEN UPTAKE

The maintenance of aerobic metabolism during exercise is critically dependent on a continued availability of oxygen at the mitochondria. The respiratory and circulatory systems operate in series to deliver oxygen to the muscles and to remove the CO_2 generated by oxidative decarboxylation (Fig. 15-2). As work load increases, oxygen uptake ($\dot{V}O_2$) must rise in compensation, or the proportion of ATP derived from anaerobic metabolism will increase. Because of the close correlation between work load and $\dot{V}O_2$, the energy requirements of specific activities can be expressed in terms of $\dot{V}O_2$ (Fig. 15-1). As work load increases, however, $\dot{V}O_2$ will eventually attain a plateau and fail to increase further (Fig. 15-3). This level of oxygen utilization is termed the maximal oxygen uptake ($\dot{V}O_{2\ max}$), and this level of work is termed the maximal aerobic power. Further increases in work load may be achieved, but only with reliance on anaerobic processes.

PULMONARY RESPONSE TO EXERCISE

Gas Exchange at Rest

The transport of O_2 from atmospheric air to exercising muscle is performed by four distinct systems in series: pulmonary ventilation, diffusion, circulation, and tissue extraction (Fig. 15-2). Pulmonary gas exchange is the transfer of O_2 from alveolar air to pulmonary capillary blood and of CO_2 from blood to alveolar air. In a steady state, the quantity of CO_2 produced by tissue metabolism equals the quantity exhaled ($\dot{V}CO_2$, ml/min, with the gas volume at standard conditions STPD). Similarly, oxygen uptake by the lungs matches oxygen utilization by tissues. The ratio of $\dot{V}CO_2$ to $\dot{V}O_2$ is the respiratory exchange ratio (R), which equals the tissue R in a steady state. The R is determined by the type of substrate utilized by the tissues. The R for pure carbohydrate metabolism is 1; for fat, 0.7; and for protein, 0.9. The R for a normal individual at rest is 0.85 (Wasserman and Whipp [2]).

The components of gas exchange are ventilation, diffusion of gas across the alveolar–capillary membrane, and chemical reactions of CO_2 and O_2 in blood. Ventilation is accomplished by the respiratory muscles, primarily the diaphragm and the intercostal muscles.

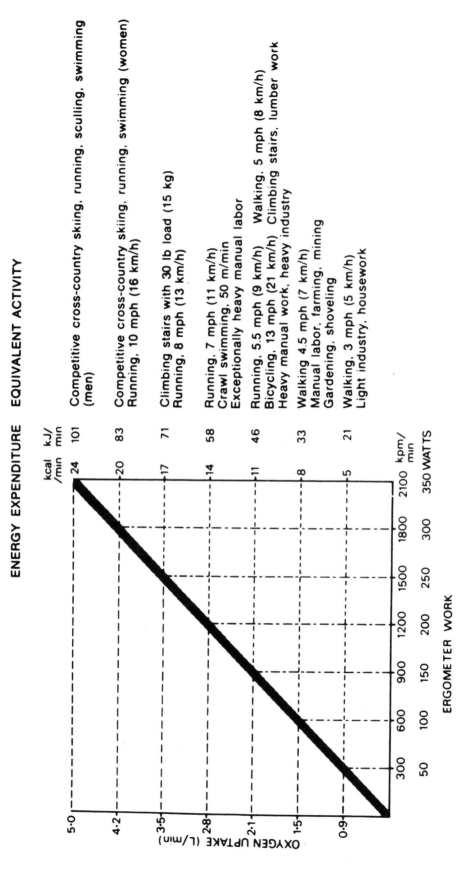

15-1 Changes in ventilation ($\dot{V}_E$), ventilatory equivalents for oxygen and carbon dioxide ($\dot{V}_E/\dot{V}O_2$ and $\dot{V}_E/\dot{V}CO_2$, respectively), and blood lactic acid concentration during progressive incremental exercise.

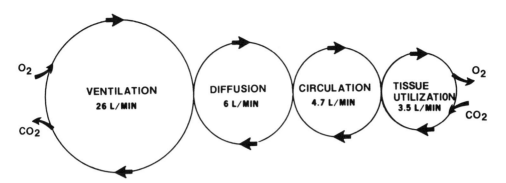

15-2   Schematic representation of O_2 and CO_2 transport. *Circles*, transport capacity of each step for O_2.

The exhaled minute ventilation ($\dot{V}_E$) is the product of tidal volume ($\dot{V}_T$) and respiratory frequency (f). The $\dot{V}_E$ is also the sum of alveolar ventilation ($\dot{V}_A$) and dead space ventilation ($\dot{V}_D$). Alveolar ventilation is the ventilation that reaches the alveolar surface and functions in gas exchange. Dead space ventilation is the ventilation distributed to the conducting airways and unperfused alveoli and is ineffective in gas exchange. The ratio of wasted, or dead space, ventilation to tidal ventilation is normally about 0.3.

Gas diffusion across the alveolar–capillary membrane occurs along partial pressure gradients. The diffusing capacity of the lung is determined in part by the thickness and the surface area of the alveolar–capillary membrane. Blood within the pulmonary capillaries functions as a sink for oxygen, and thus pulmonary blood flow is the other principal determinant of diffusing capacity. The extent to which ventilation and perfusion match across the lung also influences the efficacy of gas exchange. Thus, arterial O_2 and CO_2 tensions reflect the matching of ventilation and perfusion, as well as the diffusion of gases across the alveolar–capillary membrane.

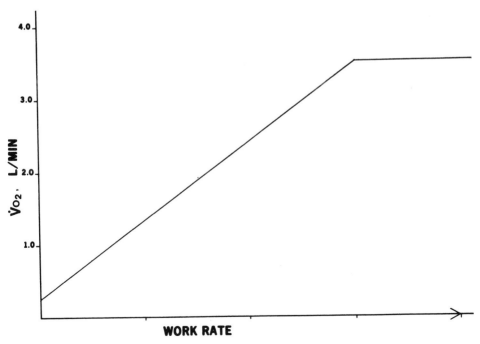

15-3   Relationship between work rate and oxygen uptake $\dot{V}_{O_2}$.

Gas Exchange During Exercise

Gas exchange varies during progressive incremental exercise in a consistent pattern (Skinner and McClellan [18]) (Fig. 15-4). At low to moderate exercise intensity (less than 50% $\dot{V}O_{2\ max}$), $\dot{V}_E$ increases linearly with $\dot{V}O_2$ and the ventilatory equivalents for O_2 and CO_2 ($\dot{V}_E/\dot{V}O_2$ and $\dot{V}_E/\dot{V}CO_2$, respectively) remain constant. Ventilation increases primarily by increasing tidal volume until 50–60% of vital capacity is reached; subsequent increases in ventilation are achieved by higher respiratory frequency. The close linkage of ventilation to exercise intensity has been attributed to the bulk flow of CO_2 from exercising muscle with resultant stimulation of either the peripheral chemoreceptors or receptors in the lung. Other factors such as stimulation of muscle mechanoreceptors and psychogenic stimuli may also have a role (Dempsey et al. [19]).

Lactic acid concentration in arterial blood remains unchanged at low to moderate work loads. Alterations in gas exchange with exercise include increased inhomogeneity of ventilation/perfusion ratios and increased alveolar–arterial oxygen tension gradients (AaDO$_2$) (Gledhill et al. [20]). However, arterial oxygen tension (P_aO_2) does not change because the median ventilation/perfusion ratio rises and alveolar oxygen tension (P_AO_2) rises secondary to increased R (Dempsey et al. [19]). Arterial CO_2 tension (P_aCO_2) also remains in the normal range.

As the exercise intensity increases to moderate levels (50–75% $\dot{V}O_{2\ max}$), $\dot{V}_E$ increases exponentially with workload, $\dot{V}_E/\dot{V}O_2$ begins a sustained increase, arterial lactate concentration rises, and P_aCO_2 and $\dot{V}_E/\dot{V}CO_2$ are unchanged. This combination of responses is designated inflection I in Fig. 15-4. When high-intensity work (greater than 75% $\dot{V}O_{2\ max}$) is achieved, $\dot{V}_E/\dot{V}CO_2$ increases, P_aCO_2 decreases, and arterial blood pH decreases (inflection II). The terminology of these changes in gas exchange with exercise has not been standardized. Most authors refer to inflection I as the anaerobic threshold (AT) when gas exchange

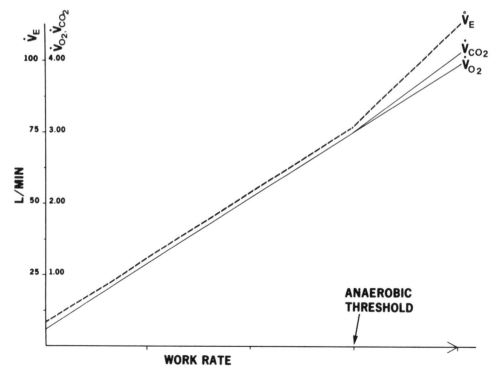

15-4 Relationship between work and rate and $\dot{V}O_2$, $\dot{V}CO_2$, and $\dot{V}_E$.

variables are considered and as the lactate threshold (LT) when arterial lactate concentrations are used to detect the inflection. The criteria for detection of AT are the inflection of ventilation and the onset of a progressive increase in $\dot{V}_E/\dot{V}_{O_2}$ without a change in $\dot{V}_E/\dot{V}_{CO_2}$; LT is the workload at which arterial lactate concentration begins to increase progressively (Brooks [21]). Inflection II is usually referred to as the threshold of decompensated metabolic acidosis (TDMA).

There is controversy about the mechanisms underlying AT and LT (Brooks [21]). Generally, AT has been attributed to the appearance of excess lactate in blood as a consequence of overproduction by exercising muscle. The inflection of ventilation and the increase in $\dot{V}_E/\dot{V}_{O_2}$ are thought to result from "nonmetabolic" CO_2 generated by buffering of the lactate by the blood bicarbonate system. This "nonmetabolic" CO_2 drives ventilation beyond the demands of the work load. Initially, the excess CO_2 is completely buffered and P_aCO_2, pH_a and $\dot{V}_E/\dot{V}_{CO_2}$ are unchanged. The TDMA is reached when the buffering capacity of the bicarbonate system is exceeded and metabolic acidosis with compensatory hypocapnia follows.

The generation of lactate from muscle was originally attributed to anaerobic metabolism in exercising muscle. However, LT may occur as a consequence of the sequential recruitment of Type 2 skeletal muscle fibers, which are richer than Type 1 fibers in the enzymes of the Embden-Meyerhoff pathway of glucose metabolism and have fewer mitochondria available for aerobic metabolism. This pattern of fiber activation results in preferential production of lactate at higher exercise intensities (Essen [22]; Vollestad et al. [23]). In addition, the correlation of AT and LT reported in several investigations may be fortuitous (Yeh et al. [24]; Gladden et al. [25]). Moreover, alterations in substrate availability have been shown to have opposite effects on AT and LT (Hughes et al. [26]). Although these issues remain unresolved, AT has been shown to be useful in determining fitness, training effect, and endurance performance (Conconi et al. [27]; Reybrouck et al. [28]; Tanaka and Matsuura [29]).

Oxygen Transport Capacity During Exercise

The respiratory and circulatory systems operate in series to deliver O_2 to exercising muscle. As described by the Fick equation, $\dot{V}_{O_2}$ is the product of cardiac output ($\dot{Q}$) and the arteriovenous oxygen content difference ($C_aO_2 - C_vO_2$):

$$\dot{V}_{O_2} = \dot{Q}(C_aO_2 - C_vO_2).$$

The respiratory system serves to maintain C_aO_2. The following analysis of oxygen transport shows that $\dot{V}_{O_2\,max}$ is not limited by the respiratory system in normal individuals.

An average-size adult male can achieve a maximum $\dot{V}_A$ of 150 L/min, which delivers 26 L of oxygen. The oxygen transport capacity of the diffusion and chemical reaction steps of gas exchange are estimated to be 6 L O_2 per minute (Johnson [30]). Circulation is the next step; maximum cardiac output is approximately 23 L/min, which delivers oxygen at a rate of 4.7 L/min. At most, 75% of this oxygen can be utilized during heavy exercise. Thus, as suggested by the Fick equation, cardiac output and muscle capacity to extract oxygen are the principal determinants of $\dot{V}_{O_2\,max}$ (Snell et al. [31]).

FACTORS INFLUENCING EXERCISE PERFORMANCE

Aging

Cross-sectional and longitudinal studies demonstrate that $\dot{V}_{O_2\,max}$ declines progressively from the maximum value attained in the late teens to early 20s at an annual rate of loss of approximately 0.4 ml/kg/min (Jones et al. [32]); this rate of loss is less for persons who remain physically active (Dehn and Bruce [33]). Performance in athletic events declines in parallel with the decrease in $\dot{V}O_{2\ max}$ (Shephard [34]).

Effects of aging on several components of the oxygen transport system contribute to the decline in aerobic power (Table 15-2) (Fitzgerald [35]). The forced expiratory volume in 1 sec (FEV$_1$), forced vital capacity (FVC), and maximum voluntary ventilation (MVV) decline progressively from peak values attained in the 20s. In many cigarette smokers, the rates of decline of these spirometric variables are increased. Increased inhomogeneity of ventilation–perfusion matching reduces the ability of the aging lung to oxygenate the blood. Ventilatory responsiveness to hypoxia and to hypercapnia also declines with aging. However, exercise ventilation is greater in elderly subjects compared to young subjects; this is most likely due to the greater inefficiency of gas exchange in the elderly (Brischetto et al. [36]). Age-related decreases in maximal heart rate and left ventricular ejection fraction reduce the maximum cardiac output that can be achieved during exercise (Port et al. [37]; Rodeheffer et al. [38]). Changes in the peripheral circulation and in skeletal muscle metabolism may contribute to the reduction in $\dot{V}O_{2\ max}$ related to aging, but their importance has not been determined. The observed decline in maximum arteriovenous oxygen difference may reflect changes in these two peripheral factors. The specific contributions of changes in each component of the oxygen transport system have not been experimentally assessed.

The decrease in maximum cardiac output with aging may also reflect diminished responsiveness to sympathetic stimulation (Rodeheffer et al. [38]). Middle-aged and elderly people respond to endurance training with increased $\dot{V}O_{2\ max}$ and anaerobic threshold (Davis et al. [39]; Yerg et al. [40]). Unlike the response in younger people, this increase results from increased cardiac output only rather than from both increased cardiac output and increased arteriovenous oxygen difference. Nevertheless, elderly subjects can safely participate in endurance training (Shephard [41]; Badenhop et al. [42]).

Training

Training is the regular performance of a work load that stresses the athlete and results in physiologic adaptation. Training activities may be loosely categorized as directed either at increasing muscle strength and anaerobic processes or at increasing endurance and aerobic processes. The former type requires brief bursts of intense muscle activity, whereas the

Table 15-2 Effects of Aging on the Components of the Oxygen Transport System

Component	Effect
Ventilation	↓ FEV$_1$*
	↓ FVC†
	↓ MVV‡
	↑ Closing Volume
Gas Exchange	↑ Ventilation-perfusion imbalance
	↓ Diffusing capacity
Control of Respiration	↓ Response to hypercapnia and to hypoxia
Cardiac Function	↓ Maximal heart rate
	↓ Stroke volume
	↓ Maximal cardiac output
Peripheral Circulation	Importance not determined
Skeletal Muscle	Importance not determined

*Force expiratory volume in 1 sec.
†Forced vital capacity.
‡Maximum voluntary ventilation.

latter type requires more prolonged submaximal activity. Because the respiratory system has a limited role in adaptation to isometric exercise, the following discussion focuses on endurance training. Both human and animal data concerning the effects of training are available. The human investigations, however, are frequently flawed by inability to separate training effects from inherent constitutional capabilities.

Performance is determined by a complex interaction between psychologic and physiologic factors. Fatigue is hypothesized to arise from lactic acid accumulation in muscle cells if the intensity of the exercise exceeds the anaerobic threshold (Hogan and Welch [10]; Mainwood and Renaud [11]); fatigue in aerobic exercise is thought to result from glycogen depletion in the working muscles (Costill et al. [7]). Endurance training postpones the development of fatigue; this effect appears to be a result of delayed onset of lactic acid accumulation (increased anaerobic thesbold) and increased $\dot{V}O_{2\ max}$ (Davis et al. [39]; Poole and Gaesser [43]). During endurance training the $\dot{V}O_{2\ max}$ increases at a weekly rate of 0.11 L/min (Hickson et al. [44]; Mikesell and Dudley [45]) until a plateau is reached. The respiratory muscles also adapt to training (Lieberman et al. [46]; Moore and Gollnick [47]; Bender and Martin [48]). However, it is unlikely that respiratory muscle fatigue is a major contributor to limitation of exercise in normal individuals. Younes and Kivinen [49] have shown that the transdiaphragmatic pressures generated during performance of $\dot{V}O_{2\ max}$ are well below the critical values associated with the development of fatigue during inspiratory muscle loading (Bellamere and Grassino [50]).

The correlation between performance and $\dot{V}O_{2\ max}$ has been established by cross-sectional studies of athletes and by longitudinal studies of untrained subjects (Conconi et al. [27]; Maughan and Leiper [1]; Reybrouck et al. [28]; Tanaka and Matsuura [29]). The $\dot{V}O_{2\ max}$ of champion endurance athletes may exceed that of untrained persons by as much as 40 ml/kg/min. Similarly, the mean $\dot{V}O_{2\ max}$ for 8 elite marathon runners was 74.1 ml/kg/min, approximately 50% greater than predicted (Pollock [51]). Although a high $\dot{V}O_{2\ max}$ is prerequisite for champion endurance athletes, the level of $\dot{V}O_{2\ max}$ is a poor predictor of performance among elite athletes. These cross-sectional investigations of $\dot{V}O_{2\ max}$ also cannot determine the relative contributions of training and of genetic endowment to the increased aerobic power of elite athletes.

Longitudinal studies of both males and females have consistently shown that $\dot{V}O_{2\ max}$ increases in untrained persons in response to a training program (Kearney et al. [52]; Hickson et al. [44]). In fact, previously fit subjects will also show improved $\dot{V}O_{2\ max}$ and endurance performance when the intensity of the training stimulus is increased (Mikesell and Dudley [45]). Those subjects with the lowest initial $\dot{V}O_{2\ max}$ sustain the greatest increments (Saltin et al. [53]).

Performance generally improves in parallel with the increase in $\dot{V}O_{2\ max}$. Although the increase in $\dot{V}O_{2\ max}$ appears to be the principal determinant of improved performance, other factors, such as improved technique and psychologic adaptation, are probably also important. The magnitude of the increase in $\dot{V}O_{2\ max}$ is determined by the intensity, duration, and frequency of the training stimulus. The minimum training regimen for achieving cardiopulmonary fitness consists of a frequency of 3 times per week, a duration of at least 20 min, and an intensity sufficient to achieve a heart rate of at least 70% predicted maximum (Sharkey [54]).

As anticipated from the Fick equation, training increases $\dot{V}O_{2\ max}$ by increasing maximum cardiac output and by increasing oxygen extraction by the muscles (Hammond and Froelicher [55]). Although training may affect some pulmonary function parameters and the pulmonary physiology of elite athletes may differ from that of normal individuals, alterations in the respiratory system do not contribute to the increasing $\dot{V}O_{2\ max}$ with training.

Increased cardiac output and increased tissue oxygen extraction contribute equally to the increase of $\dot{V}O_{2\ max}$ as follows (Rowell [56]):

Heart

1. Increased stroke volume, decreased heart rate at submaximal loads
2. Increased maximal cardiac output
3. Increased left ventricular volume and mass (Graettinger [57])
4. Increased myocardial vascularity (Thomas [58])

Skeletal Muscle (Holloszy [59])

1. Increased myoglobin content
2. Increased size and number of mitochondria
3. Increased enzymes involved in fatty acid metabolism
4. Increased glycogen synthetase activity and elevated glycogen stores
5. Increased muscle capillary density (Anderson and Henriksson [60])

Although specific relationships between skeletal muscle adaptations and increased $\dot{V}O_{2\,max}$ are not well defined, each appears to increase the capacity for aerobic metabolism (Gollnick and Matoba [61]). In fact, the enzyme adaptations are remarkably specific. For example, mitochondrial enzymes that are not involved in aerobic pathways do not increase, nor do glycolytic enzymes. Whether these adaptations occur differentially in the two human muscle fiber types is uncertain (Holloszy [59]; Gollnick [61]). Similarly, we do not know the relative importance of training and of genetic endowment in producing the increased percentage of Type 1 fibers found in endurance athletes. Short-term studies suggest that the usual training does not convert a fiber of one type to the other (Gollnick [61]). However, Type 2A fibers, a subclass of Type 2 fibers, respond to training by developing a metabolic profile that resembles that of the Type 1 fibers (Gollnick [61]).

These adaptations are linked to performance primarily through increased aerobic power and anaerobic threshold (Ivy et al. [62]). The increased cardiac reserve, increased skeletal muscle capillary density (Anderson and Henriksson [60]; Gollnick [61]), and increased myoglobin concentration facilitate oxygen delivery to exercising muscles. The trained muscle appears adapted for aerobic metabolism (Ivy et al. [62]). The increases in oxidative enzymes may allow the muscle to function more effectively at a lower tissue P_{O_2}, which would be anticipated as oxygen extraction rises. Known consequences of the muscle enzyme changes include increased glycogen stores, increased reliance on fat metabolism during exercise, and increased capacity to oxidize carbohydrates (Holloszy [59]; Gollnick [61]). Thus, for the trained athlete, submaximal exercise results in lower lactate levels and slower glycogen depletion; fatigue is delayed and endurance performance improves.

Current knowledge of training effects on the respiratory system is limited and derived largely from cross-sectional studies of athletes. The data have not conclusively established that pulmonary function of endurance-trained athletes is superior to that of untrained normal persons; published reports provide conflicting observations concerning the lung volumes and spirometric indices (Astrand and Rodahl [63]; Biersteker and Biersteker [64]). Interesting recent cross-sectional studies of endurance athletes have demonstrated decreased ventilatory responsiveness to hypoxia and hypercapnia (Bryne-Quinn et al. [65]; Scoggins et al. [66]). Relatives of these athletes displayed similar reduction of chemosensitivity (Scoggins et al. [66]). This implies that ventilatory response patterns of endurance athletes may be the consequence of familial factors rather than of training. In contrast, a study of marathoners (Mahler et al. [67]) failed to show a difference in hypoxic or hypercapnic response in the athletes in comparison with nonexercising controls. Chemosensitivity in the marathoners did not correlate with marathon performance. Respiratory drive was not changed by training previously sedentary men (Bradley et al. [68]).

The respiratory muscles, including the diaphragm, are skeletal muscles; thus, training increases their aerobic power as well as that of the limb muscles (Lieberman et al. [46]; Moore and Gollnick [47]; Bender and Martin [48]). Although maximal voluntary ventilation (MVV) has not been consistently shown to increase with training, the fraction of the MVV that can be sustained for prolonged periods does increase (Leith and Bradley [69]). In addition, the respiratory muscles can be specifically trained; one study showed that endurance training of the respiratory muscles (isocapnic hyperpnea) resulted in a 14% increase in MVV, and the proportion of the MVV that was sustainable increased from 81% to 96% (Leith and Bradley [69]). These training-related changes in the respiratory muscles may contribute to improved performance by reducing the sensation of dyspnea.

Hypertransfusion

Exercise performance may also be enhanced by hypertransfusion, or "blood doping." This technique consists of phlebotomy and storage of the blood until the hematocrit has returned to normal. Reinfusion of the whole blood or packed erythrocytes increases the hematocrit and hence the oxygen-carrying capacity. Hypertransfusion of competitive women runners was shown to increase anaerobic threshold and $\dot{V}O_{2\,max}$, although the relative anaerobic threshold was not changed (Pierucki et al. [70]). Maximal oxygen uptake and endurance time were also shown to increase after blood doping (Buick et al. [71]). The enhancement of performance lasted 16 weeks even though the hematocrit returned to normal (Buick et al. [71]). The authors speculate that the ability to train at higher intensity may explain the persistence of the effect. Buick's and other studies of hypertransfusion confirm the relationship between oxygen-carrying capacity and performance (Buick et al. [71]; Eckblom et al. [72]; Pierucki et al. [70]).

PULMONARY RESPONSE TO EXERCISE IN LUNG DISEASE

Clinical Exercise Testing

Exercise testing is usually performed by the application of either a progressively increasing work load or a constant work load. The load can be applied by a cycle ergometer or treadmill. During an exercise test, collection, measurement, and analysis of exhaled air allow the determination of tidal volume ($\dot{V}_T$), minute ventilation ($\dot{V}_E$), oxygen consumption ($\dot{V}O_2$), carbon dioxide production ($\dot{V}CO_2$), anaerobic threshold (AT), and respiratory exchange ratio (R). If arterial blood gases are measured, alveolar ventilation ($\dot{V}_A$), dead space ventilation ($\dot{V}_D$) and the alveolar arterial oxygen tension gradient ($AaDO_2$) can also be determined. Heart rate and blood pressure should also be monitored (Jones [73]).

Chronic Airflow Obstruction

Dyspnea on exertion is the most common symptom in patients with chronic airflow obstruction (CAO). Reduced expiratory flow rates in this syndrome are caused by loss of elastic recoil in pulmonary tissue as a result of emphysema and increased airway resistance because of airway narrowing and obliteration (Thurlbeck [74]). Exercise limitation in CAO correlates with the severity of the airflow obstruction (Spiro et al. [75]; Nery et al. [76]; Dillard et al. [77]). However, other factors are also important in the impairment of exercise in these patients. For example, some patients, particularly those with decreased diffusing capacity, develop worsened hypoxemia with exercise (Owens et al. [78]). Right ventricular dysfunction has also been demonstrated during exercise (Mahler et al. [79]; Light et al.

[80]). In addition, diaphragmatic fatigue, occurring early in exercise, limited performance in one study (Bye et al. [81]). Dyspnea usually occurs when the FEV_1 is less than 2 L, or approximately 50% of predicted. Exercise limitation is proportional to the severity of the airflow obstruction. Ventilation in CAO approaches the maximum level (MVV) and heart rate does not reach the maximum predicted value at maximum exercise (Nery et al. [76]).

Although the exercise performance of patients with CAO is limited, they may exercise and participate in physical training programs. A properly designed exercise program should result in improved exercise tolerance (Chester et al. [82]; Belman and Kendregan [83]). However, the mechanisms underlying the improved performance are uncertain and may differ from those in normal persons (Degre et al. [84]; Chester [82]; Belman and Kendregan [83]). Because patients with CAO are unable to achieve adequate training intensities to improve cardiovascular fitness, improvements of performance are probably attributable to enhanced exercise efficiency. Specific training of the respiratory muscles may be accomplished by repetitive breathing against a resistance device (Belman and Mittman [85]; Hsiun-Ing et al. [86]). Health professionals should use routine pulmonary function testing and measurement of exercise capacity in designing realistic programs for such patients.

Asthma

The exercise performance of patients with asthma is limited by reduced expiratory flow rates when the disease is active. Moreover, exercise-induced asthma (EIA), an increase in airway resistance that usually occurs 5–10 min after cessation of exercise, is common in asthmatics (Kawabori et al. [87]). Exercise-induced asthma has been postulated to result from increased respiratory heat exchange (McFadden and Ingram [88]) or water loss from airway epithelium (Anderson [89]). The exact mechanism by which heat flux or water loss triggers release of mediators of bronchospasm is unclear. The types of exercise most strongly associated with EIA have high aerobic demands, e.g., cycling and running. However, EIA is uncommon with swimming. The severity of EIA is directly proportional to the intensity of the exercise (McFadden and Ingram [88]).

The airway response to short-term exercise in asthma is bronchodilation during the exercise bout, with the bronchospasm occurring after cessation of exercise. Fit asthmatics have greater bronchodilation during exercise (when standardized for heart rate) than unfit asthmatics (Haas et al. [90]). This response may be due to adaptation of the fit asthmatic's airways to the effects of cooling or water loss.

Clinically, EIA may be manifest as wheezing, dyspnea, or cough during or after physical activity (Shephard [91]). The physician should consider EIA in patients whose wheezing, cough, or dyspnea is primarily associated with exercise, for example, the runner who complains of cough after a morning workout. The diagnosis should be confirmed with exercise testing. Characteristically, ventilatory measurements, such as FEV_1 and airway resistance, begin to show impairment within 5–10 min after cessation of exercise. Inhalation of sympathomimetic aerosols before exercise is the treatment of choice for EIA. These agents may improve basal pulmonary function, and in most patients they abolish EIA (Anderson et al. [92]; Eggleston et al. [93]; Sly [94]). Oral sympathomimetics and theophylline compounds are less effective (Anderson et al. [92]; Eggleston et al. [93]; Sly [94]). Cromolyn sodium may also be used, but it does not improve basal pulmonary function (Horn et al. [95]).

Interstitial Lung Disease

Interstitial lung disease limits exercise by increasing the elastic work of breathing. The lung mechanics are characterized by reduced compliance and reduced lung volumes. The degree of dyspnea correlates with the reduction in vital capacity (Burdon et al. [96]; Kelley and Daniele [97]). These patients increase ventilation during exercise testing primarily through increasing respiratory frequency, because vital capacity is reduced by the abnormal compliance (Burdon et al. [96]). The limitation of exercise performance is due to both the ventilatory impairment and to exercise-induced hypoxemia. The magnitude of the reduction of oxygen tension during maximum exercise testing correlates with the severity of the interstitial process and is a useful clinical evaluation (Kelley and Daniele [97]).

EXERCISE UNDER SPECIAL CONDITIONS

Cigarette Smoking

Tobacco smoke is a complex mixture of several thousand distinct chemical compounds. The physiological consequences are myriad, and only those relevant to the endurance athlete are mentioned here. Acute inhalation of cigarette smoke may increase airway resistance and elevate blood carboxyhemoglobin because of the high concentration of carbon monoxide in cigarette smoke. Chronic cigarette smoking may result in permanent reduction of ventilatory and gas exchange capacity. The effects on the circulatory system range from acute elevation of blood pressure and pulse rate to promotion of degenerative cardiovascular disease. Thus, the empirical observation that cigarette smokers have reduced $\dot{V}O_{2\ max}$ is not surprising (Ingemann-Hansen and Halkajer-Kristensen [98]); nor are the investigators' personal observations that endurance athletes do not smoke.

Air Pollution

Both popular literature and scientific reports have hypothesized that ambient air pollution may limit exercise performance and that high minute ventilation of the endurance athlete may place him or her at high risk for pollution effects. Air pollution is a mixture of atmospheric contaminants that can be categorized into two major types. The sulfur oxide, a particulate complex produced by the combustion of fossil fuels, affects the industrialized urban areas of the eastern and central United States. Photochemical pollution, or smog, results principally from motor vehicle emissions and predominates in metropolitan areas of the western United States.

Few data are available to support the hypothesized effects of air pollution on the endurance athlete. In Los Angeles, performance of high school cross-country track teams was adversely affected by photochemical pollution (Wayne et al. [99]). Lebowitz et al. [100] demonstrated that exercise on high pollution days decreased lung function. Similar studies of populations exposed to sulfur oxide and particulate matter pollution have not been performed. Experimental chamber exposures of exercising human subjects generally support the cited studies. Effects of pollutants, however, are usually observed only at levels severalfold above those normally encountered in ambient air. Certain people, such as those suffering from asthma, may be more sensitive to pollution.

Carbon monoxide is of particular interest for the endurance athlete beause of its effects on oxygen transport and the exposure of urban athletes to motor exhaust. Carbon monoxide limits oxygen transport by combining with hemoglobin to form nonfunctional carboxyhemoglobin and by limiting tissue oxygen availability by increasing hemoglobin affinity for oxygen. Exercise increases the rate at which hemoglobin achieves equilibrium with inhaled carbon monoxide. In young healthy men, $\dot{V}O_{2\ max}$ declines linearly as carboxyhemoglobin increases from 5% to 35%. Effects on oxygen transport have not been demonstrated at levels below 4% in healthy subjects. Patients with coronary artery disease or peripheral vascular disease, however, appear to be affected by levels as low as 2.5–3% carboxyhemoglobin. Carbon monoxide pollution severe enough to limit the maximum performance of normal individuals rarely occurs. In certain western cities of the United States the combined effects of exercise, carbon monoxide, and altitude might limit oxygen transport under unusual circumstances (National Research Council [101]).

Altitude

The partial pressure of oxygen in ambient air declines linearly with increasing altitude (Frisancho [102]). As a result, the $P_{A}O_2$ is reduced at high altitude and the oxygen transport system delivers less oxygen to tissue than at sea level (Fig. 15-2). Each step in oxygen transport is affected by altitude (Frisancho [102]; Lenfant and Sullivan [103]). Consequently, above 1600 m, $\dot{V}O_{2\ max}$ declines by approximately 5.6% per 1000 m ascent (Faulkner et al. [104]; Escourrou et al. [105]; Tucker et al. [106]). A subnormal cardiac output with exercise causes the reduction of $\dot{V}O_{2\ max}$ in both sojourners and natives at high altitude (Lenfant and Sullivan [103]; Frisancho [102]).

Rapid ascent to high altitude results in increased ventilation with respiratory alkalosis and resting tachycardia with increased cardiac output (Frisancho [102]; Lenfant and Sullivan [103]). With acclimatization, hyperventilation persists, but at a lower level than initially; resting cardiac output declines, red cell mass increases, the oxyhemoglobin dissociation curve shifts to the right, and tissue capillarization and enzymes related to oxidative metabolism increase. These adaptations result in a partial reversal of the altitude-related reduction of $\dot{V}O_{2\ max}$. Reduced maximum cardiac output continues to limit $\dot{V}O_{2\ max}$, however.

Highland natives also have polycythemia and reduced maximum cardiac output (Frisancho [102]). Their level of ventilation at high altitude is less than that of sojourners primarily because of reduced ventilatory response to hypoxia. Compared to lowlanders, highland natives have increased lung volumes and pulmonary diffusing capacity (Frisancho [102]; Lenfant and Sullivan [103]). During exercise at high altitude, highland natives have smaller $AaDO_2$ than sea level controls; during exercise at sea level the opposite is true (Cruz et al. [107]). The $\dot{V}O_{2\ max}$ of the high altitude native exceeds that of the acclimatized lowlander, unless the latter moved to high altitude during childhood (presumably before the cessation of lung growth).

The physician may be asked to advise athletes about training at high altitude. Frequently asked questions relate to the potential advantages of training and exercise at high altitude and to the potential hazards of such training. It is unclear that training at high altitude confers any benefit for performance at sea level. Several studies have been conducted in which performance and $\dot{V}O_{2\ max}$ at sea level were measured after training at high altitude (Faulkner et al. [108]; Dill and Adams [109]). The conflicting results of these studies suggest that training at high altitude probably does not significantly improve sea level performance (Smith and Sharkey [110]).

Physicians should be aware of the syndrome of acute mountain sickness (Hecht [111]; Hackett et al. [112]; Hultgren [113]; Meehan and Zavala [114]). Both lowlanders rapidly ascending to high altitude and high-altitude natives returning to high altitude are at risk. Exercise, particularly by untrained individuals, increases the risk of acute mountain sickness. The incidence of this syndrome increases with altitude and is greatest at above 10,000 feet. Manifestations include headache, central nervous system effects, dyspnea, anorexia, nausea, and vomiting (Hackett et al. [112]; Meehan and Zavala [114]). Acute pulmonary edema due to increased permeability of the alveolar–capillary membrane is another hazard of altitude exposure. Normal individuals exhibit a wide range of susceptibility to acute mountain sickness. The pathophysiology of these syndromes is related to the development of widespread increased capillary permeability as well as an exaggerated hemodynamic response to hypoxia (Meehan and Zavala [114]).

REFERENCES

1. Maughan, R.J., Leiper, J.B. 1983. Aerobic capacity and fractional utilisation of aerobic capacity in elite and non-elite male and female marathon runners. Eur J Appl Physiol 52:80–87.
2. Wasserman, K., Whipp, B.J. 1975. Exercise physiology in health and disease. Am Rev Respir Dis 112:219–249.
3. Jones, N.L. 1980. Hydrogen ion balance during exercise. Clin Sci 59:85–91.
4. Astrand, P., Rodahl, K. 1977. Textbook of Work Physiology. McGraw-Hill, New York, pp 11–34.
5. Felig, P., Wahren, J. 1975. Fuel homeostasis in exercise. N Engl J Med 293:1078–1084.
6. Idstrom, J-P, Harihara, S., et al. 1985. Oxygen dependence of energy metabolism in contracting and recovering rat skeletal muscle. Am J Physiol 249:H40–H48.
7. Costill, D.L., Sparks, K., et al. 1971. Muscle glycogen utilization during exhaustive running. J Appl Physiol 31:353–356.
8. Sahlin, K., Edstrom, L., et al. 1981. Effects of lactic acid accumulation and ATP decrease on muscle tension and relaxation. Am J Physiol 240:C121–C126.
9. Sahlin, K., Edstrom, L., et al. 1983. Fatigue and phosphocreatine depletion during carbon dioxide-induced acidosis in rat muscle. Am J Physiol 245:C15–C20.
10. Hogan, M.C., Welch, H.G. 1984. Effect of varied lactate levels on bicycle performance. J Appl Physiol 57:507–513.
11. Mainwood, G.W., Renaud, J.M. 1985. The effect of acid-base on fatigue of skeletal muscle. Can J Physiol Pharmacol 63:403–416.
12. Hickson, R.C., Rennie, M.J., et al. 1977. Effects of increased plasma fatty acids on glycogen utilization and endurance. J Appl Physiol 43:829–833.
13. Hargreaves, M., Costill, D.L., et al. 1984. Effect of carbohydrate feedings on muscle glycogen utilization and exercise performance. Med Sci Sports Exerc 16:219–222.
14. Gladden, L.B., Welch, H.G. 1978. Efficiency of anaerobic work. J Appl Physiol 44:564–570.

15. Heigenhauser, G.J.F., Sutton, J.R., et al. 1983. Effect of glycogen depletion on the ventilatory response to exercise. J Appl Physiol 54:470–474.
16. Holloszy, J.O. 1982. Muscle metabolism during exercise. Arch Phys Med Rehab 63:231–234.
17. Felig, P., Cherif, A., et al. 1982. Hypoglycemia during prolonged exercise in normal man. N Engl J Med 306:895–900.
18. Skinner, J.S., McLellan, T.H. 1980. The transition from aerobic to anaerobic metabolism. Res Q Exerc Sport 51:234–248.
19. Dempsey, J.A., Vidruk, E.H., et al. 1985. Pulmonary control systems in exercise: update. Fed Proc 44:2260–2270.
20. Gledhill, N., Froese, A.B. et al. 1978. VA/QC inhomogeneity and AaDO2 in man during exercise: effect of SF6 breathing. J Appl Physiol 45:512–515.
21. Brooks, G.A. 1985. Anaerobic threshold: review of the concept and directions for future research. Med Sci Sports Exerc 17:22–31.
22. Essen, B. 1978. Glycogen depletion of different fibre types in human skeletal muscle during intermittent and continuous exercise. Acta Physiol Scand 103:446–455.
23. Vollestad, N.K., Blom, P.C.S. 1985. Effect of varying exercise intensity on glycogen depletion in human muscle fibers. Acta Physiol Scand 125:395–405.
24. Yeh, M.P., Gardner, R.M., et al. 1983. "Anaerobic threshold": problems of determination and validation. J Appl Physiol 55:1178–1186.
25. Gladden, L.B., Yates, J.W., et al. 1985. Gas exchange and lactate anaerobic thresholds: inter- and intraevaluator agreement. J Appl Physiol 58:2082–2089.
26. Hughes, E.F., Turner, S.C., et al. 1982. Effects of glycogen depletion and pedaling speed on "anaerobic threshold." J Appl Physiol 52:1598–1607.
27. Conconi, F., Ferrari, M., et al. 1982. Determination of the anaerobic threshold by a non-invasive field test in runners. J Appl Physiol 52:869–873.

28. Reybrouck, T., Chesquire, J., et al. 1983. Ventilatory thresholds during short- and long-term exercise. J Appl Physiol 55:1694–1700.

29. Tanaka, K., Matsuura, Y. 1984. Marathon performance, anaerobic threshold, and onset of blood lactate accumulation. J Appl Physiol 57:640–643.

30. Johnson, R.L., 1973. The lung as an organ of oxygen transport. Basics Resp Dis 2(1):1–6.

31. Snell, P.G., Mitchell, J.H. 1984. The role of maximal oxygen uptake in exercise performance. Clin Chest Med 5:51–62.

32. Jones, N.L., Makrides, L., et al. 1985. Normal standards for an incremental progressive cycle ergometer test. Am Rev Respir Dis 131:700–708.

33. Dehn, M.M., Bruce, R.A. 1972. Longitudinal variations in maximal oxygen intake with age and activity. J Appl Physiol 33:805–807.

34. Shephard, R.J. 1978. Physical Activity and Aging. Year Book Medical Publishers, Chicago, pp 204–224.

35. Fitzgerald, P.L. 1985. Exercise in the elderly. Med Clin North Am 69:189–196.

36. Brischetto, M.J., Millman, R.P., et al. 1984. Effect of aging on the ventilatory response to exercise and CO_2. J Appl Physiol 56:1143–1150.

37. Port, S., Cobb, F.R., et al. 1984. Effect of age on the response of the left ventricular ejection fraction to exercise. N Engl J Med 310:1133–1137.

38. Rodeheffer, R.J., Gerstenblith, G., et al. 1984. Exercise cardiac output is maintained with advancing age in healthy human subjects: cardiac dilatation and increased stroke volume compensate for a diminished heart rate. Circulation 69: 203–213.

39. Davis, J.A., Frank, M.H., et al. 1979. Anaerobic threshold alterations caused by endurance training in middle-aged men. J Appl Physiol 46:1039–1046.

40. Yerg, J.E., Seals, D.R., et al. 1985. Effect of endurance exercise training on ventilatory function in older individuals. J Appl Physiol 58:791–794.

41. Shephard, R.J., 1978. Physical Activity and Aging. Year Book Medical Publishers, Chicago, pp 176–203.

42. Badenhop, D.T., Cleary, P.A., et al. 1983. Physiological adjustments to higher- and lower-intensity exercise in elders. Med Sci Sports Exerc 15:496–502.

43. Poole, D.C., Gaesser, G.A. 1985. Response of ventilatory and lactate thresholds to continuous and interval training. J Appl Physiol 58:115–1121.

44. Hickson, R.C., Bomze, H.A., et al. 1977. Linear increase in aerobic power induced by a strenuous program of endurance exercise. J Appl Physiol 42:372–376.

45. Mikesell, K.A., Dudley, G.A., 1984. Influence of intense training on aerobic power of competitive distance runners. Med Sci Sports Exerc 16:371–375.

46. Lieberman, D.A., Maxwell, L.C., et al. 1972. Adaptation of guinea pig diaphragm muscle to aging and endurance training. Am J Physiol 222:556–560.

47. Moore, R.L., Gollnick, P.D. 1982. Response of ventilatory muscles of the rat to endurance training. Pflugers Arch 392:268–271.

48. Bender, P.R., Martin, B.J. 1985. Maximal ventilation after exhausting exercise. Med Sci Sports Exerc 17:164–167.

49. Younes, M., Kivinen, G. 1984. Respiratory mechanics and breathing pattern during and following maximal exercise. J Appl Physiol 57:1773–1782.

50. Bellamere, F., Grassino, A. 1982. Effect of pressure and timing on human diaphragm fatigue. J Appl Physiol 53:1190–1195.

51. Pollock, M.L. 1977. Submaximal and maximal working capacity of elite distance runners. I. Cardiorespiratory aspects. Ann NY Acad Sci 301:310–322.

52. Kearney, J.T., Stull, G.A., et al. 1976. Cardiorespiratory responses of sedentary college women as a function of training intensity. J Appl Physiol 41:822–825.

53. Saltin, B., Blomqvist, G., et al. 1968. Response to exercise after bed rest and training. Circulation 38(Suppl VII): 1–78.

54. Sharkey, B.J. 1970. Intensity and duration of training and the development of cardiorespiratory endurance. Med Sci Sports Exerc 2:187–201.

55. Hammond, H.K., Froelicher, V.F. 1985. The physiologic sequelae of chronic dynamic exercise. Med Clin North Am 69: 21–39.

56. Rowell, L.B. 1974. Human cardiovascular adjustments to exercise and thermal stress. Physiol Rev 54:75–179.

57. Graettinger, W.F. 1984. The cardiovascular response to chronic physical exertion and exercise training: an echocardiographic review. Am Heart J 108:1014–1018.

58. Thomas, D.P. 1985. Effects of acute and chronic exercise on myocardial ultrastructure. Med Sci Sports Exerc 17:546–553.

59. Holloszy, J.O. 1982. Adaptions of mus-

cular tissue to training. Prog Cardiovasc Dis 18:445–458.

60. Anderson, P., Henriksson, J. 1977. Capillary supply of the quadriceps femoris muscle of man: adaptive response to exercise. J Physiol 270:677–690.

61. Gollnick, P.D., Matoba, H. 1984. The muscle fiber composition of skeletal muscle as a predictor of athletic success. An overview. Am J Sports Med 12:212–217.

62. Ivy, J.L., Withers, R.T., et al. 1980. Muscle respiratory capacity and fiber type as determinants of the lactate threshold. J Appl Physiol 48:523–527.

63. Astrand, P., Rodahl, K. 1977. Textbook of Work Physiology. McGraw-Hill, New York, pp 291–329, 391–445, 449–480.

64. Biersteker, M.W.A., Biersteker, P.A. 1985. Vital capacity in trained and untrained healthy young adults in the Netherlands. Eur J Appl Physiol 54:46–53.

65. Bryne-Quinn, E., Weil, J.V., et al. 1971. Ventilatory control in the athlete. J Appl Physiol 30:91–98.

66. Scoggins, C.H., Doekel, R.D., et al. 1978. Familial aspects of decreased hypoxic drive in endurance athletes. J Appl Physiol 44:464–468.

67. Mahler, D.A., Moritz, E.D., et al. 1982. Ventilatory responses at rest and during exercise in marathon runners. J Appl Physiol 52:388–392.

68. Bradley, B.L., Mestas, J., et al. 1980. The effect on respiratory drive of a prolonged physical conditioning program. Am Rev Respir Dis 122:741–746.

69. Leith, D.E., Bradley, M. 1976. Ventilatory muscle strength and endurance training. J Appl Physiol 41:508–516.

70. Pierucki, C., Serniak, E., et al. 1985. Effects of blood loss and blood doping on maximum O_2 uptake and anaerobic threshold in female runners. Fed Proc 44:1370.

71. Buick, F.J., Gledhill, N., et al. 1980. Effect of induced erythrocythemia on aerobic work capacity. J Appl Physiol 48:636–642.

72. Ekblom, B., Goldbarg, A.N., et al. 1972. Response to exercise after blood loss and reinfusion. J Appl Physiol 33:175–180.

73. Jones, N.L. 1975. Exercise in pulmonary evaluation. Rationale, methods and the normal respiratory response to exercise. Clinical applications. N Engl J Med 293:541–544, 647–650.

74. Thurlbeck, W.M. 1977. Aspects of

chronic airflow obstruction. Chest 72:341–349.

75. Spiro, S.G., Hahn, H.L., et al. 1975. An analysis of the physiological strain of submaximal exercise in patients with chronic obstructive bronchitis. Thorax 30:415–425.

76. Nery, L.E., Wasserman, K., et al. 1983. Contrasting cardiovascular and respiratory responses to exercise in mitral valve and chronic obstructive pulmonary diseases. Chest 83:446–453.

77. Dillard, T.A., Piantadosi, S., et al. 1985. Prediction of ventilation at maximal exercise in chronic air-flow obstruction. Am Rev Respir Dis 132:230–235.

78. Owens, G.R., Rogers, R.M., et al. 1984. The diffusing capacity as a predictor of arterial oxygen desaturation during exercise in patients with chronic obstructive pulmonary disease. N Engl J Med 310:1218–1221.

79. Mahler, D.A., Brent, B.N., et al. 1984. Right ventricular performance and central circulatory hemodynamics during upright exercise in patients with chronic obstructive pulmonary disease. Am Rev Respir Dis 130:722–729.

80. Light, R.W., Mintz, H.M., et al. 1984. Hemodynamics of patients with severe chronic obstructive pulmonary disease during progressive upright exercise. Am Rev Respir Dis 130:391–395.

81. Bye, P.T., Esau, S.A., et al. 1985. Ventilatory muscle function during exercise in air and oxygen in patients with chronic air-flow limitation. Am Rev Respir Dis 132:236–240.

82. Chester, E.H., Belman, M.J., et al. 1977. Multidisciplinary treatment of chronic pulmonary insufficiency. 3. The effect of physical training on cardiopulmonary performance in patients with chronic obstructive pulmonary disease. Chest 72:695–702.

83. Belman, M.J., Kendregan, B.A. 1981. Exercise training fails to increase skeletal muscle enzymes in patients with chronic obstructive pulmonary disease. Am Rev Respir Dis 123:256–261.

84. Degre, S., Sergysels, R., et al. 1974. Hemodynamic responses to physical training in patients with chronic lung disease. Am Rev Respir Dis 110:395–402.

85. Belman, M.J., Mittman, C. 1980. Ventilatory muscle training improves exercise capacity in chronic obstructive pulmonary disease patients. Am Rev Respir Dis 121:273–280.

86. Hsiun-Ing, C., Dukes, R., et al. 1985.

Inspiratory muscle training in patients with chronic obstructive pulmonary disease. Am Rev Respir Dis 131:251–255.

87. Kawabori, I., Pierson, W.E., et al. 1976. Incidence of exercise-induced asthma in children. J Allergy Clin Immunol 58:447–455.

88. McFadden, E.R. Jr, Ingram, R.H. Jr. Exercise-induced asthma: observations on the initiating stimulus. N Engl J Med 301:763–769.

89. Anderson, S.D. 1984. Is there a unifying hypothesis for exercise-induced asthma? J Allergy Clin Immunol 73:660–665.

90. Haas, F., Pineda, H., et al. 1985. Effects of physical fitness on expiratory airflow in exercising asthmatic people. Med Sci Sports Exerc 17:585–592.

91. Shephard, R.J. 1977. Exercise-induced bronchospasm—a review. Med Sci Sports Exerc 9:1–10.

92. Anderson, S.D., Seale, J.P., et al. 1976. Inhaled and oral salbutamol in exercise-induced asthma. Am Rev Respir Dis 114:493–500.

93. Eggleston, P.A., Beasley, P.P., et al. 1981. The effects of oral doses of theophylline and fenoterol on exercise-induced asthma. Chest 79:399–405.

94. Sly, R.M. 1984. Beta-adrenergic drugs in the management of asthma in athletes. J Allergy Clin Immunol 73:680–685.

95. Horn, C.R., Jones, R.M., et al. 1984. Bronchodilator effect of disodium cromoglycate administered as a dry powder in exercise induced asthma. Br J Pharmacol 18:798–801.

96. Burdon, J.G.W., Killian, K.J., et al. 1983. Pattern of breathing in patients with interstitial lung disease. Thorax 38:778–784.

97. Kelley, M.A., Daniele, R.P. 1984. Exercise testing in interstitial lung disease. Clin Chest Med 5:145–156.

98. Ingemann-Hansen, T., Halkajer-Kristensen, J. 1977. Cigarette smoking and maximal oxygen consumption in humans. Scand J Clin Lab Invest 37:143–148.

99. Wayne, W.S., Wehrle, P.F., et al. 1967. Oxidant air pollution and athletic performance. JAMA 199:901–904.

100. Lebowitz, M.D., Bendheim, P., et al. 1974. The effect of air pollution and weather on the lung function in exercising children and adolescents. Am Rev Respir Dis 109:262–273.

101. National Research Council, Committee on Medical and Biological Effects of Environmental Pollutants. 1977. Carbon Monoxide. National Academy of Sciences, Washington DC.

102. Frisancho, A.R. 1975. Functional adaptation to high altitude hypoxia. Science 187:313–319.

103. Lenfant, C., Sullivan, K. 1971. Adaptation to high altitude. N Engl J Med 284:1298—1309.

104. Faulkner, J.A., Kollias, J., et al. 1968. Maximum aerobic capacity and running performance at altitude. J Appl Physiol 24:685–691.

105. Escourrou, P., Johnson, D.G., et al. 1984. Hypoxemia increases plasma catecholamine concentration in exercising humans. J Appl Physiol 57:1507–1511.

106. Tucker, A., Stager, J.M., et al. 1984. Arterial O_2 saturation and maximum oxygen consumption in moderate-altitude runners exposed to sea level and 3,050 meters. JAMA 252:2876–2871.

107. Cruz, J.C., Hartley, L.H., et al. 1975. Effect of altitude relocations upon AaDO2 at rest and during exercise. J Appl Physiol 39:469–474, 1975.

108. Faulkner, J.A., Daniels, J.T., et al. 1967. Effects of training at moderate altitude on physical performance capacity. J Appl Physiol 23:85–89.

109. Dill, D.B., Adams, W.C., 1971. Maximal oxygen uptake at sea level and at 3,090-m altitude in high school champion runners. J Appl Physiol 30:854–859.

110. Smith, M.H., Sharkey, B.J. 1984. Altitude training: who benefits? Phys Sports Med 12(4):48–62.

111. Hecht, H.H. 1971. A sea level view of altitude problems. Am J Med 50:703–708.

112. Hackett, P.H., Dennie, D., et al. 1976. The incidence, importance, and prophylaxis of acute mountain sickness. Lancet 2:1149–1155.

113. Hultgren, H.N. 1979. High altitude medical problems. West J Med 131:8–23.

114. Meehan, R.T., Zavala, D.C. 1982. The pathophysiology of acute high-altitude illness. Am J Med 73:385–403.

.16.

Hematology of Sports

Toby L. Simon

Two areas of relationship exist between hematology and sports medicine and exercise. First, there is the impact of exercise on the management of a hematologic disease. Second, there is the effect of the hematologic system and the elements of the bloodstream on exercise and sports performance. In this chapter both aspects are reviewed.

EXERCISE AND HEMATOLOGIC DISEASE

In general, the subject of exercise is not of paramount importance in hematologic disease. Patients with anemia have decreased oxygen delivery to tissues and impairment in their ability to exercise and perform in sports. Most hematologic diseases are characterized by some impairment in sports performance. In polycythemia, increased red cell mass or viscosity would similarly impair performance. Patients with bleeding disorders would be at increased risk for bleeding in exercise and any contact sports. Thus, in general, this set of diseases precludes significant exercise and high-level sports performance.

Hemophilia

One example where the importance of exercise to the overall management of the disease is such that the risks must be weighed against benefit is hemophilia. Patients with hemophilia A (deficiency of clotting factor VIII) and hemophilia B (deficiency of clotting factor IX) have increased bleeding as a result of their clotting factor deficiency. Mildly hemophiliac individuals bleed only with trauma or hemostatic challenge such as surgery. Severely hemophiliac individuals, however, bleed spontaneously. The major areas of bleeding are joints and muscles. Recurrent bleeding into the joints and muscles leads to the disability of chronic arthritis. Disease in the joints predisposes to more frequent spontaneous bleeding.

Therefore, physical exercise is of great importance in increasing muscle strength. As muscle strength increases, joint support is improved. This improvement in joint support is associated with decreased hemorrhage. Therefore, in hemophilia, exercise programs are needed to ensure decreased bleeding and improve the management of the underlying disease process.

This work was supported by grants from The Blood Systems Research Foundation, National Institutes of Health grant NHLBI 5 K07 HL01252, and National Institutes of Health General Clinical Research Center grant DRR NIH 5 M01 RR 00997.

Ideal exercises for the patient with hemophilia are those that can be done without increasing the force of gravity on joints. Jogging is discouraged. Contact sports are discouraged, not only because of the force of gravity on joints and thus possible increased bleeding, but also because of injury that can occur with contact that would have greater bleeding associated with it than would be found in the patient with normal hemostasis.

The sports that are excellent for strengthening the joints without increasing bleeding are swimming and bicycling. Most hemophilia programs urge patients to swim regularly. Bicycling is somewhat less advantageous because falls may occur with bleeding episodes. However, if done with caution, it can also be recommended (Kasper and Dietrich [1]).

Simple isometric exercises play a major role. When done daily, they have been shown to improve strength and knee extension by at least one-third. It is recommended that a regular program of exercise start in early childhood and continue throughout life (Greene and Strickler [2]).

Sickle Cell Disease

Sickle cell disease is another instance in which the issue of exercise has assumed prime importance. This is a clinical syndrome in which sickled cells are found in the patient's blood. Patients are homozygous for the gene for sickle hemoglobin. Heterozygosity for the sickle cell gene results in sickle cell trait without significant clinical symptoms. The abnormal hemoglobin that sickles is rapidly destroyed, and the patients are typically anemic. The disease is most commonly found in blacks from tropical Africa but is present to a lesser extent in the Middle East. Clinical features include periodic crises in which sickling is increased with infarctions in tissue. There also may be increased hemolysis (hemolytic crisis) or bone marrow failure (aplastic crisis). Growth abnormalities, damage to the renal medulla, splenomegaly, jaundice and hepatomegaly, myocardial dysfunction, pulmonary infarctions, retinal vessel changes, cerebral vascular accidents, leg ulcers, and complicated pregnancies are seen. Patients typically have a hemoglobin between 5 and 11 g that is normochromic and normocytic with an elevated reticulocyte count. Treatment is supportive (Beutler [3]).

Obviously, in sickle cell anemia, exercise is impaired. However, because of the large number of individuals living long lives with this disease, there has been interest in whether the exercise impairment can be treated. In children with sickle cell anemia, ischemic electrocardiographic (ECG) response to dynamic cyclic exercise testing was associated with the extent of hemoglobin deficiency. Long-term myocardial ischemia was related to stress and could lead to fibrosis and decreased myocardial contractility in adults (Alpert et al. [4]).

Exercise is known to lead to hemoglobinuria and hemoglobinemia because sickle red cells are more shear sensitive. Exercise-induced hemolysis in sickle cell disease seems to be proportional to dehydrated shear-sensitive cells (Platt [5]).

Longitudinally studied hemodynamic changes induced by exercise appear to progress over time (Alpert et al. [6]). Cardiac function at rest is normal, but with maximum exercise, heart rate, cardiac output, and heart work decrease proportionately to the degree of anemia. The ischemic-exercise ECG is related to the increase in left ventricular end diastolic volume (Covitz et al. [7]).

In one study of patients treated with blood transfusion, exercise capacity was improved by transfusion, related to the hemoglobin concentration per se rather than the percent of sickle cells (Charache et al. [8]). However, a different study using exchange transfusion suggested that the greatest benefit was the increase in the percentage of normal hemoglobin rather than the actual extent of anemia (Miller et al. [9]). Thus, the relationship between exercise, anemia, and cardiac deterioration and general deterioration is not fully understood. It would appear that both anemia and the sickling phenomenon relate to the inability to sustain exercise.

Greater controversy has surrounded exercise in sickle cell trait. In these individuals who are not anemic and appear to be normal, the question is whether the trait itself predisposes to sickling under stress situations and whether individuals with the trait are unable to sustain normal exercise.

The relationship of sickle cell trait to sudden death is unknown. At present there is no proof of increased mortality due to the presence of the trait. There have been reports of death in severe training situations in which the autopsy showed signs of sickle cell crisis. If exertion results in intravascular sickling in subjects with sickle cell trait, certain pathologic consequences would follow. It is not yet clear that clinically significant sickling can be induced by physical stress (Sears [10]). Studies of football players in the National Football League in the United States have shown sickle cell trait players to perform as well as those with totally normal hemoglobin (Murphy [11]).

Four cases of sudden death in patients with trait were reported during combat training. These were thought to be related to a combination of moderate to severe exercise at altitude and dehydration (Jones et al. [12]). In ECG studies of exercise in children with sickle cell trait, no definite ischemia was found. But suggestive evidence of ischemia was found in 8.3% of those tested. Exercise was apparently safe, but the study was not conclusive (Alpert et al. [13]).

The most extensive review of the subjects, by Diggs on behalf of the Armed Forces, suggested that exercise may lead to crisis or infarctive aspects of sickle cell in trait subjects when superimposed on other major diseases. Death has been reported in underwater swimming and in hypoxic environments. (Diggs [14]). In vivo sickling and splenic infarcts have been associated with unpressurized airplanes and hypoxic environments in sickle cell trait patients. Ambient hypoxia, i.e., exercise at altitudes greater than one mile, might also relate. Infections, dehydration, alcohol or drugs, chilling, overheating, stress and muscular exertion also have been found to cause problems. Cases of sudden death usually relate to sickled red cells in the microvasculature. In addition, exercise-induced rhabdomyolysis has been found to relate to intravascular sickling. Exertional syndromes lead to hypoxia, acidity, hypo-osmolarity and hypothermia, all of which favor sickling (Diggs [15, 16]).

While sickle trait has been shown to cause no disability, military service may take stress to the limit leading to some potential problems (Diggs [17]). As a result, it was suggested that it is appropriate to have sickle cell trait individuals in sports or in military duty but that they should be excluded from being pilots, co-pilots, and navigators on military aircraft; paratroopers; crew of transport ships; deep-sea divers; or crew involved in activities with maximum stress and endurance, particularly at high altitudes (Diggs [17]). Thus, sickle cell trait seems to dispose to a rare, unexpected sickling complication with very high levels of exertion, but in general, such individuals can participate in sports and exercise up to levels of maximum stress (Diggs [17]).

PHYSIOLOGIC CHANGES RELATED TO EXERCISE

The greatest impact of hematology on exercise relates to the red blood cell (erythrocyte), because of the critical role of the red blood cell in delivering oxygen to exercising muscles.

Anemia

The blood volume affects the hematocrit and hemoglobin concentration. A number of studies have shown that blood volume increases in significant exercise, particularly marathon running over a long period of time. Most of the increase is in plasma volume (Pugh [18]; Oscal et al. [19]); however, measurements actually taken during a marathon run showed decreased plasma volume (6.5% in males, 8.6% in females) early in the race with return to baseline by 3–4 hr. In general, stable plasma volumes were found during racing (Myhre et al. [20]). There has been data showing increased blood volume in other studies, but often with a concomitant increase in red cell mass (Adner [21]). Some studies have suggested that marathon runners develop an optimal hematocrit (Sinclair and Sarelius [22]).

Thus there has been speculation about "pseudo-anemia" because of expansion of blood volume in athletes. In one study of mature athletes, blood volume and total body hemoglobin were both found to be about 20% higher in athletes than in nonathletes. It was suggested that they were, however, independently controlled (Brotherhood et al. [23]). One jogger studied, running across the United States, was found to have a decrease in plasma volume, an increase in hematocrit and red cell mass, and total blood volume remaining unchanged (Bruce et al. [24]). In general, it appears that there is an increased plasma volume in athletes due to increased sodium retention that could cause some reduction in the measure of the hemoglobin concentration or packed cell volume. This would constitute a pseudo-anemia (Lancet [25]).

True anemia caused by exercise has been suggested by a number of studies in runners and occasionally in other sports. One large study reported 4.5% of male and 7.5% of female athletes during training had low hemoglobin. They investigated serum iron as a cause of that and found that iron did not vary with hemoglobin concentration (de Wijn et al. [26]). Another large study showed that inactive persons had higher hemoglobins than those in active occupations (Adcock et al. [27]).

Sports anemia was monitored during marching in soldiers whose hematocrit and red cell counts were decreased by Day 4 of the marches with a gradual increase of hemoglobin throughout the rest of the marching period. Mean corpuscular hemoglobin concentration (MCHC) and mean corpuscular hemoglobin (MCH) were stable on exercise, but went down during recovery. Mean red cell volume (MCV) was reduced, and there was an increase in small cells in the circulation, suggesting iron deficiency (Radomski et al. [28]). Aerobic training of college women ages 19 to 21 was associated with 2.6% decrease in hemoglobin, 3.4% decrease in hematocrit, and 14.3% decrease in red cell count during training. However, with continued training, these had returned to normal by 9 weeks, suggesting many of the changes were transitory. The authors of the study hypothesized that occasionally red cell destruction increased early in training (Puhl and Runyan [29]). Swimming programs in young females have also been shown to cause higher MCV and MCH with training but without anemia (Stransky et al. [30]). One study of marathon runners starting with normal blood values during a 20-day road race showed that hemoglobin and hematocrit were down by Day 2 and continued down during the period of the race. No correlation with their performance could be found (Dressendorfer et al. [31]). However, by contrast, rowers and cyclists experienced an increase in the number of red blood cells during extensive training (Horniak [32]). In competitive swimmers ages 12 to 19, women were found to be comparable to controls, while men had slightly lower red cell counts than standard values (Willan et al. [33]).

Long-distance running has been noted to cause a number of acute changes that include rise in the hematocrit (Riley et al. [34]). In long-term periods, however, hematocrit and hemoglobin are low in runners (Bunch [35]).

Data from a comparative survey of the 1976 Canadian Olympic Team of 123 men and 64 women showed hemoglobins and hematocrits to be significantly lower than the general Canadian population. In men this was 14.7 ± 1 g, compared to 15.5 ± 1.8 g in the general population. Among the female athletes, the mean was 12.9 ± 0.7 g, compared to 13.6 ±

1.6 in the general population. In endurance sports the figures were even slightly lower: 14.1 g for men and 12.6 g for women.

Hematocrits have also been extensively studied during basic training in the military. In two courses of exercise for cadets, hemoglobin was found to fall from 16.8 to 12.8 g and 15.2 to 12.5 g, while hematocrits similarly fell from 47.1 to 38.5%, and 46.1 to 39.3%. In recovery phases there was always an increase toward initial levels (Clement et al. [36]; Lindemann [37]).

Because of this, the potential for red blood cell changes to contribute to retrogression during training has been studied. In aerobic training programs, decreased ability to perform, i.e., retrogression, tended to occur on the fifth day of training. No evidence could be found that anemia contributed (Deitrick et al. [38]).

Thus, there are a variety of data to suggest some impact of running, in particular, on hemoglobin and hematocrit during extensive training, with generally lower values, in athletes than in sedentary individuals. However, the overlap with the control group is typically considerable and the mechanism is obscure. Several possible mechanisms have been investigated, especially red cell destruction (hemolysis) and iron deficiency.

Red Cell Destruction While some studies have reported no increased red cell destruction (Brotherhood et al. [23]), a characteristic reduction in haptoglobin during peak exertion and on a chronic basis in athletes has been demonstrated, suggesting increased red blood cell destruction (DuFaux et al. [39]; Casoni et al. [40]; Magnusson et al. [41]; Ehn et al. [42]; Clement and Asmundson [43]). Some studies have quantitated increased loss of hemoglobin in the urine (Magnusson et al [41]; Jacobs and Wilson [44]).

In military recruits, haptoglobin was noted to decrease with rise in bilirubin and erythropoietin (Clement et al. [36]; Lindemann [37]). These data suggested increased red cell destruction with exercise. Myoglobin can be excreted with exercise and was observed in triathlon participants in whom the degree of mild anemia related to the finish (Thomas and Motley [45]). Presumably, hemoglobinemia, i.e., release of hemoglobin from destroyed red cells, has a similar pathogenesis to the myoglobinemia. A study in horses showed that there was a loss of red cell mass during prolonged exercise, leading to an increase in spiculated red cells (Boucher et al. [46]). Stomatocytic transformation of the red cells after a marathon has been noted in 2 subjects who were average joggers. They showed red cells of a discocyte type proportional to the hemolysis with hemoconcentration after a major run (Reinhart and Chien [47]).

Cross-country runs have also been investigated. Five out of 11 participants had rise in plasma hemoglobin of 10–18 mg/100 cc at the end of a 2.6- to 2.8-mile race. Urines were negative and the race was run in 14–18 min. When the subjects ran 4.5–5.1 miles in 28–31 min, hemoglobin levels of 17–47 mg/100 cc in the plasma were seen. Eighteen of 22 marathon runners who ran 26.2 miles had hemoglobins of 10–44 mg/100 cc hemoglobin. Four of these had hemoglobinuria. Bilirubin elevations were also seen (0.58–1.72 mg per 100 cc), and 10 had values greater than 0.8 mg/100 cc. These changes were unrelated to age, body build, position, or number of years of running, and they disappeared a few hours after the end of the run. Various lesser changes were found with walking. No changes were found with cycling. The authors concluded that there was a physiologic intravascular hemolysis with exercise, related specifically to running, that led to hemoglobin release (Gilligan et al. [48]). This phenomenon has been termed "footstrike hemolysis."

Data showed that this hemolysis involved destruction of small numbers of the oldest red cells, the ones with the highest red cell creatine. This led to a relatively increased concentration of younger red cells, which, in turn, caused a rise in the MCV. A mild reticulocytosis occurred that was not sufficient to explain the high MCV. Over time, this hemolysis could diminish the iron stores of the individuals. Thus, macrocytosis related to the hemolysis and the anemia could occur (Eichner [49]).

Osmotic fragility does not appear to be a cause, since male athletes have actually higher resistance toward hypertonic saline (Davidson [50]). Rather, this syndrome has been related to the march or exertional hemoglobinuria. Some individuals after long marching or running pass red-colored urine, which may be accompanied by nausea, abdominal cramps, aching in the back or legs, and burning on the side of the feet. This is caused by exertion in the upright erect posture. Anemia itself is uncommon and the blood loss tends to be limited to 6–40 ml. The mechanism is postulated as mechanical damage resulting in fragmentation of erythrocytes. Additional factors such as hard surfaces and shoe problems cause elimination of older cells and hemoglobinemia, a syndrome of multiple microtrauma (Davidson [50]).

Particularly in female runners, this mechanism of increased red cell destruction can lead to a stress on body iron reserves, which are mobilized to increase erythropoiesis. Usually there is no effect on the reticulocyte count. Thus, high school women who run cross-country have been found to have iron deficiency (Puhl et al. [51]).

Iron   The next most intensively investigated mechanism for so-called sports anemia is iron deficiency. Lower ferritin levels (which correlate with body iron stores) in runners compared to rowers and cyclists indicate that iron deficiency may be specific for runners (DuFaux et al. [39]). Of the 133 male ultramarathon runners studied in Italy in whom lower haptoglobins were noted, the controls were also noted to be higher in ferritin as well as hemoglobin and hematocrit (Casoni et al. [40]). Comparisons of runners and swimmers showed decreased ferritin levels in 14% of runners; however, means were comparable to those of controls. Only 2% of the controls were deficient, and no swimmers were deficient. The total iron binding capacity was also found to be higher in runners than swimmers. Ferritin was actually higher in runners than controls during the race but decreased 14 days thereafter, suggesting that training may falsely elevate iron due to plasma volume decrease and that ferritin levels need to be measured at least 14 days after intensive training. They also showed that oral iron increased iron levels in these athletes, indicating no significant malabsorption (Dickson et al. [52]). In 12 competitive distance runners studied very intensively, 6 showed mild hypochromia, 2 decreased bone marrow cellularity, 7 absent hemosiderin granules in the bone marrow, and 5 trace hemosiderin granules. The absence of bone marrow hemosiderin granules was indicative of iron deficiency. Hematocrit and hemoglobin in these competitive distance runners was lower than in controls, but none were actually anemic. Serum iron itself did not correlate with performance (Wishnitzer et al. [53]).

In a group of 86 male and 32 female nonelite runners, only 1 was found to be anemic, and that runner was not iron deficient. Runners of both sexes were low in iron (Colt and Heyman [54]). In a group of 33 women and 80 men group training by jogging, 23 were found to have latent anemia marked by small size of red blood cells suggesting iron deficiency. Poor diet correlated, and treatment led to improved performance (Hunding et al. [55]). A study of 5 female runners found that iron (not hematocrit or hemoglobin) varied specifically with the amount of fatigue experienced by the runners (Banister and Hamilton [56]). However, a study of the best male runners found none to be iron deficient (Magnusson et al. [41]).

In some cases, low iron intake, particularly in women, may contribute to the problem. In one large study in endurance runners, 26% of men and 9% of women had deficient iron intake in their diet. The mean ferritins were in acceptable range, but 21% of male runners had low saturation (suggesting iron deficiency). Thirty-two percent of men had low ferritin; 29%, low hemoglobin; and 10.5%, low saturation. Among women, 36% had low iron, 55%

had low saturation, and 82% had low ferritin, although none were truly anemic. Low haptoglobin, suggesting red cell destruction as the cause of the problem, was found in 26% of men and 9% of women. It was concluded that this red cell destruction stressed body iron stores to replace cells. Latent iron deficiency then followed (Clement and Asmundson [43]).

An extensive study of iron physiology in the setting of intense physical activity suggested that the low absorption and increased elimination combined to decrease iron stores in athletes. Mean absorption in athletes studied was 16.4%, compared with a normal of 30%. This difference was not statistically significant but was suggestive. In the bone marrow, iron was found to be absent in 5 subjects and to be at trace levels in 3 subjects studied. Total body scanning studies showed elimination of radioactive iron to be far faster in runners than in nonrunners. This suggested some mechanism of increased elimination along with some decrease in absorption that caused the problem (Ehn et al. [42]).

In a study of female high school and college cross-country runners, 18.5% were found to have iron deficiency anemia; 11%, to have iron deficiency without anemia; 22%, to have intermediate saturations of iron; 3.7%, to have other causes of anemia; and 44%, to have no problem. The authors were able to increase iron levels with supplementation in these runners. However, the effect of this on performance was not clear (Plowman and McSwegin [57]). In another study of high school female runners, the groups were divided into those on placebos, those on vitamin C to increase iron absorption, and those on actual iron supplements. Forty percent of the girls on placebo developed iron deficiency, while deficient iron stores were found in all but one of the girls not on supplements and all the girls on vitamin C. Sweat losses of iron as well as gastrointestinal and urinary loss were postulated as possible causes. The efficacy of iron supplementation in preventing iron deficiency in this group of young athletes was clear, but again the correlation with performance was not measured (Nickerson et al. [58]).

Summary: Anemia   Thus, the cause of anemia in athletes is not well understood. Clearly, there can be increased fecal loss of iron, some possible decrease of absorption, and increased iron deficiency in this population which can contribute to anemia. This iron deficiency may relate to increased iron loss, which is more significant in runners than in other athletes. It has also been suggested that increased interleukin-1 and C-reactive protein in athletes causes an acute inflammatory response that may limit erythropoiesis (Lancet [25]). Thus, decreased red cell production may combine with increased red cell loss (hemolysis). If iron is limiting, anemia would be an expected result.

With the current evidence, it seems reasonable to conclude that anemia in athletes may be a combination of pseudo-anemia caused by greater increase in plasma volumes than in red cell mass, increased red cell destruction (particularly with exercise such as jogging), and iron deficiency. The iron deficiency may have multiple causes. It relates to a dietary lack combined with increased body iron metabolism. Absorption may be low in some individuals. Female athletes normally have increased iron loss with menstrual periods, which may accentuate the problem. Nutritional deficiency such as folate and vitamin B_{12} would appear to be very unusual (Adner [21]). There may be an inflammatory response that decreases iron utilization in red cell production. More recently, gastrointestinal blood loss has appeared to be a problem that can further impact on this anemia.

Gastrointestinal Blood Loss

Another major contribution to blood loss and iron deficiency among runners is gastrointestinal blood loss. A high incidence of gastrointestinal symptoms, including diarrhea and increased defecation, has been noted among runners (Singhal and Bansal [59]). There are now studies that have documented this gastrointestinal blood loss. In a study of 24 runners,

4 (2 male and 2 female) were found to have low ferritin. Mean hemoglobin and hematocrits were lower in the group of runners than controls. Mean hemoglobin stool blood levels rose with marathon competition and peaked 54 hr after a race. They went from 1.08 ± 0.65 mg/kg to 2.25 mg/kg, a statistically significant difference. This was not caused by aspirin or nonsteroidal anti-inflammatory agents taken. The mechanism was postulated to be transient gastrointestinal ischemia. Gastrointestinal blood loss may contribute to anemia in runners (Stewart et al. [60]).

A study at the Boston Marathon found 7 of 32 runners with blood in their stools. While there was high use of aspirin and anti-inflammatory drugs in runners as a group, it did not differentiate between those who had blood in their stools and those who did not (McMahon et al. [61]). There is a further report of 3 cases of upper gastrointestinal hemorrhage in young runners due to gastritis (Porter [62]). Another author noted that bleeding has already been reported in the bladder wall with exercise-related hematuria. He postulated that there could be bowel wall bleeding as well. Of 36 runners who were all negative for blood in their stool before a race, 4 had stools that were positive, 1 tarry after a race (Papaioannides et al. [63]).

In a review by Buckman, reports of detectable gastrointestinal bleeding after marathons varied from 8% in one study to 25% in another. The last study showed that it was equal or greater than 3 g of hemoglobin per gram of stool (Buckman [64]). Thus, gastrointestinal blood loss may contribute to iron deficiency and to further anemia in runners. The extent of this in other areas of athletic competition is unknown.

Red Cell Function

Investigators have tried to determine if there is a compensatory response and increase in 2,3-diphosphoglycerate (2,3-DPG) concentration that would increase hemoglobin delivery to the tissues in long-distance runners. Such an increase would compensate for the anemia. In one study, both male and female long-distance runners were found to have a decrease in 2,3-DPG concentration after a contest for obscure reasons (Remes et al. [65]). However, another study showed that after physical training the steepness of the oxyhemoglobin dissociation curve was increased with a small increase in intraerythrocyte organic phosphates. These alterations were felt to augment oxygen extraction for a given volume of blood by up to 15% during heavy work in the trained state. Thus, an influence on the hemoglobin molecules that led to altered hemoglobin oxygen affinity and increase of oxygen extraction was found in this study (Braumann et al. [66]).

Training-dependent changes have been found in skiers, long-distance runners, and cyclists. Trained individuals had a higher P_{50} (partial pressure of oxygen at which the hemoglobin is 50% saturated), but no change in oxygen transport parameters or 2,3-DPG concentration when the red cells were adjusted for age. Exercise may have induced intravascular hemolysis, which led to a decrease in the high-density older red cells in the trained groups. This resulted in younger red cells that had a higher concentration of 2,3-DPG. These increased levels of 2,3-DPG in the remaining erythrocytes led to a training-associated decrease in the oxygen affinity of hemoglobin and an increase in oxygen delivery to the tissues. All these changes related to the mean age of the red cells, which explained the higher 2,3-DPG and the lower oxygen affinity. Selective hemolysis of the older red cells leaves the individual somewhat anemic but enriches the younger red cells, which have higher 2,3-DPG, which in turn aids oxygen extraction and performance. This may explain how runners' anemia may contribute to improved performance (Mairbaurl et al. [67]).

There is one report in women cross-country runners of increased DPG with training that may have compensated for anemia. This was seen in high school women runners, but not in college women runners (Smalley et al. [68]).

Thus, anemia is probably multifactorial in athletes. It may be compensated to some extent by 2,3-DPG elevation.

Viscosity

Another issue of interest has been the blood viscosity. Anemia with decreased blood viscosity could improve blood flow and performance. One study has shown that whole blood viscosity increases with exercise, as does plasma viscosity (Martin et al. [69]). With exercise the hematocrit increases, then decreases later. The decrease contributes to the changes in whole blood viscosity. The increase in fibrinogen in this study was less than what was expected (3–7%). That study showed that whole blood viscosity increases with maximal exercise more than can be attributed to hematocrit alone. This was due to the increase in plasma proteins. Plasma viscosity did not rise to the degree expected because fibrinogen rise was less than one usually sees with stress, and the changes in this study were independent of conditioning level, aerobic capacity, or performance (Martin et al. [69]).

Studies done in trained runners showed an increased plasma viscosity after exercise. However, enhanced fibrinolysis kept changes in this viscosity from being what might have been expected (Letcher et al. [70]).

Another study showed that tissue perfusion and oxygen delivery at rest were greater in trained runners than in controls but became similar with significant exercise (Charm et al. [71]). Viscosity is not a significant effect of running. There is less increase in fibrinogen with stress and endurance training, so that some compensatory mechanism involved in increased fibrinolysis prevents the increase in blood viscosity to the extent that might be expected and keeps it a neutral factor.

Treatment of Exercise-Induced Anemia

The paramount importance of anemia as an abnormal laboratory finding in endurance-trained athletes, in particular, suggests that treatment of this problem might improve performance. One obvious method of treatment would be nutritional supplementation. Thus, iron supplementation may have an obvious role in athletes who may have increased loss of iron stores due to intravascular hemolysis and gastrointestinal bleeding. This would allow the hematocrit (packed cell volume) to rise with the increase in blood volume with strenuous exercise.

A more direct approach would be the infusion of red blood cells. Transfusion of homologous blood involves unacceptable medical risks. Thus, transfusion therapy as a means of correction of the anemia is not warranted.

The concept of using "blood doping" to induce erythrocythemia to improve performance at a given point in time for a particular contest has become more frequently considered and is a matter of some concern. The only acceptable way to conduct such a program would be to obtain red blood cells from the athlete, store them in the frozen state for some prolonged period to allow the athlete to return to his or her normal hematocrit and hemoglobin, and then reinfuse the previously frozen red blood cells autologously. If done under appropriate medical control, this could be a safe procedure.

Whether such reinfusion is of any value is a matter of some controversy. Such a produced erythrocythemia does have a sound physiologic basis (Klein [72]). Exercise capacity is known to be related to actual oxygen uptake, which in turn is known to be related to red blood cell mass. While such an increase in oxygen-carrying capacity might be offset by increased blood viscosity, which would reduce flow, such viscosity effects are rarely of significant magnitude in hematocrits of less than 50. However, there is also some animal data to suggest that transfusion leads to increased peripheral vascular resistance and decrease in cardiac output and venous return, which might cancel out a beneficial effect.

Phlebotomy and reduced hematocrit and hemoglobin were shown to impair performance in two recent studies (Pierucki et al. [73]; Thomson et al. [74]). In both, this difference was erased by reinfusion of blood that had been removed. One study was in female runners. The study of 4 untrained males, from which 500 ml of blood had been withdrawn twice over a 2-week period and reinfused at 6 months, showed a marked decline in maximal oxygen uptake ($\dot{V}O_{2\,max}$) after donation that returned to baseline in 8 weeks and increased after blood doping by 0.5 L/min (0.2–0.6). They noted the importance of the time span between phlebotomy and reinfusion to see a significant effect. Studies were also done over 12 weeks in untrained individuals to prevent training effects. This study also sampled deep femoral venous blood, showing that the effect of the doping was truly an increased oxygen supply to tissues. Cardiac output was only up slightly, but arterial oxygen content increased to a greater extent.

Two studies gave particularly strong weight to this argument (Ekblom et al. [75]; Buick et al. [76]). In the first, 7 male physical education students were studied (a group that would not necessarily be well trained). They were divided into 2 groups, one of which had a single phlebotomy of 800 ml, leading to a hemoglobin reduction of 13% with reinfusion of stored red cells 4 weeks later. The second group had sequential phlebotomies of 1200 ml and were reinfused 24 days later. The hemoglobin had dropped 18% prior to the reinfusion. Ergometer and treadmill studies were utilized. In the first group, the maximum work time and the $\dot{V}O_{2\,max}$ increased 23% and 9%, respectively, after reinfusion. In the second group, the maximum work time increased significantly, but the $\dot{V}O_{2\,max}$ only slightly. Phlebotomy in both groups had reduced the work possible by 30%.

In Buick's double-blind studies, 11 highly trained runners were studied at different stages: 1) before phlebotomy with normal cythemia, 2) after a sham reinfusion of saline, 3) after the reinfusion of 900 ml of frozen red blood cells brought to a hematocrit of 50% by saline, and 4) after the reestablishment of the normal hemoglobin and hematocrit. Twenty-four hours postreinfusion, $\dot{V}O_{2\,max}$ and running time to exhaustion were significantly increased (5.11 to 5.37 L/min and 7.2 to 9.65 min, respectively). This effect was seen up to 7 days. At 16 weeks hemoglobin was baseline, the $\dot{V}O_{2\,max}$ was still increased, but endurance levels had returned to normal. Submaximal exercise was also improved immediately after infusion. The author concluded that the limit to aerobic activity was the transport of oxygen to muscle.

This has led to great concern that blood doping might increasingly be used by athletes, perhaps under inappropriate medical control (Williams [77]). The observed increase in the use of this procedure has caused the International Olympic Committee and the United States Olympic Committee to formally ban blood doping (Higdon [78]).

The obvious critical question is, Does blood doping work in competition—will it actually produce a true competitive edge? A double-blind control study reported on 6 highly trained male distance runners determined the effect of induced erythrocythemia. This study involved 2 phlebotomies 8 weeks apart, with red cells frozen and subjects continuing training for 11 weeks after the second phlebotomy. At the end of this period, 3 of them received autologous reinfusion of red blood cells, while 3 received a placebo infusion. A competitive race was run as a baseline prior to the reinfusion while second and third races were run 5 days after the first and a second infusion, in which subjects' infusions were crossed over. Statistical methods were applied using each individual as his own control.

This study showed a drop in the time to run a 10-km race of approximately 1 min after red cell infusion but not placebo that was statistically significant. Treadmill testing with a small number of subjects was not statistically significant for submaximal exercise. However, the trends were in the direction of improved performance. Concentration of 2,3-DPG and P_{50} were unchanged in the 2 groups, which would be expected with the use of frozen red cells. Hematocrit increase was between 5% and 6%. Thus, induced erythrocythemia in highly trained male distance runners with normal hemoglobins and hematocrits (mean 41.66% increased to 47.41%) was able to improve their performance in a competitive 10-km race. These data suggest that increasing red cell mass would improve performance (Brien and Simon [79]).

Because even autologous reinfusion of red blood cells is expensive and requires careful medical supervision, its use cannot be recommended for either training or contest. The ethical questions about it remain as well. However, these data suggest that the anemia of athletes is not a physiologic one; i.e., the performance is not improved by the lower red cell mass and in fact can be improved by returning the red cell mass either to normal or slightly above normal levels. However, red cell masses at certain high levels would involve dangers related to viscosity. The recommended approach to this is to monitor athletes for gastrointestinal, urinary, and intravascular blood loss; replete iron stores where indicated; and recommend diets with adequate iron. Prophylactic supplementation with iron in female athletes is reasonable.

White Blood Cells

Significant increase in granulocytes have been found in a number of studies (Dressendorfer et al. [31]; Horniak [32]; Priest et al. [80]). Some studies have shown a doubling. However, a large portion of the response may be negated by training. In one study the effect was seen more often in untrained individuals, among whom the increase in plasma volume was greater, along with a decreased response to isoproterenol by the granulocytes (Busse et al. [81]).

This granulocytosis is accompanied by an eosinopenia (Weber [82]), presumably due to adrenocorticotropin hormone. Lymphocyte response to phytohemagglutinin may be reduced. There appears to be a transient suppression of lymphocyte transformation. This is not seen, however, in a short run as compared to a marathon. The eosinopenia occurs in the same subjects who had increased granulocytes (Eskola et al. [83]).

Coagulation

Platelet effects appear to be somewhat complex. A number of studies have shown increased platelet count with strenuous exercise (Kishk et al. [84]; Warlow and Ogston [85]; Marley [86]; Dix et al. [87]). This response may be lost as the subject rests and appears to be a transient but significant response immediately to exercise.

The effect on platelet function is more obscure. One study showed that aggregation was increased after significant exercise (Ohri et al. [88]). A second study 24 hr after a marathon race showed the platelets had increased sensitivity to the addition of prostacycline. Presumably, this related to the activity of adenyl cyclase (Dix et al. [87]). The authors hypothesized that this was another protective effect of exercise against cardiovascular disease. Another study showed an increase in aggregation but no significant change in platelet adhesion in 24 untrained men after exercise (Warlow and Ogston [85]). No difference has been found in mean platelet volume (Kishk et al. [84]).

Theories that have been advanced concerning platelets are that there are an increased velocity of blood flow with exercise and an increased inhibition due to adrenaline and adenosine 5'-diphosphate (ADP). The exercise-induced platelet effect is short lived but measurable.

Long-term effects of exercise are very inconsistent. Some studies show decreased platelet adhesion, others do not (Marley [86]). Decrease in aggregatability to ADP has also been reported, but in the same study there was increased platelet factor IV, suggesting activation of the platelets (Knudsen et al. [89]). In this study concentrated short-run exercise increased the aggregation, but this was lost with long-term exercise such as in a marathon, a suggestion that the aggregation capacity was ultimately exhausted (Knudsen et al. [89]).

There is also a fairly consistent increase in factor VIII activity paralleled by factor VIII antigen ($75 \pm 28.5\%$) with a consequent reduction in the partial thromboplastin time ($25 \pm 6\%$) (Ohri et al. [88]). Fibrinogen increases have been reported by some (Dix et al. [87]), but not by others (Collen et al. [90]).

Fibrinolysis   Clearly, physical conditioning and exercise of various sorts augment fibrinolytic response (Williams et al. [91]; Collen et al. [90]; Mangum et al. [92]; Rosing et al. [93]; Burt et al. [94]). In a study of fibrinogen, plasminogen, and prothrombin kinetics, physical exertion by normal volunteers on a bicycle resulted in a significant shortening in the half-life of fibrinogen and plasminogen, but not prothrombin. The catabolic rates were increased. There was an increase in degradation of the alpha chain. There was a small increase in the plasmin–antiplasmin complex. The biologic significance of this was not ascertained by the study, but this paralleled an increase in fibrinolytic activity.

Another study of 44 healthy men on the treadmill for 6 min at 5% grade, 7 miles per hr or 10 miles per hr until exhausted showed a reduction in the Lee White clotting time and the recalcification time and a significant acceleration of the euglobulin lysis time, a test for fibrinolysis (Burt et al. [94]).

Other studies have shown the marked increase in the fibrinolytic activity as measured by the euglobulin lysis time (Rosing et al. [93]). In one study in which 6 elite runners and 6 nonrunners were compared, the euglobulin lysis time in the runners was short, with an increase in plasminogen (Knudsen et al. [89]). In another study (Mangum et al. [92]), the increase in fibrinolytic activity was in proportion to the intensity of the exercise, duration, and time of day. This last relates to the diurnal variation in which fibrinolytic activity is higher at 8:00 p.m. than at 8.00 a.m. Short bursts of intense exercise markedly increased the fibrinolytic activity. More prolonged exercise had a mild effect. In this study plasminogen and fibrinogen did not change significantly. Finally, the increase in fibrinolysis was also shown to accompany cold exposure as well as exercise, without a change in concentration of the fibrinogen and plasminogen components.

Summary: Coagulation   Thus, there are modest coagulation changes, particularly marked in the fibrinolytic system. These changes would not appear to impair performance. On the contrary, these may be the types of changes that cause exercise to be of benefit in reduction of risk for cardiac disease. However, the exact relationship has yet to be determined.

SUMMARY

Hematologic aspects of sports and exercise still require significant definition and study. The causes and impact of the anemia found particularly in runners need to be elucidated further. In addition, confusion exists concerning whether the findings in runners pertain to other athletes. Thus, studies in other sports are required. It is clear that hematologic changes impact on performance, and sports impact on the bloodstream.

REFERENCES

1. Kasper, C.K., Dietrich, S.L. 1985. Comprehensive management of haemophilia. Clin Haematol 14:489–493.

2. Greene, W.B., Strickler, E.M. 1983. A modified isokinetic strengthening program for patients with severe hemophilia. Dev Med Child Neurol 25:189–196.

3. Beutler, E. 1983. Sickle cell disease and related disorders. In: Williams, W., Beutler, E., et al. (eds): Hematology. McGraw-Hill, New York.

4. Alpert, B.S., Gilman, P.A., et al. 1981. Hemodynamic and ECG responses to exercise in children with sickle cell anemia. Am J Dis Child 135:362–366.

5. Platt, O.S. 1982. Exercise-induced hemolysis in sickle cell anemia: shear sensitivity and erythrocyte dehydration. Blood 59:1055–1060.

6. Alpert, B.S., Dover, E.V., et al. 1984. Longitudinal exercise hemodynamics in children with sickle cell anemia. Am J Dis Child 138:1021–1024.

7. Covitz, W., Eubig, C., et al. 1983. Exercise-induced cardiac dysfunction in sickle cell anemia. Am J Cardiol 51:570–575.

8. Charache, S., Bleecker, E.R., et al. 1983. Effects of blood transfusion on exercise capacity in patients with sickle cell anemia. Am J Med 74:757–764.

9. Miller, D.M., Winslow, R.M., et al. 1980. Improved exercise performance after exchange transfusion in subjects with sickle cell anemia. Blood 56:1127–1131.

10. Sears, D.A. 1978. The morbidity of sickle cell trait. Am J Med 64:1021–1031.

11. Murphy, J.R. 1973. Sickle cell hemoglobin (Hb AS) in black football players. JAMA 225:981–982.

12. Jones, S., Binder, R.A., et al. 1970. Sudden death in sickle-cell trait. N Engl J Med 282:323–325.

13. Alpert, B.S., Flood, N.L., et al. 1982. Responses to exercise in children with sickle cell trait. Am J Dis Child 136:1002–1004.

14. Diggs, L.W. 1984. The sickle cell trait in relation to the training and assignment of duties in the Armed Forces: I. Policies, observations, and studies. Aviat Space Environ Med 55:180–185.

15. Diggs, L.W. 1984. The sickle cell trait in relation to the training and assignment of duties in the Armed Forces: II. Aseptic splenic necrosis. Aviat Space Environ Med 55:271–276.

16. Diggs, L.W. 1984. The sickle cell trait in relation to the training and assignment of duties in the Armed Forces: III. Hyposthenuria, hematuria, sudden death, rhabdomyolysis, and acute tubular necrosis. Aviat Space Environ Med 55:358–364.

17. Diggs, L.W. 1984. The sickle cell trait in relation to the training and assignment of duties in the Armed Forces: IV. Considerations and recommendations. Aviat Space Environ Med 55:487–492.

18. Pugh, L.G.C.E. 1969. Blood volume changes in outdoor exercise of 8–10 hour duration. J Physiol 200:345–351.

19. Oscal, L.B., Williams, B.T., et al. 1968. Effect of exercise on blood volume. J Appl Physiol 24:622–624.

20. Myhre, L.G., Hartung, G.H., et al. 1985. Plasma volume changes in middle-aged male and female subjects during marathon running. J Appl Physiol 59:559–563.

21. Adner, M.M. 1984. Hematology. In: Strauss, R.H. (ed): Sports Medicine. W.B. Saunders, Philadelphia.

22. Sinclair, J.D., Sarelius, I.H. 1979. The marathon man: the physiology of the long-distance runner. NZ Med J 90:383–387.

23. Brotherhood, J., Brozovic, B., et al. 1975. Haematological status of middle- and long-distance runners. Br J Mol Med 48:139–145.

24. Bruce, R.A., Kusumi, F., et al. 1975. Cardiac limitation to maximal oxygen transport and changes in components after jogging across the US. J Appl Physiol 39:958–964.

25. "Anaemia" in athletes. 1985. Lancet 1:1490–1491.

26. de Wijn, J.F., de Jongste, J.L., et al. 1971. Haemoglobin, packed cell volume, serum iron and iron binding capacity of selected athletes during training. J Sports Med 11:42–51.

27. Adcock, E.W., Brown, J.K., et al. 1985. Haemoglobin levels in sedentary and active persons. Am J Med 78:325.

28. Radomski, M.W., Sabiston, B.H., et al. 1980. Development of "Sports Anemia" in physically fit men after daily sustained submaximal exercise. Aviat Space Environ Med 51:41–45.

29. Puhl, J.L., Runyan, W.S. 1980. Hematological variations during aerobic training of college women. Res Q Exerc Sport 51:535–541.

30. Stransky, A.W., Mickelson, R.J., et al.

1979. Effects of a swimming training regimen on hematological, cardiorespiratory and body composition changes in young females. J Sports Med 19:347–354.

31. Dressendorfer, R.H., Wade, C.E., et al. 1981. Development of pseudoanemia in marathon runners during a 20-day road race. JAMA 246:1215–1218.

32. Horniak, E. 1966. The influence of local muscle fitness upon the changes of the haemogram after a working load. Sladkovicova 11 Bratislava (Czechoslovakia) 6:244–249.

33. Willan, P.L.T., Bagnall, K.M., et al. 1981. Some haematological characteristics of competitive swimmers. Br J Sports Med 15:238–241.

34. Riley, W.J., Pyke, F.S., et al. 1975. The effect of long-distance running on some biochemical variables. Clin Chim Acta 65:83–89.

35. Bunch, T.W. 1980. Blood test abnormalities in runners. Mayo Clin Proc 55:113–117.

36. Clement, D.B., Asmundson, R.C., et al. 1977. Hemoglobin values: comparative survey of the 1976 Canadian Olympic team. Can Med Assoc J 117:614–616.

37. Lindemann, R. 1978. Low hematocrits during basic training: athlete's anemia? N Engl J Med 299:1191–1192.

38. Deitrick, R.W., Ruhling, R.O., et al. 1980. Retrogression and the red blood cell. J Sports Med 20:67–74.

39. DuFaux, B., Hoederath, A., et al. 1981. Serum ferritin, haptoglobin, and iron in middle- and long-distance runners, elite rowers, and professional racing cyclists. Int J Sports Med 2:43–46.

40. Casoni, I., Borsetto, C., et al. 1985. Reduced hemoglobin concentration and red cell hemoglobinization in Italian marathon and ultramarathon runners. Int J Sports Med 6:176–179.

41. Magnusson, B., Hallberg, L., et al. 1984. Iron metabolism and "sports anemia." I. Acta Med Scand 216:149–55.

42. Ehn, L., Carlmark, B., Hoglund, S. 1980. Iron status in athletes involved in intense physical activity. Med Sci Sports Exerc 12:61–64.

43. Clement, D.B., Asmundson, R.C. 1982. Nutritional intake and hematological parameters in endurance runners. Phys Sportsmed 10:37–43.

44. Jacobs, M.B., Wilson, W. 1984. Iron deficiency anemia in a vegetarian runner. JAMA 252:481–482.

45. Thomas, B.D., Motley, C.P. 1984. Myoglobinemia and endurance exercise: a study of twenty-five participants in a triathlon competition. Am J Sports Med 12:113–119.

46. Boucher, J.H., Ferguson, E.W., et al. 1981. Erythrocyte alterations during endurance exercise in horses. J Appl Physiol: Respirat Environ Exercise Physiol 51:131–134.

47. Reinhart, W.H., Chien, S. 1985. Stomatocytic transformation of red blood cells after marathon running. Am J Hematol 19:201–204.

48. Gilligan, D.R., Altschule, M.D., et al. 1943. Physiological intravascular hemolysis of exercise: hemoglobinemia and hemoglobinuria following cross-country runs. J Clin Invest 22:859–869.

49. Eichner, E.R. 1985. Runner's macrocytosis: a clue to footstrike hemolysis. Am J Med 78:321–325.

50. Davidson, R.J.L. 1969. March or exertional haemoglobinuria. Semin Hematol 6:150–161.

51. Puhl, J.L., Runyan, W.S., et al. 1981. Erythrocyte changes during training in high school women cross-country runners. Res Q Exerc Sport 52:484–494.

52. Dickson, D.N., Wilkinson, R.L., et al. 1982. Effects of ultra-marathon training and racing on hematologic parameters and serum ferritin levels in well-trained athletes. Int J Sports Med 3:111–117.

53. Wishnitzer, R., Vorst, E., et al. 1983. Bone marrow iron depression in competitive distance runners. Int J Sports Med 4:27–30.

54. Colt, E., Heyman, B. 1984. Low ferritin levels in runners. J Sports Med 24:13–17.

55. Hunding, A., Jordal, R., et al. 1981. Runner's anemia and iron deficiency. Acta Med Scand 209:315–318.

56. Banister, E.W., Hamilton, C.L. 1985. Variations in iron status with fatigue modelled from training in female distance runners. Eur J Appl Physiol 54:16–23.

57. Plowman, S.A., McSwegin, P.C. 1981. The effects of iron supplementation on female cross country runners. J Sports Med 21:407–416.

58. Nickerson, H.J., Holubets, M., et al. 1985. Decreased iron stores in high school female runners. Am J Dis Child 139:1115–1119.

59. Singhal, P., Bansal, I.J.S. 1984. A comparison of values for osmotic fragility of R.B.C.'s and persistence test of athletes. J Sports Med 24:230–233.

60. Stewart, J.G., Ahlquist, D.A., et al. 1984. Gastrointestinal blood loss and anemia in runners. Ann Intern Med

100:843–845.

61. McMahon, L.F., Ryan, M.J. et al. 1984. Occult gastrointestinal blood loss in marathon runners. Ann Intern Med 100:846–847.

62. Porter, A.M.W. 1983. Do some marathon runners bleed into the gut? Br Med J 287:1427.

63. Papaioannides, D., Giotis, C.H., et al. 1984. Acute upper gastrointestinal hemorrhage in long-distance runners. Ann Int Med 101:719.

64. Buckman, M.T. 1984. Gastrointestinal bleeding in long-distance runners. Ann Int Med 101:127–128.

65. Remes, K., Harkonen, M., et al. 1975. The decrease in red cell 2,3-diphosphoglycerate concentration in long distance running. J Sports Med 15:113–116.

66. Braumann, K.M., Boning, D., et al. 1982. Bohr effect and slope of the oxygen dissociation curve after physical training. J Appl Physiol: Respirat, Environ, Exercise Physiol 52:1524–1529.

67. Mairbaurl, H., Humpeler, E., et al. 1983. Training-dependent changes of red cell density and erythrocytic oxygen transport. J Appl Physiol: Respirat Environ Exercise Physiol 55:1403–1407.

68. Smalley, K.A., Runyan, W.S., et al. Effect of training on erythrocyte 2,3-diphosphoglycerate in two groups of women cross-country runners. J Sports Med 21:352–358.

69. Martin, D.G., Ferguson, E.W., et al. 1985. Blood viscosity responses to maximal exercise in endurance-trained and sedentary female subjects. J Appl Physiol 59:348–353.

70. Letcher, R.L., Pickering, T.G., et al. 1981. Effects of exercise on plasma viscosity in athletes and sedentary normal subjects. Clin Cardiol 4:172–179.

71. Charm, S.E., Paz, H., et al. 1979. Reduced plasma viscosity among joggers compared with non-joggers. Biorheology 16:185–189.

72. Klein, H.G., 1985. Blood transfusion and athletics. N Engl J Med 312:854–856.

73. Pierucki, C., Serniak, E., et al. 1985. Effects of blood loss and blood doping on maximum O_2 uptake and anaerobic threshold in female runners. Fed Proc 44:1370.

74. Thomson, J.M., Stone, J.A., et al. 1982. O_2 transport during exercise following blood reinfusion. J Appl Physiol: Respirat Environ Exercise Physiol 53:1213–1219.

75. Ekblom, B., Goldbarg, A.N., et al.

1972. Response to exercise after blood loss and reinfusion. J Appl Physiol 33:175–180.

76. Buick, F.J., Gledhill, N., et al. 1980. Effect of induced erythrocythemia on aerobic work capacity. J Appl Physiol: Respirat Environ Exercise Physiol 48:636–642.

77. Williams, M.H. 1981. Blood doping: an update. Phys Sportsmed 9:59–62.

78. Higdon, H. 1985. Blood-doping among endurance athletes. Amer Med News, Sept 27, 1985, pp 37, 39–41.

79. Brien, A.J., Simon, T.L. 1987. The effects of red blood cell infusion on 10-km race time. JAMA 257:2761–2765.

80. Priest, J.B., Oei, T.O., et al. 1982. Exercise-induced changes in common laboratory tests. Am J Clin Pathol 77:285–289.

81. Busse, W.W., Anderson, C.L., et al. 1980. The effect of exercise on the granulocyte response to isoproterenol in the trained athlete and unconditioned individual. J Allergy Clin Immunol 65:358–364.

82. Weber, H. 1971. A quantitative study of eosinopenia and other stress indices. J Sports Med 11:12–21.

83. Eskola, J., Ruuskanen, O., et al. 1978. Effect of sport stress on lymphocyte transformation and antibody formation. Clin Exp Immunol 32:339–345.

84. Kishk, Y.T., Trowbridge, E.A., et al. 1985. Platelet volume and count after severe prolonged physical effort. Thromb Res 38:439–442.

85. Warlow, C.P., Ogston, D. 1974. Effect of exercise on platelet count, adhesion, and aggregation. Acta Haematol 52:47–52.

86. Marley, W.P. 1971. The platelet and training effects. J Sports Med 16:197–201.

87. Dix, C.J., Hassall, D.G., et al. 1984. The increased sensitivity of platelets to prostacyclin in marathon runners. Thromb Haemost 51:385–387.

88. Ohri, V.C., Chatterji, J.C., et al. 1983. Effect of submaximal exercise on haematocrit, platelet count, platelet aggregation and blood fibrinogen levels. J Sports Med 23:127–130.

89. Knudsen, B., Brodthagen, U., et al. 1982. Platelet function and fibrinolytic activity following distance running. Scand J Haematol 29:425–430.

90. Collen, D., Semeraro, N., et al. 1977. Turnover of fibrinogen, plasminogen, and prothrombin during exercise in man. J Appl Physiol: Respirat Environ Exercise Physiol 42:865–873.

91. Williams, A.S., Logue, E.E., et al.

1980. Physical conditioning augments the fibrinolytic response to venous occlusion in healthy adults. N Engl J Med 302:987–991.

92. Mangum, M., Haymes, E.M., et al. 1984. Coagulation and fibrinolytic responses to exercise and cold exposure. Aviat Space Environ Med 55:291–295.

93. Rosing, D.R., Brakman, P., et al. Blood fibrinolytic activity in man. Diurnal variation and the response to varying intensities of exercise. Circ Res 27:171–183.

94. Burt, J.J., Blyth, C.S., et al. 1964. The effects of exercise on the coagulation fibrinolysis equilibrium. J Sports Med 4:213–216.

•17•

Immunology of Exercise

Laurel Traeger Mackinnon and Thomas B. Tomasi

With the recent focus on the health benefits of exercise, it is surprising that relatively little is known about how exercise influences the immune system (Mackinnon and Tomasi [1]; Simon [2]), despite an interest dating back to the early part of this century (Bailey [3]; Nicholls and Spaeth [4]; Oppenheimer and Spaeth [5]). It is generally believed (mainly by those who exercise) that exercise enhances immune function, but anecdotal statements have associated "overtraining" in athletes with increased susceptibility to infections. This chapter focuses on the role of exercise as a modulator of immune function and views exercise in the context of its relationship to other known modulators of the immune system.

EXERCISE AND INFECTION

Acute bouts of strenuous physical activity or repeated strenuous exercise are associated with increased severity of some viral and parasitic infections. Strenuous physical activity at the time of infection has been associated with increased severity of infection and paralysis from poliomyelitis in humans (Horstmann [6]; Weinstein [7]) and in experimental animal models (Levinson et al. [8]; Rosenbaum and Harford [9]). In mice infected with coxsackie B3 virus, swimming after innoculation resulted in 75 times more viremias, a 1000-fold increase in viral titers in the heart (Reyes and Lerner [10]), and more severe necrosis of cardiac muscle (Gatmaitin et al. [11]). Mice forced to swim for 6 weeks after infection with the parasite Trypanosoma cruzi exhibited more severe parasitic and cellular infiltration of the heart and increased mortality (Elson and Abelmann [12]). However, 7 days of swimming after infection with the bacterium Francisella tularensis had no effect on the severity of disease (Friman et al. [13]).

Whereas exercise after infection is often associated with susceptibility to disease, moderate exercise training prior to experimentally induced infection appears to confer resistance to some infections. In mice allowed free access to exercise wheels for 16–18 days before infection with Salmonella typhimurium, exercised mice exhibited enhanced survival rates compared to infected sedentary controls (Cannon and Kluger [14]). Similar results have been obtained with tumors. In mice, running and swimming training for 1–8 weeks before tumor implantation slowed growth of tumors (Good and Fernandes [15]; Rusch and

This work was supported in part by NIH grant AM 31448. Present address of Thomas B. Tomasi: Roswell Park Memorial Institute, Buffalo, NY 14263.

Kline [16]) and prolonged survival time after innoculation with ascites tumor (Rashkis [17]).

Because stress can modulate immune function, it is important to distinguish the effects of stress from those of exercise, although under some conditions exercise can be considered a form of stress, depending on the individual's fitness level and the intensity and duration of exercise, e.g., prolonged strenuous exercise. There are several possible ways to explain how exercise differentially affects immunity and susceptibility to infection. For example, in a healthy animal exercise training before infection may not be stressful and may enhance the immune response, whereas after infection exercise may act as additional physical stress, compromising the immune response. Another complication relates to the biphasic response of the immune system to stress; in some systems, there is initial immunosuppression followed later (several days) by immunoenhancement (Riley [18]). This may occur during the early stages of exercise training. Thus, an animal exercised for several days before infection would have entered the enhancement phase at the time of challenge, and an animal exercised immediately before or after infection might still be in the suppressive phase at the time of challenge. An alternative possibility is that inactivity imposed by a laboratory setting may represent an immunosuppressive stress to a normally active animal, and access to activity may restore immunocompetence in the uninfected animal. Following infection mice restrict spontaneous activity, so that enforced exercise after infection (when the animal does not "feel" like exercising) may add an additional immunosuppressive stress. Certainly more work with animal models is needed to understand the temporal relationship between exercise and susceptibility to infection and tumors. Human studies have not been successful in establishing an objective relationship between exercise and immunity to infection, although anecdotal statements relate "overtraining" in athletes to an increased incidence of infections (Douglas and Hanson [19]; Tomasi et al. [20]).

EXERCISE AND LYMPHOID CELLS

Leukocytes

Resting leukocyte and lymphocyte numbers are normal in marathon runners, although in one study 50% of athletes (10 of 20) had lymphocyte counts on the low side of normal (<1500 cells per mm^3) (Green et al. [21]). Those with lower counts were world-class marathoners with heavy training schedules (60–130 miles per week), suggesting that intense training may alter resting lymphocyte numbers. The lymphocyte proliferative response to T-cell mitogens phytohemagglutinin (PHA) and concanavalin A (Con A) is suppressed after endurance running (Eskola et al. [22]), so that the low leukocyte number could possibly result from the chronically suppressed capacity of lymphocytes to proliferate in response to certain stimuli.

Leukocytosis begins within the first few minutes of exercise and rises progressively with increasing work loads (Ahlborg and Ahlborg [23]). Leukocyte number begins to decrease within 10 min after stopping (Ahlborg and Ahlborg [23]), returns to baseline levels by 30 min, but increases again 120 min after maximal exercise (Robertson et al. [24]). By 24 hr postexercise, leukocyte number returns to normal (Hanson and Flaherty [25]). Such rapid changes in leukocyte numbers suggest alterations in the distribution and compartmentalization of leukocytes.

There are studies that have not found exercise-induced leukocytosis (Busse et al. [26]; Hanson and Flaherty [25]). This discrepancy may reflect differences in the severity of the exercise and state of training of the subjects. For example, Busse et al. [26] reported no leukocytosis after a training run of 13 km at 70–80% of maximum aerobic capacity ($\dot{V}O_{2\ max}$) in well-trained runners, but they did find significant leukocytosis in untrained subjects following a maximal (but shorter) run. Maximal exercise in trained or untrained subjects and submaximal exercise in untrained subjects cause leukocytosis (Ahlborg and Ahlborg [23]; Busse et al. [26]; Eskola et al. [22]; Moorthy and Zimmerman [27]; Robertson et al. [24]; Steel et al. [28]), whereas submaximal exercise in trained individuals does not (Busse et al. [26]; Hanson and Flaherty [25]). The degree of leukocytosis may be related to differences in catecholamine levels during exercise. Maximal exercise, regardless of fitness level, causes plasma catecholamine levels to increase, as does submaximal exercise in untrained individuals. On the other hand, in trained athletes submaximal exercise causes less of an increase in catecholamines. Since catecholamines induce rapid leukocytosis, the higher catecholamine levels in maximal exercise may induce leukocyte mobilization more readily than in submaximal exercise (see below).

In addition, exercise-induced leukocytosis exhibits a biphasic response, with both immediate and later increases in leukocyte number. Eskola et al. [22] and Robertson et al. [24] reported significant leukocytosis immediately after and again 2–3 hr postexercise, with leukocyte number returning to baseline levels between 45 min and 2 hr. The biphasic response may represent two different mechanisms, an immediate response mediated by catecholamines and a later one, mediated by unknown factors.

The exercise-induced increase in leukocyte number is due to increases in granulocytes and lymphocytes, although both subpopulations do not always increase equally. Eskola et al. [22] reported a 2.5-fold increase in total leukocyte number, largely due to granulocytosis after a marathon in well-trained runners. Moorthy and Zimmerman [27] found a threefold increase in total leukocyte number, with increases in both granulocyte and lymphocyte number, after a 20-mile race, in well-trained runners. The relative changes in granulocyte and lymphocyte percentages of total leukocytes also depend on fitness level: Untrained subjects generally show an exercise-induced increase in lymphocyte percentage (Hedfors et al. [29, 30]; Robertson et al. [24]; Soppi et al. [31]), whereas in trained athletes lymphocyte percentage decreases after endurance exercise (Eskola et al. [22]; Moorthy and Zimmerman [27]).

Lymphocytes

Lymphocytosis often occurs following exercise (Ahlborg and Ahlborg [23]; Hedfors et al. [29]; Moorthy and Zimmerman [27]; Steel et al. [28]; Robertson et al. [24]; Soppi et al. [31]; Yu et al. [32]). In well-trained athletes exhaustive exercise (20-mile race) increased lymphocyte number by 37% (Moorthy and Zimmerman [27]). A shorter maximal bicycle test increased lymphocyte number 74% (Ahlborg and Ahlborg [23]). Lymphocytosis also follows submaximal exercise in untrained subjects, with up to twofold increases in lymphocyte number (Hedfors et al. [29]; Landmann et al. [33]; Steel et al. [28]; Yu et al. [32]).

Some studies have not found lymphocytosis following exercise. Hanson and Flaherty [25] found a statistically nonsignificant 42% increase in lymphocyte number after an 8-mile training run at 70–75% of $\dot{V}O_{2\ max}$. Eskola et al. [22] reported no change in lymphocyte number after a marathon. It is unclear why similar exercises in well-trained athletes should yield such contrasting results. Individual variation in lymphocyte number can be large, and may explain in part the differences between studies. However, Eskola et al. [22] reported extremely low statistical variances. Individual variation in hormonal response to exercise—specifically cortisol, catecholamines, and opioid peptides—can be significant. Since these molecules are potent immunomodulators (see below), individual variation may explain in part different experimental results. Also, the time at which blood samples are taken is crucial, since lymphocytosis after exercise is transitory. Lymphocyte number begins to decrease within 10 min after cessation of exercise and returns to baseline levels by 45 min, regardless of the duration or intensity of the exercise (Ahlborg and Ahlborg [23]; Robertson et al. [24]; Steel et al. [28]). In two studies which failed to find lymphocytosis (Eskola et al. [22]; Hanson and Flaherty [25]) blood samples were taken 10 and 30 min after exercise. It is possible that these samples were taken during the time when lymphocyte number had already started to decrease.

The extent of postexercise lymphocytosis changes with training (Soppi et al. [31]). Before 6 weeks of military training, postexercise lymphocyte number increased 180% over preexercise levels; after the training program, in which $\dot{V}O_{2\,max}$ increased 5%, the postexercise increase in lymphocyte number was only 49%. Thus, moderate training is sufficient to blunt lymphocyte response to exercise. This may be related to a smaller increase in catecholamine levels during exercise as a result of training.

Exercise-induced lymphocytosis is due primarily to large increases in B-cell number, with smaller or no changes in T-cell number (Hedfors et al. [29]; Landmann et al. [33]; Moorthy and Zimmerman [27]; Steel and Evans [28]; Yu et al. [32]). The absolute number and percentage of B cells increase after exercise in both trained and untrained individuals, but the magnitude of increase is higher in untrained subjects. Absolute T-cell number may remain constant (Moorthy and Zimmerman [27]) or increase (Landmann et al. [33]; Robertson et al. [24]), but the percentage of T cells decreases, and the ratio of B to T cells usually increases.

Increases in both helper (T_H) and suppressor (T_S) T-cell numbers have been noted after exercise, and the response is greater for T_S than for T_H cells (200% vs 50% increase) (Edwards et al. [34]; Hedfors et al. [35]; Landmann et al. [33]). As a result, the ratio of T_H to T_S cells decreases approximately 20% (Landmann et al. [33]). The decrease in the T_H to T_S ratio is inversely correlated ($r = -.55$) with the increased plasma epinephrine, but not with changes in cortisol levels. Both T_H and T_S cells are regulatory cells that interact with other lymphocytes, inducing or suppressing their activities, including B-cell antibody production, T-cell cytotoxic activity, and delayed hypersensitivity. It is not known if these temporary changes in T-cell subpopulations alter immunity to infection.

Significant effects on the proliferative response of lymphocytes to mitogenic stimulation after exercise have been found. Lymphocytes taken from marathon runners at rest show normal mitogenic responses to the B-cell mitogen, pokeweed mitogen (PWM), and the T-cell mitogen PHA (Green et al. [21]). After a marathon, lymphocytes from well-trained runners show decreased response to T-cell mitogens, PHA, and Con A (Eskola et al. [22]), but a shorter run (35 min) in these same runners had no effect on the response to PHA or Con A. In untrained subjects, mitogenic responses to PWM, PHA, and Con A decrease (Hedfors et al. [29]) after submaximal exercise. More study is needed to determine how fitness level and exercise intensity and duration are related to lymphocyte proliferative capacity. If exercise can be shown to alter lymphocyte proliferative capacity, it will suggest that a single bout of exercise could exert a long-lasting (i.e., days) effect on immune function.

Whether exercise-induced changes in numbers and subpopulations of circulating lymphocytes alter any in vivo immune function in a physiologically significant manner is open to speculation. Since circulating lymphocytes represent only a small fraction of the body's total lymphocyte pool, it is possible that the changes observed in the number or types of circulating lymphocytes have little effect on immune function. Alternatively, it has been suggested that the redistribution of lymphocytes from tissues to the blood may decrease resistance to disease by removing cells from local sites of initiation of the immune response (Landmann et al. [33]).

Cytotoxic Cells

Certain types of lymphocytes are capable of cytotoxic activity by one of several mechanisms. Antibody-dependent cell-mediated cytotoxicity (ADCC) is mediated by several cell types with Fc receptors, such as lymphocytes, macrophages, and granulocytes. This cytotoxicity may be involved in defense against some microorganisms and tumors. Natural killer (NK) cells are a lymphocyte subpopulation contained within the large granular lymphocytes (LGL), capable of recognizing and killing certain tumor cells, some microorganisms, and virally infected cells. Natural killer cells can be activated by interferon but do not require expansion by prior exposure to antigens. It is thought that the ability of NK cells to mount a rapid immune response to foreign agents provides a type of surveillance mechanism.

Exercise increases both ADCC (Hanson and Flaherty [25]; Hedfors et al. [29, 30]) and NK activity (Edwards et al. [34]; Landmann et al. [33]; Targan et al. [36]). In trained runners, ADCC activity is elevated immediately after, and remains elevated for 24 hr after, an 8-mile run at 70–75% of $\dot{V}O_{2\ max}$ (Hanson and Flaherty [25]). Increased ADCC activity is proportional to the increase in K lymphocyte number after moderate bicycling (Hedfors et al. [30]).

Moderate exercise (5 min bicycling or stair climbing) or short (10–20 min) maximal exercise more than doubles in vitro NK cell activity immediately after exercise when measured by either ^{51}Cr release (Brahmi et al. [37]; Edwards et al. [34]; Targan et al. [36]) or single-cell cytotoxic (Targan et al. [36]) assays. Targan et al. [36] found no change in NK cell number, as measured by single-cell assay, with a doubling in NK cell activity after 5 min of moderate exercise. The increase in NK cell activity was due to a higher percentage of NK cells that bound target cells, a faster rate of killing, and increased recycling of killer cells. However, analysis by flow cytometry did detect a four- to fivefold increase in the number of cells expressing NK cell phenotypes, Leu 7 and Leu 11a, following moderate exercise; NK cell number declines to control levels by 1 hr after exercise (Edwards et al. [34]). Differences in methods probably account for the contrasting results: Data from the studies agree closely when similar techniques were used for NK activity (^{51}Cr release) but differ when different methods were used to identify and count NK cell number (single-cell cytotoxic assay vs monoclonal labeling of cell surface markers and flow cytometry).

Interferon (IFN) stimulates NK activity in vitro (Dempsey et al. [38]; Herberman et al. [39]; Silva et al. [40]) and further augments NK activity after exercise (Targan et al. [36]). It was suggested that IFN and exercise may increase NK activity by similar mechanisms, i.e., by increasing the number of effector-target cell interactions over time (Silva et al. [40]; Targan et al. [36]). Since IFN levels increase after exercise (Viti et al. [41]), exercise may increase NK activity via release of endogenous IFN. Interferon augmentation of exercise-stimulation of NK activity suggests that either (a) exercise and IFN stimulate NK activity via different mechanisms, or (b) if exercise stimulation of NK activity is mediated via IFN, then moderate exercise does not maximally stimulate NK activity. Further study should focus on whether IFN release and NK activity respond concomitantly to more intense exercise. In addition, interleukin-1 (IL-1), a lymphokine produced by macrophages, augments the interferon-induced stimulation of NK activity (Dempsey et al. [38]), and exercise also increases IL-1 levels (Cannon and Kluger [42]; Cannon and Dinarello [43]). It is possible that the IL-1 effect is mediated by stimulation of interleukin-2 (IL-2) by T cells, since IL-2 is known to enhance NK activity. It is not known whether exercise stimulates T cells to produce IL-2, nor whether NK cell number and/or receptors for stimulating factors (e.g., IFN, IL-2) are altered by exercise. Other factors such as prostaglandins, cyclic nucleotides, or opioid peptides, all known to enhance in vitro NK function, also may be involved.

Natural killer cells provide natural immunity against a variety of challenges, such as tumor cells and virally infected cells. Exercise, even of very short duration, activates NK cells so that the in vitro rates of killing and recycling increase for at least 3 hr after exercise (Targan et al. [36]). It is not known whether this stimulation seen in vitro also exists in vivo. However, it is possible that augmentation of NK activity is responsible for the increased survival time and decreased tumor growth observed in exercise-trained mice innoculated with tumors (Good and Fernandes [15]; Rashkis [17]; Rusch and Kline [16]). It is not known whether exercise training alters the basal levels of NK activity over time. If moderate exercise and exercise training can be shown to continually augment NK activity in the intact organism, then, theoretically, appropriate levels of exercise could be used as a means of enhancing natural immunity against infections and cancer.

Whereas moderate exercise enhances in vitro NK activity measured immediately after exercise, maximal exercise of short (10–20 min) (Brahmi et al. [37]) or long duration (2 hr) (Mackinnon and Tomasi, unpublished data) decrease NK activity measured 1–2 hr after exercise. Serum factors (e.g., IFN, IL-1, IL-2) do not appear to be involved in exercise-induced suppression of NK activity, since serum taken at various times before and after exercise have no effect on in vitro NK activity (Brahmi et al. [37]; Mackinnon and Tomasi, unpublished data). The mechanism(s) mediating exercise-induced modulation of NK function is not understood fully; it most likely involves complex interaction of several factors.

Mechanisms of Changes in Leukocyte and Lymphocyte Number

The sources of additional leukocytes and lymphocytes have not been completely identified. Factors that may contribute to leukocytosis and lymphocytosis include entry of sequestered cells into the circulation, redistribution of lymphocytes, and hemoconcentration.

Lymphocytes circulate among the blood, lymph vessels, and lymphoid organs. Release of sequestered lymphocytes into, and/or decreased efflux from, the circulation most likely contribute to exercise-induced lymphocytosis. It has been suggested that lymphocytes released during exercise come from different sites than at rest: immature cells released from bone marrow, and mature cells normally sequestered in blood vessels by laminar flow.

Using [111]indium-labeled neutrophils to track leukocyte movement, Muir et al. [44] found that leukocytes are released by the lung and taken up by the spleen during exercise. It was suggested that leukocytes normally sequestered in regions of low blood flow at rest are released into the circulation by high blood flow during exercise. Using catheters to sample from the hepatic vein, Hedfors et al. [30] found no differences between arterial and venous cell counts during exercise, indicating lymphocytes are not released from the spleen.

Lymphoid organs differ in their relative proportions of lymphocyte subpopulations; different rates of release or removal of lymphocyte subpopulations could account for altered ratios of B and T cells following exercise. Lymph flow increases during exercise (Lindena et al. [45]), redistributing lymphocytes from lymphatic to blood vessels.

Inactive or immature lymphocytes and other leukocytes may be recruited and activated during exercise. It is doubtful, however, that newly synthesized lymphocytes contribute to exercise-induced lymphocytosis. Lymphocyte proliferation requires hours, and changes in lymphocyte number are seen within minutes of starting exercise (Ahlborg and Ahlborg [23]).

Hemoconcentration occurs during prolonged exercise, and may account for a small part of lymphocytosis in some studies, since lymphocyte number is expressed per volume of blood. For example, Hedfors et al. [29] reported an increase in hematocrit from 43 to 49% after 15 min moderate bicycling. However, Moorthy and Zimmerman [27] found no hemoconcentration after a 20-mile race (most likely due to frequent water ingestion during the race), and 300% and 37% increases in leukocyte and lymphocyte number, respectively. Robertson et al. [24] corrected their data for hemoconcentration and still found lymphocytosis and leukocytosis. Because hemoconcentration is usually no more than 10%, it is unlikely that it could account for more than a fraction of the increase in leukocyte number after exercise.

CHANGES IN HUMORAL AND MUCOSAL IMMUNITY AFTER EXERCISE

Resting levels of serum immunoglobulins (IgA, IgG, IgM) are normal in well-trained endurance athletes (Green et al. [21]) and do not change after moderate exercise in trained (Hanson and Flaherty [25]) or untrained (Eberhardt [46]) subjects. Production of IgG in response to tetanus toxoid was significantly higher in runners injected 30 min after a marathon compared to sedentary controls (Eskola et al. [22]), suggesting that specific antibody response may be enhanced after exercise. More studies are needed to verify this observation with other antigens.

Serum antibody response to bacterial or viral infection is delayed or prevented in rodents forced to exercise after infection. In rats forced to swim after infection with tularemia, antibody response is delayed but reaches control values by 7 days (Friman et al. [13]). In mice forced to swim after infection with coxsackie B3 virus, no neutralizing antibodies are found in serum 3–40 days after infection (Reyes and Lerner [10]). These results may represent more of a stress response by ill animals in a life-threatening situation (swimming), than actual response to exercise.

The secretory immune system of mucosal tissues is the first barrier to colonization encountered by many microorganisms invading mucosal surfaces (Tomasi and Plaut [47]). A major mechanism by which the immune system prevents local disease is the secretion of immunoglobulins in mucosal fluids. The predominant class of antibody in secretions is IgA (Tomasi et al. [48]), which has been shown to inhibit attachment of several classes of pathogens (Tomasi and Plaut [47]). Secretory antibody levels correlate closely with resistance to respiratory illness (Liew et al. [49]). In elite endurance athletes (U.S. National Nordic ski team), resting salivary IgA levels are lower than in age-matched controls and decrease further after prolonged intense exercise (20- to 50-km race) (Tomasi et al. [20]). Tomasi et al. [20] suggested that the decrease in salivary IgA levels could be due to loss of nasal fluid, changes in the transport of mucosal immunoglobulin secreting cells, or local synthesis of immunoglobulins during competition. These changes may be related to the stress of competition, physical exhaustion, prolonged exposure to cold air, or a combination of factors. Data from this lab (Mackinnon et al., manuscript in preparation) on well-trained bicyclists after a 2-hr maximal bicycle test confirm the decrease in salivary IgA levels and show reduced salivary IgM levels as well. Levels of IgA and IgM remain depressed for 1 hr after cessation of exercise and return to preexercise levels within 24 hr. Levels of IgG are unchanged by intense endurance exercise, indicating a specific effect on secretory immunoglobulins. These tests were performed in a noncompetitive laboratory setting with controlled environment, suggesting that the secretory immune system is influenced by exercise alone. Because mucosal surface antibodies are involved in early colonization of and resistance to invading bacteria and viruses, depletion could theoretically increase susceptibility to upper respiratory infection during the first several hours after intense endurance exercise.

EXERCISE-INDUCED CHANGES IN LYMPHOKINES AND OTHER FACTORS

Interleukin-1, produced by cells of monocyte–macrophage lineage, is found in human blood after a single bout of moderate exercise (60 min of bicycling at 60% of $\dot{V}O_{2\ max}$) (Cannon and Kluger [42]). Plasma from exercised humans increases body temperature and decreases plasma iron and zinc when injected into mice (Cannon and Kluger [42]) and stimulates in vitro mouse thymocyte mitogenic response (Cannon and Dinarello [43]). Release of IL-1 has been reported to mediate a host of reactions: fever; neutrophil release from bone marrow; release of acute-phase proteins; clonal expansion of T and NK cells; B-cell proliferation; and protein degradation, cellular deposition, and amino acid oxidation in skeletal muscle (for review see Dinarello [50]).

The effects of IL-1 are thought to be protective to an infected organism, in stimulating the production of lymphocytes and immunoglobulins (by increasing IL-2 synthesis) and inhibiting replication of certain viruses and bacteria (Dinarello [50]). Release of IL-1 during exercise may be related to the increased resistance to some microorganisms after exercise training (Cannon and Kluger [42]).

Several of the changes seen with IL-1 are also seen after exercise, including elevated body temperature; neutrophil release (Ahlborg and Ahlborg [23]; Hanson and Flaherty [25]; Moorthy and Zimmerman [27]); release of acute phase proteins (DuFaux et al. [51]; Liesen et al. [52]); increased NK activity (Edwards et al. [34]; Landmann et al. [33]; Targan et al. [36]) and NK cell number (Edwards et al. [34]); lymphocytosis (Ahlborg and Ahlborg [23]; Moorthy and Zimmerman [27]; Steel and Evans [28]; Yu et al. [32]); oxidation of amino acids in skeletal muscle (Poortmans [53]); and slow-wave sleep (Shapiro et al. [54]). An area for future study is whether IL-1 mediates some of the changes in immune parameters seen during and after exercise.

Interferon stimulates NK activity in vitro (Dempsey et al. [38]; Herberman et al. [39]; Silva et al. [40]), and this stimulation is further augmented when IFN is added to NK cells from exercised humans (Targan et al. [36]). When mice swim after infection with coxsackie B3 virus, no IFN is found in serum for 24 hr after infection, and the IFN response is delayed and prolonged (Reyes and Lerner [10]). The delayed response may allow early virus replication, which could account for increased viremias and higher titres of virus in the hearts of these mice.

Complement has not been extensively studied during exercise. Moderate exercise in untrained individuals causes a modest increase in complement titre (14%), but in well-trained athletes, there are no changes in complement levels measured at rest, after exercise immediately, or 24 hr after exercise (Eberhardt [46]; Hanson and Flaherty [25]).

Acute-phase proteins (APP) are serum glycoproteins associated with inflammation, such as C-reactive protein, ceruloplasmin, α-macroglobulin, α-antitrypsin (Liesen et al. [52]). Acute-phase proteins increase following prolonged intense running (2–3 hr at 80–95% $\dot{V}O_{2\,max}$ and continue to increase for 1–4 days after exercise (Liesen et al. [52]). High APP levels probably indicate tissue damage caused by intense exercise. The increase in C-reactive protein is related to running duration but not speed. The APP response to exercise is lessened after exercise training, indicating adaptation of muscles and connective tissue.

Resting C-reactive protein levels are lower in male and female well-trained swimmers, rowers, and middle- and long-distance runners than in age-matched controls (DuFaux et al. [51]). Swimmers have the lowest values of any athletes, which is not surprising since swimming is not associated with the tissue-damaging effects seen with weight-bearing activities. The authors suggested that exercise causes two opposing influences on serum C-reactive protein: an acute stimulation resulting from tissue damage after exercise, and suppression at rest due to adaptation following training.

C-reactive protein binds to T cells and alters several T-cell functions (Mortensen et al. [55]). C-reactive protein inhibits the proliferative response of sensitized T cells and the antigen-induced production of the lymphokines migratory inhibitory factor and monocyte chemotactic factor. The high levels of C-reactive protein seen for up to 4 days after intense exercise may suppress T-cell activity, but the training-induced decrease in C-reactive protein levels may reduce this suppression. No studies have correlated exercise-induced changes in lymphocyte function with changes in C-reactive protein or other APP.

HORMONAL MECHANISMS MEDIATING EXERCISE-INDUCED CHANGES IN IMMUNE PARAMETERS

Exercise causes changes in levels of several hormones, neurotransmitters, and other metabolically active molecules, many of which are also immunomodulators. Among these substances corticosteroids, catecholamines, and opioid peptides have been implicated in stress-induced modulation of immune parameters and also may be involved in mediating exercise-induced changes in immune function. Other hormones such as corticotropin-releasing factor (CRF), adrenocorticotropin hormone (ACTH), growth hormone, prolactin, and sex hormones also may be involved, but have not been extensively studied. Few studies have focused specifically on how production and release of these substances during exercise influence the immune system. Complete understanding of exercise-induced immunomodulation must await elucidation of the complex interaction of these molecules with the neuroendocrine and immune systems.

Corticosteroid Control

Plasma cortisol levels rise during exercise, but the magnitude and time course of increase and return to baseline depend on exercise intensity and duration (Galbo and Gollnick [56]). Peak plasma cortisol is related to exercise intensity and duration. During exercise of short duration (less than 20 min at 80% $\dot{V}O_{2\ max}$), plasma cortisol rises during exercise, continues to increase, and peaks 20 min after cessation of exercise. In prolonged intense exercise (longer than 60 min), plasma cortisol increases steadily throughout and peaks at the end of exercise. In both types of exercise, plasma cortisol remains elevated for about 90 min after exercise.

Because cortisol is a suppressor of some immune parameters, particularly lymphocyte number and function, it might be expected that high plasma cortisol during exercise would decrease lymphocyte number and action. However, this does not appear to be the case, which may indicate either that the effects of cortisol on lymphocytes are different after exercise compared to at rest, or that the action of cortisol is overridden by other factors during exercise. After endurance running (marathon or 20 miles) a doubling of plasma cortisol levels is accompanied by leukocytosis, including granulocytosis and lymphocytosis (Eskola et al. [22]; Moorthy and Zimmerman [27]), and changes in leukocyte and granulocyte numbers are positively correlated to serum cortisol ($r = .87$ and $.80$, respectively). In addition, increased cortisol and postrace leukocyte number are negatively correlated to training level, i.e., miles per week ($r = -.68$ and $-.60$, respectively) (Moorthy and Zimmerman [27]). Thus, the better trained the athlete, the less the rise in serum cortisol, and the lower the exercise-induced leukocytosis.

Whereas high cortisol levels resulting from exercise are associated with increases in leukocyte and lymphocyte number, corticosteroid administration before exercise suppresses leukocytosis and lymphocytosis. In untrained men, prednisone administration (60 mg) 2 hr before 10 min of moderate exercise suppresses lymphocytosis, affecting predominantly T cells; the same dose of prednisone administered 5 hr before the same exercise suppresses both T and B cells (Yu et al. [32]). The 2-hr interval between corticosteroid administration and exercise may allow for corticosteroid suppression of lymphocytosis, whereas during exercise there may not be sufficient time for corticosteroids to cause suppression. Yu et al. [32] suggest that corticosteroids alter the equilibrium of lymphocyte distribution between the intra- and extravascular compartments by reducing the entry of lymphocytes, primarily T cells, into the circulation. Corticosteroid inhibition of T-cell entry may explain why T-cell number increases only slightly following maximal exercise, when serum cortisol levels may double. Other immunomodulating molecules released during exercise, such as catecholamines and opioid peptides, also may override the suppression by corticosteroids.

Increases in plasma cortisol levels may stimulate granulocytosis during exercise, but changes in leukocyte and lymphocyte number follow plasma catecholamine levels more closely than they do cortisol levels. Lymphocytosis may actually precede increases in serum cortisol (Robertson et al. [24]), most likely due to catecholamine stimulation, and cortisol may then act later to blunt further increases in lymphocyte number.

Adrenergic Control

Plasma catecholamine levels rise with increasing work load during exercise. Norepinephrine levels increase faster than epinephrine and are higher after short-duration exercise (less than 20 min). Epinephrine levels increase more slowly, but are higher after long-duration exercise (greater than 60 min) (Galbo and Gollnick [56]). Both epinephrine and norepinephrine peak at the end of exercise, regardless of duration or intensity, and return to baseline within 10–20 min after short exercise and 30 min after longer exercise. The lymphocyte response during and after exercise closely follows changes in plasma catecholamines, increasing at the beginning and returning to baseline within 30 min after stopping. That epinephrine induces the changes in the number and subpopulations of leukocytes and lymphocytes observed during and after exercise is supported by several lines of evidence. The rate and magnitude of leukocytosis are similar following exercise and epinephrine infusion (Muir et al. [44]). Parenteral administration of epinephrine causes leukocytosis and lymphocytosis, and B-cell number increases more than T-cell number (Eriksson and Hedfors [57]). Epinephrine infusion accelerates release of leukocytes from the lungs (Muir et al. [44]). Intramuscular or subcutaneous administration of epinephrine causes rapid leukocytosis, which persists for up to 2 hr (Crary et al. [58]; Steel et al. [59]). The leukocyte response to epinephrine, like that of exercise, is biphasic, with an early rise within minutes of injection and a later peak at 60 min (Steel et al. [59]). The rate of entry of lymphocytes following epinephrine administration (3×10^8 cells per minute) is more than sufficient to account for exercise-induced lymphocytosis (Steel et al. [59]). Furthermore, the β-blocker propranolol prevents leukocytosis and lymphocytosis during exercise, indicating at least partial β-adrenergic control (Ahlborg and Ahlborg [23]).

Lymphocytes have β-adrenergic receptors (Pochet et al. [60]), suggesting that changes in plasma epinephrine may directly influence lymphocyte activity. Lymphocyte β-adrenoreceptor density and responsiveness increase immediately following a single bout of maximal exercise in untrained subjects. Twenty-five minutes after exercise, β-adrenoreceptor density decreases to 33% below resting levels, suggesting that desensitization may occur in response to high levels of epinephrine during exercise (Butler et al. [61]). After 2 months' intense training in adolescent swimmers, receptor density (measured at rest) decreased 50% and the changes in receptor density were negatively correlated to changes in $\dot{V}O_{2\ max}$ ($r = -.89$) (Butler et al. [62]). Thus, after training, lymphocytes are less sensitive to catecholamine stimulation, presumably because of the "downregulation" of their receptors which follows repeated exposure to catecholamines during training. The decrease in the magnitude of lymphocytosis observed following training (Soppi et al. [31]) may be related to the diminished response of lymphocytes to catecholamines. In addition, it is possible that exercise training may alter the immunosuppressive effects of emotional and other forms of stress by downregulating lymphocyte β-adrenergic receptors.

Epinephrine may also regulate T-cell subpopulations during exercise, perhaps also via the β-adrenergic receptor. Plasma epinephrine levels are negatively correlated to exercise-induced changes in the ratio of T_H (T_4) to T_S (T_8) cells ($r = -.55$) (Landmann et al. [33]), and a similar decrease in the T_4/T_8 ratio is observed after subcutaneous injection of epinephrine (Crary et al. [58]). It is not known whether T_H and T_S cells differ in the number of β-adrenergic receptors and/or sensitivity to catecholamine regulation.

Exercise and Opioid Peptides

Exercise causes a rapid rise in plasma β-endorphin (β-EP) and met-enkephalin. Levels of β-EP increase within minutes of starting exercise, but return to baseline within 30 min after completing submaximal (Gambert et al. [63]) or maximal (Fraioli et al. [64]) exercise. The magnitude and time course of β-EP increases most likely are related to exercise intensity and duration, and may reflect the influence of other factors released during exercise, such as catecholamines, ACTH, and corticosteroids. Opioid peptides modulate several immune parameters, including NK activity (Aarstad et al. [65]; Faith et al. [66]; Froelich and Bankhurst [67]; Kay et al. [68]; Mathews et al. [69]; Shavit et al. [70]), ADCC (Froelich and Bankhurst [67]), leukocyte locomotion (Van Epps and Saland [71]), and lymphocyte proliferative response to mitogenic stimulation (Gilman et al. [72]). Receptors for these molecules have been found on lymphocytes, including both opioid (Wybran et al. [73]; Mehrishi and Mills [74]) and nonopioid (Hazum et al. [75]) receptors. The NH_2-terminal region of the opioid peptide molecule is involved in binding to the opioid receptor, whereas the COOH-terminal region is involved in binding to the nonopioid receptor. Only the opioid receptor is inhibited by the opioid antagonist naloxone. It has been suggested that B cells have the naloxone-insensitive (nonopioid) receptor and T cells have the naloxone-inhibited (opioid) receptor (Wybran [76]). Opioid peptides have been implicated in immunosuppression observed after stress in animal models (Aarstad et al. [65]; Lewis et al. [77]; Shavit et al. [70]). Thus, it is not unreasonable to question whether changes in circulating opioid peptides are related to certain alterations in immune parameters observed during exercise.

β-Endorphin/β-lipotrophin (β-EP/β-LT) immunoreactivity in serum increases following endurance (Carr et al. [78]; Colt et al. [79]; Elliot et al. [80]; Farrell et al. [81]; Fraioli et al. [64]; Howlett et al. [82]; Kelso et al. [83]) and resistance (Elliot et al. [80]) exercise. There is a great deal of individual variation, and β-EP/β-LT does not increase in all subjects in all exercise conditions (Colt et al. [79]; Farrell et al. [81]; Howlett et al. [82]). For example, in the same subjects running the same distance (6–12 km), β-EP levels increased in only 45% of subjects (9 of 20) after a self-paced (submaximal) run, but increased in 80% of subjects (12 of 15) after a maximal run (Colt et al. [79]). The time course of changes also varies between individuals (Kelso et al. [83]). In addition, there appear to be sex differences in the β-EP response to exercise, with untrained men exhibiting larger exercise-induced increases in β-EP than untrained women (Gambert et al. [63]).

Plasma β-EP and ACTH levels increase concomitantly during exercise and follow similar time courses in returning to baseline after exercise (Carr et al. [78]; Fraioli et al. [64]). It is not surprising that plasma β-EP, ACTH, and catecholamine levels change in concert, since β-EP/β-LT and ACTH originate from a common precursor in the pituitary (pro-opiomelanocortin), and enkephalins and catecholamines are released together from the adrenal medulla in response to stress (Hanbauer et al. [84]; Viveros et al. [85]).

β-Endorphin and met-enkephalin stimulate in vitro NK activity at physiologic concentrations (10^{-4}m and 10^{-9}, respectively) in a dose-dependent manner (Faith et al. [66]; Froelich and Bankhurst [67]; Kay et al. [68]; Mathews et al. [69]). Augmentation of NK activity is reversible with naloxone (Kay et al. [68]; Mathews et al. [69]), suggesting action via the lymphocyte opioid receptor. Single cell analysis shows that β-EP increases effector to target binding. These results are similar to what has been observed in NK cells immediately after moderate exercise (Edwards et al. [34]; Targan et al. [36]) and suggests that β-EP may mediate part of the NK cell response following exercise. However, this is in contrast to reports implicating β-EP as a mediator of reduced NK activity and immunosuppression following stress in animal models (Aarstad et al. [65]; Lewis et al. [77]; Shavit et al. [70]). Moreover, in vitro NK activity is suppressed in a dose-dependent manner after 4 days of morphine injection (Shavit et al. [70]). Exercise and stress may act upon NK activity in opposite directions via β-EP mediation in conjuction with other immunomodulating hormones such as corticosteroids and catecholamines.

β-Endorphin and met-enkephalin also stimulate in vitro and in vivo leukocyte locomotion. In vitro monocyte and neutrophil locomotion increases in the presence of physiologic concentrations of β-EP or met-enkephalin, and the increase in locomotion is prevented by naloxone (Van Epps and Saland [71]). Nonadherent cell (B and T cell) locomotion is unaffected by β-EP or met-enkephalin. In vivo infusion of β-EP into rat cerebral ventricle stimulates leukocyte migration to the ventricle. Primarily monocytes and neutrophils are involved in the observed migration, indicating that β-EP is chemotactic for monocytes in vivo as well as in vitro (Van Epps and Saland [71]). Exercise-induced leukocytosis is due to release of sequestered cells into the circulation and redistribution of cells between lymphoid tissues and the circulation. It is possible that changes in chemotactic factors, such as the opioid peptides, may initiate leukocyte movement during exercise. However, unlike monocytes, lymphocyte locomotion is not stimulated by the opioid peptides, at least not without the presence of monocytes; thus it is doubtful that the opioid peptides mediate lymphocytosis observed during exercise.

It has been suggested that the stimulating effect of opioid peptides on the immune system may at times override immunosuppression by corticosteroids (Gilman et al. [72]; Plotnikoff et al. [86]). Thus, during exercise when both opioid peptide and corticosteroid levels increase, opioid peptides may modulate the immunosuppressive effects of corticosteroids. Obviously, there is a complex interaction of various immunomodulatory molecules mediating the effects of exercise and stress on the immune system.

Recent work suggests a two-way communication between the neuroendocrine and immune systems (Blalock and Smith [87]; Smith and Blalock [88]). Under some conditions, lymphocytes appear capable of producing opioid peptides and ACTH. It has been suggested that the immune system uses these neuropeptides to communicate information on immune status to the neuroendocrine system. It is not known if exercise can induce lymphocytes to produce these neuropeptides.

In addition to chemical links between the neuroendocrine and immune systems, there are adrenergic neural connections between the sympathetic nervous system and lymphoid organs, including spleen, lymph nodes, thymus, and gut-associated lymphoid tissue (Felten et al. [89]). Nerve endings are in close proximity to lymphocytes within these tissues and lymphocytes have β-adrenergic receptors (Pochet et al. [60]), suggesting the possibility of direct communication between the sympathetic nervous system and lymphocytes. The sympathetic nervous system is active during exercise, modifying activity of several systems, e.g., the cardiovascular system. Thus, it is possible that during exercise the sympathetic nervous system modifies immune parameters directly via its neural pathways to lymphoid organs.

CONCLUSION

The term "exercise" is often used loosely to describe any type of physical activity. The physiological responses to exercise depend on the specifics of the exercise: 1) the type, intensity, and duration of the exercise; 2) the individual's age and state of training; and 3) environmental conditions. It is important to discriminate between the effects of exercise and those of stress. For example, a submaximal exercise test is more stressful in an untrained than trained individual, and maximal exercise is more stressful in a competitive event than in a laboratory setting. Since stress is known to be a modulator of immune function, careful interpretation of data is vital to distinguishing between the effects of exercise and stress. Unfortunately, it is not always possible to separate the two.

In many instances exercise and stress act in opposite directions on the immune system. For example, moderate exercise enhances but stress suppresses NK activity. Exercise causes rapid leukocytosis and lymphocytosis, while stress induces the opposite effect. After exercise there is a large increase in B-cell number and a smaller increase in T-cell number, whereas during stress T-cell number decreases dramatically and B-cell number decreases somewhat less. In general, moderate exercise is either an enhancer or neutral agent, whereas stress is often an inhibitor of immune function. That exercise and stress elicit such different responses suggests stimulus-specific mechanisms and interactions, probably involving some of the same immunomodulatory molecules.

At present, comparison of data from different studies is difficult because of widely differing exercise protocols, subjects, and experimental techniques. Longitudinal training studies correlating immune function and physical activity are certainly needed. Use of different exercise intensities and durations with individuals of varying fitness levels would be helpful in distinguishing the effects of exercise from those of stress. Understanding the relationship between exercise intensity and duration and immune function would be of interest to millions of people currently participating in programs of regular physical activity. Moreover, understanding the interaction of exercise and stress, and their combined effects on the immune system, would be important to athletes who often participate in events where both elements are present. In addition, if moderate exercise can be shown to enhance immune function, appropriate levels of exercise could have potential therapeutic value in counteracting the immunosuppression that has been reported to be associated with aging (Cooper [90]), and this in turn could influence susceptibility to diseases such as cancer that occur predominantly in the elderly.

Almost all studies described in this review have looked at the immune response to exercise in young, healthy men. It remains to be seen if exercise alters immune parameters in other populations, e.g., women, children, the elderly, and those with chronic diseases. Further study is needed to determine if the transitory changes observed immediately after exercise induce long-term modulation of the immune system.

Although many studies show that exercise alters several parameters central to immunity, it has not been shown conclusively that exercise influences resistance to disease. There are several anecdotal reports of enhanced immune function with moderate exercise training and increased susceptibility to infections with "overtraining." However, objective correlation of training or fitness levels with immune status have yet to corroborate these claims. Certainly, more work is needed at both the level of the organism to look at systemic responses to exercise and at the subcellular level to determine the mechanisms behind the observed exercise-induced changes. Finally, attention has yet to be focused on how exercise may affect immunity via other immunoregulatory factors, such as prostaglandins, cyclic nucleotides, lymphokines such as interleukin-2, B-cell growth and differentiation factors and lymphocyte surface receptors for the various lymphokines, as well as the integrated activity of subsets of lymphoid cells.

REFERENCES

1. Mackinnon, L.T., Tomasi, T.B. 1986. Immunology of exercise. Ann Sports Med 3: 1–4.
2. Simon, H.B. 1984. The immunology of exercise. JAMA 252:2735–2738.
3. Bailey, G.H. 1925. The effect of fatigue upon the susceptibility of rabbits to intratracheal injections of type I pneumococcus. Am J Hygiene 5:175–195.
4. Nicholls, E.E., Spaeth, R.A. 1922. The relation between fatigue and the susceptibility of guinea pigs to infections of type I pneumococcus. Am J Hygiene 2:527–535.
5. Oppenheimer, E.H., Spaeth, R.A. 1922. The relation between fatigue and the susceptibility of rats towards a toxin and an infection. Am J Hygiene 2:51–66.
6. Horstmann, D.M. 1950. Acute poliomyelitis: relation of physical activity at the time of onset to the course of the disease. JAMA 142:236–241.
7. Weinstein, L. 1973. Poliomyelitis—A persistent problem. N Engl J Med 288: 370–372.
8. Levinson, S.O., Milzer, A., et al. 1945. Effect of fatigue, chilling, and mechanical trauma on resistance to experimental poliomyelitis. Am J Hygiene 42:204–213.
9. Rosenbaum, H.E., Harford, C.G. 1953. Effect of fatigue on susceptibility of mice to poliomyelitis. Proc Soc Exp Biol Med 83:678–681.
10. Reyes, M.P., Lerner, A.M. 1976. Interferon and neutralizing antibody in sera of exercised mice with coxsackievirus B-3 myocarditis. Proc Soc Exp Biol Med 151:333–338.
11. Gatmaitin, B.G., Chason, J.L., et al. 1970. Augmentation of the virulence of murine coxsackie-virus B-3 myocardiopathy by exercise. J Exp Med 131:1121–1136.
12. Elson, S.H., Abelmann, W.H. 1965. Effects of muscular activity upon the acute myocarditis of C3H mice infected with Trypanosoma cruzi. Am Heart J 69:629–636.
13. Friman, G., Ilback, N-G., et al. 1982. The effects of strenuous exercise on infection with Francisella tularensis in rats. J Infect Dis 145:706–714.
14. Cannon, J.G., Kluger, M.J. 1984. Exercise enhances survival rate in mice infected with Salmonella typhimurium. Proc Soc Exp Biol Med 175:518–521.
15. Good, R.A., Fernandes, G. 1981. Enhancement of immunologic function and resistance to tumor growth in Balb/c mice by exercise. Fed Proc 40:1040.
16. Rusch, H.P., Kline, B.E. 1944. The effect of exercise on the growth of a mouse tumor. Cancer Res 4:116–118.
17. Rashkis, H.A. 1952. Systemic stress as an inhibitor of experimental tumors in Swiss mice. Science 116:169–171.
18. Riley, V. 1981. Psychoneuroendocrine influences on immunocompetence and neoplasia. Science 212:1100–1109.
19. Douglas, D.J., Hanson, P.G. 1978. Upper respiratory infections in the conditioned athlete. Med Sci Sports Exer 10:55.
20. Tomasi, T.B., Trudeau, F.B., et al. 1982. Immune parameters in athletes before and after strenuous exercise. J Clin Immunol 2:173–178.
21. Green, R.L., Kaplan, S.S., et al. 1981. Immune function in marathon runners. Ann Allergy 47:73–75.
22. Eskola, J., Ruuskanen, O., et al. 1978. Effect of sport stress on lymphocyte transformation and antibody formation. Clin Exp Immunol 32:339–345.
23. Ahlborg, B., Ahlborg, G. 1970. Exercise leukocytosis with and without beta-adrenergic blockade. Acta Med Scand 187:241–246.
24. Robertson, A.J., Ramesar, K.C.R.B., et al. 1981. The effect of strenuous physical exercise on circulating blood lymphocytes and serum cortisol levels. J Clin Lab Immunol 5:53–57.
25. Hanson, P.G., Flaherty, D.K. 1981. Immunological responses to training in conditioned runners. Clin Sci 60:225–28.
26. Busse, W.W., Anderson, C.L., et al. 1980. The effect of exercise on the granulocyte response to isoproterenol in the trained athlete and unconditioned individual. J Allergy Clin Immunol 65:358–364.
27. Moorthy, A.V., Zimmerman, S.W. 1978. Human leukocyte response to an endurance race. Eur J Appl Physiol 38:271–276.
28. Steel, C.M., Evans, J., 1974. Physiological variation in circulating B cell:T cell ratio in man. Nature 247:387–389.
29. Hedfors, E., Holm, G., et al. 1976. Variations of blood lymphocytes during work studied by cell surface markers, DNA synthesis and cytotoxity. Clin Exp Immunol 24:328–335.
30. Hedfors, E., Biberfeld, P., et al. 1978. Mobilization to the blood of human non-T and K lymphocytes during physical exercise. J Clin Lab Immunol 1:159–162.
31. Soppi, E., Varjo, P., et al. 1982. Effect of strenuous physical stress on circulating lymphocyte number and function before

and after training. J Clin Lab Immunol 8:43–46.

32. Yu, D.T.Y., Clements, P.J., et al. 1977. Effect of corticosteroids on exercise-induced lymphocytosis. Clin Exp Immunol 28:326–331.

33. Landmann, R.M.A., Muller, F.B., et al. 1984. Changes of immunoregulatory cells induced by psychological and physical stress: relationship to plasma catecholamines. Clin Exp Immunol 58:127–135.

34. Edwards, A.J., Bacon, T.H., et al. 1984. Changes in the populations of lymphoid cells in human peripheral blood following physical exercise. Clin Exp Immunol 58:420–427.

35. Hedfors, E., Holm, G., et al. 1983. Physiological variation of blood lymphocyte reactivity: T-cell subsets, immunoglobulin production, and mixed lymphocyte reactivity. Clin Immunol Immunopath 27:9–14.

36. Targan, S., Britvan, L., et al. 1981. Activation of human NKCC by moderate exercise: increased frequency of NK cells with enhanced capability of effector-target lytic interactions. Clin Exp Immunol 45:352–360.

37. Brahmi, Z., Thomas, J.E., et al. 1985. The effect of acute exercise on natural killer-cell activity of trained and sedentary human subjects. J Clin Immunol 5:321–328.

38. Dempsey, R.A., Dinarello, C.A., et al. 1982. The differential effects of human leukocytic pyrogen/lymphocyte-activating factor, T cell growth factor, and interferon on human natural killer activity. J Immunol 129:2504–2510.

39. Herberman, R.R., Ortaldo, J.R., et al. 1979. Augmentation by interferon of human natural and antibody-dependent cell-mediated cytotoxicity. Nature 277:221–223.

40. Silva, A., Bonavida, B., et al. 1980. Mode of action of interferon-mediated modulation of natural killer cytotoxic activity: recruitment of pre-NK cells and enhanced kinetics of lysis. J Immunol 125:479–484.

41. Viti, A., Muscettola, M., et al. 1985. Effect of exercise on plasma interferon levels. J Appl Physiol 59:426–428.

42. Cannon, J.G., Kluger, M.J. 1983. Endogenous pyrogen activity in human plasma after exercise. Science 220:617–619.

43. Cannon, J., Dinarello, C. 1984. Interleukin-1 activity in human plasma. Fed Proc 43:462.

44. Muir, A.L., Cruz, M., et al. 1984. Leukocyte kinetics in the human lung: role of exercise and catecholamines. J Appl Physiol 57:711–719.

45. Lindena, J., Kupper, W., et al. 1984. Enzyme activities in thoracic duct lymph and plasma of anaesthetized, conscious resting and exercising dogs. Eur J Appl Physiol 52:188–195.

46. Eberhardt, A. 1971. Influence of motor activity on some serologic mechanisms of nonspecific immunity of the organism. II. Effect of strenous physical effort. Acta Physiol Pol 22:185–94.

47. Tomasi, T.B., Plaut, A.G. 1985. Humoral aspects of mucosal immunity. In: Gallin, J.I., Fauci, A.S. (eds): Advances in Host Defense Mechanisms. Raven Press, New York, pp 31–61.

48. Tomasi, T.B., Tan, E.M., et al. 1965. Characteristics of an immune system common to certain external secretions. J Exp Med 121:101–124.

49. Liew, F.Y., Russell, S.M., et al. 1984. Cross-protection in mice infected with influenza A virus by the respiratory route is correlated with local IgA antibody rather than serum antibody or cytotoxic T cell reactivity. Eur J Immunol 14:350–356.

50. Dinarello, C.A. 1985. An update on human interleukin-1: from molecular biology to clinical relevance. J Clin Immunol 5:287–297.

51. Dufaux, B., Order, U., et al. 1984. C-reactive protein serum concentrations in well-trained athletes. Int J Sports Med 5:102–106.

52. Liesen, H., DuFaux, B., et al. 1977. Modifications of serum glycoproteins the days following a prolonged physical exercise and the influence of physical training. Eur J Appl Physiol 37:243–254.

53. Poortmans, J.R. 1984. Protein turnover and amino acid oxidation during and after exercise. In: Marconnet, P., Poortmans, J., et al. (eds): Medicine and Sport Science Vol. 17: Physiological Chemistry of Training and Detraining. S. Karger, Basel, Switzerland, pp 130–147.

54. Shapiro, C.M., Bortz, R., et al. 1981. Slow-wave sleep: a recovery period after exercise. Science 214:1253–1254.

55. Mortensen, R.F., Braun, D., et al. 1977. Effects of C-reactive protein on lymphocyte functions. III. Inhibition of antigen-induced lymphocyte stimulation and lymphokine production. Cell Immunol 28:59–68.

56. Galbo, H., Gollnick, P.D. 1984. Hormonal changes during and after exercise. In: Marconnet, P., Poortmans, J., et al. (eds): Medicine and Sport Science Vol. 17: Physiological Chemistry of Training and Detraining. S. Karger, Basel, Switzerland,

pp 97–110.

57. Eriksson, B., Hedfors, E. 1977. The effect of adrenaline, insulin and hydrocortisone on human peripheral blood lymphocytes studied by cell surface markers. Scand J Haematol 18:121–128.

58. Crary, B., Hauser, S.L., et al. 1983. Epinephrine-induced changes in the distribution of lymphocyte subsets in peripheral blood of humans. J Immunol 131:1178–1181.

59. Steel, C.M., French, E.B., et al. 1971. Studies on adrenaline-induced leucocytosis in normal man. I. The role of the spleen and of the thoracic duct. Br J Haematol 21:413–421.

60. Pochet, R., Delespesse, G., et al. 1979. Distribution of beta-adrenergic receptors on human lymphocyte subpopulations. Clin Exp Immunol 38:578–584.

61. Butler, J., Kelly, J.G., et al. 1983. β-adrenoceptor adaptation to acute exercise. J Physiol 344:113–117.

62. Butler, J., O'Brien, M., et al. 1982. Relationship of β-adrenoreceptor density to fitness in athletes. Nature 298:60–62.

63. Gambert, S.R., Garthwaite, T.L., et al. 1981. Running elevates plasma β-endorphin immunoreactivity and ACTH in untrained human subjects. Proc Soc Exp Biol Med 168:1–4.

64. Fraioli, F., Moretti, C., et al. 1980. Physical exercise stimulates marked concomitant release of β-endorphin and adrenocorticotropic hormone (ACTH) in peripheral blood in man. Experientia 36:987–989.

65. Aarstad, H.J., Gaudernack, A., et al. 1983. Stress causes reduced natural killer activity in mice. Scand J Immunol 18:461–464.

66. Faith, R.E., Liang, H.J., et al. 1984. Neuroimmunomodulation with enkephalins: enhancement of human natural killer (NK) cell activity in vitro. Clin Immunol Immunopath 31:412–418.

67. Froelich, C.J., Bankhurst, A.D. 1984. The effect of β-endorphin on natural cytotoxicity and antibody dependent cellular cytotoxicity. Life Sci 35:261–265.

68. Kay, N., Allen, J., et al. 1984. Endorphins stimulate normal human peripheral blood lymphocyte natural killer activity. Life Sci 35:53–59.

69. Mathews, P.M., Froelich, C.J., et al. 1983. Enhancement of natural cytotoxicity by β-endorphin. J Immunol 130:1658–1662.

70. Shavit, Y., Lewis, J.W., et al. 1984. Opioid peptides mediate the suppressive effect of stress on natural killer cell cytotoxicity. Science 223:188–190.

71. Van Epps, D.E., Saland, L. 1984. β-endorphin and met-enkephalin stimulate human peripheral blood mononuclear cell chemotaxis. J Immunol 132:3046–3053.

72. Gilman, S.C., Schwartz, J.M., et al. 1982. β-endorphin enhances lymphocyte proliferative responses. Proc Natl Acad Sci 79:4226–4230.

73. Wybran, J., Appelboom, T., et al. 1979. Suggestive evidence for receptors for morphine and methionine-enkephalin on normal human blood T lymphocytes. J Immunol 123:1068–1070.

74. Mehrishi, J.N., Mills, I.H. 1983. Opiate receptors on lymphocytes and platelets in man. Clin Immunol Immunopath 27:240–249.

75. Hazum, E., Chang, K-J., et al. 1979. Specific nonopiate receptors for β-endorphin. Science 205:1033–1035.

76. Wybran, J. 1985. Enkephalins and endorphins as modulators of the immune system: present and future. Fed Proc 44:92–94.

77. Lewis, J.W., Shavit, Y., et al. 1983. Apparent involvement of opioid peptides in stress-induced enhancement of tumor growth. Peptides 4:636–638.

78. Carr, D.B., Bullen, B.A., et al. 1981. Physical conditioning facilitates the exercise-induced secretion of beta-endorphin and beta-lipotropin in women. N Engl J Med 305:560–563.

79. Colt, E.W.D., Wardlaw, S.L., et al. 1981. The effect of running on plasma β-endorphin. Life Sci 28:1637–1640.

80. Elliot, D.L., Goldberg, L., et al. 1984. Resistance exercise and plasma beta-endorphin/beta-lipotrophin immunoreactivity. Life Sci 34:515–518.

81. Farrell, P.A., Gates, W.K., et al. 1982. Increases in plasma β-endorphin/β-lipotropin immunoreactivity after treadmill running in humans. J Appl Physiol 52:1245–1249.

82. Howlett, T.A., Tomlin, S., et al. 1984. Release of β-endorphin and met-enkephalin during exercise in normal women: response to training. Br Med J 288:1950–1952.

83. Kelso, T.B., Herbert, W.G., et al. 1984. Exercise-thermoregulatory stress and increased plasma β-endorphin/β-lipotropin in humans. J Appl Physiol 57:444–449.

84. Hanbauer, I., Kelly, G.D., et al. 1982. [Met^5]enkephalin-like peptides of the adrenal medulla: release by nerve stimulation and functional implications. Peptides 3:469–473.

85. Viveros, O.H., Diliberto, E.J. Jr, et al.

1979. Opiate-like materials in the adrenal medulla: evidence for storage and secretion with catecholamines. Mol Pharmacol 16:1101–1108.

86. Plotnikoff, N.P., Murgo, A.J., et al. 1985. Enkephalins: immunomodulators. Fed Proc 44:118–122.

87. Blalock, J.E., Smith, E.M. 1985. A complete regulatory loop between the immune and neuroendocrine systems. Fed Proc 44:108–111.

88. Smith, E.M., Blalock, J.E. 1981. Human lymphocyte production of corticotropin and endorphin-like substances: association with leukocyte interferon. Proc Nat Acad Sci USA 78:7530–7534.

89. Felten, D.L., Felten, S.Y., et al. 1985. Noradrenergic and peptidergic innervation of lymphoid tissue. J Immunol 135:755s–765s.

90. Cooper, E.L. (ed): Stress, Immunity, and Aging. Marcel Dekker, New York.

.18.

Oxygen Transport During Exercise at Sea Level and High Altitude

Stephen C. Wood

For healthy individuals at rest, the acquisition and transport of oxygen (O_2) are subliminal processes. However, three situations bring the importance of O_2 transport, and the discomfort of hypoxia, to conscience levels. These are cardiopulmonary disease, exposure to high altitude, and vigorous exercise. These situations involve inadequate O_2 uptake (cardiopulmonary disease), inadequate O_2 supply (exposure to altitude), and/or inordinate O_2 consumption (vigorous exercise). How the O_2 transport system adjusts to altitude and exercise is the topic of this chapter.

THE OXYGEN "CASCADE"

The transport of O_2 from the environment to tissue and of carbon dioxide (CO_2) in the reverse direction involves four processes, each of which has a variable rate. The components of O_2 supply to muscle are illustrated in Figure 18-1. They are:

1. Ventilation
2. Diffusion from alveolar gas to pulmonary capillaries
3. Circulation
4. Diffusion from tissue capillaries to the cellular sites of utilization

The two active steps, ventilation and circulation, have the most variable rates and are the most important in acute compensation for exercise or disease. In chronic (or genetic) compensation the rate of diffusion is also increased both in the lungs and muscles (see Weibel [1]). The O_2 stores (lung, hemoglobin, myoglobin) are of limited value in exercise, amounting to a total of only about 2 L in a 70-kg person (Cherniak and Longobardo [2]). However, the O_2 stores of blood and cells as well as the high-energy phosphate store adenosine triphosphate (ATP) play important roles as buffers, with ATP utilization buffered by creatine phosphate and O_2 buffered by hemoglobin.

The rate of O_2 transfer at each step may be quantified by using the equations shown in Figure 18-2. The first equation uses the variables for measuring O_2 uptake in the laboratory, i.e., ventilation of air and concentration of O_2 in the inhaled and exhaled air. Oxygen

This work was supported by National Science Foundation grants PCM-7724246 and 8300472.

STEPS IN O_2 UPTAKE

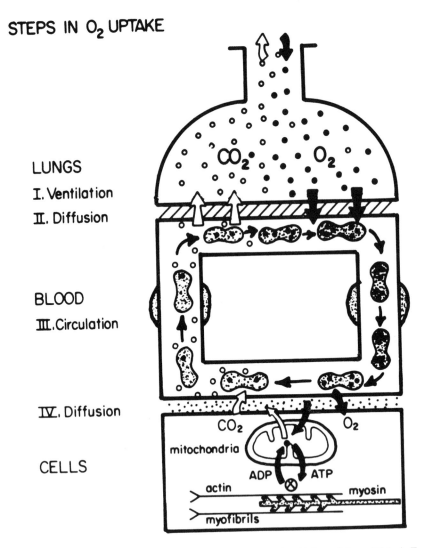

LUGS

I. Ventilation

II. Diffusion

BLOOD

III. Circulation

IV. Diffusion

CELLS

18-1 Respiratory system, indicating the four steps in O_2 uptake. (Adapted from Weibel, E. 1979. The scaling of oxygen transport in mammals. In Wood, S.C., and Lenfant, C. (eds): Evolution of Respiratory Processes: A Comparative Approach. Marcel Dekker, Inc., New York.)

transfer across the air–blood barrier (second equation) is passive, depending on the diffusing capacity (D_L) and partial pressure (PO_2) driving force. The third equation is the Fick principle, stating that O_2 delivered to tissues is the product of cardiac output (V_{blood}) and arteriovenous O_2 difference. Lastly, the rate of O_2 consumed by tissues is the product of tissue diffusing capacity (D_T) and the PO_2 difference between capillary blood and sites of tissue utilization.

These steps are in series. Therefore, under steady-state conditions, all equations give identical values of MO_2. Furthermore, the maximum O_2 uptake, measured acutely, is obviously limited by the step that has the lowest capacity to increase during exercise. It is generally accepted that for sea level- or low-altitude exercise, the limiting step is the maximum circulatory transport of O_2 (cardiac output × arterial [O_2]). However, at high altitude and during maximum exercise in athletes with very high cardiac outputs (therefore shortened transit time in pulmonary capillaries), diffusive limitations for lung O_2 transfer be-

STEPS IN O_2 UPTAKE

EQUATIONS FOR
O_2 TRANSFER

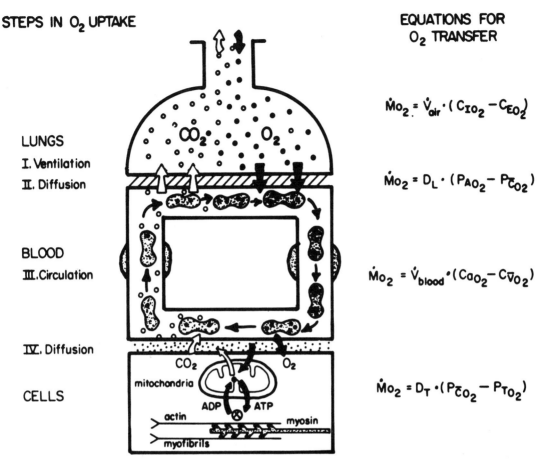

LUNGS

I. Ventilation

II. Diffusion

BLOOD

III. Circulation

IV. Diffusion

CELLS

$$\dot{M}_{O_2} = \dot{V}_{air} \cdot (C_{I_{O_2}} - C_{E_{O_2}})$$

$$\dot{M}_{O_2} = D_L \cdot (P_{A_{O_2}} - P_{\bar{c}_{O_2}})$$

$$\dot{M}_{O_2} = \dot{V}_{blood} \cdot (C_{a_{O_2}} - C_{\bar{v}_{O_2}})$$

$$\dot{M}_{O_2} = D_T \cdot (P_{\bar{c}_{O_2}} - P_{T_{O_2}})$$

18-2 Quantification of steps in O_2 transport for convective and diffusive transfer of O_2. See text for discussion.

come an important limitation (see section on oxygen transport and delivery at high altitude later in this chapter).

Variables associated with each step in O_2 transfer are presented in Figure 18-3. Each variable is also potentially adaptive to exercise-induced increases in O_2 demand or altitude-dependent decreases in O_2 supply.

OXYGEN UPTAKE

Skeletal muscle cells account for most of the O_2 uptake during rest and exercise (Hill [3]). In these and other cells, the mitochondria are the primary sites of O_2 utilization. An adequate supply of O_2 to muscle ensures that metabolic fuels are combusted to CO_2 and H_2O (Fig. 18-4). This oxidative metabolism produces 18 times as much ATP per mole of glucose as anaerobic metabolism. Adenosine triphosphate, in turn, provides energy for muscle contraction and relaxation.

With increased physical activity, O_2 consumption increases as a result of increased ATP utilization by skeletal muscles. For adults weighing about 70 kg, the O_2 uptake at rest is approximately 250 ml/min, irrespective of their athletic prowess. For untrained adults, O_2 uptake may increase 16-fold (4000 ml/min) at maximum effort; trained adults may in-

STEPS IN O_2 UPTAKE

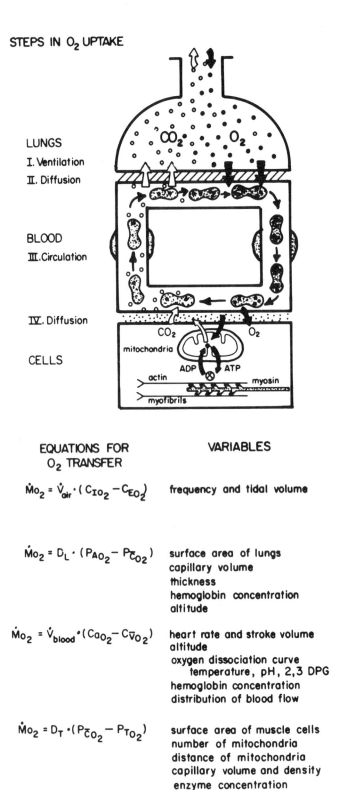

LUNGS

I. Ventilation

II. Diffusion

CO_2 O_2

BLOOD

III. Circulation

IV. Diffusion

CO_2 O_2

CELLS

mitochondria

ADP   ATP

actin   myosin

myofibrils

EQUATIONS FOR
O_2 TRANSFER

VARIABLES

$\dot{M}o_2 = \dot{V}_{air} \cdot (C_{Io_2} - C_{Eo_2})$ frequency and tidal volume

$\dot{M}o_2 = D_L \cdot (P_{Ao_2} - P_{\bar{c}o_2})$
surface area of lungs
capillary volume
thickness
hemoglobin concentration
altitude

$\dot{M}o_2 = \dot{V}_{blood} \cdot (Ca o_2 - C\bar{v}o_2)$
heart rate and stroke volume
altitude
oxygen dissociation curve
    temperature, pH, 2,3 DPG
hemoglobin concentration
distribution of blood flow

$\dot{M}o_2 = D_T \cdot (P_{\bar{c}o_2} - P_{To_2})$
surface area of muscle cells
number of mitochondria
distance of mitochondria
capillary volume and density
enzyme concentration
altitude

18-3 Main variables at each step of O_2 transfer. Each variable is a potential limit to maximum O_2 uptake.

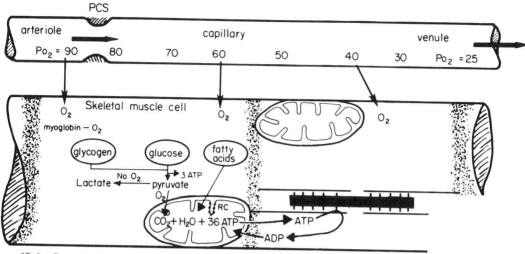

18-4   General scheme of O_2 uptake by muscle cells. Precapillary sphincters (*PCS*) vary rate of muscle capillary blood flow. See text for discussion.

crease up to 25-fold (6250 ml/min) or more. There are, however, large differences in maximum O_2 uptake between the sexes, among different types of athletes, and at various altitudes (see Table 18-1). The ability of athletes to increase their maximum O_2 uptake by training depends on the variables shown in Figure 18-3.

The relative importance of these variables will be discussed, but it is useful first to consider how a high maximum O_2 uptake is important to athletic performance. The best available data apply to distance runners. The oxygen "cost" of running is independent of running speed; i.e., O_2 uptake increases linearly with running speed and is the same for male and female runners (Fig. 18-5a). Thus, the cost of running (the slope of Fig. 18-5a) is constant at about 6.6 ml O_2/kg/min/mph. However, it should be noted that O_2 cost for improving performance in terms of time per unit distance is not a constant. Since time is the reciprocal of speed, the O_2 cost of improving running time is not linear (Fig. 18-5b). For example, to decrease running time from 10 to 8 min/mile requires an increase in O_2 uptake of about 8 ml/kg/min (from 30 to 38), but the same 2-min improvement from 7 to 5 min/mile requires an increase of about 25 ml/kg/min (from 40 to 65). Note also (Fig. 18-5) that a running speed slightly faster than 12 mph is necessary to complete a marathon in world class time. This requires an O_2 uptake in excess of 70 ml/kg/min, which is 20–30 ml/kg/min greater than the maximum O_2 uptake of untrained adults.

Table 18-1   Maximum Ventilation and Maximum Oxygen Uptake in Trained and Untrained Men and Women at Sea Level and Altitude

Age	Sex	Condition*	Body Weight (kg)	$\dot{V}_{E\,max}$ (L/min)	$\dot{V}_{O_2\,max}$ Liters/min	Ml/min/kg	Reference
33	M	UT	80.7	100	4.15	50.8	20
33	M	WCR	63.5	162	4.64	72.5	9
30	F	WCR	52.3	115	3.04	58.2	9
25	M	XCS	—	—	6.20	85.0	7
25	F	XCS	—	—	3.80	73.0	7
26	M	MC-SL	73.0	97	3.21	45.3	14
26	M	MC-5305m	73.0	145	2.26	34.4	14

*UT, untrained; WCR, world class runners; XCS, cross-country skiers; MC-SL, mountain climbers at sea level; MC-5305m, mountain climbers at altitude of 5305 meters (17,400 ft).

a

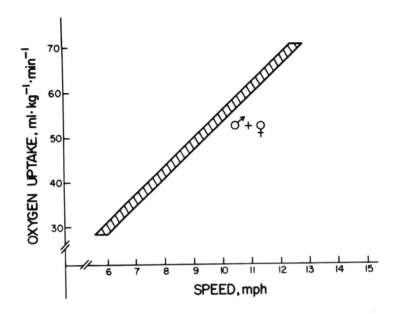

b

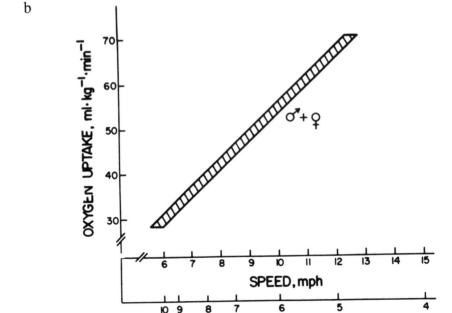

18-5 a, Oxygen uptake as function of running speed in men and women. b, Same as a, with time in minutes per mile shown on the x axis. (Redrawn from Davies, C.T.M., Thompson, M.W. 1979. Aerobic performance of female marathon and male ultra marathon athletes. Eur J Appl Physiol 41:233–245.) See text for discussion.

The importance of a high maximum O_2 uptake for competitive performance depends largely on the length of the race. In sprints and other short-distance races, the value of maximum O_2 uptake is less important, as "oxygen debts" are easily tolerated for short durations. In longer races, e.g., marathons, there is generally little or no lactic acid accumulation in trained competitors—the race is run under steady-state, aerobic metabolism. Under these conditions, there is a significant correlation between maximum O_2 uptake (measured on a treadmill) and finishing times for both male and female runners (Fig. 18-6). In a longer "ultramarathon" race, however, there is a much weaker correlation, indicating, perhaps, the importance of psychological factors.

Distribution of Blood Flow

The primary cardiovascular adaptations to exercise are an increase in total cardiac output and redistribution of blood flow to favor skeletal muscles. The change from rest to heavy work alters the proportion of cardiac output going to skeletal muscle from 15–20% to 80–85%. This redistribution of blood flow to exercising muscles is essential in assuring the increased O_2 supply during work. The O_2 uptake of muscles at maximum uptake ($VO_{2\ max}$) is about 100 times their resting O_2 uptake. With an arteriovenous O_2 difference of twice the normal, this requires a 50-fold increase in blood flow (Asmussen [4]).

The mechanism of this adaptive response to exercise has been attributed to: (a) stimulation of sympathetic vasodilator fibers resulting in an initial, even anticipatory decrease in resistance; and (b) local (auto) regulation, whereby low O_2 levels cause decreased resistance, either directly or via release of some vasodilator metabolite. More recent evidence indicates that intrinsic nerves act to maintain maximum vasodilation during muscle contraction. Intrinsic sympathetic fibers *initiate* vasodilation before contraction, assuring maximum flow at onset of contraction (avoiding early O_2 debt), and maintain maximum vasodilation during contraction. Moreover, local metabolites result in vasodilation, which persists

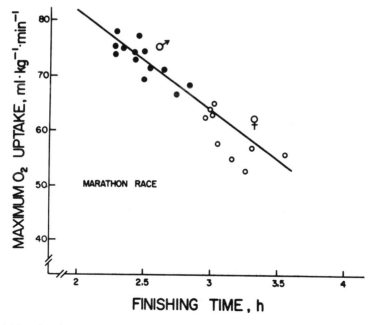

18-6 Finishing time in marathon race as function of maximum O_2 uptake for male and female runners. (Redrawn from Davies, C.T.M., Thompson, M.W. 1979. Aerobic performance of female marathon and male ultra marathon athletes. Eur J Appl Physiol 41:233–245.)

after contraction ceases, allowing repayment of an O_2 debt (Honig [5]). In addition to vaso-dilation, the increase in flow is enhanced by the recruitment of capillaries that are usually closed at rest. For example, the number of open capillaries in guinea-pig muscle increases from about 30 per mm^2 at rest to 2500 per mm^2 during exercise (Krogh [6,7]).

OXYGEN TRANSPORT VERSUS OXYGEN DELIVERY

The Fick Principle

The amount of oxygen made available to any tissue (per minute) is the product of blood flow and arterial O_2 content; i.e., systemic oxygen transport (SOT) (ml O_2/min) = Q (liters of blood/min) $\times$ CaO_2 (ml O_2/liter of blood). For a normal person at rest, SOT to all tissues is about 1000 ml O_2/min (5 L/min $\times$ 200 ml O_2/liter of blood).

The SOT determines the maximum O_2 available. However, the O_2 *delivered* (or utilized) is a more important measure. Once O_2 is transported to tissue capillaries, its utilization and uptake depend on the rate of diffusion (passive or facilitated by myoglobin). At this point it is helpful to use the Fick principle to relate the variables that determine O_2 uptake by tissues, i.e., O_2 transported in $-$ O_2 transported out, or

$$\dot{V}_{O_2} = (\dot{Q} \times CaO_2) - (\dot{Q} \times CvO_2)$$

or, since $\dot{Q}$s are equal,

$$\dot{V}_{O_2} = \dot{Q} \times (CaO_2 - CvO_2).$$

Role of the Oxyhemoglobin Dissociation Curve in Exercise

The relationship between blood O_2 content and partial pressure is described by the oxyhemoglobin dissociation curve (ODC) (Fig. 18-7). For a given ODC, the arterial (CaO_2) and the venous (CvO_2) oxygen contents correspond to a unique PO_2. The ultimate phys-

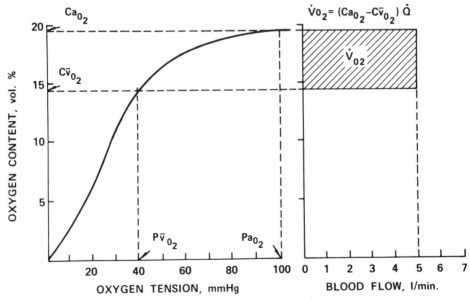

18-7 Graphic representation of the Fick principle, $\dot{V}_{O_2} = \dot{Q} \times (Ca_{O_2} - C\bar{v}_{O_2})$, showing the oxygen dissociation curve for blood. See text for discussion.

Table 18-2 Summary of Responses of Oxygen Transport System to Endurance Training

Transport System	Type of Response		
	Increased	Unchanged	Decreased
O_2 uptake	Maximum $\dot{M}O_2$	Resting $\dot{M}_2$	
Lungs	Maximum $\dot{V}E$		Ventilation at submaximal load
		Diffusing capacity	VD/VT ("dead space")
Blood	Maximum $\dot{Q}$	Maximum HR	HR at submaximal loads
	Maximum SV	Hemoglobin	Blood lactate at submaximal loads
	O_2 delivery (2,3 DPG)		Blood flow per unit muscle
Muscles	Capillary density	Efficiency of fibers	
	Oxidative enzymes		
	Mitochondria		

iologic role of the ODC is to ensure that capillary PO_2 is high enough for an adequate O_2 diffusion into tissues. Any adaptation of the shape or position of the ODC must be one that maximizes PvO_2.

Influence of the Hematocrit   One way of increasing capillary PO_2 (as reflected by PvO_2) is to have increased red cells and therefore increased O_2 capacity (and increased CaO_2). If O_2 extraction ($CaO_2 - CvO_2$) is constant, an increase in O_2 capacity (hematocrit) will result in an increased PvO_2. This is the theoretical basis for blood doping and a major component of acclimatization to mountaineering at high altitude. However, this does not seem to play a role in adaptation to exercise at sea level and is not seen in endurance runners who train at moderate altitudes (up to 7000 ft; Table 18-2).

Influence of the Position of the Oxyhemoglobin Dissociation Curve   The oxygen affinity of blood is usually quantified as the P_{50} (the PO_2 of 50% saturated blood). The P_{50} is influenced by the ODC, as shown in Figure 18-8, in which the P_{50}s are approximately 20, 27, and 30 mm Hg. The traditional view is that any factor that shifts the ODC to the left and lowers P_{50} (Curve III, Fig. 18-8) will decrease O_2 delivery, whereas a shift of the ODC to the right (Curve II, Fig. 18-8) increases O_2 delivery, and a higher P_{50} is always advantageous. However, this generalization must be qualified, particularly if arterial hypoxemia exists (Lahiri [8]). Although an increase in O_2 capacity improves O_2 delivery, an increase in P_{50} is advantageous only if arterial PO_2 exceeds a certain value and O_2 "loading" in the lung is not significantly impaired. Consequently, a high P_{50} may be detrimental during arterial hypoxemia if O_2 extraction is increased as a result of exercise or reduced cardiac output. Also, as O_2 extraction varies among different organs, so does the advantage or disadvantage of a given P_{50}.

Potent factors that alter the position of the ODC during exercise are pH and temperature. As shown in Figure 18-9, the changes in pH and temperature during exercise act together to shift the ODC to the right. At sea level in healthy people, this increases O_2 delivery to working muscles. In addition to elevated temperature and acidosis, a right-shifted ODC will result from an increase in the amount of 2,3-diphosphoglycerate (DPG) in red cells. The role of 2,3-DPG in adaptation to exercise is controversial. The results of studies at sea level on the effects of exercise on red cell 2,3-DPG levels are inconsistent. The studies

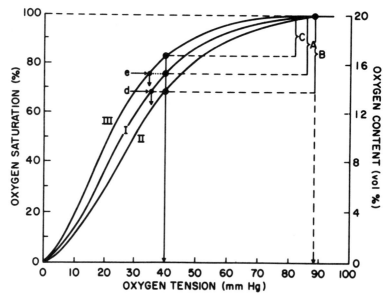

18-8 Influence of position of oxyhemoglobin dissociation curve (ODC) on O_2 extraction at normal sea level values of arterial and mixed-venous P_{O_2}. Curve I represents normal ODC in human subjects. Curve II, shift of ODC to right, increases O_2 delivery. Curve III decreases O_2 delivery (from bracket *A* to bracket *C*). (From Shappell, S.D., Lenfant, C. 1975. Physiological role of the oxyhemoglobin dissociation curve. In: Surgenor, D.M. (ed): The Red Blood Cell, Vol 2. Academic Press, New York. Reprinted with permission of the publisher.)

showing increased 2,3-DPG are almost evenly matched by those showing no change or a decrease in 2,3-DPG. When 2,3-DPG is altered and exercise capacity is examined, the results are also equivocal. At present, the best evidence indicates an insignificant effect of a left-shift mediated by 2,3-DPG in the ODC on O_2 delivery during exercise. For example, men (and rats) whose ODCs were left shifted (by 2,3-DPG depletion) showed no decrease in $\dot{V}_{O_2 \, max}$ or endurance (Wranne et al. [9]). On the other hand, phosphate loading leading to increased 2,3-DPG resulted in significantly increased $\dot{V}_{O_2 \, max}$ and anaerobic threshold in distance runners (Cade et al. [10]). The equivocal nature of the studies on 2,3-DPG and exercise probably reflects differences in experimental protocols and work levels. For example, a primary factor controlling red-cell DPG concentration is pH. Lactic acidosis would deplete 2,3-DPG, and the work levels needed to produce acidosis would depend on physical conditioning (see section on the limits of maximum oxygen uptake). Furthermore, a relatively small effect 2,3-DPG-induced change in P_{50} is expected because of the very large changes in P_{50} from temperature and pH and the high O_2 extraction of muscle.

A graphic representation of the Fick principle (Fig. 18-10) illustrates the essentials of the foregoing discussion. What happens during exercise? In this example, O_2 uptake increases to a maximum; in untrained persons the increase is about 16-fold (to 3.9 L/min). The ODC shifts to the right as a result of a decrease in pH (lactic acidosis) from 7.4 to 7.2 (middle ODC) and even farther to the right when there is an elevation in blood temperature from 37°C to 41°C. The combined factors increase P_{50} from approximately 27 to 42 mm Hg. An important concept is illustrated by the vertical lines for mixed venous P_{O_2} (Fig. 18-10). If the Pv_{O_2} remained at resting value of 36 mm Hg, the increase in P_{50} would almost double the O_2 extraction. However, actual extraction exceeds this, and actual Pv_{O_2} decreases to about 20 mm Hg. At this P_{O_2} the ODCs converge and the effect of the large change in P_{50} on extraction is greatly reduced.

Although the shift in the ODC has a more limited effect on Cv_{O_2} at low values of

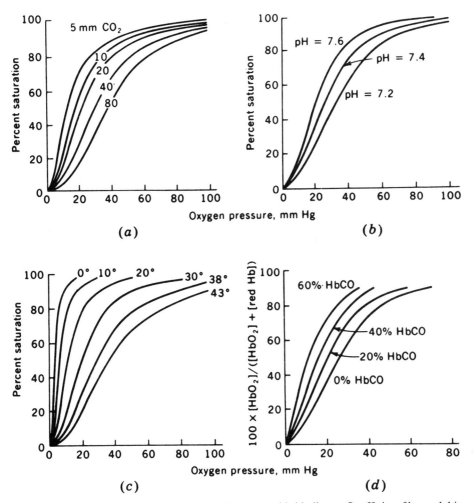

18-9 Effects of P_{CO_2}, pH, temperature, and carbon monoxide binding on O_2 affinity of hemoglobin. (From Astrand, P.O., Rodahl, K. 1977. Textbook of Work Physiology, 2nd Ed. McGraw-Hill Book Co., New York. Reprinted with permission of the publisher.)

$P_{v}O_2$, the adaptiveness of the increased P_{50} is clear when the effect on cardiac output is considered. The actual cardiac output at $\dot{V}_{O_2 max}$ is approximately 21 L/min (Fig. 18-10), but without a shift in the ODC the required cardiac output would be approximately 30 L/min, beyond the capacity of most people. A portion of the 1979 and 1980 endurance runs (28.5 miles) along the crest trail of the Sandia Mountains (near Albuquerque, New Mexico) was held at the altitude of 10,500 ft (Fig. 18-10, arrow), and most of the course is at about 9000 ft. At this level of hypoxemia ($P_aO_2 = 58$ mm Hg), the right-shifted ODC loses its advantage because "loading" of O_2 in the lungs is impaired more than the "unloading" of O_2 in muscle is increased.

Sex Differences The smaller $\dot{V}_{O_2 max}$ of women athletes in comparison with men in the same sport persists when corrected for body size (Table 18-1). Part of the reason for this difference (Fig. 18-11) is that women athletes begin with a lower O_2 capacity (less hemoglobin) and lower arterial O_2 content. Thus, although the relative O_2 extraction increases with $\dot{V}_{O_2}$ almost equally in women and men, the amount of O_2 delivered and the arteriovenous O_2 difference are much higher in men. Consequently, assuming a lower limit of

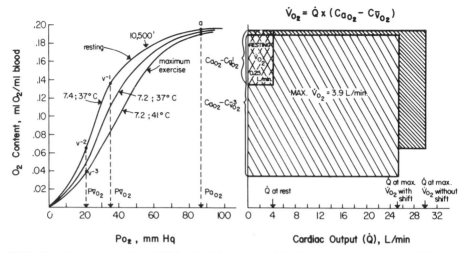

18-10 Graphic representation of Fick principle at rest and during maximum exercise. Shift of oxy-hemoglobin dissociation curve to right occurs as a result of decreased blood pH (if lactic acid accumulates) and increased blood temperature. Values for flow, O_2 contents, and partial pressures represent normal values for a healthy man at rest. O_2 uptake of 5 liters/min $\times$ 50 ml O_2/liter = 250 ml O_2/min. *Arrow,* approximate Pa_{O_2} at altitude of 10,500 ft.

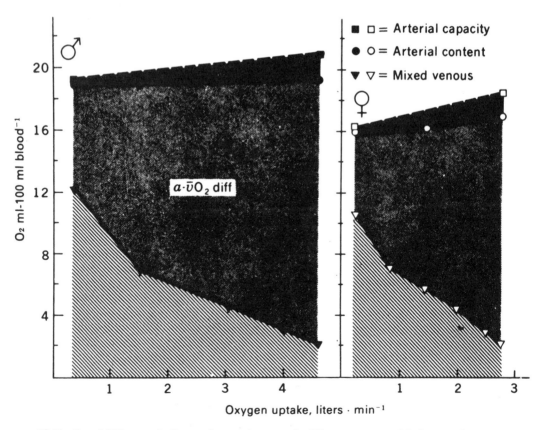

18-11 Sexual differences in O_2 capacity, arteriovenous O_2 difference at rest and during exercise up to maximum. (From Astrand, P.O., Rodahl, K. 1977. Textbook of Work Physiology, 2nd Ed. McGraw-Hill Book Co., New York. Reprinted with permission of the publisher.)

mixed venous O_2 content of 2 vol %, men have an O_2 uptake of approximately 4.5 L/min compared with 2.8 L/min for women. The role of this relative anemia in accounting for sex difference in $\dot{V}O_{2\,max}$ has not been proved. However, data for men from experiments on blood removal and reinfusion ("doping") (Fig. 18-12b) suggest that the quantity of O_2 transported to tissues *is* a main factor limiting $\dot{V}O_{2\,max}$. Preliminary data for female runners show a significant effect of blood loss (1–2% Hct decrease) and blood doping (1–3% Hct increase) on $\dot{V}O_{2\,max}$ (Pierucki et al. [11]). An important problem for future research is to determine the *optimum* hematocrit (see below) for female athletes. Is it lower than that of men and, if so, why?

Limits of Maximum Oxygen Uptake

Maximum O_2 uptake is unquestionably important to success in most types of athletic performance (see Fig. 18-6). There is also no doubt that endurance training can increase $\dot{V}O_{2\,max}$. The important questions are how this occurs and what limits $\dot{V}O_{2\,max}$.

Most evidence suggests that circulatory or metabolic factors limit maximum aerobic capacity. The principle circulatory limitation is the maximum SOT, i.e., $\dot{Q}_{max} \times CaO_2$. The previous discussion on women athletes and the evidence presented in Figure 18-12 support this argument. Figure 18-12a shows the effects of hypoxia (HbCO) and hyperoxia (high O_2) on transported O_2 during maximum running and the resulting effect on maximum O_2 uptake. The effect on breathing high O_2 (50% O_2) is attributed to an increase in dissolved O_2 delivered to tissues and not to an enhanced O_2 diffusion rate in the lungs. For example, inhalation of 25% O_2 enhances diffusion by increasing the alveolar to capillary PO_2 gradient, but there is no increase in $\dot{V}O_{2\,max}$. However, diffusion limitation may be an important factor at altitude.

Related evidence is shown in Figure 18-12b. Acute blood loss (lowering O_2 capacity) causes a sharp drop in both maximal work time (time to exhaustion during a standardized maximal run) and $\dot{V}O_{2\,max}$. Conversely, reinfusion of the packed red cells after 28 days (when O_2 capacity had returned to control values) caused a sharp increase (to supernormal values) in both measures. It is curious that analogous, but longer term, increases in hematocrit due to altitude acclimation do not have the same effect in improving $\dot{V}O_{2\,max}$ after return to sea level (Astrand and Rodahl [12]; Cerretelli [13]). As hematocrit increases, whether by blood doping or natural erythropoiesis, so does blood viscosity. A point is reached (optimum hematocrit) where further increases in hematocrit cause a decrease in cardiac output that more than offsets the increase in O_2 capacity. Thus, the product of blood flow and O_2 content (SOT) is reduced.

The value of the optimum hematocrit is not well documented under in vivo conditions. There is evidence that it increases with exercise up to values of 50–60% (Gaehtgens et al. [14]). There is also evidence that mountaineers acclimated to high altitude may, in spite of their polycythemia, not have hematocrits above the optimum for O_2 delivery. Horstman et al. [15] tested the hypothesis that bloodletting would improve performance of mountaineers. They found, however, that reducing the hematocrit of 9 subjects from 53 to 48% resulted in a decrease in $\dot{V}O_{2\,max}$ in spite of an increase in maximum cardiac output. Training does increase $\dot{V}O_{2\,max}$, and the most obvious effect of training is an increase in cardiac output. This, in turn, is due primarily to an increase in stroke volume. Training is also known to increase muscle capillary density, the concentration of oxidative enzymes (Saltin and Rowell [16]), and the volume of muscle mitochondria (Weibel [1]). Evidence that the mitochondrial content of muscle cells is the rate-limiting step in $\dot{V}O_{2\,max}$ is quite persuasive when different species or individuals of different work capacities are compared (Weibel [1]). Other responses of the O_2 transport system to endurance training are summarized in Table 18-2.

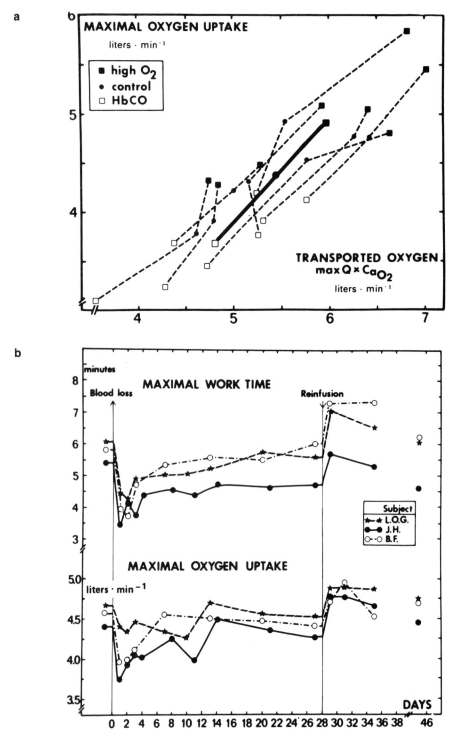

18-12 a, Effect of transported O_2 on maximum O_2 uptake during maximum running of 8 subjects. Transported O_2 was lowered by inducing 15% carboxyhemoglobin and raised by adding 50% O_2 to inspired air. b, Effects of 800 ml blood loss and reinfusion of packed cells in maximal work time (time to exhaustion during maximal running) and maximal O_2 uptake. (From Ekblom, B., Goldbarg, A.N., Gullbring, B. 1972. Response to exercise after blood loss and re-infusion. J Appl Physiol 33:175–180. Reprinted with permission of the publisher.)

Anaerobic Work

If delivery of O_2 to working muscles is inadequate, there is increased lactate formation from anaerobic metabolism and generation of an "oxygen debt." Most runners associate "exhaustion" with excessive lactic acid, although a study by Hill and Lupton [17] clearly showed that subjective "exhaustion" could occur without lactate accumulation.

The level of blood lactate during muscular work depends on: a) the rate of lactate formation, b) the rate of lactate utilization in cells, and c) the rate of diffusion of lactate into blood. The intensity of work required for lactate accumulation is variable, but it is an excellent index of fitness (Fig. 18-13). Lactate accumulation occurs with moderate work in heart patients. In sedentary but otherwise normal people, lactate accumulates when O_2 uptake reaches approximately 1.2 L/min. For an 80-kg person, this corresponds to a jogging speed of 5.7 km/hr or 17.5 min/mile. In contrast, a trained person may show no lactate accumulation until O_2 uptake reaches 2.5 L/min, equivalent to a jogging speed of approximately 9 min/mile. The speeds at which lactate accumulates are more impressive for trained runners. Many marathon racers had little or no blood lactate at the finish; the highly trained distance runners could utilize up to 90% of $\dot{V}O_{2\ max}$ for 30 min with only moderate lactate accumulation (Costill [18]). For most people, lactate accumulation begins at approximately 70% of $\dot{V}O_{2\ max}$.

OXYGEN TRANSPORT AND DELIVERY AT HIGH ALTITUDE

Oxygen Availability

One factor that brings oxygen demand from subliminal to consciousness is high altitude. At moderate altitudes hypoxia-induced hyperventilation usually remains subliminal. For ex-

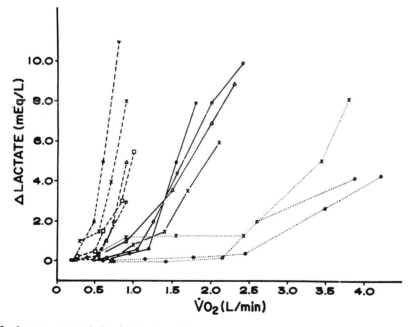

18-13   Lactate accumulation in blood at different levels of work in heart disease patients (*dashed lines*), sedentary normals (*solid lines*), and trained athletes (*dotted lines*). (From Wasserman, K., Whipp, B.J. 1979. Exercise physiology in health and disease. Am Rev Respir Dis 112:219–249. Reprinted with permission of the publisher.)

ample, normal $PaCO_2$ at an altitude of 5000 ft is about 36 mm Hg, compared with approximately 40 mm Hg at sea level. Most people become aware of a hypoxic drive to breathe at an altitude of 9000–11,000 ft. Although the fraction of oxygen is constant at about 21%, the inspired PO_2 (PIO_2) falls with falling barometric pressure (P_B) according to the equation:

$$PIO_2 = (P_B - 47) \times 0.21,$$

where 47 is the vapor pressure of water at normal body temperature. The effect of altitude on P_B and PIO_2 is illustrated in Figure 18-14. Alveolar (PAO_2) is determined by PIO_2, $PACO_2$, and the respiratory exchange ratio (R) according to the equation:

$$PAO_2 = PIO_2 - PACO_2/R.$$

The importance of hyperventilation in altitude adaptation is emphasized when PAO_2 is calculated for the summit of Mt. Everest (altitude 8848 m; 29,200 feet). This summit, the highest point on earth, is by provocative coincidence the highest altitude attainable by man. It was first reached by Messner and Habeler without supplemental O_2 in May 1978. Barometric pressure at this altitude is approximately 250 mm Hg. Thus, PIO_2 would be $(250 - 47) \times 0.21 = 43$ mm Hg. If $PACO_2$ and R remained at sea level values (i.e., no hyperventilation), PAO_2 would be the impossible value of

$$PAO_2 = 43 - 40/0.8 = -7 \text{ mm Hg.}$$

The observed survival of humans breathing air at this altitude is possible only by a drastic reduction of $PACO_2$ by hyperventilation. The 1981 American Medical Research Expedition to Mt. Everest obtained alveolar gas samples on the summit. They found a mean $PACO_2$ of 7.5 mm Hg (see West [19]). This degree of hyperventilation, an essential corequisite of a successful ascent to the summit, provides a PAO_2 of about 30 mm Hg. This,

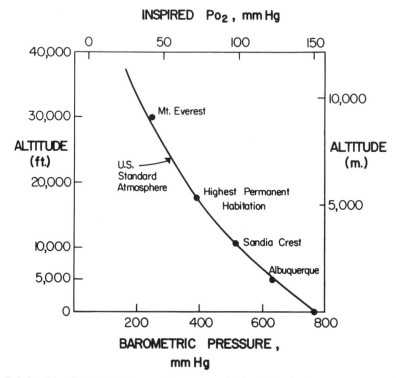

18-14 Relationship of altitude to barometric pressure (PB) and inspired oxygen pressure (PI_{O2} = (PB − 47) × 0.21).

however, is not enough, since without a long period of acclimatization, a PAO$_2$ of 30 would render normal persons unconscious.

The Oxygen "Cascade" at High Altitude

The drop in PO$_2$ at each step of O$_2$ transport becomes much less as altitude increases. The decrease in the first drop (PIO$_2$ − PAO$_2$) reflects the increasing degree of hyperventilation as altitude increases. The second drop in PO$_2$ (PAO$_2$ − PaO$_2$) also decreases as arterial oxygenation begins to occur on the steeper portion of the ODC. However, because the driving pressure for diffusion (PAO$_2$ − PCO$_2$) is vastly reduced (from a PO$_2$ of approximately 60 mm Hg at sea level to approximately 11 mm Hg at 29,000 ft), there is a substantial diffusion limitation on Mt. Everest, even at rest. Similarly, the reduced drop in blood PO$_2$ (PaO$_2$ − PvO$_2$) reflects the fact that tissue O$_2$ delivery is occurring on the steep portion of the ODC.

The Fick Principle at High Altitude

The graphic representation of the Fick principle in Figure 18-15 presents data (Pugh [20]; Pugh et al. [21]) on O$_2$ transport at high altitude and emphasizes the crucial importance of increased O$_2$ capacity in adaptation to altitude. Indeed, after acclimation to an altitude of 5800 m (19,000 ft), the arterial O$_2$ content at rest and during light work (300 kg/min) is (at 70% saturation) the same as or slightly higher than the preacclimation sea level value (97% saturation). For the O$_2$ uptake of 0.91 at this work rate, the O$_2$ delivery and cardiac output is the same at sea level and 5800 m.

At the higher work rate of 900 kg/min (equivalent to running about 5.5 mph), Vo$_2$ is 1.96 L/min and the effects of altitude are pronounced. Arterial saturation decreases, presumably as a result of diffusion limitation, causing a smaller O$_2$ extraction than at sea level. This was the highest work rate for which adequate data were available. Maximum heart rate

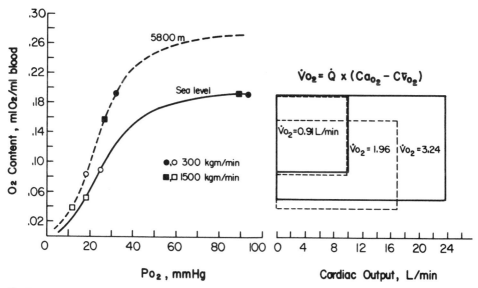

18-15 Graphic representation of Fick principle during light (300 kg/min), moderate (900 kg/min) $\dot{V}_{O_2}$ = 1.96 liters/min, and heavy (1500 kg/min) work at sea level and at 5800 m altitude. The $\dot{V}_{O_2}$ of 1.96 liters/min corresponds to a work level of 900 kg/min at 5800 m. See text for discussion. (Based on data in Pugh, L.G.C.E. 1964. Cardiac output in muscular exercise at 5800 m (19,000 ft). J Appl Physiol 19:441–447.)

decreases at altitude, apparently as a result of increased parasympathetic tone and direct effects of hypoxia on the sinoatrial node (Cerretelli [13]). This accounts for the reduction in maximum cardiac output since maximum stroke volume is not affected by altitude.

Most of the evidence points to a circulatory limit of $\dot{V}O_{2\ max}$, i.e., the maximum O_2 transport ($\dot{Q}_{max} \times CaO_2$). Studies in which subjects breathing O_2-enriched air show an increase in $\dot{V}O_{2\ max}$ indicate that the oxidative capacity of muscles exceeds the O_2 transport capacity of blood. At high altitude, diffusion limitation may also play a role in limiting $\dot{V}O_{2\ max}$ because arterial saturation and CaO_2 decrease as work rate increases. This would result from both a decrease in transit time of red cells in pulmonary capillaries and a decrease in the (alveolar–capillary) PO_2.

The decrease in $\dot{V}O_{2\ max}$ at high altitude is usually due to a decrease in both $\dot{Q}_{max}$ and CaO_2. The upper portion of a curve illustrating $\dot{V}O_{2\ max}$ at different barometric pressures (Fig. 18-16) is relatively flat, but there are significant diminutions of athletic performance at moderate altitudes. For example, there were no world records established in endurance events in the Olympic games held in Mexico City ($P_B = 580$ mm Hg). The predicted $\dot{V}O_{2\ max}$ on Sandia Crest would be only 80% of the sea level value. Extrapolation of this curve suggests that $\dot{V}O_{2\ max}$ would be zero at P_B of approximately 240 mm Hg. On the summit of Mt. Everest ($P_B = 250$ mm Hg) the $\dot{V}O_{2\ max}$ would be only 3–4 ml O_2/min/kg, roughly the basal $\dot{V}O_2$. Cerretelli [13] made an interesting observation (Fig. 18-16) in his study on factors limiting O_2 transport on Mt. Everest. He found that even when subjects were breathing 100% O_2 at P_B of 390 mm Hg, they were unable to attain the preexisting sea level $\dot{V}O_{2\ max}$ in spite of a 40% increase in hematocrit and a limited reduction in maximum cardiac output ($\dot{Q}_{max}$). He speculated that this could be explained by the increased viscosity of the blood, which would alter the microcirculation such that blood (and O_2) would bypass the resistance blood vessels in muscle.

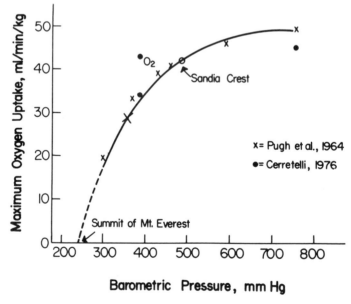

18-16 Relationship between maximum O_2 uptake and barometric pressure. See text for discussion. (Based on data from Pugh, L.G.C.E. et al. 1964. Muscular exercise at great altitudes. J Appl Physiol 19:431–440; and Cerretelli, P. 1976. Limiting factors to oxygen transport on Mt. Everest. J Appl Physiol 40:658–667.)

Oxygen Dissociation Curve During High-Altitude Exercise

For a given work rate, more lactic acid is produced at high altitude than at sea level. On the other hand, acute altitude-induced hyperventilation will produce respiratory alkalosis. Thus, the role of acid-base balance in O_2 transport is complex. In addition, the advantage or disadvantage of a left or right shift of the ODC depends on altitude and arterial PO_2. Therefore, the familiar and advantageous right shift of the ODC during exercise at sea level could be maladaptive at high altitude. Whether or not a right shift of the ODC occurs as a result of increased 2,3-DPG depends primarily on blood pH. A decrease in pH inhibits overall glycolytic rate and 2,3-DPG phosphatase, causing a depletion of 2,3-DPG. Alkalosis has the opposite effect by activating 2,3-DPG mutase, causing accumulation of 2,3-DPG. The redox potential of the red cell, reflected by the ratio of lactate to pyruvate, is also a key factor. In hypoxia, as the lactate/pyruvate ratio increases, 2,3-DPG levels decrease.

As previously noted, there is little agreement on the role of 2,3-DPG-induced shifts in the ODC as an adaptation to exercise at sea level (Thomson et al. [22]). The picture is equally cloudy at high altitude. In a recent study of marathon racing at 1600 m altitude, 2,3-DPG and P_{50} were found to increase in the slower finishers, but not in the runners with times under 3:20 (Wood et al. [23]). In two endurance runs along the crest of the Sandia Mountains (altitude 7000–10,650 ft) all runners ($n = 40$) who did not become acidotic had an increase in P_{50}, whereas those who were acidotic at the finish ($n = 7$) had a decrease in P_{50}. The changes in P_{50} were related to the degree of acidosis and the consequent changes in red cell 2,3-DPG (Wood and Hoyt, unpublished observations). Because of the low PaO_2 during much of the run, it is not certain that runners with increased 2,3-DPG benefited by the right-shifted ODC, although the right shift in ODC offsets the effect of alkalosis, which has an opposite effect. Clearly, much more work is needed to elucidate the role of ODC and its modulators in the adaptation to exercise at sea level and high altitude.

REFERENCES

1. Weibel, E.R. 1985. The Pathway for Oxygen. Harvard University Press, Cambridge, MA.
2. Cherniak, N.S., Longobardo, G.S. 1970. Oxygen and carbon dioxide stores of the body. Physiol Rev 50:196–243.
3. Hill, A.V. 1922. The maximal work and mechanical efficiency of human muscles and their most economical speed. Am J Physiol 56:19–26.
4. Asmussen, E. 1965. Muscular exercise. In: Fenn, W.O., Rahn, H. (eds): Handbook of Physiology (Vol. 2). American Physiological Society, Washington, D.C., p 943.
5. Honig, C.R. 1976. Mechanisms of circulation metabolism coupling in skeletal muscle. In: Grote, J., Reneau, D., et al. (eds): Oxygen Transport to Tissue (Vol. 2). Plenum Publishing, New York, pp 623–639.
6. Krogh, A. 1919. The supply of oxygen to the tissues and the regulation of the capillary circulation. J Physiol 52:457–474.
7. Krogh, A. 1936. The Anatomy and Physiology of Capillaries. Yale University Press,, New Haven, CT.
8. Lahiri, S. 1975. Blood oxygen affinity and alveolar ventilation in relation to body weight in animals. Am J Physiol 229:529–536.
9. Wranne, B., Nordgren, L., et al. 1974. Increased blood oxygen affinity and physical work capacity in man. Scand J Clin Lab Invest 33:347–352.
10. Cade, R., Conte, M., et al. 1984. Effects of phosphate loading on 2,3 diphosphoglycerate and maximal oxygen uptake. Med Sci Sports Exer 16:263–268.
11. Pierucki, C., Serniak, E., et al. 1985. Effects of blood loss and blood doping on maximum O_2 uptake and anaerobic threshold in female runners. Fed Proc 44:1370.
12. Astrand, P.O., Rodahl, K. 1977. Textbook of Work Physiology (2nd Ed). McGraw-Hill, New York.
13. Cerretelli, P. 1976. Limiting factors to oxygen transport on Mt. Everest. J Appl

Physiol 40:658–667.

14. Gaehtgens, P., Kreutz, F., et al. 1979. Optimal hematocrit for canine skeletal muscle during rhythmic isotonic exercise. Eur J Appl Physiol 41:27–39.

15. Horstman, D., Weiskopf, R., et al. 1980. Work capacity during 3 week sojourn at 4,300 m: effects of relative polycythemia. J Appl Physiol: Respir Environ Exer Physiol 49:311–318.

16. Saltin, B., Rowell, L.B. 1980. Functional adaptations to physical activity and inactivity. Fed Proc 39:1506–1513.

17. Hill, A.V., Lupton, H. 1923. Muscular exercise, lactic acid and the supply and utilization of oxygen. J Med 16:135–171.

18. Costill, D.L. 1970. Metabolic responses during distance running. J Appl Physiol 28:251–255.

19. West, J.B. 1983. Climbing Mt. Everest without oxygen: an analysis of maximal exercise during extreme hypoxia. Respir Physiol 52:265–271.

20. Pugh, L.G.C.E. 1964. Cardiac output in muscular exercise at 5,800 m (19,000 ft). J Appl Physiol 19:441–447.

21. Pugh, L.G.C.E., Gill, M.B., et al. 1964. Muscular exercise at great altitudes. J Appl Physiol 19:431–440.

22. Thomson, J.M., Dempsey, J.A., et al. 1974. Oxygen transport and oxyhemoglobin dissociation during prolonged muscular work. J Appl Physiol 37:658–664.

23. Wood, S.C., Schade, D.S., et al. 1979. Marathon racing at 1600 m altitude: effects on red cell 2,3 DPG and hemoglobin-oxygen affinity. Fed Proc 38:1050.

SECTION 5
Locomotion and Sports

•19•

Ocular Injuries
in Athletic Activities

William Selezinka

Increasing emphasis on athletics in schools and in communications media and the resulting surge in the numbers of persons engaging in exercise and body conditioning have led to an increased number of ocular injuries. Eye safety in athletics through preventive measures, public education, and design of protective eye devices has been emphasized, but eye injuries still occur (Pashby [1]). Some of these are unavoidable, others are due to carelessness or refusal to wear protective devices; nevertheless, three out of four people fear blindness more than any other illness except cancer (Research to Prevent Blindness, Inc. [2]). This is significant when one considers that 75% of sensory input is through the eye. Ophthalmologists treating ocular trauma see a substantial number of cases that result from recreational activities.

Eye injuries should not be ignored, because, initially, they may appear deceptively mild (irritation and some tearing, slightly blurred vision, or transient double vision). If associated with head injury, however, the symptoms may be attributed to central disturbances of the visual system when both central and peripheral injuries coexist. A superficial injury of the eye or surrounding structures may be the outward sign of a more severe contusion of the eye itself. An obvious severe injury of the lids or globe should be managed by an ophthalmologist. In other, less severe injuries, the examining physician should perform a thorough eye examination (Wilkinson [3]). Practical knowledge of management of ocular injuries is important for early correct diagnosis and treatment. This may prevent worsening of the injury and possible subsequent blindness (Morin [4]).

Between 2% and 4% of the population have unilateral amblyopia, so among 1 million sports participants, 20,000–40,000 can be expected to have varying degrees of unilaterally impaired vision (Pashby [5]). In these people, injury of the normal eye may be tragic. A survey of eye injuries in ice hockey participants indicates that 15% became legally blind, and the highest number occurred in 11- to 15-year-olds (Pashby [6]). Another study showed that 16 of 38 eye injuries required hospitalization of the victims, 12 of whom needed follow-up care for late complications from angle recession, subluxated lens, traumatic cataract, and retinal detachment. Some even required enucleation (Vinger [7]). One-half of traumatic retinal detachments were legally blind even after successful surgery (Antaki et al. [8]), and 31%–44% had less than 20/40 vision. In racquetball, tennis, and squash, up to one-half the injuries required hospitalization, mostly due to hyphema (Easterbrook [9]). Many eye injuries have peripheral retinal tears and detachments. Some of these can be repaired if treated early. Others have central retinal damage. In squash the likelihood of eye injury is not reduced even in an experienced player (Seelenfreund and Freilich [10]). Thorough ophthalmologic examination is urgent for all sports-injured eyes.

MANAGEMENT OF OCULAR TRAUMA

Good records are essential. Notes are made of how the eye was injured and whether glasses, contact lenses, or a protective device was worn. Previous eye injury, disorder, or systemic disease (e.g., bleeding disorder) that might affect management or outcome should be noted (Levin and Bell [11]). Signs and symptoms such as decreased vision, diplopia, and pain should be recorded.

It is always important to check visual acuity. This can be done with a Snellen chart or a Rosenbaum near-vision card (Fig. 19-1) held 14 inches from the eyes, which should be individually tested. In a presbyope, near vision is tested with bifocals or reading glasses. If only finger-counting or hand-movement vision exists, the distance at which this is possible is noted. Care is taken to indicate whether the patient has light perception (LP). If he or she also detects the direction from which the light is coming (light projection—LP), then it is recorded as LP & LP, as light perception is required to detect light direction. No light perception (NLP) is recorded when the eye is totally blind, which may be the case in an optic nerve avulsion or in a fracture of the optic nerve canal in which the nerve is severed. Vision should be measured with spectacle correction or, if the glasses are broken, with a pinhole and a Snellen chart. Visual fields should be examined by confrontation (Fig. 19-2).

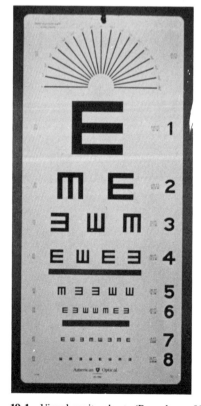 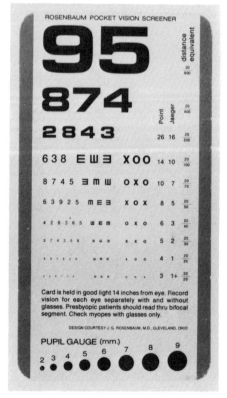

19-1 Visual acuity charts (Rosenbaum Vision Screener).

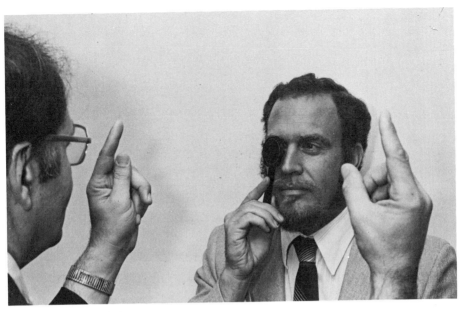

19-2 Confrontation field.

The extent of ecchymosis, chemosis, and conjunctival hemorrhages is recorded (Fig. 19-3), and preceding infection of the periorbital skin, lids, conjunctiva, or tear sac is noted. Ocular motility is checked in all directions of gaze and diplopia is looked for with a red glass. Restricted eye movements may indicate extraocular muscle entrapment in a bony orbital fracture. The orbital rim is palpated, and cutaneous sensation below the eye is tested. One should feel for lid crepitus from subcutaneous emphysema, usually originating from a fractured paranasal sinus. Displacement of the globe should be noted and measured if an exophthalmometer is available. Auscultation for orbitocranial bruit should also be done.

Depth and location of lid lacerations, especially if they involve the nasolacrimal system or the canthal tendons, should be noted. If present, they require the attention of an ophthalmic surgeon to reconstruct proper tear drainage, equal-sized eye apertures, and a good cosmetic result by a three-layer closure.

Pupil size, shape, and equality, and reactions, including the results of the swinging penlight test for a possible Marcus Gunn pupil (usually from an optic nerve injury), are recorded.

The swinging penlight test is useful in the detection of pupillary afferent fiber defects. It consists of shifting a light back and forth from pupil to pupil, allowing approximately 5 sec at each eye to observe for dilatation of the pupil. In a normal eye, the illuminated pupil may redilate slightly. In the affected eye, however, pupillary redilatation during illumination is proportional to the severity of the conduction defect in the injured optic nerve (Paton and Goldberg [12]).

Actual pupillary size may be measured in millimeters with a pupil scale on a Rosenbaum chart. It is especially important to note a pupil dilated from trauma to the sphincter or ciliary ganglion, or a constricted pupil from traumatic iritis or Horner's syndrome, secondary to accompanying neck or brachial plexus injury. A "teardrop" pupil usually indicates iris entrapment in a corneal or scleral laceration.

One notes if a hyphema is present and if there is an iridodialysis or iridodonesis (a tremulous iris because of loss of support from a subluxated or dislocated lens).

Finally, a loupe or slit lamp (which many hospital emergency rooms now have) should be used to check for corneal abrasions, foreign bodies, and hyphema. The slit lamp helps in

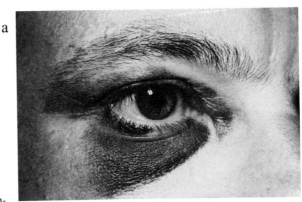

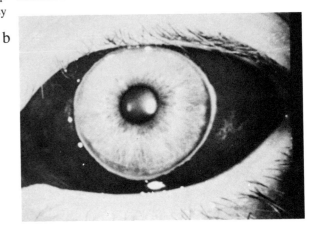

19-3 Ecchymosis (a) and subconjunctival hemorrhage (b). (Courtesy of University of Michigan)

assessing the anterior chamber for microscopic hyphema, traumatic iritis, and the state of the lens—i.e., its location and whether or not there is a traumatic cataract. The anterior vitreous can also be examined for red blood cells, which may be present from a peripheral retinal tear. At the same time, the intraocular pressure can be measured if the cornea is intact.

Systematic ophthalmoscopic examination after athletic injuries should include the optic nerve, retinal vessels, choroid, macula, and peripheral retina. An indirect ophthalmoscope is best for visualizing peripheral retinal dialysis or tears, hemorrhages, or retinal edema through a dilated pupil. This should be done soon after injury, as vitreous blood may later spread and obscure the retina. Central retinal edema (commotio retinae) is very common in contused eyes, and it can best be seen with the red-free light of the ophthalmoscope. It should be noted that more mistakes are made by not looking than by not knowing. Many eye injuries receive delayed, inadequate, or misguided treatment. Therefore, a methodical, thorough examination and proper treatment are essential.

All extraocular injuries must have an intraocular examination.

X-ray examinations of the orbits, facial bones, and, when indicated, skull and optic nerve canals should be made in contusion injuries or if an intraocular or intraorbital foreign body is suspected. In some cases, a CAT scan may be useful, and documentation by photography is also often helpful. The clinical evaluation of an injured eye may be difficult because of the patient's tendency to squeeze the eye shut and to blink vigorously as a result of photophobia and intense lacrimation. The examination should, therefore, be performed in subdued light. Some of the blepharospasm may be overcome by the use of local anesthetic. This should not be used indiscriminately, nor should it be given for self-medication at home, as a severe (chemical) keratitis may result from its overuse. After the lids are relaxed and open, one can measure visual acuity. If the lids are still closed, they can be retracted gently by hand or with a small lid retractor. At the same time, the cornea should be inspected for abrasions, lacerations, and foreign bodies. If examination cannot be done, one should gently apply an eye patch and send the patient to an ophthalmologist or hospital as soon as possible.

DECREASED VISION IN INJURED EYES

Decreased vision after eye injury may result from trauma to various ocular structures. In severe lid injury resulting in massive swelling and/or blood on the cornea, vision is impaired. A hyphema, dislocated lens, or traumatic cataract may also be responsible. Commotio retinae (macular edema) or hemorrhages of the retina resulting from a direct blow may decrease vision, and choroidal rupture in the macular area or between the macula and the optic nerve also impairs vision. A central retinal artery or vein occlusion from direct compression of these vessels by orbital hemorrhage may decrease vision or cause total visual loss. Retinal detachment and vitreous hemorrhage are other causes. Lastly, cortical blindness (patient may be unaware of blindness) may result from a blow, usually to the back of the head, such as occurs in contact sports. Various causes of visual loss must, therefore, be considered in evaluating the injured eye.

LID INJURIES

The extent of lid injuries should be ascertained. At the same time, the eye itself must also be examined. Tetanus prophylaxis should be given if indicated, as for lacerations and avulsions of other body parts. Simple lid lacerations need meticulous primary repair. Many oculoplastic ophthalmic surgeons recommend the use of a microscope for better approximation of the various layers and for removal of microscopic foreign bodies within the wound. Each anatomic lid layer (skin, orbicularis muscle, and tarsus-palpebral conjunctiva) should be repaired separately (Fig. 19-4). Because of the abundance of skin in the lid vicinity, large skin defects can be closed by undermining and sliding skin over the more fixed, deeper layers. Skin grafts may be obtained, if needed, from the area behind the ear.

Fat in the laceration, orbital septum perforation, and a deep injury in the eyelid could involve the eyeball (Fig. 19-5). An absent lid fold (in non-Orientals) or blepharoptosis may point to traumatic dehiscence of the levator palpebrae muscle, which requires repair by an ophthalmologist. However, soreness or photophobia can cause partial "protective ptosis," which disappears when the irritation subsides.

Medial and, particularly, lateral canthal tendon damage is frequent in trauma and should be identified and repaired. Lacerated lid margins require proper reapposition at the gray line and the use of 7-0 or 9-0 silk for suturing. A continuous strip of tarsus at least 3 mm wide should be left at the margin. These injuries should be treated by an ophthalmologist.

The lacrimal duct canaliculus may be transected in lacerations near the medial canthus. This also requires meticulous repair with fine silicone tubing (Fig. 19-6). Dental malocclusion and facial bone fractures may be associated with a nasolacrimal duct tear between the tear sac and nose.

Marked lid ecchymosis from a direct blow often results because of good blood supply to the area. Orbital or subconjunctival hemorrhage and even proptosis may also be present.

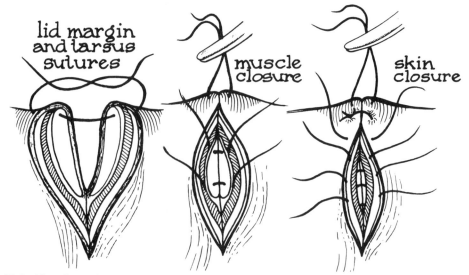

19-4   Three-layer closure of full-thickness lid laceration.

Hemorrhage may spread subcutaneously across the midline from one eye to the other or may extend to the cheek and jaw over 24–48 hr. The spread is of no consequence, except that it may indicate coexisting serious orbital injury. For example, ringlike periorbital blood may indicate skull fracture. An orbital floor fracture is often associated with inferior orbital and lower lid ecchymosis and anesthesia of lateral skin of the lower lid, side of the nose, and cheekbone because of involvement of the infraorbital branch of the trigeminal nerve. Orbital roof fracture may present as ecchymosis of the upper lid and subconjunctival hemorrhage, the blood spreading along the levator muscle, and downward under the conjunctiva.

The treatment of lid ecchymosis is similar to that of contusions elsewhere. At first, cold compresses are used for 24–48 hr. This may be changed to warm compresses later. Sunglasses are worn for cosmetic reasons.

Enlarged submaxillary and preauricular nodes may indicate infection. The lymphatic drainage from the temporal third of the lids is to the preauricular nodes and the nasal two-thirds drains to the submaxillary lymph nodes.

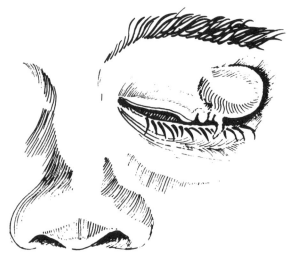

19-5   Orbital fat protruding through lid laceration.

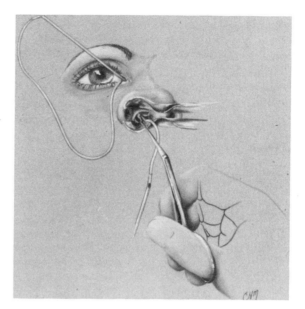

19-6 Canaliculus repair. (Courtesy of A. Perry, La Jolla, CA)

ORBIT INJURIES

The orbital rim protects the eye from blows by objects larger than the rim circumference. An anterior orbit blow causes serum and blood release into the lids and surrounding tissues, forcing eyelid closure. Mild to severe proptosis and even ophthalmoplegia may result from orbital hemorrhage. Anesthesia of skin served by the supraorbital and infraorbital nerves occurs if they are involved in fracture margins. Diplopia and impaired upward gaze often result from inferior rectus and inferior oblique muscle entrapment in an orbital floor fracture (Fig. 19-7). Subcutaneous emphysema, which may be seen on X-ray, can cause lid crepitus and indicates medial orbital wall (ethmoid sinus) fracture. Systemic antibiotics should be given to these patients because of the possibility of orbital cellulitis due to organisms entering from the paranasal sinus. When orbital fractures are present, straining (heavy lifting) and nose-blowing should be avoided. Orbital roof fractures may cause cerebrospinal fluid rhinorrhea. Plain X-ray films of the skull, orbits, and sinuses miss many fractures of this

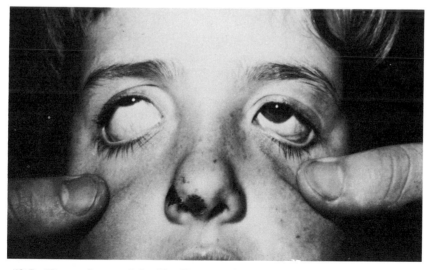

19-7 Blowout fracture, left orbit. (Courtesy of University of Michigan)

type. Tomography or computerized axial tomography correlated with clinical findings is often required for identification of orbital fractures (Fig. 19-8).

The timing of surgery is important. Delay of up to 10 days may be required for edema to subside, but surgery should be done before fibrosis begins. Early repair may be justified if there is obvious enophthalmos, X-ray proof of the fracture, and the patient is undergoing surgery for another facial injury. Postoperative complications can occur. Many cases do not require surgery. Postoperative complications include enophthalmos, limitation of vertical gaze, lower lid ectropion, trichiasis, postoperative cellulitis, dacryocystitis, extrusion of implant, and even postoperative visual loss from surgical trauma to the optic nerve or from orbital hemorrhage.

CONJUNCTIVAL AND CORNEAL INJURIES

Commonly seen conjunctival trauma leads to subconjunctival hemorrhage. Most of the time, specific treatment is not indicated. If the hemorrhage is severe, with chemosis, eye closure may not be possible. When this occurs, application of an ointment to the eye, and coverage with adhesive transparent kitchen wrap protects the cornea until the lids can be closed again (Fig. 19-9). An ice pack may help to reduce swelling. Associated injuries are of more concern. Severe chemosis may indicate an intraorbital foreign body, scleral rupture, and invisible conjunctival perforation—associated with an invisible scleral perforation, an orbital fracture, or a carotid-cavernous fistula. Therefore, careful avoidance of pressure on the eye during examination is essential to prevent prolapse of the intraocular contents through a possible hidden scleral wound. Foreign bodies removed from *perforating* conjunctival injuries should be cultured for bacteria and fungus even though perfora-

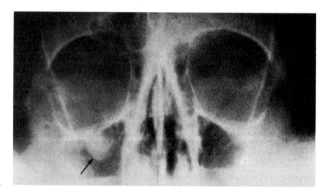

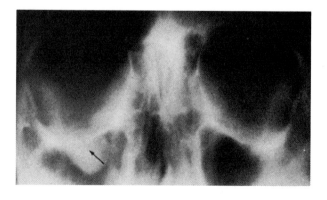

19-8 Plain X-ray film of blowout fracture (top) and tomography (bottom) for comparison. (Courtesy of Dr. Hanafee, University of California, Los Angeles)

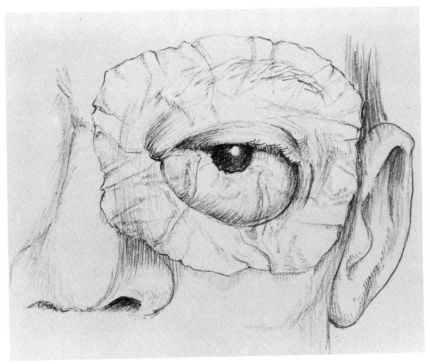

19-9   Adhesive transparent kitchen wrap protects excessive chemosis.

tions seldom become infected and usually heal rapidly. Conjunctival lacerations longer than 1 cm are repaired, or if they are contaminated and extensive, they require débridement. Traction on the plica semilunaris by sutures should be avoided, and Tenon's fascia should not be caught in wound edges, nor should conjunctival epithelium be trapped subconjunctivally.

Corneal abrasions are painful. Because of tearing, severe pain, and lid spasm, clinical examination is difficult and can be assisted by use of topical anesthetic and an oblique light. A sterile fluorescein paper strip stains areas of corneal epithelial loss. If a fluorescein strip is not available (avoid aqueous fluorescein solutions, which may harbor *Pseudomonas* after the bottle has been opened), a light directed at suspected damage may reveal corneal abrasions. When the light is moved parallel to the iris, the corneal defect may be seen as a shadow on the iris opposite to the light (Fig. 19-10). The upper lid is everted to check for foreign bodies that may be responsible for the abrasion (Selezinka [13]) (Fig. 19-11). Dry cotton swabs should not be used on the eye. However, a saline-moistened cotton swab may be used to remove foreign bodies from the corneal surface. Corneal abrasions are managed by the instillation of antibiotic and mydriatic drops, followed by snug application of two pads to the injured eye. The cul-de-sac accommodates only one drop of medication; therefore, the time of application of the two medications is spaced and the punctum occluded with tissue or cotton ball for 30 sec before patching. If healing is slow or there is doubt, an ophthalmology consultation should be obtained. Steroid-containing medications are not indicated for corneal abrasions because an occult herpetic infection of the cornea could spread.

Hard contact lenses should be removed soon after severe facial injury if this can be done easily before the lids swell (Selezinka [13]). Corneal and corneoscleral lacerations are the domain of the experienced ophthalmic surgeon. These may be present with iris prolapse and give the pupil a teardrop shape. Surgery should be performed as soon as possible.

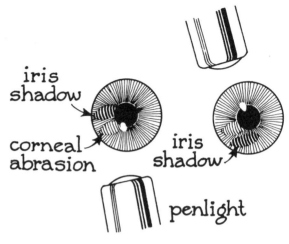

19-10 Shadow cast on iris by corneal abrasion.

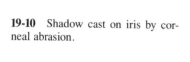

CONTUSIVE INJURIES

In contusion, the anterior segment may be involved, causing a hyphema (Fig. 19-12). The hyphema may layer inferiorly or fill the entire chamber. Approximately 20% rebleed. Between 25% and 50% eventually result in 20/40 vision or less. Therefore, an ophthalmologist's care is essential (Paton and Goldberg [12]). Patients require hospitalization, biomicroscopy, and applanation tonometry for daily intraocular tensions, to record deterioration resulting from multiple areas of eye damage. In addition, approximately 7% of patients develop glaucoma in later years because of angle recession produced by the trauma (Fig. 19-13). Somnolence is the hallmark of hyphemas, particularly in young people; the possibility of coexisting head injury must be excluded.

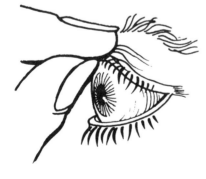

19-11 Everting upper lid.

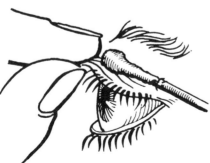

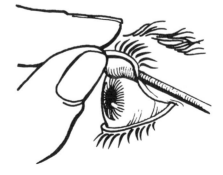

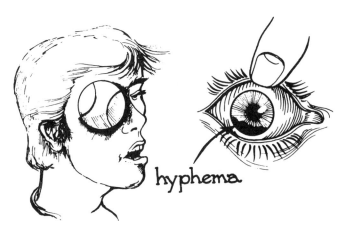

19-12 Hyphema.

Traumatic mydriasis from rupture of the iris sphincter results in permanent pupillary deformity. The lens may be dislocated and produce visual changes or develop a cataract.

Scleral rupture with intact conjunctiva commonly occurs at the limbus and may not be easily visible. The rupture is usually arc-like and opposite the impact site but near the rectus muscle insertion on the nasal side (Fig. 19-14). Marked localized hemorrhagic chemosis and a hyphema are always present. The lens may be dislocated subconjunctivally through the rupture site. Surgical intervention is necessary.

The presence of a vitreous hemorrhage should be considered when the "red reflex" is lost and an ophthalmoscopic view is hazy or bloody. It signifies damage to the retina, choroid, or ciliary body. Treatment consists of bed rest. An old vitreous hemorrhage may eventually need vitrectomy.

Central retinal edema (commotio retinae) is common after direct blows. Initially, vision decreases as edema increases, and then it gradually improves. Return to normal depends upon the extent of the injury. Perimacular pigmentary changes eventually occur. In boxers, recurrent contusive injury may cause persistent edema, with macular cyst or hole formation and loss of central vision (Fig. 19-15). Chronic edema after a single injury may produce the same bad results. Central retinal edema appears as a whitish, cloudy discoloration. Comparison with the uninvolved eye using a red-free ophthalmoscope light aids in diagnosis. An Amsler grid shows irregular lines.

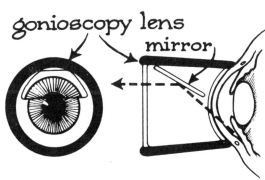

19-13 Angle recession.

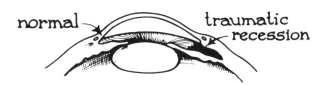

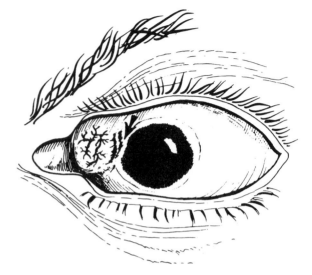

19-14 Scleral rupture at limbus.

Retinal hemorrhages, edema, and exudates may result from a direct blow to the eye, a blow to the back of the head, or from contrecoup injury. Retinal detachment may occur as a result of a tear in the extreme peripheral retina (Cox et al. [14]; Weidenthal and Schepens [15]). It is estimated that 15% of all detachments result from trauma. Retinal dialysis may occur immediately after trauma (Fig. 19-16). About 80% of retinal detachments become symptomatic within 2 years of trauma, although the detachments usually occur soon after injury. Floating black specks, a persistent cobweb in the peripheral visual field, and light flashes are symptoms that make one suspicious of detachment. Ophthalmoscopy shows a billowy grayish retina that may shift as the patient moves the eye. Traumatic detachments occur near the ora serrata in 59.4% of cases, and 9.1% are of the posterior type (Cox et al. [14]). The ora serrata type progresses insidiously until the macula is involved, and is seen primarily in young people after sports accidents. Surgical intervention is indicated. *All* orbital contusive injuries need careful indirect ophthalmoscopy to prevent eventual visual loss.

In sports the frequency of ocular injuries can be summarized as follows (adapted from Rousseau [16]):

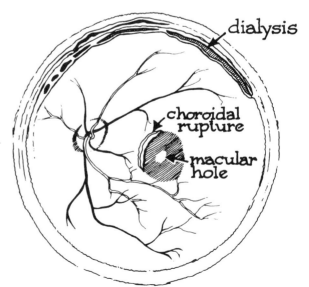

19-15 Schematic of traumatic retinopathy.

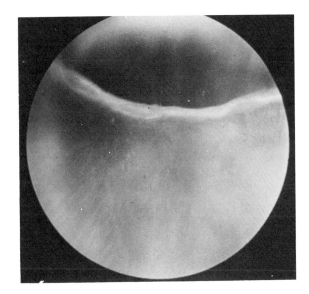

19-16   Retinal dialysis.

Hockey	31.0%
Sporting equipment (BB, darts, etc.)	19.3%
Transport (bicycle, snowmobile, etc.)	16.5%
Racquet sports	10.3%
Baseball, etc.	8.2%
Golf, fishing, boxing, skiing, basketball	14.3%

Sports cause significant eye injuries. Physicians need to impress sports participants of the need to prevent eye injury by the use of protective devices or by game rule changes. Recognition of a variety of eye injuries in athletics and subsequent proper management by the primary physician is important. Thorough examination and good records aid in treatment. The risk of visual loss from an unrecognized serious eye injury is high. Therefore, it behooves the physician to realize that more mistakes are made by not looking than by not knowing.

REFERENCES

1. Pashby, T.J. 1977. Eye injuries in Canadian hockey. Phase II. Can Med Assoc J 117:671–678.
2. Research to Prevent Blindness, Inc. Annual Report. 1977. New York.
3. Wilkinson, C.P. 1976. Injury in the vicinity of the eye. In: O'Donoghue, D.H. (ed): Treatment of Injuries to Athletes, 3rd Ed. W.B. Saunders Co., Philadelphia, pp 130–132.
4. Morin, D.J. 1978. Primary management of ocular trauma. Can Med Assoc J 118:305–307.
5. Pashby, T.J. 1975. Eye injuries in Canadian hockey. Can Med Assoc J 113:663–674.
6. Pashby, T.J. 1979. Eye injuries in Canadian hockey. Phase III. Can Med Assoc J 121:643–644.
7. Vinger, P.F. 1976. Ocular injuries in hockey. Arch Ophthalmol 94:74–76.
8. Antaki, S., Labelle, P., et al. 1977. Retinal detachment following hockey injury. Can Med Assoc J 117:245–246.
9. Easterbrook, M. 1978. Eye injuries in squash. Can Med Assoc J 118:298–305.
10. Seelenfreund, M.H., Freilich, D.B. 1976. Rushing the net and retinal detachment. JAMA 235:2723–2776.
11. Levin, D.B., Bell, D.K. 1977. Traumatic retinal hemorrhages with angioid streaks. Arch Ophthalmol 95:1072–1073.
12. Paton, D., Goldberg, M.F. 1976. Management of Ocular Injuries. W.B. Saunders Co., Philadelphia.
13. Selezinka, W. 1979. Eye injuries. In: Ryder, S.M. (ed): To Help You Save

Lives. Rescue Publications, Scottsdale, pp 33–34.

14. Cox, M.S., Schepens, C.L., et al. 1966. Retinal detachment due to ocular contusion. Arch Ophthalmol 76:678–685.

15. Weidenthal, D.T., Schepens, C.L. 1966. Peripheral fundus changes associated with ocular contusion. Am J Ophthalmol 62:465–477.

16. Rousseau, A.P. 1979. Ocular trauma in sports. In: Freeman, H. M. (ed): Ocular Trauma. Appleton-Century-Crofts, New York, pp 353–361.

•20•

General Surgery and Sports Medicine

William R. Schiller

Many athletic injuries are primarily orthopaedic in nature, but minor problems may be referred to a general surgeon. These include not only soft-tissue injuries, but also those involving thoracic and abdominal viscera. In addition, general surgeons may be asked to diagnose and manage surgical illnesses unrelated to injuries in athletes. The most common injuries of athletes are lacerations and contusions. Blisters, abrasions, and calluses also cause discomfort and loss of competitive edge in many sports.

SOFT-TISSUE INJURIES

Contusion

Injury from being struck by another participant or by a piece of equipment is inevitable in a variety of contact sports. Although abrasion or laceration of overlying skin may occur, the common denominator of contusions is bleeding into soft tissues; the severity of this is directly proportional to the force applied. Blood from small vessels dissects into tissue planes, causing the appearance of diffuse bruising rather than presenting a localized hematoma. This type of bleeding usually does not result from injury to larger vessels. Much morbidity (bruising) results from the large quantity of blood that extravasates and dissects into the tissue planes. Painless function is regained faster when extravasation is minimized. Measures that limit the effects of bruising include cold pack application—usually a dry, protected ice bag—to the injured part. This procedure causes vasoconstriction and minimizes bleeding into the injured site. Although rebound vasodilatation may occur after cold application, it can be limited by continued use of the cold pack until the injury is stable, usually 24 hr following injury. Thereafter, when further bleeding is less likely, warmth can be applied locally to decrease discomfort. Localized cutaneous injury from the cold application can be prevented by placing a layer of material such as a pantleg between the ice bag and the skin (Fig. 20-1). Moreover, keeping the area dry decreases the likelihood of cold injury. Compression of the injured area with a woven elastic bandage over the ice bag to hold it in place further limits bleeding. Finally, elevation of the injured part minimizes swelling. Rest for the acutely injured part is beneficial, but athletes should be encouraged to maintain

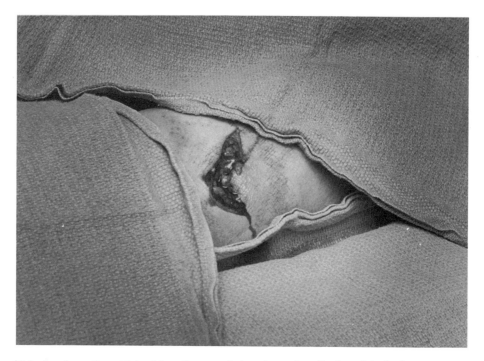

20-1 Leg laceration with bruising after wound cleansing and application of sterile drapes.

general conditioning by exercising uninjured body parts. Graded activity may be resumed when pain and swelling are gone. The use of a contused area should be regulated so that pain and/or swelling does not recur. If either becomes apparent, the athlete is exercising the injured part too soon or too vigorously and should limit its use. This general program should allow a return to full athletic capability over the ensuing week.

Hematomas

Subcutaneous hematomas are common in participants of contact sports. Small hematomas resorb with appropriate padding and should be allowed to do so. Larger, more localized hematomas resolve more quickly if aspirated one or more times. Diffuse hematomas within muscle bundles are difficult to aspirate, but localized hematomas are usually removed easily with a syringe fitted with a large-bore needle. Drainage of hematomas by incision should be resisted unless they are infected. Incising hematomas converts a trivial wound into a serious open wound that takes a long time to heal, causing restriction of active participation in sports. Needle aspiration of hematomas should be preceded by proper antiseptic skin preparation to prevent introduction of pathogenic bacteria into the wound.

Lacerations

Small lacerations are frequent on the athletic field, and those that penetrate the skin should be sutured, since primarily closed wounds heal more rapidly with less scarring than those that are allowed to heal secondarily. Minor lacerations not involving deeper structures can be sutured in the locker room, but larger ones should be cared for in the emergency department. After the wound has been cleansed thoroughly with soap and water, sterile drapes are applied (Fig. 20-2). Many athletes feel that they are obliged to accept sutures without local anesthetic. However, a better and more meticulous repair can be done with local anesthetic

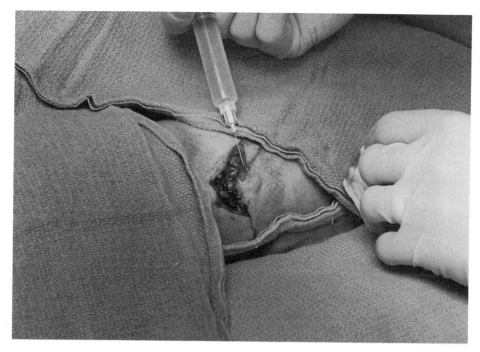

20-2 Clean wound being infiltrated with local anesthetic solution prior to primary suture repair.

use, and players will appreciate the afforded comfort (Fig. 20-3). It is unpleasant, ineffective, and unnecessary to suture a writhing, grimacing athlete for purely "macho" reasons. If activity is resumed, a protective dressing, often including a splint, should be used over the healing laceration until a mature scar has formed. In lacerations of the hands, this is especially important since repeated trauma causes inflammation in the healing wound. Lacerations in certain areas of the body require special attention:

Eye When lacerations occur around the eye, the eye itself should also be examined. When facial lacerations are being treated, the eyebrow should never be shaved. The likelihood of infection is not increased if eyebrows are left, and the risk that they will not regenerate to a normal configuration is eliminated. The possibility of a facial fracture underlying a laceration should be kept in mind. Closure of these wounds to restore anatomical layers using fine sutures is the technique of choice.

Ear Ear lacerations must be treated with care if the cartilage, which is especially susceptible to infection, is involved. Cartilage infection may cause loss of substance and result in ear deformity. Aseptic techniques and thorough cleansing must be meticulously performed prior to wound closure with fine sutures. The cartilage should be reapproximated to its anatomic position with fine, soluble suture. Overlying skin can then be closed in a separate layer, using 6–0 nylon sutures. A splinting dressing will then support and maintain the normal shape of the ear during healing. The ear should be padded, inside protective headgear, until healing is complete.

Hematoma formation between the skin and auricular cartilage, causing a painful "cauliflower ear," is a well-known injury in wrestlers. The clinical setting for this injury is as follows: The victim is held tightly around the head and either attempts to, or does in fact withdraw from the grip of the opponent, causing contusion and shearing of the ear. The hematoma must be drained for maximal restoration of contour through a small skin incision

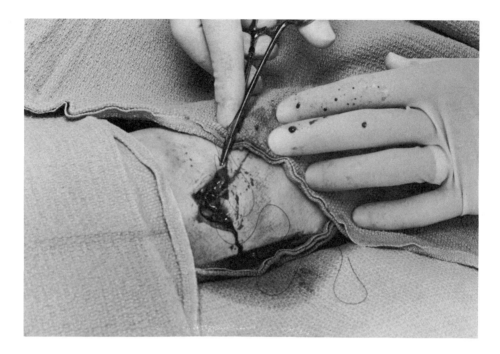

20-3 Closure of the wound using sterile technique and fine suture material. A protective dressing is applied after the wound edges are reapproximated.

under local anesthesia. The underlying cartilage should be avoided, and several incisions may be necessary to completely evacuate the clot. The ear must then be encased in a splinting dressing. One should warn athletes with this injury that residual deformity may occur. More attention should be paid to preventing the injury through use of proper headgear.

Tongue or Lip A bitten tongue or lip is another common injury that may either be self-induced or result from a blow to the mouth by an opponent. Tongue lacerations are best closed with absorbable sutures in layers, under local anesthesia. If the tongue is not sutured, a nodule of tissue, frequently bitten accidentally by the patient, will result. Prompt healing can be expected if repaired properly. Lip lacerations are common in many sports and should be closed in layers so that the orbicularis oris is reapproximated, as well as the overlying mucous membrane and skin. Careful attention must be paid to realigning the vermilion lip border so that normal contour is restored. Careless suturing of the vermilion border, with resultant offset after recovery, is not acceptable.

HAND INJURIES

Hand injuries are relatively frequent and include superficial abrasions, lacerations, and injury of underlying tendons and bones. Fingernails are commonly avulsed, partially or totally, or a blow to the finger may cause a subungual hematoma. If the avulsed fingernail is partially attached, it is best replaced on the nailbed. A proper dressing over the repositioned nail is needed and the finger should be protected until the nail regrows. Only completely avulsed nails should be discarded, and the nailbed in this case should be covered with a sterile, nonadherent dressing. Occasionally a laceration involves the nail without avulsion. This should be treated as any other laceration, with reapproximation of tissue planes and a sterile dressing. Subungual hematomas are painful because of increased pressure caused by blood between the nail and nailbed. The throbbing pain can be incapacitating even to a stoic athlete. Treatment is drainage through a hole drilled in the nail. A hot paper clip may be used to melt a small hole in the nail to allow the underlying blood to escape. In most cases, this can be done painlessly without local anesthetic. Drainage provides instantaneous relief of pain. A fracture of the underlying distal phalanx is commonly present with subungual hematomas; therefore X-ray examination of the finger is recommended. This injury is not usually a cause of prolonged disability, and most athletes promptly return to full activity, especially if damage has not occurred to the underlying phalanx. Hand injuries may involve more than the overlying skin. Therefore, examination of nerve and tendon function is necessary when lacerations are deep. If these structures are clinically involved, the injury should be treated by a surgeon with a special expertise in hand injuries. A final good result is often related to proper early management, so the team physician must be alert to the possibility of complicated hand injury. Fractures of hand bones may occur either from direct involvement in athletic events or from an altercation, commonly seen in hockey games. Fifth metacarpal fracture from such incidents may cause residual hand and finger deformity if not cared for properly. With metacarpal fracture, the hand must be carefully examined for teeth marks, for the human bite is prone to infection. Careful cleaning of the laceration is, therefore, important. Consideration should be given in each case as to whether primary or delayed closure of the human bite wound is the safer management. Most surgeons give antibiotics to victims of human bites.

NECK INJURIES

Neck injuries may involve associated damage to the cervical vertebrae and underlying spinal cord. Those who complain of neck pain after an injury should be carefully evaluated for contusion of cervical musculature or more serious injuries, such as vertebral fractures. If the diagnosis is not clear, the athlete must have cervical spine X rays and neurologic evaluation. Poorly conditioned athletes who take unexpected falls are especially vulnerable to cervical vertebral injuries. Indications of injury to these vital structures require neurosurgical consultation. Less devastating is neck contusion, which may produce a hematoma in the cervical musculature. This can be managed as for any other contusions, but attention should be given to assuring an adequate airway, since a large hematoma may produce tracheal-compression. Injuries to the larynx must also be considered. An athlete who is struck in the neck and then has hemoptysis should be suspected of sustaining airway injury, which requires prompt treatment to avoid or remedy airway obstruction.

THORACIC INJURIES

Serious intrathoracic injuries are not common in athletes, since impact forces to the well-protected thorax are not sufficient to produce visceral injury. Exceptions are jockeys and race car drivers, who may be subjected to considerable force against the thoracic cage in the event of an accident. In contact sports, however, athletes commonly complain of painful contusions of the lower rib cage. Although the ribs are seldom fractured, these injuries produce considerable morbidity because of pain. When ribs are fractured, athletes often have difficulty breathing and will subsequently refrain from all-out effort because of fear of repeating the injury. Contused areas may involve the cartilaginous portions of the ribs, which do not heal rapidly. Prompt recovery is probably most assured if the athlete continues general conditioning but is withdrawn from actual contact until chest pain begins to subside. Rib fractures are painful and inhibit respiratory excursion of the involved hemithorax. Chest examination may reveal splinting, which produces a noticeable difference in respiratory excursion between the sides. The fracture site is tender, so crepitation of the fracture edges should not be attempted in making the diagnosis. Management includes exclusion of injury to underlying organs (hemothorax or pneumothorax). The presence of subcutaneous air may be a good clinical indication of pneumothorax. Attempted taping of broken ribs is usually not satisfactory and only inhibits respiratory effort without affording protection or pain relief. The most common intrathoracic injury is simple pneumothorax, which is usually associated with a rib fracture and produces an inordinate amount of dyspnea. The pneumothorax is visible radiographically, and treatment is placement of a chest tube. A small pneumothorax may resorb without a chest tube, but faster resolution occurs when air is aspirated via a properly placed tube connected to water-seal drainage. Occasionally, rib fractures are associated with free blood in the pleural cavity either with or without pneumothorax. The hemothorax may be detectable only by chest X ray even though the rib fracture is obvious clinically. The blood should be removed by tube thoracostomy, for it takes considerable blood to produce an abnormality on the chest film. Most severe intrathoracic injuries, cardiac contusion, and great vessel injury are seen in association with automotive trauma and not athletic events.

Foreign-body aspiration occurs occasionally in athletes. They should not have objects in their mouths (chewing gum or tobacco) on the playing field. The techniques for removal of aspirated objects are well standardized, but prevention is certainly the best and least embarrassing method of dealing with this problem.

INJURIES OF ABDOMINAL MUSCULATURE

Abdominal wall contusions are common and should be treated in the same manner as contusions elsewhere on the body. They are painful and may require prolonged convalescence before maximal activity is again possible.

Hernias should be repaired during the off season when possible. Most surgeons do not allow significant weight-lifting or other physical stress until 6 weeks after hernia repair. At that time, the tensile strength of the wound should be about 90% of normal. Most athletes can resume conditioning training at that point, within limits of discomfort. Activities that cause discomfort should be temporarily stopped until it is certain that no harm is being done to the wound. Gradual increase to normal activity without discomfort should be the rule. Weight-lifters, who generate tremendous strain on the abdominal wall, require special care. Gradual resumption of effort seems to be the safest policy.

Acute appendicitis requiring appendectomy is a common affliction of young people. Most surgeons remove the appendix through a transverse lower abdominal incision, which heals readily and is strong in uncomplicated cases. Wound strength is from the overlying abdominal wall musculature, which is merely split and not divided during surgery. These patients may resume some conditioning activities 3 weeks after surgery or whenever the wound becomes painless. Contact sports should not be allowed for approximately 6 weeks after appendectomy.

INTRA-ABDOMINAL INJURIES

Intra-abdominal injuries are relatively uncommon in contact sports because the forces generated are of low kinetic energy. Although a blow to the abdomen may produce a painful contusion or intramuscular hematoma, injuries to underlying viscera are exceptional.

Athletes suspected of having sustained an intra-abdominal injury should be thoroughly examined as soon as possible. This may include laboratory tests to detect bleeding or peritonitis. The organs most commonly injured from blunt trauma are the liver and spleen, because of their considerable size and partial fixation to the abdominal wall. Both organs are soft and vulnerable to laceration by external forces. The injured athlete may show signs of peritoneal irritation, such as rebound tenderness, localized abdominal wall tenderness, or pain in the shoulder, which are suggestive of diaphragmatic irritation. Diagnostic peritoneal lavage may be useful in some instances.

Bowel injuries may be associated with a torn mesentery and intra-abdominal bleeding. A blowout bowel perforation, leading to generalized peritonitis, can also occur. Increasing abdominal pain, rigidity, and rebound tenderness may evolve as peritonitis develops. Those patients who have signs of intra-abdominal bleeding or peritoneal irritation should be transported to an appropriate medical facility and considered for surgery to control bleeding and repair injured organs.

Injury of certain viscera is not associated with much peritoneal reaction. This applies to retroperitoneal organs, kidneys, urinary bladder, pancreas, and duodenum. Patients with genitourinary injuries commonly have hematuria, which should be investigated if it persists for more than a few hours or produces grossly bloody urine. These patients need urinalysis and perhaps even contrast X rays of the genitourinary system. Contused or minimally lacerated kidneys are usually treated conservatively with bed rest, fluids, and antibiotics, but bladder rupture is more serious. A small retroperitoneal bladder injury can be treated by Foley catheter drainage for 7–10 days, but an intraperitoneal bladder rupture requires surgical closure. Athletes should empty the bladder prior to competition since this may prevent bladder injuries.

GENITAL AND URETHRAL INJURIES

Women are usually spared genital injuries, although occasionally female athletes sustain a severe mons pubis hematoma. This can be treated conservatively, or if the hematoma is large, aspiration may be required.

Men are more prone to genital injuries, hence the requirement for protective gear. In spite of precautions, contact sports participants are occasionally hit in a way that produces severe testicular injury. Actual testicular fragmentation may occur. This causes immediate and severe pain. On examination, marked swelling is evident, but outright disruption of the testis may not be apparent. With testiculular rupture, operative intervention to restore tunica continuity is necessary. After surgery, a support should be worn for comfort and to promote healing. Hormone production by injured testes continues normally, and unilateral injuries do not cause loss of fertility, although bilateral injuries may cause infertility.

The female urethra is short and almost immune from blunt injury. The male urethra is much longer and therefore vulnerable. Injuries to the urethra usually cause severe perineal pain and swelling. Urethrography should be performed to rule out urethral injuries when athletes report severe perineal trauma associated with bleeding from the meatus. Minimal urethral disruptions may be treated with an indwelling catheter. Complete urethral tears require a suprapubic cystotomy tube with subsequent repair after swelling and hematoma resolve.

Male athletes, like the rest of the male population, are susceptible to hydrocele and varicoceles. These should be repaired in the off-season, and proper support should be worn afterwards. Surgical repair does not compromise ability after the operative discomfort and swelling subside.

MINOR INJURIES

Abrasions

Rubbing of equipment against body parts occurs in almost all sports. The resulting injury depends on the equipment and body part. One of the simplest injuries is skin abrasion, which results from a tight strap. This can be prevented with proper padding. Treatment consists of keeping the involved area clean, using a topical antibiotic, and frequent dressing changes. Although abrasions are uncomfortable, they cause minimal disability.

Calluses

A more chronic injury, which usually occurs on the feet but may also be seen on the hands, is callus from repeated minor stresses. Keratin buildup occurs at the point of contact. Sharp excision of the callus usually results in pain in the area from which the callus was removed. Thus, it is preferable to treat calluses by shaving with an emery board and softening with a lanolin-based ointment. It is possible, when acute stress is superimposed on the usual chronic forces over a callus, for a blister to form within or under the callus. Blister therapy takes precedence over long-term treatment of the callus.

Blisters

Blisters occur when friction is centered over more or less unyielding skin, such as that on the palms and soles. Easily movable skin is more resistant to blistering. Blisters can be induced by prolonged exercise in poorly fitting or new shoes. Shoes, especially, tend to cause blistering because they provide abrasive contact points, warm the skin, and make evaporation of sweat difficult. Slightly moist and warm feet are more susceptible to blistering than cold feet that are either perfectly dry or are very slippery and wet. Blisters on hands and fingers are caused by gripping athletic equipment (tennis rackets) for long periods, allowing friction stresses.

It has been found experimentally that little heat is generated by the force sufficient to produce a blister, so that blistering is not a thermal injury. Typically, the cleft formed by a blister is in the epidermis above the basal cells and usually involves the granular cell layer. Blister fluid forms after the cleft develops, and the rate of accumulation is related to capillary pressure in the adjacent microcirculation. Blister fluid is similar to serum although electrolytes are somewhat lower and calcium content is significantly less. Small amounts of serum proteins are present in the fluid, but fibrin and fibrinogen are usually absent. Immunoglobulins occur in small quantities, and abnormal proteins (myeloma protein) are detectable in blister fluid.

Prevention—the best blister management—is not always possible. Intact blisters should be aspirated but not unroofed. If the blister is aspirated within 24 hr, the chance that the epidermal layer will again stick to the blister bed is approximately 85%. If the blister is aspirated three times, usually 2, 6, and 12 hr during the first 24 hr, the chance that the blister's top will stick to the base is over 90%. Local application of an antibiotic ointment and a protective pad are helpful. Blisters that stick again to the base will do so within 4 days. Withdrawal from athletic events for approximately this time, but with maintenance of general conditioning, is the usual management.

Many blisters are already unroofed by the time they are discovered and are, therefore, more painful. The treatment in this case consists of keeping the area clean, application of antibiotic ointment, and a protective dressing. Blisters usually heal in 4–5 days. Shoe padding protects the healing blister of the foot and prevents recurrence.

Burns

Trivial burns may be inflicted by hot water, electrical appliances, and cigarettes. Skin that is healing from a burn is very susceptible to other minor injury. The newly generated epithelium does not tolerate shearing forces and should be protected from athletic pads and contact with helmet inner linings. An ear recovered from a burn should be well padded from the minor trauma of protective headgear. A freshly healed burn does not tolerate sunlight well and should be protected from it by clothing or by an effective sunscreen.

Warts

Warts can be difficult, especially when they affect the soles of the feet. The temptation to excise plantar warts should be resisted, for a painful wound, worse than the original problem, usually results. Warts may be effectively treated by metatarsal arch bars and the use of mild desiccating agents, such as trichloroacetic acid, applied only to the wart, with removal of the chemical within an hour. Warts resolve slowly, but with proper foot support and avoidance of radical measures, continued athletic participation is possible.

Hemorrhoids

Acute hemorrhoids are painful when prolapsed and may cause itching. Athletes should avoid constipation, which aggravates prolapse. Advice about drinking adequate water and use of a stool softener usually alleviates the discomfort. Acutely prolapsed hemorrhoids are best treated with a hypertonic poultice (saturated magnesium sulfate solution), which dramatically reduces the edema. Acute hemorrhoidal thrombosis produces a painful anal nodule that can be incised under local anesthesia for thrombus evacuation.

Pilonidal Sinus

Pilonidal sinuses may be asymptomatic. Many, however, eventually become infected, causing a very tender, swollen, inflamed area in the intergluteal fold. An infected pilonidal sinus should be unroofed under local anesthesia. Pus and debris, such as hair, should be removed. A clean wound will heal by secondary intention. With proper cleanliness and padding to the area, prolonged disability does not usually result from the treatment.

Furuncles

Acute furuncles, localized and very painful, are found in hair-bearing areas. Warm soaks may help to localize the infection. Rapid resolution after incision and drainage under local anesthesia can be expected. Furuncles are almost always caused by staphylococci. When cellulitis or lymphangitis is present, the patient should be given an antistaphylococcal antibiotic for a few days. The drained furuncle heals quickly by secondary intention and usually causes minimal difficulty.

Trauma to Nipples

Female athletes in particular may develop irritated, tender, bleeding nipples if they participate without supportive garments. This is well known in joggers (joggers's nipples) and can be prevented or treated by use of a proper brassiere or emolient ointment applied before prolonged exertion.

·21·

Orthopaedic Aspects of Sports Medicine

Barry R. Maron

COMMENTS ON ATHLETIC INJURIES

1. All physical complaints should be considered seriously. The athlete believes he or she has an injury, and the physician should assume a serious disorder is present until proven otherwise. The diagnosis of a psychosomatic condition is made by exclusion.
2. The athletic personality is special. The physician must believe the patient can achieve certain athletic goals, and the physician should do all possible to help in this endeavor.
3. Deterioration in an athletic performance should be investigated to exclude physical or psychologic reasons. A coach who is aware of a player's change in performance should bring this to the physician's attention.
4. An injured joint should be evaluated soon after injury. Most information about the joint and the severity of the injury can then be obtained before swelling, reactive spasm, and guarding occur.
5. Loose joints do not become tighter with time. Developmentally lax ligaments should be protected, and post-traumatic joint laxity should be evaluated. Evaluation of the opposite uninjured extremity usually gives some measure of the looseness and suggests developmental or post-traumatic disorders.
6. An acutely injured extremity should be splinted immediately; failing this, it should be examined and then splinted.
7. The use of X rays should not be spared. An X-ray film, once taken, must be correctly interpreted. If there is any doubt, help should be obtained from a radiologist or orthopaedist.
8. All injured extremities should have immediate and short-term follow-up examination of sensory, motor, and vascular status. Swelling after 4–6 hr can cause significant damage to nerves, blood vessels, and musculature.
9. The obvious extremity injury may not be the only one. Careful evaluation is advisable for all the joints above and below the injured area. If a long bone fracture (femur, tibia, fibula, radius, and ulna) is found, an X-ray film of the joint proximal and distal to the fracture should be obtained. A fracture of a forearm could have an associated dislocated radial head. A fractured femur could have an associated fracture or dislocation of the hip.

10. Dislocated joints should be gently reduced as soon as possible. Ideally, an anesthetic should be used for reduction. Muscle relaxation from the anesthetic will decrease the stress of muscle action upon the joint and prevent injury to joint surfaces during reduction.

11. Qualifying sprained joints by degrees (first degree, second degree, third degree) encourages a detailed examination. If there is instability, it is best described by either degrees of opening at the joint surface or by the number of millimeters of joint opening or bone displacement. This allows the physician or subsequent physicians examining the same joint to use common language.

12. Decisions on the open or closed treatment of ligament injury should be made early. Operative treatment, possible for the first 7–10 days, is more ideal within the first 24–36 hr.

13. The ideal treatment of the athlete is a return to anatomic and functional normality. Coordination and mechanical advantage that enable participation in athletics may depend on anatomic restoration.

14. Steroids are antianabolic. When applied locally by injection they may impede healing by stopping the first stage, the inflammatory response. If they are injected for tendon inflammation, they should be applied around the tendon and not into the tendon. Steroids should not be injected into acute ligament injuries (sprains). Their use orally for 5–6 days in tapering doses is safer than local injection, and the beneficial effects on healing can be similar. If steroids are used locally, the region into which they are injected should be protected from all but minor stresses for 21 days.

15. Vitamin C does not necessarily prevent the common cold, but it is important in maintaining the structural integrity of collagen in ligaments and tendons. Increased doses of vitamin C used for 14 days after injury can be helpful in healing.

16. Muscle rehabilitation should start immediately after injury. Muscle contractions may be painful, as a result either of direct injury or of joint stresses caused by muscle activity. Both flexor and extensor muscles controlling the joint should be moved by isometric contraction first and then isotonic contractions as the situation improves. Galvanic electrical stimulation of the muscle can help contractions and maintain muscle function. Transcutaneous nerve stimulators, by blocking some pain perception and allowing muscle rehabilitation to proceed, are helpful after injury.

17. A slipped capital femoral epiphysis in adolescents can have dire consequences if the diagnosis is missed. Persistent hip or knee pain should be evaluated by X ray, including comparison examination of the opposite extremity. Bilateral slipped epiphyses are not uncommon, however, and it should be kept in mind that both sides may have the same appearance on X-ray films and be pathologic (i.e., bilateral slipped epiphyses).

18. It should always be assumed that a "sprained" knee joint is a complex problem involving more than one ligament, a meniscus, or even a bony structure. The joint may have been dislocated and at examination is already in a reduced state. Stability and peripheral vascular and peripheral nerve function should be examined. A missed knee dislocation with associated arterial damage can cause loss of a limb. Collateral circulation around the knee may initially mask major arterial damage.

19. A bone scan can be helpful in diagnosing a stress fracture when X-ray studies are normal and pain in a bone area exists.

20. Some forearm fractures have an associated dislocation or subluxation of the radial head (Monteggia's fracture). Always examine the elbow carefully and x-ray it.

THE ATHLETIC PERSONALITY

The complete and successful treatment of an athlete requires that the physician understand the athletic personality. The athlete is anxious to perform physically and is "tuned in" to even minor imperfections in body functions. He or she seeks answers to questions about symptoms that may not have a physiologic basis. A sullen and introverted response to an athletic injury can also be expected. Encouragement, in order to keep recovery capabilities within the athlete's reach, is necessary. Reassurance is vital to help the athlete keep faith in returning to the original or an alternative sport. The patient's belief in self and his or her athletic abilities must be shared by the physician with the same enthusiasm to maintain rapport with the patient. The athlete's motivation to get well is great, but a lack of rehabilitation "programs" may delay recovery and there may be excessive stresses of the injured part. Diversions from the injury are necessary, and part of each day should be occupied by physical therapy that is both treatment and diversion. If the injury is not severe but does prevent participation in one sport, substitution of another less stressful activity for a time is suggested. For example, a runner with a foot injury could swim or ride a bicycle until the foot has recovered. Coaches, teammates, teachers, friends, and physician must coordinate their efforts to counteract anticipated depression accompanying serious injury.

INJURY EVALUATION

The acute injury gives the examining physician an advantage:

1. The history is recent and the mechanism of injury will be recounted in detail.
2. The earlier a patient is seen after an injury, the easier it is to examine the injured part. There is less edema and pain, and therefore less guarding by the patient, soon after the injury.

Chronic and recurring symptoms demand detective work to find their cause:

1. Careful history
    a) Onset of symptoms: Was there a specific injury? Were symptoms associated with preparticipation warm-up? What was the duration of play before symptoms began? Can symptoms be predicted or induced by certain activities? What is the duration and frequency of the symptoms? Has there been treatment? What has been the response to treatment (e.g., ice, heat, salicylates, rest)? What other injuries have occurred in the past?
    b) Other medical problems: Has patient ever experienced arthritis, other joint disorders, collagen diseases, metabolic disorders? What has been the family medical history? Has the patient urinary or eye discomfort to suggest Reiter's syndrome? Has there been exposure to gonorrhea?
2. Detailed examination, including, if possible, evaluation of the patient's performance in sports or during simulated sporting activities.

INJURY PREVENTION

The best treatment for injuries is prevention. Not all sports are safe for all people. Some will have to be advised to change sports. Others will need counseling regarding their proper place in sports. This counseling should take into consideration the following factors:

1. Injury history
2. Joint mobility
3. Muscle power
4. Ligamentous stability
5. Developmental anomalies
6. Body type (mesomorphic; ectomorphic; endomorphic)
7. Motivation for participation

Generalizations cannot be made, and the patient must be studied. For example, someone with spondylolysis or spondylolisthesis, whether symptomatic or not, would be vulnerable to injury in gymnastics or a collision sport such as football. A distance runner who has been treated for recurrent knee effusions and pain needs help in assessing his or her place in running.

O'Donoghue [1] stresses conditioning and instruction programs. These should include:

1. Proper techniques for the particular sport
2. Protective equipment
3. Calisthenics
4. Endurance training
5. Weight training

Vulnerable parts of the body should be protected with taping and orthotic supports.

SPRAINS AND STRAINS

A sprain (ligament injury) and strain (muscle-tendon unit injury) will be part of most injuries. The problem may be acute, with local hemorrhage and swelling from sudden excess stress. The injury may be chronic (recurring) from overuse and associated with pain and limitation of motion with little swelling. Careful examination is necessary to define: 1) functional loss; 2) joint stability; 3) degree of tissue damage. Treatment depends upon grading of the injury and functional loss. Grade I (first-degree) and Grade II (second-degree) injuries are usually associated with little functional deficit and need only protection until spontaneous healing. During healing, the affected muscles should be subjected to isometrics and progressive resistive exercises. This should be carried out until symptoms subside and there is return of confidence and performance.

Grade III injuries (third-degree) are usually associated with significant joint instability or muscle destruction. These injuries may need surgical repair of ligaments or muscles. The decision on operation should be made early before fibrosis and contractures occur.

COMMON ACUTE SPINAL INJURIES

Neck Injuries

It is not possible fully to evaluate neck pain on the athletic field. Minor neck symptoms may be associated with major spinal injuries (i.e., spinal fractures or spinal subluxations). Patients with acute neck injuries should be given undivided attention at the scene, even if progress of a sporting event is delayed. The sequence of evaluation and treatment should be as follows:

1. Interview the patient if he or she is conscious. Assess what active function is present in arms and legs. Be certain to note all motor function dependent on intact innervation by the brachial plexus and sciatic nerve.
2. Examine motor function. Look for clonus, plantar responses, and sensory deficits.
3. Support the head with sandbags. Do not try to remove a helmet. Be certain that the airway is patent. It may be necessary to use bolt cutters to remove the face mask from a football helmet without moving the head.
4. Palpate bony prominences for tenderness and instability. Keep the injured patient in the same position until it is established that it is safe to move him or her at all. If establishing an airway by moving the patient into the supine position, be certain that head movement is done slowly. At the same time, speak to the patient and apply gentle traction to the head. Keep track of the conscious patient's ability to move the extremities.
5. Do not ask the patient to turn the head or to flex or extend the neck. Do not passively move the neck. Many times the patient will be turning his or her own head when first seen, removing, at least temporarily, doubt about motion capabilities. There must be enough assistance available to move the patient to the stretcher. The entire spine should be supported while gentle axial traction is maintained on the neck and lower extremities.
6. Transport the patient to a hospital or office for full X-ray evaluation.

Many patients present neck symptoms when sitting or walking. Their evaluation should be similar, taking full precautions. A collar can be placed around the neck for protection, or the patient can be examined supine. Plain X-ray films may not always be adequate and special studies may be necessary (tomogram, CT scan, or special views). Full support of the injured area must be contained until all serious damage to the cord has been excluded.

Major neck injuries can progress rapidly, and deterioration in function of the cord can be irreversible.

When it is safe to do so, flexion, extension and lateral X-rays can be helpful. Always insist on full cervical X-ray pictures, especially to show the C6-7 and C7-T1 levels. Swimmer's views and tomograms are sometimes necessary to see the lower cervical area. The CT scanner can give valuable diagnostic information.

If acute neck symptoms have subsided following treatment and the skeletal evaluation is normal, then early reevaluation is necessary if they recur.

Stretch Injuries to the Brachial Plexus

The "burner" or "stinger" described by some football players occurs in the neck and shoulder after head or shoulder contact. Shoulder girdle depression, together with neck extension or deviation away from the depressed side, can cause tension and stretching of the brachial plexus. Neurologic function should frequently be evaluated in such patients. They should be advised on strengthening shoulder girdles and neck muscles. These players should also use protective neck rolls during contact or collision sports. Advice should be given as to vulnerability of the brachial plexus to serious injury if continued collisions occur. A small number of players with such complaints will develop selective brachial plexus lesions and functional deficits in the upper extremities.

Neck Sprains

Various ligaments may be torn by flexion, extension, or rotatory forces. Second- and third-degree injuries are important and potentially deadly. A high level of suspicion by the examiner is necessary to diagnose major sprains. X-ray films are mandatory to assist in making the proper diagnosis.

1. Flexion injuries

   Symptoms: The patient with neck pain will resist active flexion, rigidly holding the neck in extension to the point of fatigue.

   Signs: Exquisitely tender posterior interspinous structures may be found by palpation. The patient will not rotate the head to the side.

   Treatment: A collar or brace support is applied to prevent flexion of the neck. When symptoms subside, cervical isometrics can begin. Six to 8 weeks are needed for healing a ligament.

Avulsions of the spinous process, subluxations, or dislocations may occur without fracture of the vertebral body or vertebral lamina. The degree of muscle spasm, the limitation of motion, and the history will help in arriving at the correct diagnosis. If dislocation has occurred, all motion of the neck is resisted.

   Minor sprains must be protected until fully evaluated and until all symptoms subside. The patient may be symptomatic for 3–8 weeks, depending on the severity of injury. Injured ligaments in the neck are vulnerable to reinjury, especially before complete healing has occurred.

2. Extension injuries

   Symptoms: Extension injuries cause varying degrees of anterior pain and tenderness in the neck. Extension of the head is painfully avoided.

3. Rotational injuries

   Symptoms: These patients usually present minor pain and limited motion if seen after the injury. As spasm increases over 24 hr, the head will be rotated to the injured side and be kept slightly flexed. If subluxation has occurred, motion will be even more limited and spasm will be more acutely prominent. The appearance of the patient is similar to that of a person with a "wry neck," with the head rotated so the chin is upward and toward the opposite side (O'Donoghue [1]). The sternocleidomastoid muscle will be tight on the involved side.

4. Subluxation

   Symptoms: Some people are loose-jointed or habitual "neck poppers." They may have subluxation from even minor injury with no acute damage to the ligamentous structures themselves. Reduction of the subluxation reverses most symptoms immediately. The athletic future of these people excludes contact sports. The first subluxation without residual damage should be protected for 6–8 weeks; no sports participation is allowed.

Treatment for neck sprains depends on the severity of the injury. In general, a soft collar, analgesics, ice massage to reduce spasm and pain, and heat applications alternating with the use of ice are indicated. Traction at home or in a hospital is helpful. Muscle relaxants and local injections of anesthetic agents relieve discomfort. Oral cortisone in tapering doses for 2–6 days helps resolve local swelling.

COMMON ACUTE INJURIES OF THE DORSAL AND LUMBAR SPINE

Sprains and strains in the region of the dorsal and lumbar spine may present symptoms and signs similar to those of neck sprains: 1) pain; 2) limited motion away from the injured side; 3) muscle spasm in the region; and 4) tilting of the torso toward the injured side. Treatment begins with rest in bed with the hips and knees flexed over pillows or bolsters. At home, a suitcase with a pillow placed on it can be used as leg support. Ice massage to the area and local anesthetic injections into trigger points, with or without hyaluronidase, may be added. The injection of an anesthetic agent can be repeated if successful. On rare occasions, cortisone may be tried mixed with the anesthetic injection. However, if cortisone is to be used at all, the oral route in tapering doses over 4–6 days is preferable.

Traction and orthotic supports are occasionally helpful. Braces, corsets, and body jacket casts, although unpleasantly warm and heavy, are supportive if used for several days or weeks. Fractures and dislocation of the dorsal and lumbar spine may occur and can be seen on X-ray studies.

Vulnerability to injury may occasionally be predicted from spinal contours. The hyperlordotic person is vulnerable to extension stresses. The kyphotic person is more vulnerable to flexion stresses in the dorsal area and to extension stresses in the lumbar area. It is not unusual to find compensatory increased lumbar lordosis in association with a dorsal kyphosis.

Fractures of the transverse processes (Fig. 21-1) should be treated as sprains, or strains. Failure of union is not uncommon but is usually not a source of discomfort.

Fractures in the region of the pars interarticularis (spondylolysis) may be acute, but they are usually developmental in origin and are brought to attention by an injury. The diagnosis is made by X-ray study (Fig. 21-2). A bone scan is helpful in deciding treatment and prognosis. A hot scan at the spondylolysis area suggests "healing" is possible and can be treated by prolonged body casting (plaster body jacket with or without one thigh included in the cast) or by bracing. If the scan is cold, treatment is as for a sprain. Symptoms may not fully subside, and there is vulnerability to reinjury. Recurring symptoms are a common nuisance. It is often necessary to restrict sports and recommend surgical treatment.

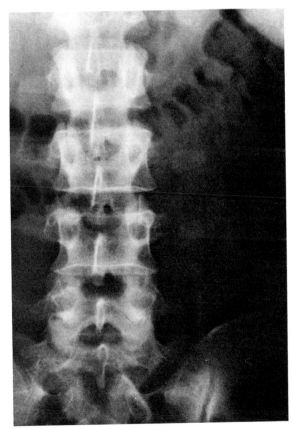

21-1 Anteroposterior view of lumbar spine shows displaced fractures of transverse processes of L3–4 and an undisplaced fracture of transverse process of L5.

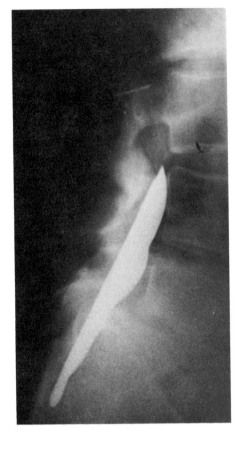

21-2 Lateral myelogram of lumbar spine, showing spondylolisthesis defect, Grade I at L5–S1. Pantopaque column is relatively displaced as it passes from L5 to S1 segment.

Disc Lesions

Lumbar disc injuries with degeneration or rupture are important. Symptoms may mimic strains or sprains but are usually associated with radiation of pain to the hip, buttock, or extremity. The signs are similar to those of sprains, but there will usually be sciatic tension signs, sensory deficits, motor weaknesses, and reflex changes. Muscle atrophy may be present.

Disc lesions in the dorsal spine usually present with pain or sometimes lower extremity weakness or clumsiness. In cervical disc lesions, symptoms are similar to those of a sprain or a strain, but they are associated with persistent, usually radicular, pain along one of the brachial plexus dermatomes. Weakness, sensory deficits, and reflex changes in the upper extremity may or may not be present.

The diagnosis of a disc lesion is made in part by exclusion after treatment failure for sprains and strains. Once neurologic localizing signs are present, the diagnosis is usually apparent. Tests to confirm the levels of the disc lesions are usually performed, once the decision is made to proceed with surgery. They include electromyography, epidural venography, myelography (Figs. 21-3, 21-4), and CT scan. Persistent or recurring swelling of the articular facet joint or joint of Luschka in the neck may cause radicular symptoms by pressure on nerve roots.

Disc lesions of the dorsal and lumbar region can be treated in similar fashion to sprains and strains. Bed rest in the position of comfort or in hip-flex-knee-flex position decreases nerve root tension and will allow swelling to subside around the roots. After several days, the patient's discomfort is relieved or improved. Anti-inflammatory drugs, with bed rest,

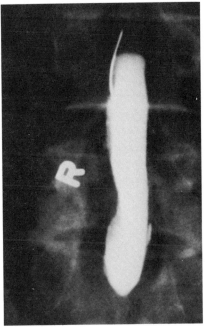 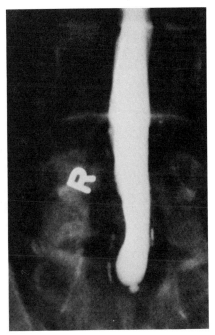

21-3 In anteroposterior view of myelogram, large filling defect at level of L5–S1 (*right*) suggests that a herniated nucleus pulposus fragment has entered spinal canal and is deflecting nerve roots.

are helpful. If oral cortisone is used in tapering doses over 5–7 days, precautions should be taken to minimize irritative effects upon the gastrointestinal tract. Regular meals, antacids between meals, and cimetidine (300 mg) three times daily for the duration of the oral anti-inflammatory therapy are recommended.

Changes in bladder or bowel habits immediately after the onset of symptoms or even later in the course of disc disease are serious complications. Pressure from a herniated disc or extruded disc fragment may cause bladder or bowel dysfunction, or both. Early careful evaluation is essential to determine 1) rectal sphincter tone, 2) the bulbocavernosus reflex, and 3) sensation in the region of the genitalia and perineum. This is a medical emergency and demands immediate relief of pressure on nerve roots to preserve bowel and bladder function.

Compression Fractures of the Dorsal and Lumbar Spine

Acute fractures in this area present severe pain. The pain may be accompanied by neurologic deficits in the lower extremity or distal to the lesion (i.e., sensory loss, muscle weakness, reflex changes). Occasionally the pain may be minor and may be erroneously attributed to a sprain or strain.

Dorsal and Lumbar Injury

The patient is usually in the supine position but is occasionally seated with severe back pain in association with the signs that have been cited. There may also be a loss of bowel sounds. Undivided attention should be given immediately at the scene. If involuntary bowel or bladder evacuation has occurred, there has usually been a major insult to the central nervous system (i.e., concussion, seizure, spinal cord injury). In addition to concentrating on the

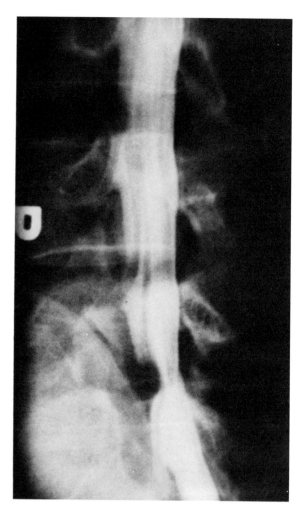

21-4 Oblique view of myelogram shows larger defect at level of L5–S1 (*right*) that is typical of a large herniated nucleus pulposus in spinal canal, pressing on a nerve root.

area of symptoms in the back, a full neurologic evaluation should be carried out, including cranial nerves and peripheral nervous system. The sequence of evaluation and treatment is as follows:

1. Interview the patient. Assess active function in arms and legs by noting movements at first contact.
2. Observe motor function by asking patient to voluntarily move toes, ankles, and knees. If there is no visible motion, palpate muscles to see if there is a flicker of motor response. Look for clonus, plantar responses, and sensory deficits. Gently palpate the spine by slipping a hand underneath the back and moving the fingers gently down the spinous processes. Fracture areas with intact sensation are extremely tender on palpation. Keep the injured patient in the original position until it has been determined that moving the patient will be safe. There should be enough personnel available to support the entire spine while moving the patient.
3. Transport the patient to a hospital or office for full evaluation by X-ray films.

When major neurologic deficits are not present and the patient is ambulatory and functional, flexion and extension lateral X-ray views are helpful in diagnosing residual instability in the spinal column. Sometimes tomographic motion studies are necessary to detect motion at the center of vertebral bodies. This motion is often easier to measure than that noted on plain flexion and extension views or on plain lateral bending films of the spine.

The sprain or strain of the back that remains symptomatic for 10 days or longer and is associated with percussion tenderness should be studied by X ray to detect the presence of compression fractures. X-ray findings may not give information about the age of the wedging or compression. In this situation, bone scan may be helpful. The scan will usually be "hot" in areas of recent fractures at least 12 hr old. The increased uptake of the radioisotopes may persist for 90 days or until there has been complete healing and maturation of tissues.

Always consider Scheuermann's disease (juvenile osteochondrosis) in evaluating an injured spine. This developmental epiphysitis will cause developmental kyphosis. It may be difficult on X-ray studies to separate developmental from post-traumatic wedging of the vertebrae.

THE SHOULDER

The shoulder is a ball-and-socket joint. The ligaments surrounding the shoulder are designed to limit movement, but they do not maintain the joint surfaces in apposition. The humerus can be separated from the glenoid passively. The joint is protected by an arch formed by the coracoid process, the acromion, and the coracoacromial ligament (Gray [2]).

Common Acute Shoulder Injuries

1. Contusion of the shoulder tip
   Symptoms: The patient will present difficult abduction pain at the tip of the shoulder (deltoid region) even with slight active motion; passive motion is full with minimal discomfort.
   Signs: There is tenderness at the tip of the shoulder, with bruising and tissue swelling; the ability to abduct the shoulder from the neutral position with or without resistance depends upon the degree of injury.
   X-ray studies: These are usually normal.
   Testing: Infiltration with a local anesthetic agent in the region of tenderness and maximal pain should be tried. If pain is relieved, then the rotator cuff is either intact or in continuity, and abduction of the arm from the neutral position against resistance will be good or excellent. With a moderate or large tear in the rotator cuff or a significant hematoma in the surrounding tissues beyond the area of anesthetic infiltration, abduction will not improve with local anesthesia.
   Differential diagnosis: The possibilities to consider are: 1) contusion or 2) rotator cuff injury.
   Treatment: Ice, a sling, rest, gradual physiotherapy exercises, and oral enzymes are recommended. If, after anesthesia, good abduction of the shoulder is possible, then 21 or preferably 28 days should be allowed for the healing of rotator cuff and surrounding tissues. If abduction after anesthetic infiltration remains weak, and this weakness persists for 14–21 days, then a shoulder arthrogram should be obtained to assess the degree of rotator cuff damage. Large and small tears with persistent functional deficit should be surgically repaired.
2. Acromioclavicular (AC) pain
   History: The patient reports striking the shoulder tip during a fall.
   Symptoms: Pain is present at the AC joint with any motion of the shoulder; there is swelling or deformity of the AC joint region; motion of the shoulders induces snapping at the AC joint area.

Signs: Tenderness is elicited over the AC joint. Clicking or subluxation of the clavicle is induced by palpation on movement of the shoulder and subluxation of the acromion downward with passive application of weight to the involved extremity. There is also apparent subluxation of the lateral tip of the clavicle upward during normal standing, and hypermobility of the clavicle on passive stress of the lateral tip upward.

X-ray studies: Anteroposterior X-ray films are made of the shoulder while the extremity is weighted or while the patient holds onto an immovable object and tries to lift it (Fig. 21-5). There may be hypermobility of the lateral tip of the clavicle (riding cephalad above the acromion). Fracture of the lateral tip of the clavicle may be present. Irregularities or sclerosis of the acromioclavicular joint should be noted.

Differential diagnosis: The following disorders should be considered:

a. Acute separation of the acromioclavicular joint
b. Synovitis of the acromioclavicular joint

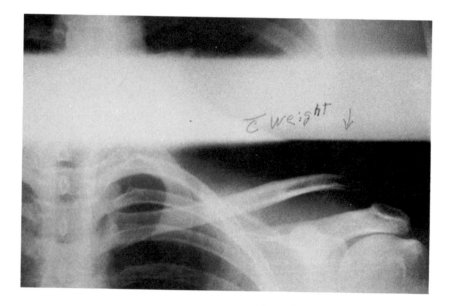

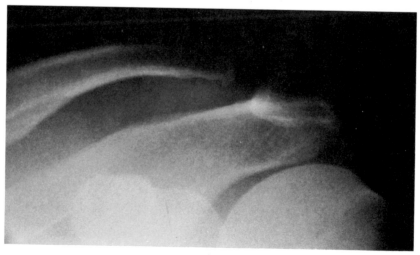

21-5 X-ray films of shoulder acromioclavicular separation. Lateral end of clavicle is superior to articular edge of acromion.

c. Acromioclavicular degenerative arthritis aggravated by recent injury

d. Fracture of the lateral clavicle

In a first-degree acromioclavicular separation, minimal displacement of the clavicular relation to the acromion is found. Third-degree separation shows complete displacement of the clavicle upward from the acromion either with or without applied stress. Also in third-degree separation there is a tear of the acromioclavicular and the coracoclavicular ligaments.

Treatment: Sling rest is helpful. A Kinney-Howard sling splint for severe grade II and grade III separation is recommended along with anti-inflammatory drugs or enzymes orally. Local anesthetic injection may help, but no steroid should be injected. Surgery may be needed in third-degree lesions, to insure stability by removal of the articular disc and repair of the ligaments. Resection of the lateral tip of the clavicle is sometimes performed together with other stabilizing measures.

3. Anterior dislocation of the shoulder

Symptoms: The arm is usually held by the opposite hand in slight abduction and external rotation. Pain occasionally radiates along branches of the brachial plexus.

Signs: Passive adduction or internal rotation is strongly resisted. The acromion is prominent, and the humeral head can be felt anterior to the acromion and adjacent to the coracoid process. Occasionally the humeral head is located inferior to the glenoid fossa, which can be palpated. The acromion is then more prominent than with a simple anterior dislocation. Posteriorly, the absence of the humeral head is noted by contour and on palpation. The posterior glenoid rim is prominently palpable.

The examiner should check for brachial plexus deficits, and should document impaired nervous function at the time of initial evaluation. The circulatory status will be noted by the appearance of nail beds and palpation of the radial pulse.

X-ray studies: Anterior and inferior displacement of the humeral head (Fig. 21-6) will be evident, as well as a fracture, if one has occurred (Fig. 21-7).

Treatment: Attempted reduction should be gentle. If circumstances are not ideal, the patient must be transferred to adequate facilities for reduction of the dislocation. A skilled examiner may attempt on-site reduction after documenting the patient's pre-reduction neurovascular status, but the possibility should be considered that a fracture might coexist with the dislocation. Reduction under general anesthesia is the most gentle technique, allowing minimal stress to joint surfaces while muscle relaxation is maximal. X-ray documentation before and after reduction is recommended.

Reduction techniques:

a. Gentle axial traction alone is used, with countertraction in the form of a sheet around the upper chest held by an assistant pulling in the opposite direction.

b. The patient is prone, with a weight hanging on the arm and the pectoral region raised on a support fashioned from towels or a small bolster. This allows gravity to do the reducing as the muscles relax by fatigue.

c. If the Kocher maneuver is employed, the arm is abducted and externally rotated; adduction and external rotation are then used; internal rotation is the final maneuver. All movements are performed with gentle axial traction at the elbow with one hand, while the wrist is supported on the physician's other hand.

d. When the straight overhead technique is used, the patient is supine. The physician inspires confidence by explaining the plan. Slowly, but steadily and actively, the patient's hand is moved over the shoulder until it touches the sheet just behind the patient's head. The elbow is kept flexed. Gentle pressure is applied to the humeral head, backward and upward with one hand while the other hand guides the arm into flexion overhead. Reduction will be followed by relief of discomfort and easy, active motion of the shoulder joint.

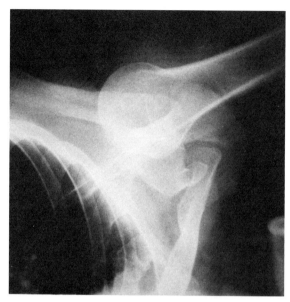

21-6 Inferior dislocation of shoulder; luxation erectae type.

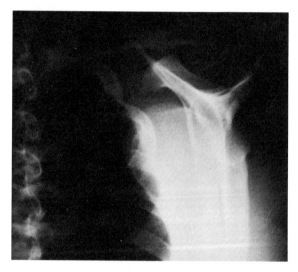

Lateral view of shoulder with anterior inferior dislocation of humeral head. Head of humerus displaced anterior to juncture (*Y*) of scapular spine, coracoid process, and body of the scapula.

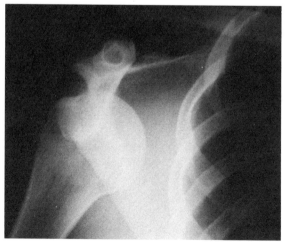

Anterior inferior dislocation of shoulder.

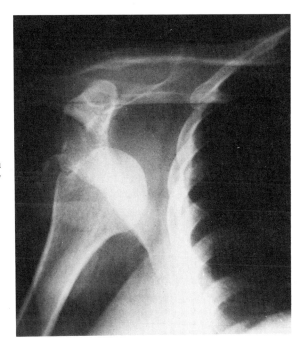

21-7 Anterior inferior dislocation of shoulder with greater tuberosity fracture.

General anesthesia, intravenous diazepam, or intravenous narcotics are helpful and recommended to ensure gentle manipulation.

Additional injuries found by X-ray studies must be dealt with. Avulsion fractures of the glenoid or fractures of the greater tuberosity or humeral neck may be associated with dislocation of the shoulder. Rarely, the tendon of the long head of the biceps will bowstring across the joint and prevent reentry of the humeral head into the joint area. The post reduction treatment is immobilization by:

1. Sling with a woven elastic wrap around the chest, arm, and forearm, preventing external rotation;
2. Commercial shoulder immobilizer; or
3. Commercial sling and swathe.
    The first episodes of anterior shoulder disclocation should be treated by immobilization, in the hope that healing and reestablishment of normal stability will occur. This takes at least 4 weeks. Gradual range-of-motion exercises should then be tried, starting with gravity exercises and progressing to passive and active overhead mobilization. Internal rotation exercises are important to regain shoulder mobility posteriorly. This motion is commonly forgotten. The patient should hold a doorknob with the problem hand and turn away from the treated arm, utilizing body momentum for internal rotation in a posterior direction.
4. Posterior dislocations of the shoulder
    The diagnosis can be missed even after X-ray films have been made, unless the existence of a posterior dislocation has been considered.
    Symptoms: The shoulder is painful and there is inability to actively rotate the shoulder externally. Occasionally the pain radiates to the tip of the shoulder, along the distribution of the axillary nerve.
    Signs: The arm is held rigidly in internal rotation. Passive motion is strongly resisted. The coracoid process is more prominent than usual and the humeral head can be felt posterior to the acromion. The glenoid fossa can be easily palpated anteriorly. Careful

examination is necessary, with attention to circulation and neuromuscular function at the elbow, wrist, and hand.

X-ray studies: The X-ray films can easily be misinterpreted. If there is doubt, the involved shoulder should be compared with the normal side. A tangential view of the scapula and axial view of the shoulder are helpful. On the tangential view, the humeral head should center at the junction of the scapular spine, glenoid, and acromion projections. Fractures of the glenoid or proximal humerus may accompany this dislocation.

Treatment: Definitive treatment depends upon coexisting fractures. Some fractures need open reduction. Ideally, reduction is attempted under general anesthesia. Gentle axial traction with countertraction by a sheet around the chest and forward pressure to the humeral head with gentle external rotation of the humerus may be successful. Muscle relaxation and analgesia require at least intravenous diazepam or a narcotic. Immediate reduction in the field can be accomplished by a skilled manipulator, but all precautions should be taken (see section on anterior dislocations).

Postreduction management is immobilization for at least 3 weeks, and preferably 4 weeks for the first dislocation. Gravity exercises and increasing range of motion begin after immobilization. The arm can be immobilized in neutral position or in external rotation by means of a modified plaster spica. This type of bandage allows shortening of the posterior capsular distance between the humeral head and the glenoid and may insure more stable healing.

If the dislocation (anterior or posterior is a recurrent one, then immobilization should be only long enough for relief of symptoms. It is improbable that a recurrent dislocation will become more stable with prolonged immobilization after each episode (see section on common chronic or recurring shoulder symptoms later in this chapter).

Fractures of the Humerus

The treatment of fractures of the humerus depends upon location of the fracture, displacement of the segments, and associated nerve or vascular injury. The objective in teenagers and older athletes is to obtain close anatomic reduction and full return of function. Therefore, treatment usually entails one or all of the following at different stages after the injury:

1. Sling and swathe immobilization
2. Hanging cast
3. Coaptation splints
4. Side-arm or over-the-head skeletal traction
5. Open reduction with internal fixation

Open reduction with internal fixation is rarely necessary, but on occasion, nerve exploration, blood vessel repair, or repair of unacceptable shortening or malunion is desirable.

Axial forces applied to the shoulder or direct or rotational forces applied to the proximal humeral region can cause the immature humerus to slip off the proximal humeral epiphysis (Figs. 21-8, 21-9). Treatment is reduction without excessive manipulation. The young, immature, proximal humerus will remodel with time if rotational alignment is good. Occasionally anatomic reduction may be obtained under general anesthesia, and the repair is held in place with a percutaneous transfixing pin. A shoulder spica can be applied, with the arm overhead in the "Statue of Liberty" position, with the cast extending to the wrist or palm.

In fractures of the humerus, careful documentation of the status of the neurovascular structures of the extremity is necessary. Blood flow and neural function must be closely

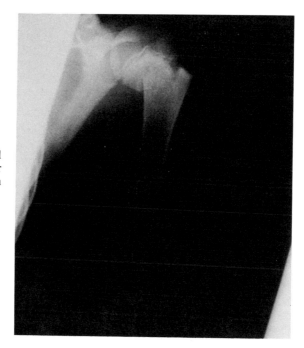

21-8 Epiphyseal slip of proximal humeral epiphysis, anteroposterior view. Arm is in external rotation under anesthesia.

observed for 72 hr. Injuries to the brachial plexus are not uncommon in association with fractures of the humerus. Injury to the radial nerve may also occur frequently.

Common Clavicular Injuries

Sternoclavicular Sprains   The sternoclavicular joint is a double arthroidial joint. It is formed by the sternal end of the clavicle, the upper and lateral part of the manubrium sternae, and the cartilage of the first rib.

Symptoms: Pain and swelling are present at the medial (sternal end) of the clavicle.
Signs: Tenderness is felt in the area of swelling, and there is fluctuation of the medial end of

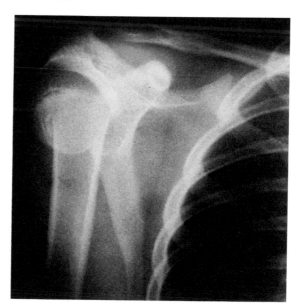

21-9 Proximal humeral epiphysis slip with shoulder in internal rotation under general anesthesia.

the clavicle on gentle pressure to the bone of the clavicle. Manipulation of the clavicle outward (anteriorly) will show hypermobility of the medial end.

X-ray studies: Subluxation or dislocation may be evident, but it is very difficult to isolate this joint by routine X-ray films. Tomograms may be necessary if documentation is required. A CT scan will also show this area well.

Treatment: Partial tears (first-degree and second-degree) should be treated with ice, rest, and a sling until tenderness subsides. Complete tears (third-degree) involve the sternoclavicular and the costoclavicular ligaments. These are treated by surgical reduction and stabilization.

Many third-degree lesions are missed because of local swelling and minimal deformity. They become manifest later with discomfort and functional limitations.

In posterior dislocations, the medial end of the clavicle is displaced behind the manubrium sternae and locked in that position. Such dislocations will present the same symptoms and, on occasion, swelling of the extremity because of pressure upon major vessels. Posterior dislocation is treated immediately by gentle manipulation of the clavicle forward, preferably under a general anesthesia. Some dislocations will reduce spontaneously and present with a lax sternoclavicular joint and the findings that have been discussed.

Shaft Fractures of the Clavicle Most shaft fractures of the clavicle are treated with a figure-eight splint and a sling support on the injured side. Occasionally, a plaster figure-eight splint is applied to maintain reduction. A plaster splint is no better and no more secure than a soft figure-eight appliance. It is usually not necessary to reduce clavicular fractures surgically except to treat a rare nonunion. Nonunions usually occur in fractures previously reduced surgically. Even comminuted fractures with displaced and rotated butterfly fragments have healed with splinting. If the fragment causes tenting of the skin, the bony protrusion is removed surgically under local anesthesia after healing has occurred.

Acute open reduction and internal fixation may be necessary in cases with a fracture of the clavicle on the dominant side, in athletes involved in throwing or racquet sports. Athletes have special mechanical advantages in the shoulder girdle, which they use with precision. Shortening or slight malrotation of the clavicle can change performance unpredictably.

Some lateral clavicle fractures are treated as a grade III acromioclavicular separation. A Kinney-Howard acromioclavicular splint may be tried. If this splint is successful, X-ray films show acceptable reduction with the splint in place. The splint must be worn day and night for at least 4 weeks. Open repair is occasionally necessary.

For lateral fractures distal to the coracoclavicular ligamentous attachments with intact ligaments, a sling is used for support until swelling and pain subside. Gradual motion can then be started.

After reductions at the shoulder or clavicle, X-ray studies should be obtained to document the status of the bones after manipulation. If doubt exists about shoulder girdle structures, the films should be sent for consultation to a radiologist or orthopedist. Second opinions of X-ray studies may stimulate thoughts on the ideal treatment of athletes.

Common Chronic or Recurring Shoulder Symptoms

Bateman [3] has made some critical evaluations and commentaries about shoulder problems.

1. Subdeltoid or subacromial pain
    Symptoms: The patient suffers aching pain at rest and there is painful and limited range of motion of the shoulder joint.

Signs: Tenderness is present anterior to the acromion or laterally under the deltoid muscle at the greater tuberosity of the humerus. There is pain with greater than 80° abduction. Pronation or supination against resistance is painless.

X-ray studies: X-ray films may show calcification in the region of the rotator cuff or capsular structures.

Differential diagnosis: Among the causes, the following should be considered: 1) tendinitis of the rotator cuff; 2) subacromial bursitis; 3) subdeltoid bursitis; 4) brachial plexus stretch injury; and 5) thoracic outlet syndrome.

Treatment: Initially, a sling, ice, salicylates, and anti-inflammatory drugs are used. Later, local anesthetic injections may be given. Active motion and gravity-assisted passive motion should be encouraged while the anesthetic is effective. Repetitive ice massage helps relieve discomfort and muscle spasm. Oral steroids in tapering doses for 5–7 days are often helpful. Local anesthetic injection can be repeated after 10–14 days, but steroids should not be given again for at least 3 weeks, with no more than three repetitions.

2. Posterior or lateral shoulder pain

   Sport: Football, hockey, or any other sport in which frequent falls and trauma to the deltoid region occur may result in shoulder pains.

   Signs: The victim suffers tenderness of the deltoid muscle; there is function (abduction of 15° against resistance); range of motion is full, but passive.

   Differential diagnosis: Possible causes include hematoma of the deltoid muscle and myositis ossificans.

   Treatment: The hematoma should be aspirated and a local anesthetic agent injected. A sling should be applied and the patient should rest. Ice applications intermittently for 42–72 hr will help. Isometric exercises and pendulum exercises may be used as healing begins.

3. Recurrent pain at the start of throwing or serving in tennis

   Signs: The patient experiences tenderness of the greater tuberosity of the humerus and under the tip of the acromion.

   Differential diagnosis: The following disorders should be ruled out: 1) rotator cuff tendinitis; 2) subacromial bursitis; 3) subdeltoid bursitis.

   Treatment: Throwing frequency should be decreased; salicylates or other anti-inflammatory drugs may be given. Ultrasound treatment and occasionally a diuretic will reduce local swelling.

   After the season, local steroid injections around the tendon and into the bursa can be tried while the joint is rested; pendulum and isometric exercises should continue. Local anesthetic injections alone, without the steroid mixture, can be used. Immediately after the local anesthetic injection, 5- to 7-day tapering doses of oral cortisone derivative can be used to reduce inflammation.

   X-ray studies may show calcified areas in the region of the rotator cuff (Fig. 21-10). Injections can be made into these areas with the use of fluoroscopy to guide the needle. Large-bore needles are useful for puncturing and aspirating the soft calcium deposits. Recurrent pain should be evaluated by arthrogram to exclude a tear in the rotator cuff (Fig. 21-11). Sometimes surgery is necessary to repair a cuff tear or release the coracoacromial ligament to stop impingement of the humerus against it.

4. Recurrent shoulder dislocations should be assessed for surgical stabilization.

5. Pain at the end of throwing and serving in tennis

   Signs: Tenderness is experienced at the posterior glenoid rim.

   Differential diagnosis: Possible causes are the following: 1) tendon insertion tear (long head of the triceps); 2) tear of the posterior capsule; 3) posterior osteophytes.

   Treatment: The arm and shoulder should have rest in a sling; anti-inflammatory drugs,

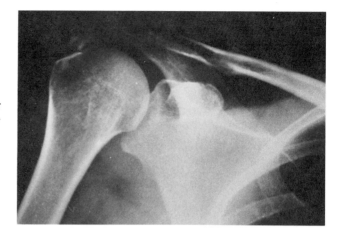

21-10 Calcification in rotator cuff of shoulder in calcific tendinitis of rotator cuff.

ultrasound, and ice massage will help to alleviate pain. A slow return to hard throwing or serving should be made over several weeks. Surgical removal of an osteophyte or loose fragment within the joint may be necessary.

6. Gradual loss of motion of the shoulder with pain during almost all movement
   Signs: There is loss of some posterior internal rotation and abduction in forward flexion with anterior, lateral, and posterior tenderness at the glenoid rim. Crepitus and stability can be assessed under general anesthesia.
   X-ray studies: Films may show notching of the humeral head posteriorly; osteophytes of the genoid rim may be present; an osteophyte at the inferior aspect of the humeral head may be present; the humeral head may be distorted.
   Diagnosis: Post-traumatic osteoarthritis is the likely cause.
   Treatment: Anti-inflammatory drugs will help, as will active range-of-motion exercises, minimal passive range-of-motion exercises, and heat application. Gentle manipulation of the joint under anesthesia may be necessary, depending on individual circumstances.

7. Anterior shoulder pain
   Signs: Tenderness is present, and sometimes snapping or crepitation in the bicipital groove. There is some anterior pain with external rotation of the arm while the arm is held abducted 45° and pain with supination of the forearm against resistance. Bateman [3] noted that anterior shoulder pain is frequently found in underhand pitching, bowling, or overhand throwing activities.

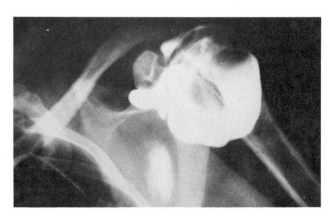

21-11 Arthrogram of shoulder, showing tear in rotator cuff with extravasation of contrast material (Conray) out of joint capsule and into subacromial bursa.

Differential diagnosis: The following causes should be considered: 1) bicipital tendinitis; 2) dislocating biceps tendon; 3) subscapularis tendinitis; 4) impingement of the coracoacromial ligament on the biceps tendon; 5) rotator cuff tears; 6) shoulder subluxation.

X-ray studies: Films may show a shallow bicipital groove and/or calcification in the rotator cuff tendon. Arthroscopy of the shoulder joint and subacromial space can help define the cause of pain and assist in its treatment.

Treatment: Rest in a sling is advisable, as are anti-inflammatory drugs and physical therapy. Occasionally surgery is needed to repair the transverse humeral ligament or to transfer the long head of the biceps tendon or apply tenodesis.

8. Scapular pain, especially at the medial border

   Associated Sports: The shot-put, discus, javelin may induce scapular pain.

   Signs: Tenderness is experienced along the medial border of the scapula; there may be crepitation and local muscle spasm

   Diagnosis: A muscle tear at the medial scapular attachment (rhomboid muscle) or tendinitis of the parascapular region may be the cause.

   Treatment: Ice massage, sling, rest, local anesthetic injections, ultrasound or other heat may bring relief. Oral steroids with local anesthetic injections can be utilized. Steroid administration should be tapered over 5–7 days.

   Comments:
   a. Intra-articular fractures should be surgically restored to anatomic continuity.
   b. Long immobilization of the elbow may be associated with permanent loss of motion. Ideally, motion is started early, while control of fracture segments is still maintained. Sometimes internal fixation is necessary to accomplish this.
   c. Epiphyseal injuries not readily apparent on plain X-ray films may occur in the immature elbow. Views of the opposite elbow will facilitate meticulous comparison of the anatomic structures on both sides. Small calcific areas in ectopic sites may indicate an epiphyseal fracture, with avulsion of a portion of bone adjacent to the nonosseous cartilaginous portion of the growth center. X-ray findings should be correlated with clinical swelling, tenderness, and functional deficits.
   d. Myositis ossificans or calcification of the elbow joint capsule is not predictable. If surgery is to be carried out, it should be done within the first 24 hr or after 21 days to minimize complications.

The Dislocated Elbow

Dislocation of the elbow is an emergency. Whenever possible, an X-ray film should be obtained prior to treatment to show associated fractures. Without X-ray facilities, treatment can be instituted by skilled manipulation.

Treatment: Ice and a splint are applied immediately. Neurovascular function of the wrist, hand, and antecubital region should be assessed. Additional injuries should also be assessed (especially to the shoulder, wrist, and hand). If the patient is treated at the scene: 1) The radius and ulna are moved gently into alignment by palpation. 2) The elbow is gently extended with one hand at mid forearm or wrist while the other hand is above the elbow. Simultaneously traction is applied at the wrist or hand. If tolerance of pain allows, reduction will occur. Multiple attempts at reduction should not be made. If reduction fails, the patient is transported for X-ray films and reduction under anesthesia. Anesthesia decreases stresses at the articular surface of the elbow joint during reduction maneuvers.

Elbow Sprains and Strains

First and second degree sprains and strains with little loss of function need only protection, muscle-controlling isometric exercises, gentle range of motion, and progressive resistive exercises until symptoms subside and full function and confidence return.

Third-degree sprains rarely need more than supportive care. Occasionally a complete collateral ligament tear will require surgical repair. Early controlled motion is ideal after operative or nonoperative treatment.

A dislocated elbow is, in fact, a severe third-degree sprain. Evaluation of the collateral ligaments of the elbow joint after the dislocation has been reduced may rarely show ligamentous instability of a degree to warrant surgical correction.

Elbow sprains can be associated with tears of capsular structures. Initially the joint may be painful but with decent range of motion. Gradually pain-free contracture with limitation of motion may develop. In some patients, X-ray studies 3 weeks after injury may show calcification of the capsule. The treatment is gentle, active, controlled motion of the elbow. After tissue matures, gradual stretching can be accomplished through both active and passive motion.

Chronic, Recurring Elbow Symptoms; Medial and Lateral Joint Pain

These symptoms are called "tennis elbow," epicondylitis, or tendinitis.

Sport: Racquet and throwing sports most commonly cause recurrent symptoms.

Signs and symptoms: Grip is painful, and there is tenderness at the attachment to the epicondylar ridge of the humerus of the common extensor, or common flexor tendon mass. Pain is felt with wrist extension or wrist flexion against resistance at the respective tendon attachment sites at the elbow. There may be weakness of dorsiflexion at the wrist if the lateral region is involved. Lack of full extension of the elbow joint is common.

X-ray studies: The films are usually normal, but there may be calcium deposits along the epicondylar ridge.

Treatment: Rest in a sling or splint, ice massage, and salicylates are recommended. A short course of oral steroids may be tried if symptoms persist; local anesthetic injection may be used later. An elastic clasp band (tennis elbow band) applied at the proximal forearm just distal to the common tendon insertions relieves stress at the attachment sites. As a last resort, operations have been successful. These operations vary from muscle slides (a type of muscle lengthening) to tendon lengthening procedures. Occasionally, entrapment of a branch of the radial nerve has been the source of pain.

Warning Signs at the Elbow

Lack of full extension is a common elbow sign. When perceived in pre-teenage children, it should be a reminder to observe and evaluate the joint carefully. Myostatic contractures of the elbow flexors can result from overuse of the joint, starting with myositis of the common flexor-pronator group as a result of dynamic overload. The condition then goes on to static contractures.

Valgus deformity of the elbow may be a serious sign in the pre-teenager. Irritation of the medial humeral condyle or, more importantly, of the capitellum can result in osteochondritis dissicans or ischemic necrosis (Panner's disease) with resulting growth disturbances. Such abnormalities have been seen in children overusing the arm in throwing sports. If diagnosed early, the treatment should include: 1) rest; 2) change of sport; 3) alternation of sports; 4) gentle active stretching; 5) physical therapy with heat; 6) salicylates; 7) ice massage after usage.

At times, orthopedic surgery is helpful. Osteotomies or débridements can relieve pain, restore carrying angle, and improve function. Occasionally osteochondral fragments occur within the joint. They can be treated by surgical replacement into their normal anatomic sites or by removing them from the joint.

FOREARM AND WRIST INJURIES

Contusions, sprains, strains, and fractures are the most common injuries to this part of the body.

Forearm Fractures

Fractures of the radius and ulna usually present a deformity with exquisite tenderness at the fracture site (Fig. 21-12). Treatment is with splinting and ice application, then transportation for X-ray films and reduction or casting, as necessary.

If marked angulation is present and the circulation or motor function is significantly impaired, immediate reduction of the forearm bones can be performed by a skilled manipulator at the scene.

Before any reduction, the neurovascular status should be documented. After reduction has been performed, sensation, circulation, and motor capabilities of the wrist and hand should be reexamined and documented. A splint or cast should be applied; the extremity should be elevated (wrist higher than elbow and elbow higher than heart level); and ice should be applied for 24–36 hr.

Forearm compartment pressure syndromes may result from swelling within muscle compartments that causes ischemia and muscle necrosis. The swelling can be prevented by anticipating a pressure syndrome; splints applied to the wrist and forearm should allow for swelling. A skilled examiner should evaluate the extremity at frequent intervals and note changes in the neurovascular status. Pain should be controlled by ice, aspirin, and splinting. Narcotics should not be used because they mask the pain of incipient muscle ischemia. The fingers should be almost fully extendable, actively or passively, with only minimal discomfort at the fracture site. Sensation to all dermatomes of the hand should be intact.

Two-point discrimination should be tested and compared with the uninjured hand. Any impairment is an indication of possible increasing pressure in the forearm or at the wrist. Capillary filling response of the nailbed should be good when compared with the uninjured

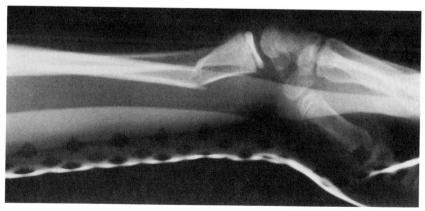

21-12 X-ray film of wrist, showing dorsally displaced fracture fragment of the distal radius in a 12-year-old boy.

extremity. The thumb should oppose the middle finger and index finger with good pinch power. The cast should not hinder thumb motion during this test. The fingers should abduct and adduct with strength sufficient to hold a piece of cardboard between the fingers.

The flexor retinaculum forms the carpal tunnel on the volar aspect of the wrist covering the flexor tendons and the median nerve, and the tunnel can become edematous and press upon the median nerve. The ulnar nerve can become involved in a similar fashion in the ulnar canal of Guyon at the wrist. This is a canal at the distal end of the forearm, through which the ulnar artery and nerve pass to the hand (Spinner [4]). Neurologic deficits in the dermatomes of the median and ulnar nerves will suggest pressure problems. Blockage of conduction of motor or sensory impulses to the hand will be detectable by electrodiagnostic tests. If carpal tunnel or Guyon tunnel syndromes develop and do not respond to elevation of the limb for several hours, further treatment should be considered. Injections of a local anesthetic agent mixed with dexamethasone and hyaluronidase can be used locally with some success. Pressure syndromes are treated by surgical decompression. Injections themselves may temporarily increase the pressure within tight compartments and should not be tried by those with little experience.

Death of muscle is not reversible but is preventable. Most hospitals are equipped with arterial pressure monitoring devices. These can be adapted to measure compartment pressures by comparison with the uninjured limb or by absolute values. Once a syndrome is diagnosed, the treatment is surgical release of the compartment. One should err in releasing a normal compartment rather than in temporizing with a swollen compartment.

Arterial injuries occur at fracture sites. If pulses are not palpable, a Doppler flowmeter should be used. Nailbed filling of capillaries is checked with the arm elevated and arm dependent. Filling and emptying of the veins on the dorsum of the hand are checked by forearm positioning, but swelling of the forearm at the fracture site may prevent such observations.

The adolescent with a forearm fracture needs excellent reduction. Do not hesitate to use open reduction if closed reduction has been less than ideal. It is very difficult for a good athlete to adapt to a poorly functioning forearm that is the result of a malunion of forearm bones. Note: Some forearm fractures have an associated dislocation or subluxation of the radial head (Monteggia's fracture). The elbow should be seen on X ray and any radial abnormality treated.

Wrist Injuries

The wrist joint is a condyloid articulation. Proximally located are the distal end of the radius and undersurface of the articular disc between the radius and ulna. Distally are the navicula, the lunate, and the triangular bone (triquetrum) (Gray [2]).

Sprains, contusions, and fractures are common injuries of the wrist. The painful swollen wrist should be splinted and then evaluated by X-ray studies. The neurovascular status should be assessed immediately and again at reasonable intervals for the subsequent 24 hr. *Carpal bone fractures or carpal fracture with associated intercarpal dislocation can easily be missed.*

Marked swelling and limitation of motion out of proportion to a "minor injury" or neurovascular impairment should lead to the suspicion of intercarpal dislocation.

Wrist trauma can cause a carpal tunnel syndrome or swelling within the tunnel of Guyon.

Negative results on X-ray studies, with tenderness at the "snuffbox" over the carpal scaphoid bone, suggest a fracture of the scaphoid. The wrist and thumb should be splinted for 14–21 days and then reevaluated clinically and by X-ray films to visualize the scaphoid fracture. This fracture deserves special comment. The healing time in a cast can be greater than 3 months. Some fractures go on to nonunion despite early casting. Some fractures remain undiagnosed and are treated as a sprain for several weeks. Initial treatment for a scaphoid fracture is a long arm-to-thumb spica cast with the forearm in neutral position. Some physicians use only a short arm-to-thumb spica cast. A few incorporate the index and middle fingers into the long cast for more rigid immobilization.

Small chip fractures of the distal end of the scaphoid may be treated as a sprain, with soft immobilization only, until symptoms subside, even though there is the possibility of a fibrous union of that small fragment.

Occasionally an X-ray film will reveal a fracture of the carpal scaphoid bone that already has arthritic changes in and around the radial carpal joint when the diagnosis is finally made. Other missed fractures will have cystic or avascular changes in the carpal scaphoid bone when they are eventually recognized.

The treatment of carpal scaphoid fractures must be individualized. Sometimes early open reduction and internal fixation are recommended. At other times the treatment is staged. Initially a soft wrap is utilized and the patient is allowed to engage in usual activities while internal fixation and bone grafting is planned for a later date. Staging treatment must be done with the informed consent of the patient.

Forced dorsiflexion or forced palmar flexion can cause various degrees of epiphyseal injuries in the immature wrist (Fig. 21-13). If there has not been complete separation or

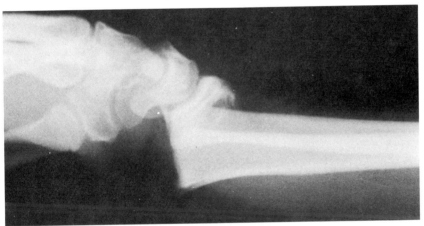

a

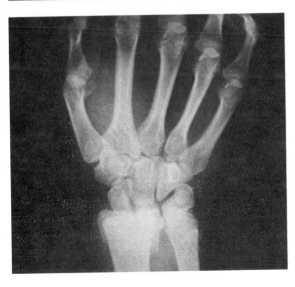

21-13 Anteroposterior (a) and lateral (b) views of wrist in a 14-year-old roller skater. There is dorsal displacement of the distal radial epiphysis (epiphyseal slip).

b

displacement of the growth area, X-ray films may be normal. A swollen wrist with exquisite fracture-type tenderness and significant functional impairment should be considered a fracture and treated as such until proved otherwise. X-ray studies of the uninjured wrist for comparison should be made and compared. The epiphyseal injury will commonly show at least some widening of the epiphyseal line. The only X-ray sign of a slipped epiphysis might be a small, displaced portion of bone at the periphery of the growth line. An inexperienced examiner might conclude that an avulsion fracture has occurred and miss the more serious growth-plate injury.

Treatment for epiphyseal injuries should be immobilization until complete healing. Displacements should be reduced under ideal conditions and as gently as possible, with the aid of appropriate anesthesia. The prognosis for growth will vary, depending on the severity of the epiphyseal trauma. These injuries are graded clinically by the location and extent of the fracture line into the epiphysis and by the degree of compression forces necessary to injure the growth center.

The final measures for sprains and fractures around the wrist include protection during periods of vulnerability and include: 1) taping, 2) elastic wrap or leather gauntlet, and 3) commercial splinting.

Avascular necrosis of the carpal lunate bone and early, arthritic changes in the wrist bones will give pain. The best treatment is early recognition and protection from stresses that may cause further injury to the wrist. Later the care, including surgical measures, must be individualized.

COMMON HAND INJURIES

Stress to the Carpal-Metacarpal Joint of the Thumb

Initially, thumb injury is treated with a splint, and the patient is transported for X-ray studies. The hand is examined for fractures, subluxation, or dislocation. The degree of stability is assessed, and a local anesthetic injection is given to relieve guarding, if necessary. Treatment must be individualized. If no fracture or subluxation is found, a splint is applied, with the proximal phalanx of the thumb included. Some fractures in this area may need open fixation of fragments and repair of soft tissues.

Sprain of the Metacarpal-Phalangeal Joint of the Thumb

Gentle stress should be applied to check for joint stability. Local anesthetic injections will facilitate stability evaluation and allow accurate recording of the degree of instability. X-ray films should be obtained while stress is applied to the medial collateral ligament and then the lateral collateral ligament to document the instability. Clinical and X-ray film comparisons can be made with the opposite extremity.

Severe instability due to torn collateral ligaments found after injury should be surgically repaired. Occasionally, avulsion fractures are associated with instability; these can be repaired by internal fixation. Small articular fractures that are not displaced and are associated with minimal or no instability can be treated by casting. Acute injuries without instability should be protected by a splint or cast extending from the distal segment of the thumb to above the wrist, with the hand and wrist in neutral position. Protection should be continued until tenderness subsides, usually after 3 weeks. Later, spica figure-eight taping should be used for at least an additional 3 weeks. Tape protection is offered for all future activities that might injure the thumb again.

Sprains of the Interphalangeal Joints of the Fingers

Ligament injuries at this level can vary from minor to complete tears of the collateral ligaments, volar capsular plate, or a central slip of the extensor mechanism, with dislocation.

Treatment must be individualized after X-ray studies to examine the degree of stability, and review of the mechanism of injury. Some unstable joints will need open repair of the ligament or fracture fixation. A dislocated interphalangeal joint should be gently reduced and splinted. The position of splinting varies and depends on the mechanism of injury and the areas of instability. Mobilize interphalangeal joint injuries early, usually on the first day after injury if 1) the collateral ligaments are intact, 2) no fracture fragments or only a small volar avulsion fragment is noted with minimal or no displacement, and 3) the central slip of the extensor apparatus allows full, active extension.

If these conditions are found, a "buddy-taping" system is recommended: The injured finger is taped to an adjacent finger. A splint is also applied for part of each day, with encouragement to remove it several times a day so that the joint can be moved.

Avulsion of the Extensor Tendon

Avulsion of the extensor tendon from the distal phalanx (also called mallet finger or baseball finger) can occur with or without avulsion of a small fragment of bone from the extensor surface of the distal phalanx. Avulsion occurs at the tendon insertion. Most such injuries can be treated by a small volar splint across the distal interphalangeal joint, with the joint in hyperextension. Open reduction and internal fixation are indicated when a large fragment is avulsed or an early postsplinting X-ray film shows persistence of the bony fragment in a dorsally displaced position.

In some cases, percutaneous pinning across the extended distal interphalangeal joint can be carried out. If there is excellent extensor function at the distal interphalangeal joint, and good 15°–25° active flexion despite the presence of a large displaced fragment, splinting alone is sometimes the best treatment.

Despite treatment, there may still be persistent tenderness or fullness at the insertion of the tendon on the dorsum of the distal phalanx.

There may also be persistent extensor lag (mallet deformity). Operative treatment may lead to limitation of flexion at the distal interphalangeal joint, even though the extensor lag has been reduced or corrected. Careful evaluation of the patient's functional needs for the hand is necessary. If the distal interphalangeal joint becomes stiff and flexion is lost, serious impairment may occur.

Fractures of the Metacarpal Bones and Phalanges

These fractures are considered individually after X-ray studies and clinical evaluation (Fig. 21-14). Special attention should be given to epiphyseal injuries in children. After the initial evaluation and treatment, patients should be seen for follow-up two or three times per week until healing occurs, to insure that proper rotation and alignment are maintained. Children heal rapidly, and malpositions must be corrected while fracture motion still exists.

Nerve and Vascular Injuries

Direct trauma to the palm or wrist that is simultaneous with hyperextension can injure the palmar arterial arch, ulnar artery, and median or ulnar nerves. These injuries should be kept in mind when a swollen wrist or hand is undergoing examination. If blood vessels have been injured, there will usually be point tenderness over the involved arteries. Commonly, vascu-

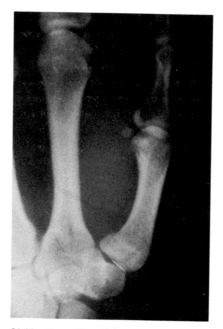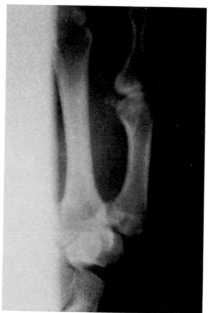

21-14 X-ray film of first metacarpal bone, showing minimally displaced intra-articular fracture of base of first metacarpal bone.

lar injury occurs in the region of the hamate bone at the ulnar border of the hand, in the vicinity of the tunnel of Guyon.

The circulation to the nails or fingers can be checked by Allen's test. This is performed by having the patient elevate the hand and clench the fist, to exsanguinate the hand. While the fist is clenched, the examiner's fingers are applied to occlude the radial and ulnar arteries. The patient's hand is then opened and pressure is released one vessel at a time. If the hand blushes as blood enters it, then the vessel is patent.

RIB CAGE INJURIES

Rib fractures usually present with painful respirations. The chest should be inspected to note the presence of decreased inspiratory excursion. Palpation will define areas of exquisite fracture-type tenderness and subcutaneous emphysema. Auscultation may reveal impaired ventilation and also the presence of subcutaneous emphysema. Percussion may be dull, as a result of bleeding into the peripleural space. Supportive care depends upon respiratory impairment until chest and rib X-ray films can be obtained. Sternochondral and costochondral injuries should be suspected when pain and tenderness are present in these areas.

Treatment consists of ice, local anesthetic injection, and an elastic binder for temporary pain relief. The physician should ascertain that the patient's respirations are not significantly impaired by the binder. Evaluation of the chest must be complete, for any force violent enough to fracture or dislocate ribs can cause intrathoracic injury.

Some sternochondral or costochondral injuries need open repair. Others present chronically with the sensation of snapping, pain, and instability. Chronic injuries often need surgical treatment.

A painful chest area, with or without clinical signs of tenderness or instability, needs exact localization of pain distribution. Selective intercostal nerve blocks may help in localizing the level of discomfort.

Rib fractures may be present with initially negative X-ray films. Reliance on symptoms and clinical findings is thus important. The conclusion that a fractured rib is present often can be based on symptoms only. Follow-up X-ray studies at 3–4 weeks will usually show fracture callus.

Radicular pain from an injured dorsal spine can radiate along the distribution of an intercostal nerve. The spine must be completely evaluated when symptoms or signs of rib injuries are being treated.

INJURIES TO THE STERNUM

The sternum may suffer contusions, sprains, dislocations, and fractures. The physician should palpate and localize tender areas over the sternum. X-ray studies are less important in this region. It is difficult to see sternoclavicular or even costosternal relationships on plain X-ray films. Tomograms or CT scans will help identify injuries.

Dislocations of the manubrium sterni can occur. Usually reduction is spontaneous, and the patient presents with pain, tenderness, and shallow respirations. Dislocations that do not spontaneously reduce usually involve the body of the sternum. They are depressed and associated with anterior prominence of the distal edge of the manubrium. These dislocations should be reduced under general anesthesia. Open reduction is sometimes necessary.

Fractures or subluxations involving the sternum can be associated with intrathoracic injuries resulting from the same force, and cause progressive impairment of function. Close evaluation in the hospital for 24–48 hr is recommended after a proven dislocation of the sternum.

COMMON INJURIES TO THE PELVIS AND HIP

Contusions and Strains

Contusions and strains are the dominant injuries of the pelvis. The most important contusion is called a "hip pointer." A hematoma forms at the point of contact along the iliac crest. The best prevention is the use of appropriate protective padding. Once a hip pointer occurs, treatment consists of ice applications, compression, and local injection of a long-acting anesthetic agent and hyaluronidase. Ultrasound is also helpful. The deep structures are not usually involved.

Strains vary in degree, depending on the extent of tearing of a tendon insertion away from the iliac bone. The common aponeuroses of the external oblique muscles can be torn completely from the iliac crest. Occasionally distraction or compression stresses to the immature pelvis will cause an epiphyseal injury. This will show on an X-ray film as widening of the growth apophysis of the iliac bone. This injury is similar to an avulsion fracture in which a separation occurred at the cartilaginous growth area instead of bones being torn from the parent bone (O'Donoghue [1]).

Major tears of the aponeuroses present with guarding and difficulty in straightening the torso. There is localized tenderness. Treatment is determined by the degree of tear. Most will respond to supportive treatment and no strenuous activities until symptoms subside. Abdominal binders or tight adhesive taping is helpful. Occasionally, surgical repair will be necessary to restore anatomic continuity of tissues. If the normal aponeurotic planes are reestablished surgically, there is less morbidity.

A large segment of scar tissue in the torn aponeuroses or immature fascial tissue in the region of the tearing is often painful when stressed. Surgical repair prevents pathologic scar tissue formation. For most contusions and deep hematomas in the vicinity of the pelvis, ice is applied for 15–30 min separated by 30-min intervals. This procedure is continued for the first 24 hr after injury. Ice can then be used periodically for a week to relieve symptoms and encourage deep drainage of the resolving hematoma.

Pelvic Fractures and Sprains

Fractures of the pelvis are not uncommon in sports. They result usually from compression of the iliac wing, either by a lateral force or by an anterior force. The ischium and pubic bones are also vulnerable to hard, direct pressure. More frequent, but still uncommon, are avulsion fractures of the anterosuperior iliac spine or ischial tuberosity. Unusual, violent muscle contractions of the sartorius and tensor fasciae latae in jumping or running sports can avulse the anterior iliac apophysis (O'Donoghue [1]).

Forced hip flexion with the knee extended can apply stress to the common origin of the hamstrings at the ischial tuberosity. This injury can be seen in hurdlers and other track and field athletes. Straddle injuries can lead to avulsion of the common adductor tendon from the pubic bone, with or without a small bone segment. Forced extension and internal rotation of the hip can cause injuries to the iliopsoas muscle, leading to an avulsion of the lesser trochanter. X-ray studies are necessary for diagnosis.

Clinical Findings Exquisite tenderness is present at the fracture site. There is pain with contraction of the involved muscle and relief on relaxation. Holding the extremity passively in the position achieved by maximal contraction of an involved muscle relieves tension on that muscle. For example, the sartorius muscle is at rest with hip flexion, knee flexion, and external rotation of the hip joint. The adductor muscles are at rest when the thighs are together in adduction. The hamstring muscles are at rest when the knee is flexed and the hips are slightly extended while the patient is lying sideways.

Treatment The treatment for avulsion injuries around the pelvis is usually ice, rest, and occasionally casting of the involved extremity in the position of least stress on the involved muscle. Widely separated fractures can be treated by surgical reattachment and internal fixation. Late surgical treatment is possible if the patient remains symptomatic, but it is less satisfactory because of muscle shortening and intrinsic scar formation. These make reattachment of the avulsed area difficult.

Fractures of the sacrum can escape diagnosis and heal while treated as a contusion. X-ray films of the sacrum should be obtained, especially if disability is excessive for a "contusion." The athlete and coach can then better plan the future, once the true nature of this injury is recognized. Full healing of the sacrum is important before allowing stress to the region.

Sprains in the pelvic area are common, especially at the sacroiliac region. *(A disc lesion can present presacral or sacroiliac pain also.)* Acute sprains in this region are associated with tenderness. Lumbosacral disc herniations may cause pain or pressure or a burning discomfort, but otherwise palpation is negative. The sacroiliac joint can be stressed in a side-lying (decubitus) position. Rocking of the sacroiliac joint occurs if the hip on the side against the table is held hyperflexed while the opposite hip is passively extended. Pain in this position is not always diagnostic of sacroiliac irritation. This test should be part of the general examination that includes hip-roll stressing, straight-leg raising, and compression and separation of the iliac wings. All these maneuvers apply stress to the sacroiliac joints. A neurologic evaluation of the lower extremities is also necessary in order to determine, especially, sciatic tension signs, reflex changes, sensory deficits, and motor weaknesses. Discrepancy in leg length should be noted by accurate measurement from the umbilicus to the medial malleolus or from the anterosuperior iliac spine to the medial malleolus.

Stress injuries to the perineum can cause severe sprains of the pubic symphysis. Unless actual separation of the bones has occurred these respond to simple, supportive measures, which include rest, ice, and avoidance of thigh abduction. Injuries to the urethra or bowel can occur from the same injuries to the perineum. Voiding should be tested and rectal examination carried out. Urinalysis and cystogram may be necessary to assess the injury completely. Consultation with a urologist or gynecologist may be necessary.

Fractures and Dislocations Around the Hip Joint

Proximal fractures of the femoral neck, intertrochanteric or subtrochanteric region present severe pain and inability to bear weight (Fig. 21-15). If displacements have occurred, these will be (in the supine position) external rotation deformity of the involved extremity and resistance to internal rotation or flexing of the leg. Initial treatment is splinting of the extremity, utilizing the opposite extremity or a broomstick. Definitive treatment is traction or surgical fixation.

Acute anterior dislocations of the hip present with fixed deformity in flexion and external rotation. Attempts at passive internal rotation are met with resistance and cause marked discomfort. Posterior dislocation of the hip presents with fixed flexion, adduction, and internal rotation (Fig. 21-16). Attempts to move the hip are met with pain and resistance.

In the adolescent, the "sprained hip" may represent a slipped capital femoral epiphysis (Fig. 21-17). Occasionally this presents pain in the knee (especially the medial aspect of the knee). Objective examination reveals a normal knee but limited hip motion, especially internal rotation and flexion. This is a not uncommon abnormality in overweight adolescents.

In general, X-ray studies are important in hip injuries. Tomograms or CT scans may be necessary to show an otherwise invisible fracture or osteochondritis dessicans within the

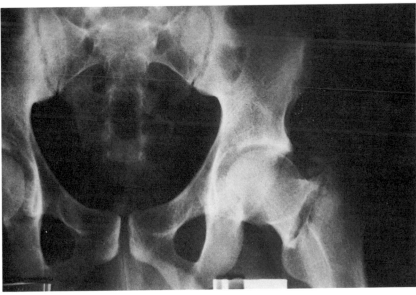

21-15　X-ray film of hip, showing minimally displaced fracture at base of femoral neck in a 25-year-old patient injured while skiing.

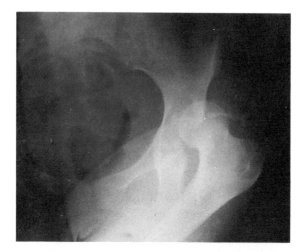

21-16a Posterior dislocation of hip, with a fracture of posterior wall of acetabulum (*top*). Reduced fracture of hip, with posterior fragment of acetabulum still displaced (*bottom*).

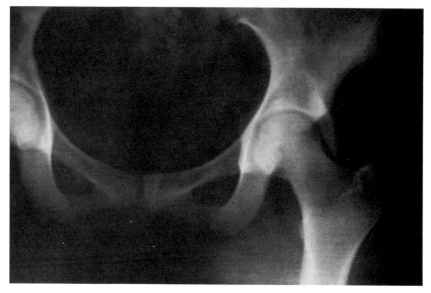

hip joint. If a slipped capital femoral epiphysis is found on one side, the other side should be examined also. The asymptomatic side should be observed at intervals thereafter to detect an early slip.

Treatment for slipped capital femoral epiphysis is usually internal fixation. Treatment for hip dislocations is closed reduction under general anesthesia.

COMMON ACUTE INJURIES TO THE THIGH

Contusion

A contusion of the thigh presents swelling and often discoloration in the region of the bruise. Palpation defines the area of muscle or subcutaneous hematoma. Treatment varies, but no definitive measure will prevent organization and calcification rather than absorption of the hematoma.

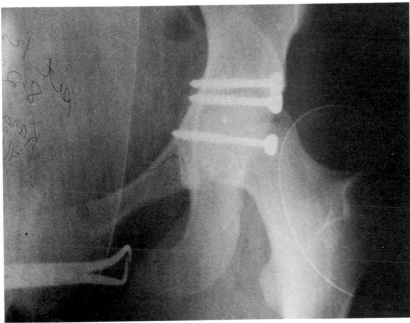

21-16b Postoperative film showing screw fixation of posterior wall of acetabulum and reduced hip joint.

Treatment may include the following steps:

1. Rest, by splinting or crutches and ice applications. (The rest period should extend for the duration of symptoms and while painful isometric contractions persist. Oral enzymes are utilized to facilitate hematoma breakdown and absorption. Later, physical therapy and heat are helpful.)
2. Aspiration of the hematoma, injection of a local anesthetic agent, and hyaluronidase solution to aid hematoma absorption.
3. Regional nerve blocks once or twice daily for 2 or 3 days to relieve spasm and allow pain-free hip and knee motion and isometric muscle contractions. (The blocks are used in conjunction with ice applications and supportive analgesics.)

Contusions, treated early, will do well. If treatment is started after 72 hr, the patient may have a greater tendency to scar formation or calcification in the region of the hematoma.

Muscle Tears

Hamstrings, quadriceps, or adductor muscles can tear partially or completely. Initial treatment is ice and compression wrap. For complete tears, early repair of the muscles should be done before muscle shortening and fibrosis occurs. Sometimes local or general anesthesia is necessary to assess fully the degree of muscle damage.

Partial tears should be protected for 4–6 weeks to allow complete healing before returning to athletics.

Rarely, isolated fascial tears can occur without muscle damage. The tear allows bulging (herniation) of the muscles through the rent in the fascia. Small bulges can be painful. If symptoms persist, surgery is indicated to enlarge the rent in the fascia, dissipate the forces of herniation, and render the area asymptomatic.

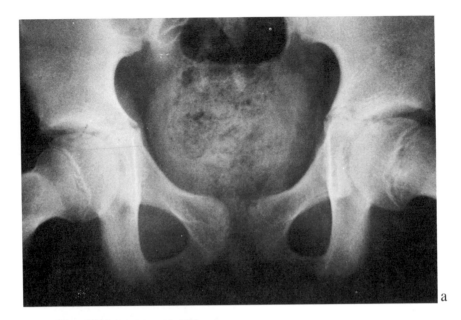

a

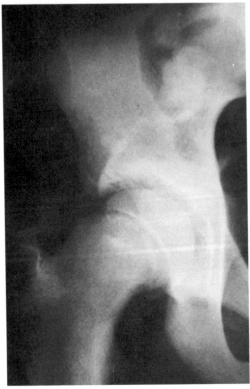

b

21-17 Frog lateral (a) and antero-posterior (b) views of hip in 11-year-old female with Grade I slippage of capital femoral epiphysis.

Femoral Shaft Fractures

Fractures of the femoral shaft are initially treated by splinting and ice application. Definitive treatment requires hospitalization.

Be aware that thigh compartment syndromes can develop from swelling within the thigh. Pressure assessments can be made with commercial pressure meters and decompression performed as necessary.

MYOSITIS OSSIFICANS

This unpredictable calcification of injured muscle requires varied treatment (Fig. 21-18). The ectopic bone must fully mature before it is removed. Maturation takes 9–12 months and can be monitored by bone scan. The calcified area should not be more active than the other bone. Once maturation has occurred, the bone can be removed surgically with less likelihood of recurrence. Diphosphonates or irradiation may be used to decrease recurrence of myositis ossificans. These measures are considered experimental and need fully informed consent.

KNEE INJURIES

The knee joint is a hinge joint or ginglymus joint, but is more complex because of its rotational capacity. The articular surfaces of the femur and tibia are connected by ligaments (Gray [2]):

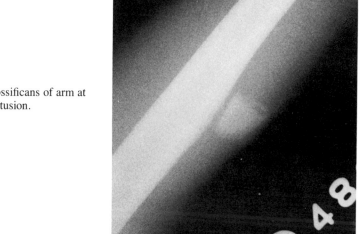

21-18 Myositis ossificans of arm at site of muscle contusion.

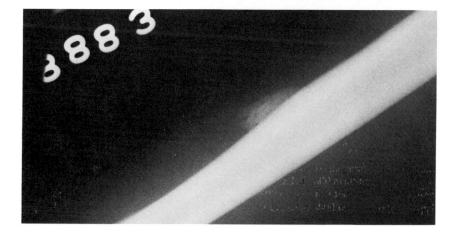

1. Medial and lateral capsular ligaments
2. Ligament of the patella
3. Oblique popliteal ligament
4. Arcuate popliteal ligament
5. Tibial collateral ligament
6. Fibular collateral ligament
7. Anterior cruciate ligament
8. Posterior cruciate ligament
9. Medial and lateral menisci
10. Transverse ligament
11. Coronary ligaments

Sprains at the Knee

Medial Injuries   These involve the medial capsular ligament. The mid one-third of the ligament (medial collateral ligament) has a deep and a superficial layer. First-degree tears will cause pain and limited motion ("stiff knee"). On examination, there is tenderness along most of the course of the ligament from the adductor tubercle to just below the joint line. A tear of the medial meniscus can coexist with injury to the medial collateral ligament.

A second-degree tear can compromise a complete tear of the deep layer and a partial tear of the superficial portion or a partial tear of both segments. Instability may be minimal when valgus stress is applied to the knee while the knee is flexed 15°–20°.

Third-degree tears are complete tears, involving both superficial and deep layers of the medial collateral ligament. These sprains allow opening of the mid joint line with valgus stress when the knee is in flexion of 15°–20°. The normal laxity of the joint can be noted by testing the uninjured knee. X-ray documentation is important. Films should be obtained to show the degree of joint line opening with valgus stress. In third-degree tears, swelling of tissues surrounding the joint may be minimal. The disruption of the capsular structures allows diffusion of inflammatory exudates into the surrounding tissues. There will not usually be a joint effusion.

The ability to open the medial joint line with valgus stress while the knee is fully extended (0° of flexion) implies posterior cruciate insufficiency or a tear.

It is rare to have a "simple" ligament injury to the knee. Usually, there are injuries to at least two other major knee structures. Careful and systematic examination should be performed to assess fully the extent of injury.

Lateral Injuries   These injuries involve the lateral capsular ligament. Varus knee stress can tear the capsule or avulse a bone fragment from the tibia or femur. These fragments can be seen on plain films of the knee or varus stress films. Signs will include tenderness of the lateral joint line with some lateral opening of the joint when there is varus stress with the knee flexed 15°–30°. Avulsion of the lateral-collateral ligament and biceps femoris muscle attachment from the fibular head can occur from the same type of force. Swelling may be minimal, as a result of the severity of tearing and diffusion of blood into soft tissues. Documentation of the varus laxity should be made by varus stress X-ray studies. Peroneal nerve injuries can occur in association with lateral ligament disruption.

The more severe the ligament injury, the less pain is felt with stress examination of the ligament. Minor tears are more painful and are associated with more guarding to prevent the stress of the examination. If an acute peroneal palsy is present, the implications must be discussed with the patient. Most peroneal palsies recover with time, but some do not. Stretch injuries or tears of the nerve should be diagnosed early and repaired or decompressed by utilizing microscopic techniques. Electromyographic studies early and late after injury are important to evaluate function fully.

Cruciate Ligament Injuries   Forced hyperextension, forced internal rotation of the thigh upon a planted foot with a flexed knee, or sudden hyperflexion with posterior directed stress can cause tears of either or both cruciate ligaments. These are severe injuries, associated with immediate pain and instability. The patient usually cannot walk unassisted. The degree of instability will be determined by the severity of ligament involvement. It should be noted that there is rarely a simple injury to the ligaments of the knee. Always assume that cruciate ligament injury is complex, involving other knee structures as well. An on-the-spot examination will give most information before swelling, pain, spasm, and guarding make assessment difficult.

Knee Examination

Inspection   Attitude of the knee should be determined. Is it flail? Is it held flexed, or is it lying fully extended with valgus or varus attitude? What is the color of the foot or leg? Is there joint swelling with obliteration of normal contours? Is the patella floating (ballottable)? Is the kneecap in its normal anatomic position?

Palpation   Is the pedal pulse present? Is sensation normal? Are active toe and ankle motion normal with good strength? The heel should be gently lifted to note hyperextension at the knee. The joint line should be palpated to note tender areas above and below or just at the joint line. Is there tenderness at the fibular head? With the knee straight, valgus or varus stress is applied and joint opening noted. The degree of opening (in millimeters) is estimated and recorded. A Lachman anterior drawer sign is elicited with the knee fully extended by gently applying anterior force below the knee (pulling leg forward) and counterforce posteriorly above the knee. The patient is requested to flex the knee slowly while a hand supports the popliteal region. With the knee flexed 15°–20°, valgus and varus stresses are applied to check stability and note joint openings medially or laterally. The posterior drawer sign should be checked with the knee flexed. Gentle force is applied posteriorly (pushing leg backward) just distal to the joint to determine whether the tibia moves posteriorly in relation to the femur.

Similarly, the Lachman drawer sign is rechecked with the patient supine and the involved extremity on the side of the examiner. With the patient's knee held between full extension and 15° flexion and slight external rotation at the hip, the femur is stabilized with one hand while firm pressure is applied to the posterior aspect of the proximal tibia in an attempt to translate it anteriorly (Torg et al. [5]).

The anterior drawer sign is again checked with the knee flexed almost to 90° and the leg held first internally and then externally rotated at the knee. If the anterior drawer sign is abolished by forced internal rotation, this implies that the posterior cruciate ligament is intact. If anterior drawer is present with external rotation the implication is that the anterior cruciate ligament is torn.

If a tibia is posteriorly displaced due to a posterior cruciate ligament laxity or tear, the anterior drawer maneuver will bring the tibia to its normal position. This can be misinterpreted as a positive anterior drawer sign.

Rotational instability can be noted by eliciting a pivot shift (anterior lateral) or posterior lateral drop off. With the patient supine, the knee should be flexed 90° and supported with one hand under the thigh just above joint and the second hand under the upper leg; the thumb should be under the fibula head. The knee is extended slowly by the examiner as the thumb under the fibula rotates the leg inward. With instability present the leg will shift forward at the anterior lateral joint line. Flexion of the knee to 90° will reduce the shift.

Posterior lateral rotational instability can be shown by suspending the leg by the heel. Recurvatum at the knee and posterior lateral drop off of the tibia at the joint line can be seen and felt.

The popliteal, posterior tibial, and dorsalis pedis pulses should be palpated. The hands are moved slowly across the hamstrings medially and laterally to check for swelling, tenderness, and spasm. The condyles are gently palpated in the supracondylar region of the femur to note crepitation, bony irregularities, and exquisite fracture tenderness.

A developmentally "tight joint" may have a cruciate ligament injury with no clinical instability.

After the initial examination has been completed, the extremity is splinted until definitive treatment, X-ray studies, or further examination under anesthesia can be performed. If the injury is not examined within 6 hr, guarding and spasm will prevent adequate assessment. Spinal or general anesthesia may be necessary to define the injury fully. A subtle posterior cruciate injury can be missed. Clues to the presence of a posterior cruciate lesion are as follows:

1. Straight posterior laxity (posterior drawer sign).
2. Valgus opening of the medial jointline with the knee fully extended. (Examination will further define whether there is an acute straight instability or rotational instability at the knee.)
3. Failure to stop an anterior drawer sign with forced internal rotation of the tibia.

Acutely Swollen Knee

Joint effusion appearing immediately after an injury is due to blood accumulation within the joint (hemarthrosis). Hemarthrosis is a significant injury. The patient will be unable fully to extend and lock the knee. There will be a limp and, very likely, assistance in walking will be needed. Because the joint has contained the blood within, the likelihood of an acute third-degree tear of the capsular ligament is less. Third-degree tears will allow diffusion of blood into soft tissues outside the joint. Possible causes of an acute hemarthrosis are as follows:

1. Meniscus tear (medial or lateral)
2. Anterior cruciate tear
3. Dislocation or subluxation of the patella
4. Synovial pinching or tearing
5. Osteochondral fracture

Treatment   After examination has established the diagnosis, the joint is aspirated under aseptic conditions, and frequent reevaluation is necessary. X-ray studies should be obtained as soon as pain tolerance allows. When possible, X-ray studies should include anteroposterior views; 45° flexion lateral view; tunnel view; skyline view of the patella; and weight-bearing anteroposterior view. Oblique views may help reveal avulsion fractures from the articular margins. Arthrography and arthroscopy should be considered in the first 24 hr after injury for precise diagnosis. If there are clear indications of instability, surgery becomes necessary and arthrography can be avoided. Arthroscopy may precede the surgical procedure if there is no evidence of capsular tearing (which could cause extensive soft-tissue swelling from fluid extravasation). At surgery a thorough joint examination should also be done.

The surgical objective is to reestablish anatomic continuity of torn structures and restore stability to the knee.

Patellar Dislocation or Subluxation

Some knees are more vulnerable to lateral displacement of the patella because of developmental variations, such as: 1) genu valgum, 2) patella alta, 3) vastus medialis insufficiency, 4) increased quadriceps angle (Q-angle), and 5) externally pointing patellae.

Acute Patellar Dislocation or Subluxation

Many patellar dislocations or subluxations will spontaneously reduce, and the patient will have a swollen, painful knee. On palpation, there is a hemarthrosis and tenderness at the medial capsule. Efforts to move the patella laterally, while gently, passively extending the knee will be met with resistance and anxiety. Because of the hemarthrosis, the knee cannot flex past 60°–80°, nor can it be extended beyond 15° flex position.

The history is often that the patella shifted or snapped with an associated sudden pain, causing a fall. A careful history may reveal similar, but less severe previous episodes.

A patient with recurrent dislocations may present only with a swollen knee, without tenderness along the medial capsule or vastus medialis. In such patients, soft tissues have already been stretched from prior episodes and were not significantly injured during the last, acute injury.

Patellar dislocations can cause a chondral or osteochondral fracture of the articular surface of the patella or of the lateral femoral condyle. X-ray films should be obtained at the initial evaluation and after reduction.

A patella presenting in a dislocated lateral position must be reduced. It is best to use general anesthesia or, alternatively, to fill the joint, under sterile conditions, with local anesthetic solution in addition to a regional block of the femoral nerve. The anesthetic allows minimal forces to the articular surface of the patellofemoral joint during reduction. After spontaneous or therapeutic reduction the joint hematoma should be aspirated, ice should be applied, and the knee splinted. Isometric exercises should begin immediately. Some acute capsular tears are best treated by surgical repair to decrease the chance of recurrence.

If an osteochondral fracture is seen on X-ray films, surgery should be performed to assess the damage, replace or remove the fragments, and repair torn soft tissues.

Systematic examination for associated ligamentous injuries should always be performed, as outlined. Attention should not be focused only at the obvious kneecap injury while an associated ligamentous tear with potential instability is missed.

Bursitis of the Knee

All the bursae around the knee can become acutely swollen or inflamed. The bursae are as follows:

1. Suprapatellar
2. Prepatellar
3. Superficial infrapatellar
4. Deep infrapatellar
5. Anserine
6. Semimembranous
7. Bursa at the head of the fibula

8. Bursa between the fibula collateral ligament and the popliteus tendon
9. Bursa between the lateral gastrocnemius head and the lateral femoral condyle
10. Bursa just anterior to the popliteus muscle

Treatment

1. Warm compresses
2. Aspiration, culture, and gram stain of the aspirate
3. If no infection is found, local steroid injection
4. Short immobilization if necessary

Bursitis can occur from direct contusion or overuse due to rubbing of the bursa during athletic activity.

It is necessary to distinguish between a deep infrapatellar bursitis and an irritation of the patellar fat pad. Hyperflexion of the knee will increase pressure within the bursa but not in the fat pad. Passive or active knee extension will stress the fat pad but will not usually increase pressure in the bursa. The relatively superficial position of the bursa makes it easier to compress it on palpation and cause pain. It is more difficult to compress the fat pad palpably (O'Donoghue [1]).

Injuries to Menisci

The medial meniscus is injured more commonly than the lateral meniscus. The coronary ligament connects the meniscus medially to the tibia and to the medial one third of the capsular ligament. Laterally there is no capsular attachment of the meniscus; only the coronary ligament attaches to the tibia. Because of more adherence to collateral structures medially, the medial meniscus is more vulnerable to injury. Peripheral tears of the menisci in or near the coronary ligament potentially heal with time if stress to the area is decreased. A tear within the substance of the meniscus will be prevented from healing by local stresses and a poor blood supply in this region. Tears may be longitudinal, oblique, and transverse. Meniscus lesions that cause recurring pain or recurrent locking of the joint are detrimental to the joint. Such functional impairment may cause destruction of areas of articular cartilage and can predispose the knee to ligamentous injury by increasing its vulnerability to trauma.

Menisci are useful weight-bearing cushions and stabilizing elements in the knees. The function of the knee joint is more effective with the menisci intact. When the meniscus is injured, causing joint effusion, unreduced locking, recurrent locking, or pain at the joint line with activity, orthopaedic evaluation and treatment may be necessary.

The acutely injured meniscus may present as one of the following:

1. A locked knee (unable to extend fully and unable to flex fully)
2. A swollen knee (hemarthrosis)
3. Joint-line tenderness in the vicinity of the meniscus tear

The patient's history will often show previous "catching" episodes, knee sprain or knee effusions (water on the knee). The knee should be systematically examined, as for sprain. Blood should be aspirated and the knee reexamined. A locked knee can be reduced by skilled manipulation with or without a general anesthetic. Weight-bearing should not be allowed until the joint is movable again. The locked knee is not protected during weight-bearing. Weight-bearing causes impingement of the tibial cartilage surface against the femoral cartilage surface rather than the usual gliding of the cartilaginous surface. The true stability of the knee (especially the status of the anterior cruciate ligament) cannot be determined while the knee is "locked."

Diagnosis of Acute Meniscus Problems

It is best to assemble as much information as possible about an injured knee within the first 24 hr. This will allow a definitive decision about knee stability and whether ligament repair will be necessary. The following situations should be checked:

1. If the knee is not locked, or if it can be unlocked without anesthesia, the joint is examined as it is for sprains, discussed earlier in this chapter, and signs of meniscus hypermobility are noted. If there is no instability, but signs of meniscus tear are found, an arthrogram (Fig. 21-19) and arthroscopy will further define the problem.
2. If the arthrogram shows no lesions of the meniscus, then treatment is supportive (splint, isometric exercises, progressive resistance exercises, gradual range-of-motion activities, and follow-up in 1 week).
3. If the arthrogram shows a tear in the meniscus, with the substance of the meniscus and the cruciate system apparently intact, then treatment is individualized. There is no urgency to remove a torn meniscus, so long as the knee is not locked. Supportive care is necessary, however, with a splint, crutches, isometric exercises, and gradual range-of-motion exercises. Weight bearing may be permitted in some cases, and the patient is followed up in 1 week. Arthroscopy will be helpful.

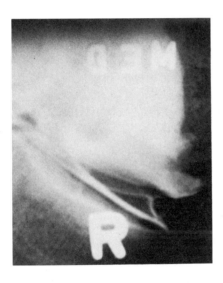

21-19 Arthrography of medial compartment of knee shows anterior (a), posterior (b), and midvertical (c) tearing of medial meniscus, in which contrast material flowed between body of meniscus and its peripheral attachment. The tear is complete, of bucket-handle type, and is unstable, with a tendency for central portion to be displaced into joint, causing locking or knee buckling.

a

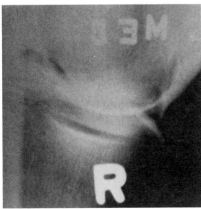

b

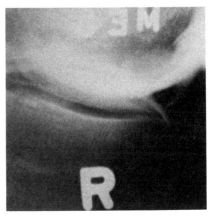

c

4. If the arthrogram shows absence of the cruciate ligament, examination under anesthesia, arthroscopy, and surgery may be necessary.
5. If there is repetitive pain and locking, in association with positive results on an arthrogram, arthroscopy and surgery are performed.
6. If anesthesia is necessary to unlock the knee, arthroscopy is performed; definitive surgery often follows.
7. Many physicians are using diagnostic and operative arthroscopy to definitively treat meniscus pathology early.

Chronic Meniscus Lesion

Patients suffering chronic problems of the meniscus present a history of the knee "giving way," "catching," or locking, in association with recurrent effusions (water on the knee). Quadriceps atrophy will often be noted by comparison with the opposite side at a fixed-distance point above the knee joint. Squatting may be difficult. The cutting maneuver or pivoting maneuver may cause pain or snapping. Joint-line tenderness in the area of a meniscus tear is usually found. This must be differentiated from tenderness along the entire medial collateral ligament, which is seen with a sprain of the ligament. A sprain of the medial collateral ligament may coexist with a meniscus lesion.

The McMurray maneuver, the Apley grind test, or the Apley distraction test can reproduce symptoms by causing the meniscus to move at the tear.

The McMurray test is used to diagnose a lesion of the posterior or mid third segment of the meniscus. The patient is supine, and the knee is flexed maximally toward the buttock. One hand steadies the knee, and the other hand holds the heel. To test the lateral meniscus, the leg is turned with internal rotation, and slight varus stress is applied. To test the medial meniscus, the leg is externally rotated while slight valgus stress is applied. While the knee is forcibly rotated, the leg is extended slowly. A painful click will be felt and sometimes heard as the meniscus moves in and out of its normal position or the femoral condyle moves over an irregularity in the meniscus.

The Apley grinding test is performed while the patient is lying prone. The knee is flexed 90° and rotated while a compression force is applied. This causes pain if a meniscus is torn.

The Apley distraction test is performed while the patient is prone. The examiner holds the patient's thigh on the table with his own knee, then applies rotation and distraction to the patient's knee. Pain indicates that a ligament rather than the meniscus has been injured (Helfet [6]).

Treatment of a symptomatic, isolated meniscus lesion should include consideration of the following points:

1. The athletic objectives of the patient
2. The stability of the knee before meniscus surgery (rotatory instability of the knee may be increased by removal of the meniscus)
3. Frequency of pain, catching, or swelling
4. Partial meniscus excision with intact peripheral rim
5. The status of the articular cartilage (as noted on X-ray studies and by arthroscopy) to determine whether the meniscus is reparable
6. The possibility of treating torn segments by operative arthroscopy
7. Loose bodies within the knee joint

The presence of loose fragments on X-ray films and their anatomic relationships may allow correlation with clinical instability. Avulsion fracture fragments usually, but not always, necessitate surgical repair of an involved ligament. Common avulsion fracture sites are the following:

1. Tibial spine (anterior cruciate ligament)
2. Posteromedial aspect of the femur (posterior cruciate ligament)
3. Tibial tubercle (patellar tendon insertion)
4. Lateral rim of tibial plateau (lateral capsular ligament)
5. Inferior tip of patella (patellar ligament insertion)
6. Upper pole of patella (quadriceps insertion point)

Patellofemoral Arthralgia

In patellofemoral arthralgia (also called chondromalacia of the patellofemoral articulation), pain on the articular surface of the kneecap is difficult to cure. It is probably the most common knee complaint in practice and occurs more often in females. Symptoms are caused by areas of surface irregularities of the patella alone or of the patella and the femoral groove.

Symptoms

1. Pain at anterior aspect of knee with walking or running
2. Anterior pain on descending stairs, squatting, or ascending stairs
3. Recurrent effusion, depending upon activity
4. Crepitation (the feeling of grating), as knee is actively flexed and extended
5. Rarely, symptoms at rest

Signs

1. Crepitation as patella is passively moved within femoral groove while pressure is simultaneously applied
2. Easy lateral subluxation of patella with lateral stress
3. Pain and recurrence of symptoms with passive movement of and simultaneous pressure to patella within the femoral groove
4. Pain with contraction of quadriceps as patella is held in groove (patella inhibition test)
5. Quadriceps angle (Q-angle) greater than $10°$, often $15°-20°$
6. Tenderness on palpation of lateral patellofemoral ligament. (This can be elicited in supine position. It is more easily done while patient is prone. The patella is gently moved out of the femoral groove while pressure is applied to lateral soft-tissue attachments of kneecap.)
7. Genu valgum deformity
8. External tibial torsion with external rotation of tibial tubercle
9. Femoral anteversion combined with external tibial torsion (malalignment syndrome)

The articular pathology should be graded by both clinical assessment and by arthroscopic evaluation. Grade I is softening of the articular surface. Grade II is fissuring of the articular surface. Grade III is fragmentation of the articular surface. Grade IV is eburnation or hard, bony exposure with loss of articular cartilage.

X-ray Signs

1. Patella alta
2. Shallow femoral groove

3. Shallow patellar articular angle
4. Tilting of patella on skyline view

Treatment

1. Development of strong quadriceps and hamstring muscles by isometric exercises and progressive resistive exercises
2. Avoidance of stair climbing and squatting whenever possible
3. Small doses of aspirin on a regular basis
4. Pull-on elastic knee support or restraining brace for patella
5. Orthotic inserts to alter stress at knee by balancing foot
6. Surgery as a last resort, utilizing realignment measures; shaving and drilling; elevation of tibial tubercle; resurfacing; or patellectomy

Osteochondritis Dissecans of Knee Joint

This osteochondral defect (bone and cartilage fragment) is usually localized to the lateral articular edge of the medial femoral condyle. The fragment is usually not displaced or is only minimally elevated from the surrounding articular cartilage. Rarely, it has been noted in other areas of the articular surface of the knee joint. The etiology of osteochondritis dissecans is not known, but vascular compromise and trauma have been suggested. It presents as a painful knee. Symptoms are associated with running, kicking (especially side kicks and cross-over kicks, common in soccer). Objective findings may be minimal: 1) joint effusion; 2) pain on placing the heel of the symptomatic leg on the opposite knee in a cross-knee fashion and passively forcing external rotation at the hip.

The diagnosis is made by X-ray studies (Fig. 21-20) (especially the tunnel view of the knee). The joint surface can be inspected by arthroscopy.

Treatment   The patient's age, symptoms, and the degree of elevation and separation of the fragment from articular cartilage determine the type of treatment. The preteenager can be treated with casting, splint, and isometric exercises, with reasonable chances of healing. Older patients will need individual considerations. Symptomatic lesions in older patients are usually removed surgically. Some fragments may be held with internal fixation pins or suture material.

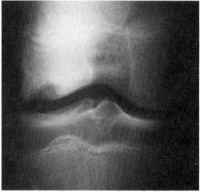 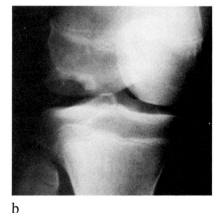

a   b

21-20   Anteroposterior (a) and oblique (b) views of knee, showing large osteochondritis dissecans defects in articular surface of lateral femoral condyle.

Osgood-Schlatter Disease

The symptoms of Osgood-Schlatter disease occur in the immature knee and can be due to inflammation of the deep infrapatellar tendon bursa or to irritation or fragmentation of the anterior proximal tibial epiphysis (epiphysitis).

The patient presents activity-induced discomfort and tenderness, localized to the tibial tubercle. The symptoms usually subside after epiphyseal closure and tissue maturation in the region of the tibial tubercle. On rare occasions, symptoms persist into adulthood and are associated with the persistence of bone or cartilage fragments in the region of the tibial tubercle.

Treatment

1. Decreasing activities to tolerance
2. Ice applications to tibial tubercle before and after activities
3. Strengthening quadriceps and hamstring muscles
4. Use of knee-immobilizing splint periodically to rest knee while isometric exercises are continued for quadriceps and hamstrings
5. On rare occasions, an injection of local anesthetic agent with steroids into region of patellar tendon insertion
6. Surgical removal of fragments of epiphysis (to be done only after bone has matured) (This procedure can cause premature anterior tibial epiphyseal closure with a resulting recurvatum deformity of the knee.)

Recurrent Knee Joint Effusion

The cause of the effusion must be sought systematically by the following means.

1. A check for mechanical reasons (chondromalacia, meniscus lesions, knee instability, and loose bodies)
2. Aspiration of fluid for analysis (cell count, mucin clot test, crystals, uric acid level, complement and enzyme studies)
3. Blood tests (sedimentation rate, rheumatoid factor, antinuclear antibodies, uric acid levels, HLA-B27)
4. Culture of aspirate (routine aerobic and anaerobic organisms, acid fast organisms, fungus, and brucella)

Treatment   Therapy should be directed at etiology. If no diagnosis is made, symptomatic treatment and maintenance of function should be instituted:

1. Immobilization with splint or cast
2. Isometric and progressive resistive exercises
3. Oral anti-inflammatory drugs (aspirin, acetominophen, and newer anti-inflammatory medications)
4. Rare steroid injection if tuberculosis and other infections have been excluded
5. Outpatient saline washout with 1000–2000 cc saline run through joint by irrigation tubes
6. Diagnostic arthrography and arthroscopy to search for mechanical causes or to obtain synovial biopsy

Minor Knee Symptoms

Lateral joint-line pain associated with distance running can be caused by bursitis, popliteal tendinitis, iliotibial band irritation, meniscus tears, or meniscus cysts. These can be treated by rest, ice massage, gradual increase in running tolerance by decreasing distances, and increasing sprinting. Rarely, local injections of an anesthetic agent, with or without a steroid preparation, can be tried. A podiatric evaluation with foot balancing sometimes solves the problem.

Complete Dislocation of the Knee

Tibial-femoral dislocation is, fortunately, an uncommon injury in athletes. Before examination there has usually been spontaneous reduction of the dislocation. On occasion, the patient has already been splinted and is ambulatory on crutches at the time of the examination. The knee should be systematically evaluated, and sensory function and circulation distal to the knee should be carefully examined. If, after the examination, the clinical assessment is that of anterior and posterior cruciate ligamentous tears, then it may be assumed that dislocation of the knee has occurred. It is imperative to assess and follow carefully for 24–36 hr the blood supply to the involved extremity. It is not uncommon for trauma to the popliteal vessel to allow good blood flow initially and then for obstruction of flow to occur after several hours. The collateral circulation around the knee may often carry enough blood to the foot and ankle, which remain pink with good capillary supply to the nailbed and palpable dorsalis pedis and posterior tibial pulses. It is important to quantitate the pulses by comparison with the opposite extremity and by correlation with the patient's blood pressure.

Doppler flow studies or arteriograms are worthwhile during the first 24 hr to document patency of the popliteal vessel and an uninjured trifurcation (peroneal artery, posterior tibial artery, and anterior tibial artery).

Treatment of the dislocated knee is surgical, to establish anatomic continuity of torn structures. If vascular compromise is discovered, vessels should be repaired by a vascular surgeon and the knee stabilized by temporary internal or external fixation until the repaired vessels have healed.

In the immature knee, the same force that would cause a dislocation can lead to a major displacement (slippage) of the proximal tibial epiphysis. If the shaft of the tibia is displaced posteriorly, the popliteal artery can be injured (Fig. 21-21). With this injury, the knee ligaments are usually not torn.

COMMON LEG INJURIES

Compartment Syndromes

Overuse can cause swelling within leg compartments. The anterior and lateral compartments are frequently involved. This disorder is common in runners. It can also occur with leg contusion or fractures of leg bones. The patient usually presents with pain after running. The pain will respond to ice and rest. Sometimes the swelling within the compartment does not subside before causing signs of neurovascular compression: weakness of dorsiflexion or in extension of the large toe, or decrease in peroneal muscle function and hypalgesia in the first web space or over the entire dorsum of the foot. Rarely, the posterior or deep intermediate compartments can be involved, causing weakness of plantar flexion, flexion of the large toe and lateral toes, and hypalgesia along the distribution of the posterior tibial and plantar nerves on the sole of the foot.

If the condition is seen while in the acute stage, the diagnosis can be made by pressure studies from within the compartment and by comparing results with the opposite side (see section on Forearm Fractures earlier in this chapter).

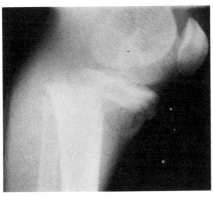 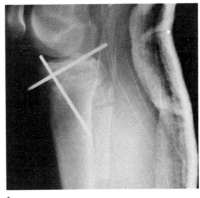

a   b

21-21 (a) Epiphyseal slip of proximal tibial epiphysis. Distal segment displaced posteriorly, causing arterial injury. Arterial repair was necessary in this case. (b) Postreduction film, showing pin fixation of epiphysis to maintain stability while arterial repair and healing occurred.

Treatment If a compartment syndrome has been documented by pressure studies and if compression of neurovascular structures compromises function, then surgical release of the fascial covering may be necessary. The deep intermediate compartment is decompressed by removing a portion of the fibula.

Shin Splints

A pain syndrome of multiple causes, usually localized to the anterolateral aspect of the leg or posteromedial aspect of the calf and associated with overuse of the extremity is known as "shin splints." Sometimes relatively little activity may induce the symptoms. The syndrome is most common in long-distance runners.

Several theories have been proposed to explain shin splints:

1. Stress fractures of the tibia or fibula
2. Partial tear of the muscle fascia of the gastrocnemius or posterior tibial muscle
3. Compartment syndrome
4. Stretch irritation of branches of the peroneal nerve because of muscle swelling or repetitive muscle contraction
5. Periostitis of the fascial attachment to the tibia

X-ray Studies Occasionally stress fractures of the tibia or fibula are seen in the region of symptoms. "Looser zones" may be noted. If so, follow-up X-ray studies should be made at 6-week intervals until these defects either resolve or show signs of callous formation, indicating a stress fracture had been present. A bone scan may be helpful.

Treatment Treatment varies with the etiology. If no one cause can be found, the treatment includes one or more of the following steps:

1. Gentle stretching of both anterior and posterior musculature (especially the calf, heel cord, and hamstring)
2. Ice massage or ice packs before and after activities
3. Gentle, progressive resistive exercises to build muscle tone (especially the dorsiflexors of the foot)

4. Gradual build-up of endurance in running or jumping sports
5. Regular use of salicylates taken just before or during sports (Some athletes improve with this regimen.)
6. Repetitive ultrasound application
7. Taping and elastic wrap of the calf, with padding over involved muscles
8. Holistic approaches, including acupuncture and vitamin and calcium supplements (There are no data to support this therapy.)
9. Long rest or change of sports (This procedure may be helpful and protective of the muscle compartments.)
10. Release of anterior and lateral compartments in runners with persistent symptoms (There is no documentation of the efficacy of this treatment.)

Muscle Tears

The most common tear occurs usually medially or centrally in the gastrocnemius fascia. The plantaris muscle tendon unit can also tear, but this is more often suspected than it actually occurs. The treatment is supportive (ice, elevation, crutches, gradual weight bearing, elastic stocking). Occult venous thrombosis can occur after injury. Increased swelling or pain should be studied by venography or phlebography.

COMMON ANKLE INJURIES

The ankle joint is a hinge. The joint is composed of the lower end of the tibia, the tibial malleolus, the fibular malleolus, and the dome of the talus. These bones are connected by the 1) deltoid ligament, 2) calcaneofibular ligament, 3) anterior and posterior talofibular ligaments, and 4) articular capsule (Gray [2]).

Sprain

Acute soft-tissue injuries of the ankle are usually the result of inversion stress to the anterolateral capsule and to the lateral collateral ligament. With the inversion stress, there is internal rotation and plantar flexion of the foot in relation to the leg. This causes tearing of the anterolateral capsule and swelling and partial tearing at the origin of the muscle mass of the short extensor muscles of the toes. There is also tearing of the fibulocalcaneal ligament (lateral collateral ligament of the ankle). The injury to the collateral ligament can be of first to third degree.

The patient presents a swollen, painful ankle; the tenderness and swelling are mostly on the anterolateral and direct lateral aspects. Occasionally there is swelling of the medial joint line in the vicinity of the deltoid ligament. A hematoma will rapidly dissect along tissue planes of the foot, causing ecchymotic discoloration in many areas.

The history is important. The patient may describe many prior, similar sprains, each one with symptoms and signs.

Clinical Examination   First-degree injury shows no signs of instability on anterior or posterior draw stress (draw sign) or with inversion stress. The instability of second- and third-degree injuries will depend on the amount of tissue tearing.

X-ray Studies   The X-ray films may reveal an avulsion fracture of the tip of the lateral malleolus (Fig. 21-22) with associated fractures of the medial malleolus or distal fibula.

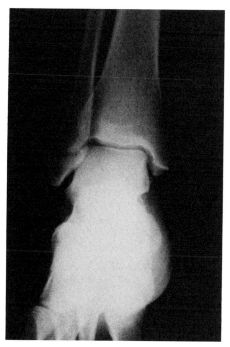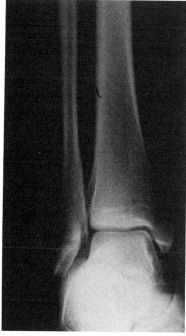

21-22 Anteroposterior view of ankle showing minimally displaced fracture of distal fibula at level of tibial-talar joint line.

There may be calcifications in soft tissue that suggest old and recurrent ligamentous trauma. Inversion stress films should be obtained to record the amount of talar tilt. A comparison should be made with the opposite ankle, though it is not uncommon for both ankles to have been involved in recurring sprains so that stress X-ray studies show bilateral laxity.

Ankle arthrograms are helpful in some instances to assess the extent of ligament damage. Bone scan and ankle arthroscopy can assess the joint status in working up acute or chronic ankle pain.

Treatment The type of care is determined by stability. A stable and minimally swollen ankle with no signs of recent fracture or dislocation requires 1) elevation, 2) ice, 3) soft ankle wrap (sheet wadding or cotton covered with an Ace bandage or covered with an Unna paste boot), and 4) use of crutches to avoid bearing weight.

After 5–7 days a heavy pull-on elastic stocking, elevation of the foot most of the time, some weight bearing with the use of a cane or crutches as necessary, will help to encourage ankle motion. Swimming is good ankle exercise. The patient should regularly do isometric and progressive resistive exercises for calf and anterior leg muscles.

If swelling is marked and the ankle is clinically stable, the balloon distention effect can mask instability temporarily. Severely swollen ankles should be casted or splinted, with the foot in neutral position. Elevation of the leg should be encouraged, and the leg reevaluated in 7–10 days.

Treatment of the unstable ankle is individualized. Many recreational and professional athletes have unstable ankles because of recurrent lateral and anterolateral tissue tears that have not been surgically treated. Decent function with an unstable ankle is possible, provided supportive taping or above-ankle shoes are utilized. Lateral or anterolateral injuries that cause ankle instability can be treated as follows:

1. The first episode associated with anterolateral or straight varus (inversion) instability without fractures requires the use of a cast for 3–6 weeks, or the torn ligaments should be surgically repaired.
2. Acute lateral or anterolateral injury, with a past history of recurrent similar injuries and associated instability, should be treated with ankle taping; pull-on elastic ankle support; and crutches or a cast for 7–10 days. Surgical treatment might necessitate reconstructive measures to create anterior and lateral stabilizing elements.
3. The first episode of lateral or anterolateral injury associated with instability can be treated with a pull-on elastic support or with taping alone, provided the swelling is not severe and the patient is cooperative and will utilize crutches. Starting early ankle motion while participating in progressive resistive and isometric exercises for calf and anterior compartment structures is essential. This treatment requires the patient's informed consent and knowledge of alternative therapies.

The application of a short walking cast to the leg is a good standby for treatment. However, the cast can cause increased morbidity, including stiffness of the ankle and phlebitis as a result of the immobilization.

Late reconstructive measures for chronic and recurring anterolateral and lateral ankle instability are successful. A choice in treatment programs short of surgery is therefore possible at an early time. Closed treatment, however, cannot predict that healing of the torn capsule and ligamentous structures will be good. Periarticular disarray of torn ligaments may never allow end-to-end joining of ligamentous structures, and fibrous bridging strong enough to give the ankle stability may not be possible. The athlete and the family, in the case of minors, should help in deciding treatment choice.

Medial ligament injuries (deltoid ligament) are less common. Third-degree tears of this ligament are associated with complete instability on eversion or valgus stress to the ankle. X-ray studies and palpation will document the condition. The draw sign may not be present with anterior and posterior stress in the neutral position of the foot. Treatment for third-degree deltoid ligament lesion is surgical repair. Most likely this ligament will be displaced between the medial malleolus and the talus, preventing adequate healing despite immobilization. Third- and second-degree tears are treated as lateral injuries.

Tears of the Achilles Tendon

Injuries to the Achilles tendon deserve special comment. This muscle tendon unit stabilizes the lower extremity. Partial or complete tear of the Achilles tendon can be diagnosed by careful systematic evaluation. The patient will complain of weakness on plantar flexion of the foot or inability to stand upon the toes of the involved foot only.

On examination there will be swelling, tenderness, and sometimes a palpable defect where the tendon is torn. When the patient is in the prone or kneeling position, complete discontinuity of the Achilles tendon can be shown when the calf muscle is squeezed. In response to this maneuver, the foot should slightly plantar flex, or at least the Achilles tendon at the point of attachment to the calcaneous should become prominent. Failure of this response implies a complete tear of the Achilles tendon.

To assess the degree of tear, infiltration with local anesthetic solution into the area of tenderness and hematoma relieves pain and allows active plantar flexion of the foot against resistance if minimal first- or second-degree tearing of the tendon has occurred. The power of plantar flexion can be compared with the opposite extremity.

Treatment Treatment for complete ruptures of the Achilles tendon in an athlete is surgical repair. Nonoperative treatment can be utilized, but the patient must understand that morbidity is prolonged and function of the gastrocnemius-soleus tendon complex may in the end be inadequate for athletic demands. Nonoperative treatment for complete tears of the Achilles tendon is a long leg cast with the knee flexed 15°–20°, and the foot plantarflexed at the ankle. The cast should be worn for at least 6 and preferably for 8–10 weeks. Alternative treatments for partial tears include crutches, no weight bearing, but isometric exercises for the calf. Restrictive taping can be used for partial tears.

Peroneal Tendon Subluxation or Dislocation

When this injury is acute, it may be confused with an ankle sprain. Forced dorsiflexion and eversion of the foot during sports can tear the retinaculum surrounding the peroneal tendons, and the long peroneal or short peroneal tendon can then move out of its normal groove behind the lateral malleolus. If the foot is brought into plantar flexion and inversion, the tendons will usually reduce.

X-ray Studies The X-ray films may show an avulsion fracture in the region of the distal fibular, but usually only soft-tissue swelling is present, without bony abnormality in this region.

Diagnosis and Treatment If the diagnosis is suspected, local anesthetic infiltration with sterile technique will allow painless reproduction of the injury and permit the tendon to slip free of its normal groove passively during dorsiflexion and eversion of the foot. The treatment is operative repair of the retinaculum or deepening of the peroneal groove, depending upon the findings at surgery.

Nonoperative treatment is supportive. A felt pad to fit over the peroneal tendons is placed under taping, or a plaster cast is applied over the felt to maintain the position of the tendons for at least 21, but preferably 28, days. During this time the foot should not be brought into eversion without a cast, and the patient should not bear weight.

The Recurring Problem Treatment for chronic subluxation or dislocation of the peroneal tendons is usually surgical reconstruction of the retinaculum or deepening of the peroneal groove behind the lateral malleolus. Supportive taping with a felt pressure pad over the tendons has been successful on occasions. If the movement at the ankle is strong, however, external supporting will not suffice.

Osteochondral Fractures

The most common location for osteochondral fragment lesions at the ankle are the superomedial or superolateral aspects of the talus. The possibility that these lesions exist within the ankle joint should be kept in mind when an ankle injury in the acute or chronic phase is being evaluated. Sometimes the first X-ray films will not show the fragments because the fragments have not displaced from the bony bed and no bone resorption has occurred at the fracture line. Follow-up X-ray films at 14–21 days will usually show the defect.

X-ray studies of the ankle should include anteroposterior and lateral and oblique views. True mortise views can be taken with the foot in maximal plantar and maximal dorsiflexion to show different areas of the talar dome. Suspicious areas in the talus on plain films can be evaluated more closely by tomograms or CT scan.

Osteochondral fracture should be suspected if morbidity after a "sprain" is excessive (Fig. 21-23).

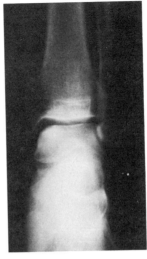 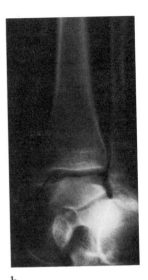

a   b

21-23 Anteroposterior (a) and oblique (b) views of ankle, showing osteochondritis dissecans of superior and medial aspect of talus.

Treatment The osteochondral fracture fragment can be removed by surgery, or if circumstances permit, the segment may be replaced. Often there will be no bony involvement, only a surface cartilage lesion. Arthroscopic techniques can be used to assess the joint and remove loose fragments and smooth rough areas.

Fractures Around the Ankle

Treatment of fractures in the vicinity of the ankle demands individualization (Fig. 21-24). Because of the weight-bearing and built-in rotational components of the joint, anatomic restoration of structures is important. Failure to obtain this can seriously affect weight-bearing relationships between the tibia and talus, causing serious mechanical consequences and early degenerative arthritis.

Even slight displacement of fractured segments of the lateral malleolus can affect the support and rotation of the talus.

COMMON FOOT INJURIES

Many foot problems of athletes are direct results of developmental variations of the lower extremity. The stresses upon the foot most often result from static alignment and dynamic relationships among the hip, knee, and ankle. For example, femoral anteversion, genu valgum, genu varum, and tibial torsion all will have direct effects on foot function.

Developmental changes within the foot are very often a consequence of proximal forces. The low-arched foot (flat foot) or the high-arched foot (cavus foot) will often predispose athletes to symptoms during activity.

Sprains of the Foot

Any foot ligament can be torn by repetitive stresses or forced torsion of the foot. Ligamentous injuries will vary in location and can be classified into first-, second-, or third-degree sprains, as elsewhere in the body. A third-degree sprain is a complete dislocation between bones connected by the affected ligaments. In the mid and hind foot, the subtalar and midtarsal joints can be involved in third-degree sprains. The only symptom or sign may be a

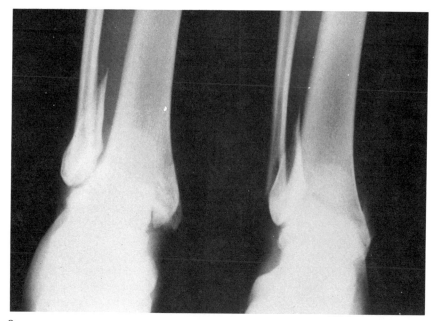

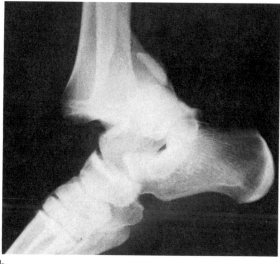

21-24 (a) Anteroposterior view of fracture dislocation of right ankle. There is a fracture through distal fibula, above syndesmosis and fracture of posterior tibial plafond, with posterior dislocation of talus. (b) Lateral view of trimalleolar ankle fracture with dislocation of talus seen above.

swollen foot. Violent high-torque injuries can cause tarsal-metatarsal dislocations. X-ray studies are important in evaluating a swollen foot to assess bone and joint relationships.

Treatment of Acute Injuries　Ice, elevation, and supportive wrap are all helpful. The wrap may be sheet wadding or cotton roll covered by muslin or roller gauze and finally covered by a woven elastic (Ace) wrap, with minimal pressure within the elastic wrapping.

The markedly swollen foot demands an accurate check of the neurologic status of all branches of the plantar and peroneal nerves and of the posterior tibial dorsalis pedis pulses and capillary filling of nail beds. It is not uncommon for a swollen foot to lead to a compartment syndrome of the foot. This can destroy the plantar musculature by circulatory compromise. The potential for compartment syndrome is greater if a third-degree sprain has occurred. The treatment of compartment syndrome is surgical release.

Sprains involving the plantar ligament deserve special comment. With weight bearing, stress is automatically applied to the span of the plantar ligament. Treatment for plantar ligament sprains is initially ice, elevation, and avoidance of weight bearing by using crutches. Local anesthetic injections and hyaluronidase sometimes disperse the hematoma and promote early healing. Ultrasound applied daily for 10–14 days is sometimes helpful in dispersing inflammatory fluids. When symptoms subside, protective taping should be applied to decrease distraction stress on the plantar surface of the foot. After the injury has recovered, an arch support is good protection. Sometimes, supportive taping must be applied indefinitely to prevent recurrence.

Sprains of the foot with weight bearing at the transverse metatarsal arch can cause recurring symptoms after an acute injury. Initial treatment is by rest and avoidance of weight bearing until symptoms subside. During the rest period, isometric and isotonic exercises of the foot can be carried out: curling the toes and picking up small objects with the toes to maintain good muscle function. Supportive taping should be utilized in a circumferential fashion at the level of the metatarsal heads. This may prevent recurrences. Orthotic inserts in the shoe to support the longitudinal and the transverse arches are also helpful.

Acute lateral ligament injuries are treated by ice and taping. During healing, lateral heel and sole wedges decrease tension on the lateral ligaments by lessening inversion stress.

Neuromas of the Feet

Irritation of nerves can occur at any point in the foot. Shoes can rub superficial sensory nerves, causing symptoms. Loss of static intermetatarsal ligamentous and muscular support can cause stress upon digital nerves or proximal branches of the plantar nerve as they pass between the metatarsal heads. Irritation occurs frequently at the junction of the medial and lateral plantar nerves, in the regions of the third and fourth metatarsal heads. This irritation is referred to as a Morton's neuralgia.

Symptoms Intermittent (shocklike) recurring pain or tingling along the lateral aspect of the distal foot, especially the adjacent sides of the third and fourth toes. If sudden pressure is applied to the transverse intermetatarsal arch, pain can radiate to the web space between the third and fourth toes.

Signs Compressing the foot around the transverse arch will reproduce the pain. Pressure by the thumb applied to the space between the third and fourth metatarsal heads will often reproduce symptoms also. Hypalgesia may be found between the third and fourth toes and in some cases hyperpathia in the same region.

X-ray Studies The X-ray films are often normal. Special studies in weight bearing will usually show the absence of the transverse arch.

Treatment Balancing of the foot is important. Longitudinal and intermetatarsal arch support proximal to the metatarsal heads is often helpful. Occasionally local injection of an anesthetic will give relief for a long period of time. A metatarsal bar on the shoe can distribute the force of the weight away from the metatarsal heads. Cortisone injections can be tried with some reservation. They may cause subcutaneous tissue atrophy and increase symptoms. Surgical treatment is a last resort and is often curative. However, caution must be used. Scar tissue is produced by surgery, and early weight bearing may cause prolonged morbidity from repetitive irritation of scar tissue.

Bursitis and Blister Problems

Overuse of the foot, with irritation from the shoe, will frequently cause blisters and irritation of various bursae. Commonly affected bursae are those between the skin and the calcaneous and at the Achilles tendon insertion (O'Donoghue [1]).

Bony prominences on the plantar aspect of the foot (especially the metatarsal heads) can lead to painful callosities in the unbalanced foot. This is especially true if the transverse arch is inadequate, leading to excessive stresses. Treatment is foot-balancing techniques and counter-pressure pads to decrease stress. Injections of steroids and local anesthetics into the bursae can be tried. However, they can cause atrophy of subcutaneous tissues. Ice massage should be utilized for acute pain, and ultrasound helps disperse inflammatory fluids. Blisters may be aspirated and coated with tincture of benzoin. The blister area may then be surrounded by a "doughnut" of thin felt to avoid pressure.

Fractures of the Foot

Comments

1. Most nonarticular fractures of the phalanges of the toes can be treated by taping to an adjacent, uninjured toe (Fig. 21-25). Supportive cotton or felt should be placed between the toes. Toe fractures needing reduction can be manipulated with or without anesthetic before taping. Documentation of the fracture by X-ray studies before and after manipulation is important.
2. Undisplaced fractures of metatarsal bones can be treated with supportive care. If the patient is more comfortable without a cast, using crutches alone, this is acceptable. Motion of the toes and bathing or swimming during convalescence is beneficial. Follow-up X-ray films at 7–10 days and then again in 3 weeks to check alignment of the fracture segment is important. If the patient is unreliable or, for convenience, needs a cast support, then a short-leg walking cast will usually suffice (Fig. 21-26).
3. Fracture at the base of the fifth metatarsal bone (dancer's fracture or Jones's fracture) is best treated with casting until healing occurs. The development of nonunion of this fracture is increased if cast support is not utilized.
4. Stress fracture can occur in any of the metatarsal bones but usually involves the second, third, and fourth metatarsals at the metatarsal neck region. Fractures may occur with repetitive trauma, such as running, or occasionally in an athlete who overuses the foot.

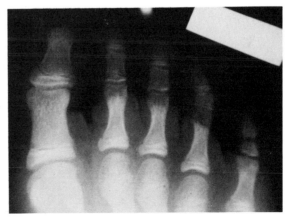

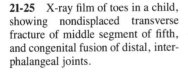

21-25 X-ray film of toes in a child, showing nondisplaced transverse fracture of middle segment of fifth, and congenital fusion of distal, interphalangeal joints.

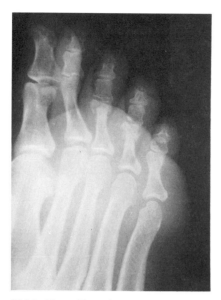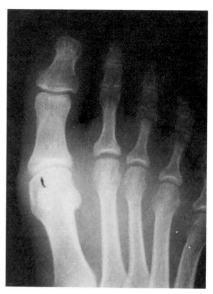

21-26 X-ray films of foot, showing comminuted but minimally displaced fractures of distal ends of proximal phalanges of third and fourth toes.

If the initial X-ray films are negative but fracture tenderness exists in the symptomatic area, the foot should be treated as for a metatarsal fracture and followed by reexamination with X-ray studies and further clinical evaluation in 14–21 days. At that time fracture callus should be present or the absorption of bone at the fracture line will make the diagnosis.

5. Fracture dislocation of the midfoot may not be readily apparent on routine films, and only by comparison with the other foot can the dislocation be noted (Fig. 21-27).
6. Anatomic reduction is preferable. Malunion of the metatarsal bones can change the stresses at the metatarsal heads, causing painful callosities or midfoot discomfort.
7. When necessary, surgical pin fixation of acute foot fractures should be used. Intraarticular fractures can result in painful spurring, deformity, and degenerative arthritis.
8. Painful joints as a result of malunion or arthritic changes may need reconstructive measures, such as joint fusion or excisional arthroplasty.

Developmental Variations Affecting Function

If symptoms are in the foot, examination from the waist down, at least, is necessary to evaluate the "whole" athlete. If the symptoms are in the hip, examination should be from the neck down. If examination is restricted to the area of pain only, the cause of the problem may be missed.

The body will adapt to structural variations. There may be a limit, however, to how long effective function with adaptations will continue. The examiner should note the following points:

1. Are the joints lax or tight? Can the elbow hyperextend? Can the knee hyperextend (back knee)? Can the thumb be brought back against the forearm?
2. Is there structural or functional scoliosis? Does the patient stand in a slouched fashion or erect? Is there hyperlordosis (sway back) with prominent buttocks?
3. Are there tight hamstrings? Can the patient easily touch the toes with knees extended?
4. Is there hip flexion contracture? Is the tightness due to a tight iliopsoas or to a tight rectus femoris? Are there structural abnormalities on X-ray films of the hips?

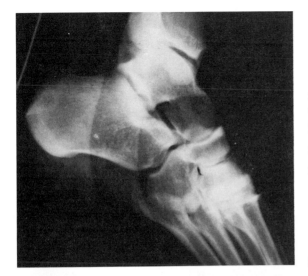

a

21-27 (a) Lateral view of midfoot dislocation. Tarsal-metatarsal joints are dislocated, and first metatarsal bone is displaced dorsally. (b) Midfoot dislocation of tarsal-metatarsal joints shows widening of joint space between first metatarsal and first cuneiform bones.

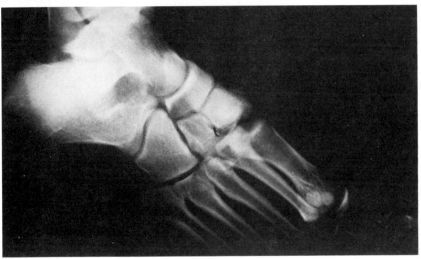

b

5. Is the walk toe-in (pigeon-toed) or toe-out (duck walk)? Do the kneecaps point forward or inward during gait?
6. Is there increased stability by internal rotation of the hip? Can the patient sit comfortably in the "squat sprawl" position (knees on the floor, hips internally rotated and buttocks resting on the heels)?
7. Are there genu valgum (knock-knee) or tibia vara (bowleg) deformities?
8. Is there internal tibial torsion or external tibial torsion?
9. Is there excessive heel valgus or foot pronation? Are there bunion deformities?

All the foregoing questions should be answered in deciding the causes of symptoms. Pain is often caused by compensatory stresses in response to malalignment.

Tight muscles should be stretched gently and regularly. Posture exercises should be encouraged to decrease lumbar lordosis stresses. A lower extremity malalignment syndrome should be treated from proximal to distal. Most fixed deformities in the lower extremities can be corrected or improved only by muscle reeducation and orthotic appliances in the shoes. Occasionally, surgical measures can be used to realign an extremity, but the basic defects must first be defined.

In younger patients, developmental problems have a better prognosis. The "kinetic chain" from proximal to distal can be altered in the growing child by stretching, muscle education, and orthotic devices. Once deformities are fixed and adaptations have occurred, the problems are more difficult to solve.

The exact cause of osteochondritis is yet to be found. Freiberg's disease of the second metatarsal head in teenagers and Sever's disease of the calcaneal apophysis in preteenagers could be related to compensatory stresses in these regions. Osgood-Schlatter disease likewise could be secondary to developmental forces on the patellar ligamentous insertion. The treatment of all these bony changes is supportive. Splinting, taping, orthotic pads, or crutches are utilized until symptoms subside. Occasionally surgery is utilized in the older patient.

RETURNING TO SPORTS AFTER INJURY

The decision on whether an athlete should return to a particular sport is the responsibility of his or her physician. It may rest upon consultation between on orthopaedist, neurosurgeon, family physician, team physician, and team coach. Some injuries lead to vulnerability for reinjury in that sport. The athlete must then consider a change. "Athletic performance" should be the primary consideration. The athlete must have confidence in his or her ability in the chosen sport. Physicians and coaches must feel that the patient's physical capability will allow safe continued participation. Objective testing should be obtained before return with isokinetic measuring methods of extremity musculature. This method compares the injured extremity with the opposite extremity or with its preinjury capabilities. Before contact sports are undertaken a coach should spend time with the individual athletes to assess performance and effectiveness in the field. When necessary, protective equipment such as braces, pads, or taping should be designed for the athlete to protect vulnerable areas.

REFERENCES

1. O'Donoghue, D.H. 1970. Treatment of Injuries to Athletes (2nd ed.). W.B. Saunders Co., Philadelphia, pp 11–33, 405, 442, 446, 493, 671.
2. Gray, H. 1959. Anatomy of the Human Body, C.M. Goss, ed (27th ed.). Lea & Febiger, Philadelphia, pp 356, 360, 366, 380, 390.
3. Bateman, J.E. 1969. Shoulder injuries in the throwing sports. In: Symposium on Sports Medicine. C.V. Mosby Co., Saint Louis, pp 87–96.
4. Spinner, M. 1972. Injuries to the Major Branches of Peripheral Nerves of the Forearm. W.B. Saunders Co., Philadelphia, p 114.
5. Torg, J.S., Conrad, W., et al. 1976. Clinical diagnosis of anterior cruciate ligament instability in the athlete. Am J Sports Med 4(2):84–91.
6. Helfet, A.J. 1963. Management of Internal Derangements of the Knee. J.B. Lippincott Co., Philadelphia, p 80.

·22·

Thermography in Sports Medicine

William B. Hobbins

BASIC THERMOGRAPHY

Thermography records surface temperature. As compared to a thermistor or skin thermometer, thermography can measure large territories of skin temperature simultaneously. There are two major methods of recording thermography. One is electronic and the other is liquid crystal sheets. These methodologies will record surface temperature to .1°C.

The cholesteric sheets (liquid crystal) are composed of mylar, with a coating of Australian sheep fat that has been encapsulated and quantified for its specific temperature response. As a cholesterol crystal is heated, it contracts and twists. This causes a color change to refracted light projected at 45° when observed at 90°. The colors go from red to yellow to green to blue. Blue is the hottest. These can be measured to .1°C.

The electronic measurement of surface temperature is performed by liquid nitrogen refrigeration of substances that, when exposed to infrared radiation, create intrinsic electrical disturbances. Such signals can be refined and projected to video screens for quantification and documentation. This methodology of heat recording was developed during the 20th century and refined for nighttime gun sight during the Korean War. It is used as a high-altitude spy plane recording device and is presently used as a national and international weather satellite, recording temperatures at the world surface.

SKIN TEMPERATURE AND NEURAL CONTROL

The importance of recording the surface temperature of the human surface was recognized by Hippocrates. He correlated health and illness to these observations. In the 19th century, the internal temperature was correlated with human conditions and the surface temperature was thought less significant.

The human surface temperature is primarily the result of the state of relaxation of the dermal microcirculation. The microcirculation of the dermis controls the major skin function, the thermal regulation of the body. The skin is the largest organ of the body, accounting for 30% of the body's weight and using a fourth of the body's blood volume.

The skin's major function is thermal regulation. Its other functions are perception of environmental sensations and alarm systems (pilomotor). The sudomotor function is an auxiliary thermal regulative intensifier.

There are two neural controls of this thermal regulatory mechanism. One is through the postganglionic fibers of the nervous system. The other is the alpha receptor in the microcirculation of the dermis. The postganglionic fibers, with their specific territories of skin temperature control, are formed in the 36th-day embryo. Each somite contributes to this circulation.

Because the human core temperature is warmer than the environment, it is necessary for the skin circulation to remain vasoconstricted to prevent the core heat from flowing to the surrounding environment (entropy). Thus, this primary sympathetic function is central to survival by thermal regulation.

To understand thermography, one must review the neural control of this thermal regulation. The preganglionic sympathetic cell bodies, which originate between T1 and L2 in the lateral column territory, are regulated by more central hypothalmic control. By way of descending fibers, preganglionic cell bodies in the spinal cord are controlled neurohormonally by the hypothalmus. (Decerebrate animals continue to control their thermal regulation spinally by the preganglionic cell bodies.) The preganglionic cell axons (myelinated— white rami) exit through the ventral ramus of the spinal nerves, from T1 to L2, to interconnect with as many as 100 postganglionic cell bodies. The exact location of the controlling preganglionic cell body for a given postganglionic cell is not known. The mediator at the synapses of the preganglionic axon and the postganglionic cell body is acetylcholine. In the normal resting state, the postganglionic cell body and axon vasoconstrict the distal vascular bed. Modulation of preganglionic fibers and of neurotransmitters (acetylcholine) at the postganglionic cell body, will alter postganglionic function. The postganglionic cell body and axon influence alpha receptors in the dermal circulation (Fig. 22-1). Circulating noradrenaline and adrenaline are activators for these receptors (Schmidt and Thews [1]). These substances cause vasoconstriction. The major mechanism for thermographic observation is the postganglionic fiber in its relationship to the alpha receptor.

The human surface temperature is symmetrical and with mostly only a .2°C difference between the two sides (Uematsu [2]), but a .6°C difference between sides is a significant abnormality.

SYMPATHETIC NERVOUS SYSTEM

22-1   Dermal vasomotor control.

SOMATIC CUTANEOUS REFLEXES

Muscles, joints, synovium, and bones do not generate heat that is reflected to the skin. When such organs produce heat, it is transmitted centrally and raises core temperature (Appenzeller [3]). This in turn affects the surface temperature to maintain body temperature. This is contrary to the work of Randall and Hertzman [4].

Extensive work has shown that no temperature change occurring deeper than .5 cm can be seen on the surface (Vermey [5]). Nilsson [6] implanted thermistors in the arms of students and confirmed this finding. Heat produced deeper is carried away by the circulation to the body core. Personal study of professional athletes running on a treadmill showed cutaneous vasoconstriction with no evidence of underlying muscular thermal energy reflected to the surface [7].

The importance of thermography in sports or in training lies in the muscles, joints, ligaments, and bones which have an embryonic somatocutaneous referral area (Figs. 22-2 and 22-3). When nociception occurs in a somatic organ, the perception of pain is projected cutaneously to specific projection areas (Kellgren [8]; Head [9]; Richter [10]).

These referred cutaneous areas are warm and the "referral" cutaneous hot spots have decreased or absent sympathetic vasoconstrictor function (Green et al. [11]). Thus, the resultant vasodilation brings more warm blood from the body core to these areas, causing increased temperature.

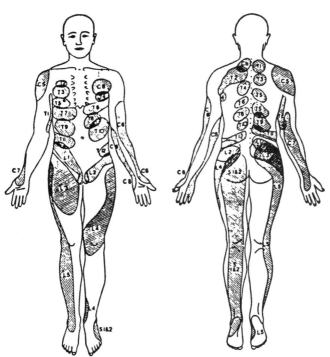

22-2 Maps showing the segmental reference of deep pain resulting from stimulation of interspinous ligaments. The numbers identify the region to which pain was referred from injecting hypertonic saline into the cervical (C), thoracic (T), lumbar (L), and sacral (S) ligaments. The segmental zones resemble but are not identical to the dermatones. (From Kellgren [8].)

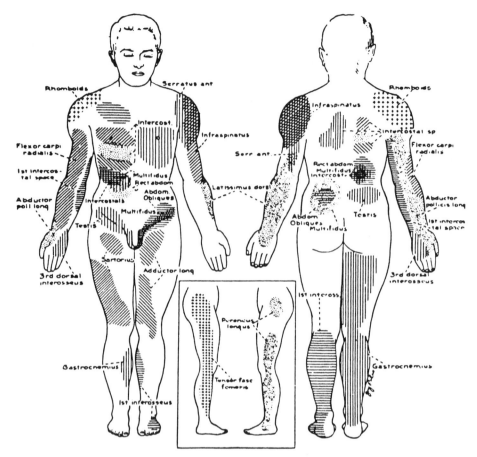

22-3 Maps showing the reference of pain resulting from stimulation of various muscles by injecting hypertonic saline. (From Kellgren [8].)

VALUE IN SOMATIC INJURY

Muscular injuries are the most common after osseous or articular lesions. The thermal content in the referred cutaneous areas was the best predictor of functional recovery, and thermography can be used to decide on resumption of athletic activities.

Symmetrical isothermic findings allowed early return to practice. Hyperthermia was related to severity of injury when measured quantitatively, and the rate at which hyperthermia disappeared after injury was best correlated with the athlete's return to full performance. Measurements of strength, range of motion, or even pain did not correlate as well as thermal signal (Schmitt and Guillot [12]).

Regional hypothermia was the most unexpected and most important finding in study of French national soccer players (Schmitt and Guillot [12]). Nondermatomal territorial hypothermia was a systemic defense mechanism against injury. It was detected in a small percentage of athletes upon entering the training room after injury. One out of 10 sprained ankles would show such vasoconstriction (Fig. 22-4). These were different vasomotor responses and were associated with a poorer prognosis for rapid return to activity.

These vasoconstrictor responses to injury have been termed reflex sympathetic dysfunctions and are associated with intense pain greater than similar injuries. Athletes dis-

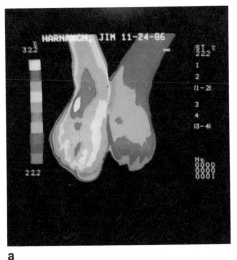 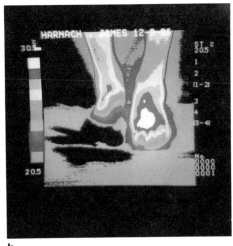

22-4 (a) Electronic thermogram of left sympathetic vasoconstriction after ankle–foot injury. (b) Follow-up thermogram after lumbar sympathetic block with complete relief of symptoms.

playing such responses will take longer to return to full performance. Measuring the territorial area of injury for the presence or absence of heat and determination of severe vasoconstriction, with loss of normal surface heat, is therefore important. Thermographic examination of a recent injury allows a sports manager to estimate the severity of the injury, monitor its evolution, and estimate the time of healing and eventual resumption of activity.

Lelik [13] has attempted to predict, with the use of liquid crystal strips, the various thermal responses of every joint of the body. The various collateral ligaments, cruciate ligaments, and cartilages produce different thermal patterns in specific areas. Devereaux et al. [14] showed that pain in front of the knee is common in athletes; this is often called patellofemoral arthralgia, but it is difficult to prove that the pain arises in that joint. Thermograms of 30 athletes clinically considered to have patellofemoral arthralgia were compared with those of a similar number of unaffected athletes matched for age and sex. A comparison was also made with thermograms of two older groups of 30 patients with knee involvement from either rheumatoid arthritis or osteoarthritis.

Twenty-eight of the athletes with patellofemoral arthralgia had a diagnostic pattern on thermography. The anterior knee view showed a rise in temperature on the medial side of the patella, and the medial knee view showed that this temperature rise referred from the patellar insertion of the vastus medialis into the muscle itself (Fig. 22-5).

Page-Thomas [15] of the Addenbrook Hospital in Cambridge has looked at the pattern of joints and their heat emission in health as well as after injury. They identified patterns of heat that are present over normal knees, elbows, wrists, shoulders, and ankles. In the presence of inflammation or injury, these patterns are altered or lost because of the abnormal skin blood flow. Ring and others have found changes in arthritis [16], similar findings in epicondylar disease of the elbow (tennis elbow) [17], and stress fractures of the feet [18] (Fig. 22-6), fibulas, and hands.

The largest contribution of thermography to sports medicine and to physical medicine and rehabilitation is a differential diagnosis of pain. Major issues in injury are undiagnosed pain, defense posturing of the injured body, and direct neurological involvement, either central or peripheral [19].

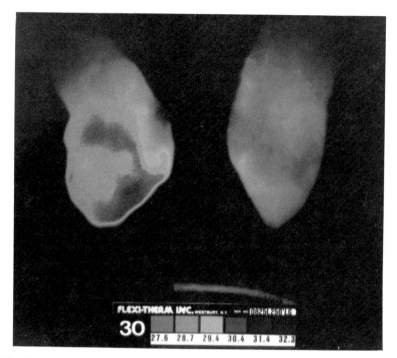

22-5 Liquid crystal thermogram of anterior knees. Right patellofemoral arthralgia—tendon vastus medialis.

METHODOLOGY

The thermographic exam in a sports medicine or pain laboratory must be performed under controlled conditions of environmental temperature, and the control of drafts and radiation heat from lights, equipment, and windows is also important. Thermography is best performed with only modest clothing so as to invoke a primary defensive response in the major surface of the body. This then contrasts the abnormal area at an ambient temperature of 68–70°F. It is possible, however, in the ordinary examining room or locker room to take the liquid crystal thermographic detectors and to make preliminary observations. With this information, it can be determined whether to use ice packs for hyperthermia or if the injured area is cold, heat for vasodilatation is indicated.

When performing a thermogram, the entire cutaneous territory of a given area is reviewed. For an injured hand or wrist, the C6, C7, and C8 peripheral nerves distribution in their entire length should be imaged, starting at the spine and proceeding to the hands. The same process applies to injuries to the lower extremity. The examination is carried out from the lumbar area to the foot, reviewing all surfaces of the involved extremities. All surfaces of the contralateral extremity are examined. The thermal image of the human body is one of symmetry (Uematsu [2]; Feldman and Nickoloff [20]). Asymmetry in normal individuals between any given territory is no greater than .4°C. These larger differences between sides occur in the most distal extremities, such as thumbs or toes, whereas the forehead has less than .1°C difference from right to left.

It is essential to learn the normal patterns of the human emission in order to ascertain abnormal or asymmetrical status. There is a distinct pattern for each and every territory; e.g., the knees are colder than the thighs, the lower legs anteriorly are generally warmer

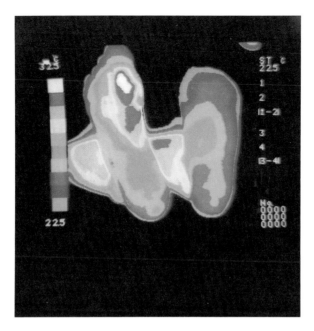

22-6 Electronic thermogram of stress fracture right second metatarsal (motorcyclist). White area is the warmest.

than the thighs. The thenar eminence is warmer than the hypothenar eminence, and the palm of the hand is generally warmer than the fingers. The hands are generally colder than the forearms, and the forearms are colder than the upper arms. The upper arms are colder than the trunk. When this pattern is lost in a cephalocaudad direction, either in the extremity or trunk, it is significant and an explanation must be sought.

DISCUSSION

The three most important contributions of thermography to sports medicine are:

1. Detection of undetermined hypersympathetic reflex, shown as severe cold area (sympathetic dysfunction).
2. Thermal demographic qualification and qualification of injury, confirming the somatic pathology. This supplies a good basis to follow progress and affirm recovery for future activity.
3. Direct neurogenic involvement can be demonstrated and differentiated from soft tissue injury.

Of the three, the vasoconstrictive process is the most important. This is an overlooked process that needs early treatment to prevent more permanent disability. The use of whirlpools, massage, stellate and lumbar sympathetic blockades, and various other methods to release this severe vasoconstriction is essential in many sports injuries, especially when the athlete's complaints are out of proportion to the injury.

CONCLUSION

Thermography (surface heat) has been correlated with the presence of pathology for centuries. The use of thermography in evaluating sports injuries can help the physician subclassify the pathophysiology and differentiate between severe vasoconstrictive and hyperthermic referred conditions, thus providing direction for additional neuromusculoskeletal workup.

Thermography is an observation of autonomic function. Autonomic function of skin temperature can be a signal from somatic nociception. Somatic nociception is a direct result of misuse or disuse or traumatic disruption and must be quantified early for possible treatment.

REFERENCES

1. Schmidt, R.F., Thews, G. 1983. Human Physiology. Springer-Verlag, New York, pp 114–120.
2. Uematsu, S. 1985. Symmetry of skin temperature comparing one side of the body to the other. Thermology 1:4–7.
3. Appenzeller, O. 1986. Clinical Autonomic Failure. Elsevier Press, New York, pp 53–57.
4. Randall, C.T., Hertzman, W.E. 1959. Vascular convection heat from active muscle to overlying skin. J Appl Physiol 14:207.
5. Vermey, G.F. 1975. The stimulation of the skin temperature by means of a relaxation method. Phys Med Biol 20:384–394.
6. Nilsson, S.K. 1975. Skin temperature over an artificial heat source implanted in man. Phys Med Biol 20:366–383.
7. Hobbins, W.B., Klein, K. 1987. Cutaneous blood flow during exercise and cooling down; George Washington University Medical School symposium. Submitted for publication.
8. Kellgren, J.H. 1937–1938. Observation on referred pain arising from muscle. Clin Sci 3:176.
9. Head, S. 1893. Brain 4:1–158.
10. Richter, C.P. 1929. Nervous control of electrical resistance of the skin. Bulletin of Johns Hopkins University 45:56–74.
11. Green, J., Reilly, A., et al. 1986. Sympathetic skin response abnormalities correlated with abnormal infrared thermogram in patients with low back pain and radiculopathy. Academy of Neuro-Muscular Thermography. Clin Pro, Modern Medicine, New Jersey, pp 89–92.
12. Schmitt, M., Guillot, Y. 1984. Thermography and muscular injuries in sports medicine. In: Ring, E.F.J., Phillips, B. (eds): Recent Advances in Medical Thermology. Plenum Press, New York, pp 439–445.
13. Lelik, F. 1983. The sports injuries and contact thermography. Initial 4:2–3.
14. Devereaux, M.D., Parr, G.R., et al. 1986. Thermographic diagnosis in athletes with patellofemoral arthralgia. Bone Joint Surg. 68-B:42–44.
15. Salisbury, R.S., Parr, G.R., et al. 1984. Heat distribution over joints: The normal and abnormal pattern. In: Ring, E.F.J., Phillips, B. (eds): Recent Advances in Medical Thermology. Plenum Press, New York, pp 453–458.
16. Dieppe, P.A., Ring, E.F.J., et al. 1984. Thermal patterns of osteoarthritic knees and hands. In: Ring, E.F.J., Phillips, B., (eds): Recent Advances in Medical Thermology. Plenum Press, New York, pp 459–462.
17. Binder, A.I., Parr, G., et al. 1984. Thermography of tennis elbow. In: Ring, E.F.J., Phillips, B. (eds): Recent Advances in Medical Thermology. Plenum Press, New York, pp 513–517.
18. Devereaux, M.D., Parr, G.R., et al. 1984. The diagnosis of stress fractures in athletes. JAMA 252:531–533.
19. Hobbins, W.B. 1982. Thermography and pain. In: Gautherie, M., Albert, E. (eds): Biomedical Thermology. Alan R. Liss, New York, pp 361–375.
20. Feldman, F., Nickoloff, E. 1984. Normal thermographic standard for the cervical spine and upper extremities. Skeletal Radiol 12:235–249.

•23•

Muscle Testing for Sports

Vivian H. Heyward

The importance of muscular fitness for successful performance in sports has led to widespread use of weight training and physical conditioning programs to supplement the skills training of athletes. Understanding how to assess various components of muscular fitness can be useful to the coach, athletic trainer, and sports physician in the following ways: 1) to evaluate the athlete's potential for a particular sport or position within that sport, 2) to plan a supplementary program of weight training and physical conditioning to improve muscular fitness and performance, 3) to pinpoint muscular imbalances that lead to an increased risk of injury, and 4) to determine loss of muscle function due to injury.

In this chapter, tests and performance norms that can be used to assess various components of muscular fitness for athletes are presented. Factors that influence muscular fitness, as well as problems associated with muscle testing, are discussed.

DEFINITION OF TERMS

Three important components of muscular fitness are strength, endurance, and power. Strength is the ability of a muscle group to exert maximum contractile force against resistance. Muscular endurance is the ability of that muscle group to exert submaximum force for extended periods of time. Power, or the rate of doing work, is a function of strength and speed (power = force × velocity). Often in athletics, the term "explosive strength" is used to describe muscular power. The extent to which each of these components is needed for successful performance is highly specific to the sport. For example, high jumping requires leg strength and power, whereas a high level of muscular endurance is needed for long-distance running.

In addition to determining the physical demands of the sport, a number of important factors must be considered when selecting tests to assess the athlete's strength, muscular endurance, or power. First, the muscle groups and the type of muscle contraction used in the performance must be identified. The type of muscle contraction may be static or dynamic, depending on the resistance encountered. When the resistance is immovable, the muscle contracts statically (or isometrically). In other words, the change in muscle length is minimal (iso = same; metric = length), and there is no visible movement at the joint. When there is visible joint movement, the muscle is contracting dynamically.

The specific type of dynamic contraction (concentric or eccentric) depends on the magnitude of the muscle force and the resistance. When the force exceeds the resistance, the muscle will shorten as it moves the bony lever (concentric contraction). When the resistance exceeds the muscle force, the bony lever will rotate in the opposite direction as the muscle lengthens and exerts tension (eccentric contraction). Eccentric contraction produces a braking force that decelerates rapidly moving body segments and resists gravitational acceleration during the movement. In the past, the term "isotonic contraction" (iso = same; tonic = tension) was used to describe both concentric and eccentric muscle contraction. In actuality, however, there are large fluctuations in muscle force throughout the range of motion, even though the external resistance or weight being raised or lowered stays the same. This fluctuation in muscle force is due to the change in muscle length and angle of pull as the bony lever is moved (Kreighbaum and Barthels [1]). As a result, the term "dynamic" is more widely accepted to describe the concentric and eccentric contractions of a muscle group.

Isokinetic contraction is a special type of dynamic muscle contraction in which the speed of contraction is controlled mechanically so that the limb rotates at a predetermined velocity (e.g., 60°/sec). Isokinetic contraction involves maximum contraction of the muscle group at a constant speed throughout the entire range of motion. Electromechanical or hydraulic mechanisms vary the resistance so that it matches fluctuations in muscle force due to the changing muscle length and angle of pull. Thus, with the aid of isokinetic exercise devices, the muscle group encounters variable maximum resistances throughout its complete range of motion.

ASSESSMENT OF MUSCULAR FITNESS

Strength, muscular endurance, and power are measured using dynamometers, cable tensiometers, force platforms, isokinetic devices, and constant resistance or variable resistance exercise machines. The selection of the test instrumentation depends on the type of test (strength, endurance, or power), the muscle group being evaluated, and the type of muscle contraction (static, dynamic, or isokinetic). In addition, certain practical factors such as transportability of equipment, time allotted for testing, ease of test administration, and availability and expense of equipment should be taken into consideration. Sources for muscle testing equipment are included at the end of this chapter in Table 23-8.

Assessing Static Muscle Function

Although most sports are dynamic in nature, it may be desirable, for certain sports or events, to evaluate strength and muscular endurance during static contractions of muscle groups. In gymnastics, for example, successful performance of an iron-cross maneuver on the stationary rings is highly dependent on the static strength and endurance of the shoulder abductors/adductors and elbow flexors/extensors. Likewise, strength and endurance of the grip-squeezing muscles are important in sports such as tennis, squash, and racquetball. When the body or sports implement must be maintained in a stationary position either momentarily or for extended periods of time, a certain degree of static strength and endurance is a prerequisite for successful performance. Static strength and endurance can be measured using dynamometers, cable tensiometers, and electromechanical devices.

Dynamometers, Test Protocols, and Norms   A handgrip dynamometer and back/leg dynamometer can be used to measure static strength and endurance of the grip-squeezing muscles and leg and back muscles. The handgrip dynamometer measures forces between 0 kg and 100 kg in 1-kg increments, whereas the back and leg dynamometer measures forces ranging between 0 lb and 2500 lb in 10-lb increments. Both dynamometers are spring devices that move the indicator needle on the dial an amount corresponding to the force applied to the instrument.

Prior to measuring grip strength or endurance, the handgrip size of the dynamometer is adjusted to a position that is comfortable for the individual. Alternatively, a caliper can be used to determine an optimum grip size (Montoye and Faulkner [2]). To measure static grip strength, the individual stands erect with the arms at the sides. With the forearm in a neutral position and the dial facing away from the body, the individual squeezes the handle as hard as possible without moving the arm. Three trials, with a 1-min rest between trials, are administered for each hand. Static grip strength is measured as the maximum force registered on the dial.

To assess the static endurance of the grip-squeezing muscles, the subject is instructed to squeeze the handle as hard as possible for a 60-sec period. The force is recorded every 10 sec. The greater the endurance, the less the rate of decline in force. The relative endurance score is the final force divided by the initial force multiplied by 100. An alternative static endurance test requires the individual to maintain a submaximum force level that is a designated percentage of his or her maximum voluntary contractile strength (e.g., 60% MVC). The relative endurance score is the amount of time that this tension level is sustained. The subject must watch the dial of the dynamometer to monitor the appropriate force level during the test.

To assess static leg strength, the subject stands on the platform of the back and leg dynamometer. The knees are flexed to an angle of 130°–140°, with the trunk kept erect. The crossbar is held using a pronated grip, and the chain is adjusted so that the handbar lies across the thighs. As the knees are slowly and vigorously extended, the indicator needle on the dial moves a corresponding amount. The maximum indicator needle remains at the peak force achieved. This score is then converted to kilograms. Usually two to three trials are administered with a 1-min rest between trials.

The back and leg dynamometer also is used to assess static back strength. Standing on the platform with the knees fully extended and the trunk erect, the individual grasps the handbar using a pronated grip for the right hand and a supinated grip for the left hand. The handbar is positioned across the thighs and is pulled upward using the trunk extensor muscles. The shoulders are rolled backward during the pull. The maximum score, as indicated on the dial, is converted to kilograms. Two trials are administered with a 1-min rest between trials.

Norms for these dynamometric tests for men and women are presented in Table 23-1. The right grip, left grip, leg strength, and back strength scores are totaled to determine the overall static strength score. Before adding the scores, however, the leg and back strength scores must be converted from pounds to kilograms. The total strength score is divided by the body weight (in kilograms) to determine the relative strength.

Cable Tensiometry   The static strength of approximately 38 different muscle groups throughout the body can be measured using cable tensiometry, which consists of a tensiometer, steel cables, strength table, wall hooks, straps, and a goniometer. The cable is attached to the wall or table hooks, and the other end is attached to the body segment being tested, using a strap. The cable is always positioned at right angles to the bony lever. After the tensiometer is positioned on the tightened cable, the individual is instructed to pull as hard as possible. The force exerted on the cable depresses the riser of the tensiometer, and the indicator needle registers the maximum force produced. Forces ranging between 0 lb and 400 lb can be measured using large tensiometers. For a more precise and accurate assessment of forces ranging between 0 lb and 100 lb, a smaller tensiometer is used.

The standardized testing procedures, as described by Clarke and Clarke [3], should be followed carefully. Since static strength is specific to the joint angle and muscle group being

Table 23-1 Static Strength Norms

Classification	Left Grip (kg)	Right Grip (kg)	Back Strength (kg)	Leg Strength (kg)	Total Strength	Strength/ BW (kg)
Men						
Excellent	>68	>70	>209	>241	>587	>7.50
Good	56–67	62–69	177–208	214–240	508–586	7.10–7.49
Average	43–55	48–61	126–176	160–213	375–507	5.21–7.09
Poor	39–42	41–47	91–125	137–159	307–374	4.81–5.20
Very Poor	<39	<41	<91	<137	<307	<4.81
Women						
Excellent	>37	>41	>111	>136	>324	>5.50
Good	34–36	38–40	98–110	114–135	282–323	4.80–5.49
Average	22–33	25–37	52–97	66–113	164–281	2.90–4.79
Poor	18–21	22–24	39–51	49–65	117–163	2.10–2.89
Very Poor	<18	<22	<39	<49	<117	<2.10

From Heyward, V. 1984. Designs for Fitness. Burgess Publishing Co., Minneapolis. Reprinted with permission of the publisher.

tested, cable tensiometer test batteries usually include three to four different sites to provide an adequate estimation of overall static strength. A goniometer is used to measure the specified joint angle for each test item. Test batteries for males (9 years old to college age) include the following three items: shoulder extension, knee extension, and ankle plantar flexion strength. For senior high school and college women, the test battery includes shoulder flexion, hip flexion, and ankle plantar flexion strength. Norms for these test batteries are provided elsewhere (Clarke [4]; Clarke and Monroe [5]).

Electromechanical Devices   If a high degree of precision is needed, electromechanical systems can be used to assess static strength and endurance of muscle groups. Linear voltage differential transformers and strain gauges can be used to transform the applied mechanical force to an electrical voltage. This change in voltage is recorded and parameters such as peak force, rate of force production, and time to peak force can be extracted from the recorded output. The system can be designed to test the static strength and endurance of many muscle groups. Due to the expense, these electromechanical devices are not very practical. The degree of sophistication afforded by these instruments, however, is well suited for research purposes.

Assessing Dynamic Muscle Function

Dynamic strength, muscular endurance, and power can be assessed using constant resistance or variable resistance exercise modes. With the constant resistance mode, the resistance that the muscle encounters does not vary with the changing mechanical and physiologic advantage of the musculoskeletal system. The maximum weight that can be moved through the full range of motion is no greater than the weight that can be lifted at the weakest point in the range. Equipment such as free weights, dumbbells, and some stations of the Universal Gym Machine provide a constant resistance.

To overcome this shortcoming, exercise machines have been designed that vary the resistance during the movement. These variable resistance exercise machines have a moving connection between the point of force application and the resistance. As the weight is lifted, the mechanical advantage of the machine decreases and more force must be applied to continue the movement. These machines attempt to compensate for the changing mechanical advantage of the muscle during the movement. They do not compensate, however, for the decreased physiologic advantage that occurs as the muscle shortens during the movement. Nautilus and Cybex make a complete line of variable resistance machines that can be used to test dynamic muscle function. These include abdominal, rotary torso, hip/back, hip abductor/adductor, leg curl, leg press, leg extension, pullover, double chest, neck, shoulder, compound arm curl, and multiexercise machines. Some models of the Universal Gym Machine also provide variable resistance at the bench press, leg press, and shoulder press stations.

Dynamic Strength Test Protocols and Norms Typically, dynamic strength is measured by determining the maximum weight that can be lifted for one complete repetition of a movement. This is known as the "1-RM value" and is obtained through trial and error. After a successful attempt at a given weight, the subject should rest 2 to 3 min before trying to lift a heavier weight. Usually, the weight is increased 5–10 lb for each trial. Pollock et al. [6] recommend using the Universal Gym Machine to determine the 1-RM strength of four muscle groups: bench press, standing press, arm curl, and leg press. Performance norms for men and women are based on bodyweight (Table 23-2).

Another test battery has been devised that evaluates the 1-RM value as a percentage of the individual's body weight (Table 23-3). The six test items are bench press, arm curl, lateral pull-down, leg press, leg extension, and leg curl. For each exercise, the 1-RM value is divided by the body weight to determine the strength/body weight ratio, and the corresponding point value is noted. The overall strength is assessed by totaling the points accumulated for each exercise.

Dynamic Muscular Endurance Test Protocols and Norms The individual's muscular endurance is highly dependent on strength. Therefore, most muscular endurance tests are designed so that the athlete performs as many repetitions as possible using a weight that is a designated percentage of the 1-RM strength value for that exercise. Another method uses a weight that corresponds to a percentage of the athlete's body weight. This method is less desirable, however, since a larger body weight does not always reflect a larger muscle mass.

To date, there are no good performance norms for evaluating dynamic muscular endurance. Pollock et al. [6] recommend using a weight that is 70% of the 1-RM for each exercise. They suggest that the average person should be able to complete 12–15 repetitions

Table 23-2 Optimal Strength Values (in Pounds) for Various Body Weights, Based on the 1-RM Test

Body Weight (lb)	Bench Press		Standing Press		Curl		Leg Press	
	Male	Female	Male	Female	Male	Female	Male	Female
80	80	56	53	37	40	28	160	112
100	100	70	67	47	50	35	200	140
120	120	84	80	56	60	42	240	168
140	140	98	93	65	70	49	280	196
160	160	112	107	75	80	56	320	224
180	180	126	120	84	90	63	360	252
200	200	140	133	93	100	70	400	280
220	220	154	147	103	110	77	440	308
240	240	168	160	112	120	84	480	336

Note. Data collected on Universal Gym apparatus. Information collected on other apparatus could modify results.

From Pollock, M.L., Wilmore, J.H., 1978. Health and Fitness Through Physical Activity. John Wiley & Sons, New York. Reprinted with permission of the publisher.

Table 23-3 Strength/Body Weight Ratios for Selected Dynamic Strength Tests

Bench Press	Arm Curl	Lateral Pull-down	Leg Press	Leg Extension	Leg Curl	Points
Men						
1.50	.70	1.20	3.00	.80	.70	10
1.40	.65	1.15	2.80	.75	.65	9
1.30	.60	1.10	2.60	.70	.60	8
1.20	.55	1.05	2.40	.65	.55	7
1.10	.50	1.00	2.20	.60	.50	6
1.00	.45	.95	2.00	.55	.45	5
.90	.40	.90	1.80	.50	.40	4
.80	.35	.85	1.60	.45	.35	3
.70	.30	.80	1.40	.40	.30	2
.60	.25	.75	1.20	.35	.25	1
Women						
.90	.50	.85	2.70	.70	.60	10
.85	.45	.80	2.50	.65	.55	9
.80	.42	.75	2.30	.60	.52	8
.70	.38	.73	2.10	.55	.50	7
.65	.35	.70	2.00	.52	.45	6
.60	.32	.65	1.80	.50	.40	5
.55	.28	.63	1.60	.45	.35	4
.50	.25	.60	1.40	.40	.30	3
.45	.21	.55	1.20	.35	.25	2
.35	.18	.50	1.00	.30	.20	1

Total Points	Strength Fitness Category
48–60	Excellent
37–47	Good
25–36	Average
13–24	Fair
0–12	Poor

From Heyward, V. 1984. Designs for Fitness. Burgess Publishing Co., Minneapolis. Reprinted with permission of the publisher.

at that intensity. The competitive athlete, however, should be able to complete 20–25 repetitions.

Dynamic Muscular Power Tests and Norms   At present, there are few practical tests that yield valid and objective measures of dynamic power. In the past, performance tests such as the sitting shot put, medicine ball throw, vertical jump, standing long jump, and sprints were used to assess upper and lower body power. These tests, however, are not recommended to assess muscular power, since their validity has not been established (Considine [7]).

In addition, it is not easy to measure muscular power using conventional constant resistance exercise equipment. Because power is a function of force and velocity, both the magnitude of the weight and the speed of the movement must be measured. Accurate measurement of the speed of movement, however, is difficult, time consuming, and expensive. Typically, high-speed cinematography is used to record the performance and to determine both the distance that the weight is moved and the movement speed through frame-by-frame analysis of the film. There is an experimental device, however, that attaches to a standard weight stack (Wilmore [8]). The device, a microprocessor, measures the lapsed time and the distance that the weight travels, thereby computing the power (force × distance/time). When this device becomes readily available, it should facilitate accurate and rapid assessments of dynamic muscular power.

Force platforms can be used to assess leg power during jumping events. The force applied to the platform and the time of force application can be recorded to the nearest 0.1 sec. The power is calculated using the following equation (Considine [7]): $P = 1/8F \times gT^2 - T_2$, where F = body weight of subject, g = gravitational acceleration, T = total elapsed airborne time, and T_2 = length of time force is applied.

Margaria et al. [9] devised a practical test to measure leg power. This test, as modified by Kalamen [10], involves running upstairs, three steps at a time, as quickly as possible. A switchmat is placed on the third and ninth steps, and is used to trigger a timer that records the elapsed time to the nearest .01 sec. Power is computed using the following equation: $P = W \times D - T$, where P = power (kg-m/sec), W = body weight of athlete (kg), D = vertical distance (m) for six steps (between third and ninth steps), and T = elapsed time (sec). Performance norms have been established based on age, sex, and fitness level of the individual (Table 23-4).

Assessing Isokinetic Muscle Function

Isokinetic dynamometers provide an accurate and reliable assessment of the athlete's strength, endurance, and power. One major advantage of using isokinetic equipment is that the dynamometer keeps the speed of limb movement at a constant preselected velocity. An increase in muscular force results in increased resistance rather than increased acceleration of the limb. Thus, fluctuations in muscle force are matched by an equal counterforce or resistance. This capability is known as "accommodating resistance" and is produced electromechanically by controlling the velocity of movement during the contraction. Since it has been documented that the muscle group is capable of generating less force at faster speeds of contraction (Coyle et al. [11]; Gregor et al. [12]; Lesmes et al. [13]; Scudder [14]; Thorstensson et al. [15]), speed settings for isokinetic strength, muscular endurance, and power tests have been recommended (Table 23-5). Another advantage of isokinetic dynamometers is that muscular function, at speeds of movement that closely simulate those used during the actual sports performance, can be evaluated using the speed control feature of these devices.

Table 23-4 Norms for Margaria-Kalamen Leg Power Test

	Men				
	Age Group (years)				
Classification	15–20	20–30	30–40	40–50	Over 50
Poor	Under 113	Under 106	Under 85	Under 65	Under 50
Fair	113–149	106–139	85–111	65–84	50–65
Average	150–187	140–175	112–140	85–105	66–82
Good	188–224	176–210	141–168	106–125	83–98
Excellent	Over 224	Over 210	Over 168	Over 125	Over 98
	Women				
	Age Group (years)				
Classification	15–20	20–30	30–40	40–50	Over 50
Poor	Under 92	Under 85	Under 65	Under 50	Under 38
Fair	92–120	85–111	66–84	50–65	38–48
Average	121–151	112–140	85–105	66–82	49–61
Good	152–182	141–168	106–125	83–98	62–75
Excellent	Over 182	Over 168	Over 125	Over 98	Over 75

Note. Units of measurement are kg-m/sec.

Based on data from Margaria, R., Aghemo, I., et al. 1966. Measurement of muscular power (anaerobic) in man. J Appl Physiol 21:1662–1664; and Kalamen, J. 1968. Measurement of maximal muscular power in man. Unpublished doctoral dissertation, Ohio State University, Columbus.

Table 23-5   Recommended Speed Settings for Isokinetic Muscle Testing (in Degrees/Second)

Joint Actions	Strength	Endurance and Power	
		Nonathletes and Female Athletes	Male Athletes
Shoulder			
Extension/Flexion	60°	180°	240° or 300°
Abduction/Adduction	60°	180°	240° or 300°
Int./Ext. Rotation	60°	180°	240° or 300°
Elbow			
Extension/Flexion	60°	180°	240°
Forearm			
Pronation/Supination	30°	120°	180°
Wrist			
Extension/Flexion	30°	120°	180°
Hip			
Abduction/Adduction	30°	120°	180°
Extension/Flexion	30°	120°	180°
Int./Ext. Rotation	30°	120°	180°
Knee			
Extension/Flexion	60°	180°	240°
Tibial Rotation	30°	120°	180°
Ankle			
Plantar/Dorsiflexion	30°	120°	180°
Inversion/Eversion	30°	120°	180°

From Cybex. 1980. Isolated Joint Testing and Exercise. Cybex. A division of Lumex, Inc., Ronkonkoma, N.Y.

Isokinetic Equipment   The Cybex II is an isokinetic dynamometer that measures muscular torque production of the shoulder, elbow, forearm, wrist, hip, knee, and ankle joints at speeds varying between 0° and 300°/sec. The resulting torque output, along with range of motion data, is recorded on a dual channel recorder.

Other isokinetic devices made by Cybex include the bench press, leg press, Orthotron, and Kinetron II. The Orthotron is similar to the Cybex II but lacks the recording capability. However, it can still be used effectively for testing and evaluating muscle function. For purposes of exercise training and rehabilitation, the Orthotron is better suited than the Cybex II, since it is more durable and less expensive. Kinetron II is designed especially for rehabilitation of the lower limb. Hydrafitness makes a complete line of variable speed/variable resistance exercise units that accommodate both the speed and strength of the individual. The Omnitron system may be used to assess knee extension/flexion, shoulder overhead press/lat pull, chest press/row, abdominal flexion, and trunk extension.

Isokinetic Strength Test Protocols   Standardized test protocols and guidelines have been recommended by the Cybex manufacturer for assessing muscle function. Isokinetic strength is measured as the peak torque (ft-lb, kg-m, or N-m) at speeds of either 30° or 60°/sec depending on the joint action and muscle group being tested (Table 23-5). Prior to testing, two submaximum practice trials are administered to familiarize the athlete with the equipment and testing procedure. This is followed immediately by three maximum contractions in both directions (e.g., pronation/supination or flexion/extension). When the Orthotron is used to measure isokinetic strength, the speed is set at either 2½ (30°/sec) or 3 (60°/sec).

Isokinetic Endurance Test Protocols   To assess the isokinetic endurance of the muscle group, repetitive maximum effort trials are used. Endurance is measured as the number of successive repetitions performed before the torque reading decreases to 50% of the initial maximum torque value. The athlete with greater muscular endurance will be able to maintain torque levels above this level for a longer time, thereby completing a greater number of repetitions. Appropriate speed settings range between 120° and 180°/sec for nonathletes and female athletes and between 180° and 300°/sec for male athletes (Table 23-5).

Isokinetic Power Test Protocols Power is a function of force and velocity and is measured by the maximum torque produced through the range of motion at a fast contractile velocity. The speed of movement varies between 120° and 300°/sec depending on the joint action and athletic classification of the individual. After two submaximum practice trials, the athlete is instructed to perform three maximum effort contractions in both directions (e.g., adduction/abduction). Power is measured as the peak torque (ft-lb or N-m) achieved in each direction of joint rotation. Alternatively, power can be measured using a digital work integrator that is attached in series to the Cybex II instrumentation system. This device integrates the area beneath the torque–time curve; thus, an accurate assessment of the total work accomplished during the movement is provided. In addition, power can be measured as the product of force and velocity using the following equation: $P = T \times V/57.29$, where P = power (ft-lb), T = torque; V = speed of movement (°/sec), and 57.29 is a constant.

Isokinetic Norms Performance norms have not been firmly established to evaluate isokinetic strength, endurance, and power of athletes. Relative strength and power norms, expressed as percentage of the individual's body weight, are presented in Tables 23-6 and 23-7.

Meaningful comparisons of means and standard deviations reported in the literature for maximum torque, endurance, and power output are not readily made, since standardized testing procedures concerning the velocity of the movement, limb position, and muscle group tested were not always followed. In general, the following observations are warranted based on data reported in the literature:

Table 23-6   Relative Strength Norms for Cybex Testing

	Percentage of Body Weight					
	Age Group (years)					
Muscle Group	<18	18–35	36–45	46–55	56–65	>65
Women						
Quads	85	90	85	80	75	70
Hamstrings	55	60	55	50	45	40
Plantar Flexors	30	35	30	25	20	15
Dorsi Flexors	5	10	5	3	2	1
Invertors	15	20	15	10	5	2
Evertors	10	15	10	5	1	0.5
Shoulder Flexors	20	25	20	15	10	5
Shoulder Extensors	40	45	40	35	30	25
Men						
Quads	95	100	95	90	85	80
Hamstrings	60	65	60	55	50	45
Plantar Flexors	35	40	35	30	25	20
Dorsi Flexors	10	15	10	5	3	1
Invertors	20	25	20	15	10	5
Evertors	15	20	15	10	5	1
Shoulder Flexors	30	35	30	25	20	15
Shoulder Extensors	50	55	50	45	40	35

From Western Region Manager, Cybex, Ventura, CA 93006

Table 23-7 Relative Power Norms for Cybex Testing

| | Percentage of Body Weight | | | | | |
| | Age Group (years) | | | | | |
Muscle Group	<18	18–35	36–45	46–55	56–65	>65
Women						
Quads	60	65	60	55	50	45
Hamstrings	40	45	40	35	30	25
Plantar Flexors	15	20	15	10	8	6
Dorsi Flexors	3	8	3	2	1	0.5
Invertors	8	13	8	5	3	1
Evertors	6	11	6	3	2	1
Shoulder Flexors	12	17	12	10	7	5
Shoulder Extensors	30	35	30	25	20	15
Men						
Quads	65	70	65	60	55	50
Hamstrings	45	50	45	40	35	30
Plantar Flexors	20	25	20	15	10	5
Dorsi Flexors	5	10	5	2	1	0.5
Invertors	10	15	10	5	3	2.5
Evertors	7	12	7	2	2	1
Shoulder Flexors	15	20	15	10	5	3
Shoulder Extensors	35	40	35	30	25	10

From Western Region Manager, Cybex, Ventura, CA 93006

1. The overall isokinetic strength, as measured by the maximum torque produced during isokinetic bench press and leg press exercises, is significantly greater for men than for women, even when differences in body size are controlled statistically. This is predominantly due to a difference in upper body strength rather than lower body strength (Hoffman et al. [16]).

2. The isokinetic bench press and leg press strength of men is significantly greater than that of women athletes (basketball and volleyball), even when differences in body size are statistically controlled (Morrow and Hosler [17]).

3. Isokinetic strength decreases as the speed of movement (0° to 300°/sec) increases for normal, healthy men (Lesmes et al. [13]; Scudder [14]); habitually active men (Thorstensson et al. [15]); competitive male athletes (Coyle et al. [11]); and competitive female athletes (Gregor et al. [12]).

4. Isokinetic power, measured as the product of maximum torque and angular velocity increases as the speed of joint rotation increases for normal, healthy men and women (Perrine and Edgerton [18]), and male and female athletes (Coyle et al. [11]; Gregor et al. [12]).

5. The rate of decline in torque production during an isokinetic endurance test is directly related to the initial isokinetic strength (Clarkson et al. [19]; Patton et al. [20]). In other words, high-strength individuals tend to have less isokinetic endurance (a faster rate of fatigue and greater loss of strength) than do low-strength individuals.

MUSCLE FIBER TYPES AND PERFORMANCE

In humans, two distinct fiber types have been identified based on contractile characteristics and histochemical myofibrillar ATPase activity of skeletal muscle. Type 1 is fast-twitch (FT) fibers; they have a faster contraction time, higher force production capability, greater anaerobic capacity, and a more rapid rate of fatigue than do Type 2, slow-twitch (ST), fibers.

Thus, FT fibers are highly recruited in and better suited for strength and power performances. Slow-twitch fibers, on the other hand, have a greater aerobic capacity, slower contraction time, and a slower rate of fatigue, making them well suited for endurance activities (Clarkson et al. [21]; Costill et al. [22, 23]; Dons et al. [24]; Gregor et al. [12]; Komi et al. [25]; Prince et al. [26]; Thorstensson et al. [27]).

When muscle fibers are classified on the basis of both myofibrillar ATPase and SDH activities, three fiber types are identified: 1) fast-twitch-glycolytic (FG), 2) fast-twitch-oxidative-glycolytic (FOG), and 3) slow-twitch-oxidative (SO) (Prince et al. [26]). The FOG fiber is an intermediate fiber type. It has an oxidative capacity that is greater than that of the FG fiber but less than that of the SO fiber. However, the contractile characteristics of the FOG are similar to that of the FG fiber.

In many research laboratories, muscle biopsies are taken routinely as a part of the athlete's physiological profile. Data indicate that there is a tendency for strength and power athletes, such as weight-lifters, sprinters, and jumpers, to have a predominance of FT fibers. Endurance athletes such as long-distance runners and cross-country skiers tend to have a greater percentage of ST fibers. There is, however, variability in fiber type between athletes within a given sport or event (Edstrom and Ekblom [28]; Komi [29]; Prince et al. [26]), as well as intraindividual variation in the muscle groups of each athlete (Clarkson et al. [30]; Elder et al. [31]).

These observations have stimulated research into muscle fiber type and sports performance in an attempt to predict an athlete's potential for a given sport. These efforts have focused on 1) the degree to which fiber type distribution is genetically determined; 2) the influence of aerobic training and weight training on fiber type distribution, relative fiber size (FT/ST ratio), and muscle metabolism of fiber types; 3) the importance of fiber type and size to the strength, muscular endurance, and power capabilities of the athlete; and 4) the prediction of fiber type composition from physical performance measures.

Influence of Heredity and Training on Fiber Type

Results of research indicate that fiber type distribution is genetically determined. For males and females, respectively, heredity accounts for 99.5% and 92.5% of the variability in fiber type (Komi et al. [32]). It has been confirmed that the percent fiber distribution does not change as a result of endurance, anaerobic, or weight training (Alen et al. [33]; Costill et al. [22]; Dons et al. [24]; Gollnick et al. [34]; Hakkinen et al. [35]; Komi et al. [36]). Although FT to ST fiber interconversions do not occur, data suggest that interconversions within FT fibers are possible due to weight training (FOG to FG conversion) and aerobic training (FG to FOG conversion) (Prince et al. [26]).

With regard to fiber size, there is evidence that supports greater hypertrophy of FT fibers due to weight training (Hakkinen et al. [35]; Komi et al. [36]; Prince et al. [26]; Thorstensson et al. [37]). In addition, comparisons of relative size of FT and ST fibers of power and endurance athletes show that power athletes tend to have a greater relative size of the FT fibers (Tesch and Larsson [38]). The FT fibers of endurance athletes are smaller, while the ST fiber size of endurance athletes is similar to that of power athletes (Clarkson et al. [21]; Edstrom and Ekblom [28]; Tesch and Larsson [38]). This same trend has been observed for both female and male athletes, although the size of the ST fibers relative to FT fibers tends to be greater for females than for males (Gregor et al. [12]).

Recent research has focused on changes in muscle fiber size and fiber number due to weight training. Using a combination of computed tomography scanning and muscle biopsy techniques, the total cross-sectional area of a muscle and the average cross-sectional area of individual muscle fibers can be measured (Schantz et al. [39]). Results indicate a high positive correlation between these two variables for both trained and untrained subjects (Mac-

Dougall et al. [40]; Schantz et al. [39, 41]. The number of muscle fibers is estimated by dividing the muscle cross-sectional area by the average fiber area. There is large interindividual variation in the number of fibers for untrained subjects and elite body builders (MacDougall et al. [40]). It appears that fiber number does not differ significantly for either males and females (Schantz et al. [41]) or trained and untrained subjects (MacDougall [40]).

The increase in total cross-sectional area of muscle resulting from weight training is most likely explained by hypertrophy of existing muscle fibers rather than an increase in the number of muscle fibers (MacDougall et al. [40]). Thus, it is very likely that athletes who have inherited a large number of muscle fibers will possess a greater potential for muscle hypertrophy.

Relationship of Fiber Type to Muscular Performance

The importance of fiber type to muscular performance has been studied extensively. The following summary is based on a review of research dealing with the relationship of fiber type to strength, muscular endurance, and power.

It has been noted that the percentage of FT fiber distribution is not significantly related to the static (isometric) strength of the knee extensors (Clarkson et al. [19, 42]; Gregor et al. [12]; Nimmo and Maughan [43]). Komi et al. [25], however, observed a statistically significant but low correlation ($r = .38$) between percentage of FT fibers and relative, static leg strength. Clarkson et al. [21], concluded that the relationship of fiber type and static strength depends on the muscle group studied and the type of athlete. They reported that the correlation between percentage of ST fibers in the vastus lateralis and static knee extensor strength was significant for power athletes ($r = .80$) but not significant for endurance athletes ($r = .63$). In contrast, the percentage of ST fibers in the gastrocnemius was noted to be negatively related to the static strength of the ankle plantar flexors for power athletes ($r = -.94$).

Percent fiber distribution is not related to dynamic strength (1-RM) of the knee extensors (Dons et al. [24]). However, Dons et al. reported after 7 weeks of strength training, the correlation between the increase in strength per unit of cross-section of the muscle and the percentage of FT fibers was .80.

A number of investigators have reported significant correlations between percentage of fiber type and isokinetic strength for high angular velocities in excess of 115°/sec (Coyle et al. [11]; Nygaard et al. [44]; Thorstensson et al. [15, 27]. These correlations range between .44 and .81. Schantz et al. [41] reported no significant relationship between fiber composition and torque production at angular velocities between 30° and 180°/sec. Gregor et al. [12] compared the isokinetic strength of the knee extensors at three different speeds of movement. National-caliber female track and field athletes were divided into two groups, those having greater than and those having less than 50% ST fiber distribution in the vastus lateralis. Gregor et al. [12] noted that the maximum torque of the >50% ST group was significantly less than that of the <50% ST group at all speeds of movement (96°, 192°, and 288°/sec). In addition, the relative fiber size (FT/ST area) was significantly related to torque production at all three speeds. Thorstensson et al. [15] also observed that the maximum speed of isokinetic contraction was significantly related to percentage of FT distribution ($r = .50$) and to relative area of FT fibers ($r = .50$).

When field tests such as the Margaria Leg Power Test and the Sargent Jump Test are used to assess power, dynamic leg power is not related to percentage of fiber type (Campbell et al. [45]). However, Bosco and Komi [46] reported that subjects who have a high percentage of FT fibers tended to be better in squatting vertical jump performance on a force platform. The FT percentage was significantly related to the average force ($r = .52$) and mechanical power ($r = .52$). Similarly, Nilsson et al. [47] noted that percentage of FT fibers was significantly related to isokinetic power assessed as the work per unit of time. Likewise, Coyle et al. [11] reported that the isokinetic power, measured as relative peak torque, was significantly greater for the FT group ($>50\%$ FT) than for the ST group ($<50\%$ FT) at velocities of 115°, 200°, 287°, and 400°/sec.

There has been little work done on the influence of fiber type on static and dynamic muscular endurance. In one study, Dons et al. [24] observed that percentage of fiber distribution is not related to performance on a variety of tests used to assess static and dynamic muscular endurance of the knee extensors. Clarkson et al. [30] reported that a higher percentage of ST fibers was associated with a slower rate of fatigue during static exercise of the plantar flexors of endurance and power athletes. The authors were unable, however, to demonstrate a similar relationship for the knee extensors. In isokinetic exercise, a higher percentage of FT fibers appears to be linked to a faster rate of fatigue and less isokinetic endurance (Thorstensson and Karlsson [48]).

Significant correlations between percentage of FT fibers and relative decline in peak torque ($r = .75$), work ($r = .64$), and power ($r = .73$) have been reported for knee extensors (Nilsson et al. [47]). In contrast, Clarkson et al. [19] were unable to support those observations. The authors suggested that the lack of relationship between fiber type and isokinetic endurance was most likely due to the limited sample size used in their study ($N = 8$).

Prediction of Muscle Fiber Type

The ability to predict muscle fiber composition from performance measures would eliminate the need for muscle biopsies, and the trauma and expense of the procedure could be avoided. However, researchers have been unsuccessful in predicting fiber type from performance measures such as bicycle ergometer power tests, Sargent Jump Test, and maximum oxygen consumption tests (Campbell et al. [45]).

PROBLEMS ASSOCIATED WITH MUSCLE TESTING

A number of factors can influence the measurement of strength, muscular endurance, and power. Each of these factors, listed below, should be controlled to ensure valid, reliable, and objective assessments of muscle function whenever possible.

1. No single test can be used to assess overall strength, muscular endurance, or power. These factors are highly specific to the muscle group, type of muscular contraction (static, dynamic, or isokinetic), the limb position, joint angle tested during static tests, and the speed of movement during isokinetic tests. To evaluate a specific muscle function, it is recommended that a test be selected that matches the requirements of the performance. For example, in high jumping the coach or trainer should assess the dynamic strength and power of the hip, knee, and ankle extensor muscle groups of the take-off leg, using patterns and speeds of movement that closely simulate those used during the high-jumping performance.
2. To assess total body strength, a minimum of three measures should be taken, due to the highly specific nature of strength. The test battery should include measures of abdominal, upper body, and lower body strength.
3. Strength and power measurements are influenced by body size and body composition. These scores, therefore, should be expressed in relative, as well as absolute terms. The performance should be evaluated relative to lean body weight or total body weight,

Table 23-8 Sources for Muscle Testing Equipment

Product	Manufacturer's Address
Cable Tensiometer (static)	Pacific Scientific Co. Inc. Anaheim, CA 92803
CAM II (variable resistance)	Keiser 220 Division Northfield, MN 55057
Cybex II, Orthotron, Kinetron II (isokinetic) and Eagle (variable resistance)	Cybex 2100 Smithtown Ave. Ronkonkoma, NY 11779
Free Weights (constant resistance)	York Barbell Co. Box 1707 York, PA 17405
Handgrip Dynamometer (static)	C.H. Stoelting Co. 424 North Homan Ave. Chicago, IL 60624
Leg/Back Dynamometer (static)	Nissen Corp. Cedar Rapids, IA 52406
Nautilus (variable resistance)	Sports/Medical Industries P.O. Box 1783 Deland, FL 32720
Omnitron System (variable speed/ variable resistance)	Hydrafitness P.O. Box 599 Belton, TX 76513
Total Gym (variable resistance)	Total Medical Systems 7161 Engineer Rd. San Diego, CA 92111
Universal Gym Machine (constant and variable resistance)	Kidde Box 1270 Cedar Rapids, IA 52406
Versa-Gym (constant resistance)	Versatile Fitness Equipment Inc. 798 Holbrook Ave. Simi Valley, CA 93065

especially if between-group comparisons (e.g., male versus female athletes or football versus basketball players) are to be made.

4. Absolute measures of muscular endurance are dependent on the strength of the individual. Therefore, it is recommended that tests that are proportional to maximum strength or to lean body weight of the athlete be used to assess muscular endurance.

5. When administering strength, muscular endurance, and power tests, standardized procedures should be followed. Factors such as body position of the athlete, joint angle, speed of movement, number of practice and performance trials, and the way in which the function is measured (best trial versus average of trials) should be noted.

6. Strength, muscular endurance, and power tests require maximum effort on the part of the athlete. Therefore, factors that influence maximum performance need to be controlled. These include time of day of testing, sex of the experimenter and subject, temperature, humidity, altitude, sleep, drug usage, and motivation of the subject. To control motivation, each subject should be treated in a similar manner by the experimenter. This means that the instructions, verbal encouragement given during the test, and knowledge of results given either during or after the test should be standardized.

7. Assessing the athlete's potential for a given sport or event is hampered by a lack of performance norms. Strength, muscular endurance, and power norms need to be established for male and female athletes in all sports.

REFERENCES

1. Kreighbaum, E., Barthels, K.M. 1985. Biomechanics: A Qualitative Approach for Studying Human Movement (ed. 2). Burgess Publishing Co., Minneapolis, MN.

2. Montoye, H.J., Faulkner, J.A. 1964. Determination of the optimum setting of an adjustable hand grip dynamometer. Res Q 35:29–36.

3. Clarke, H.H., Clarke, D.H. 1963. Developmental and Adapted Physical Education. Prentice-Hall, Englewood Cliffs, NJ.

4. Clarke, D.H. 1975. Exercise Physiology. Prentice-Hall, Englewood Cliffs, NJ.

5. Clarke, H.H., Monroe, R.A. 1970. Test Manual: Oregon Cable Tension Strength Test Batteries for Boys and Girls from Fourth Grade Through College. University of Oregon, Eugene, OR.

6. Pollock, M.L., Wilmore, J.H., et al. 1978. Health and Fitness Through Physical Activity. John Wiley & Sons, New York.

7. Considine, W.J. 1971. A validity analysis of selected leg power tests, utilizing a force platform. In: Cooper J.M. (ed): Biomechanics. The Athletic Press, Chicago.

8. Wilmore, J.H. 1982. Training for Sport and Activity: The Physiological Basis of the Conditioning Process. Allyn and Bacon, Boston.

9. Margaria, R., Aghemo, I., et al. 1966. Measurement of muscular power (anaerobic) in man. J Appl Physiol 21:1662–1664.

10. Kalamen, J. 1968. Measurement of maximal muscular power in man. Unpublished doctoral dissertation. Ohio State University, Columbus.

11. Coyle, E.F., Costill, D.L., et al. 1979. Leg extension power and muscle fiber composition. Med Sci Sports Exerc 11:12–15.

12. Gregor, R.J., Edgerton, V.R., et al. Torque-velocity relationships and muscle fiber composition in elite female athletes. J Appl Physiol 47:388–392.

13. Lesmes, G.R., Costill, D.L., et al. 1978. Muscle strength and power changes during maximal isokinetic training. Med Sci Sports 10:266–269.

14. Scudder, G.N. 1980. Torque curves produced at the knee during isometric and isokinetic exercise. Arch Phys Med Rehabil 61:68–73.

15. Thorstensson, A., Grimby, G., et al. 1976. Force-velocity relations and fiber composition in human extensor muscles. J Appl Physiol 40:12–16.

16. Hoffman, T., Stauffer, R.W., et al. 1979. Sex differences in strength. Am J Sports Med 7:265–267.

17. Morrow, J.R., Hosler, W.W. 1981. Strength comparisons in untrained men and trained women athletes. Med Sci Sports Exerc 13:194–198.

18. Perrine, J.J., Edgerton, V.R. 1978. Muscle force-velocity and power-velocity relationships under isokinetic loading. Med Sci Sports 10:159–166.

19. Clarkson, P.M., Johson, J., et al. 1982. The relationships among isokinetic endurance, initial strength level, and fiber type. Res Q Exerc Sport 53:15–19.

20. Patton, R.W., Hinson, M.M., et al. 1978. Fatigue curves of isokinetic contractions. Arch Phys Med Rehabil 59:507–509.

21. Clarkson, P.M., Kroll, W., et al. 1980. Maximal isometric strength and fiber type composition in power and endurance athletes. Eur J Appl Physiol 44:35–42.

22. Costill, D.L., Coyle, E.F., et al. 1979. Adaptations in skeletal muscle following strength training. J Appl Physiol 46:96–99.

23. Costill, D.L., Daniels, J., et al. 1976. Skeletal muscle enzymes and fiber composition in male and female track athletes. J Appl Physiol 40:149–154.

24. Dons, B., Bollerup, K., et al. 1979. The effect of weightlifting exercise related to muscle fiber composition and muscle cross-sectional area in humans. Eur J Appl Physiol 40:95–106.

25. Komi, P.V., Rusko, H., et al. 1977. Anaerobic performance capacity in athletes. Acta Physiol Scand 100:107–114.

26. Prince, F.P., Hikida, R.S., et al. 1976. Human muscle fiber types in power lifters, distance runners, and untrained subjects. Pflugers Arch 363:19–26.

27. Thorstensson, A., Larsson, L., et al. 1977. uscle strength and fiber composition in athletes and sedentary men. Med Sci Sports 9:26–30.

28. Edstrom, L., Ekblom, B. 1972. Differences in sizes of red and white muscle fibres in vastus lateralis of musculus quadriceps femoris of normal individuals and athletes. Relation to physical performance. Scand J Clin Lab Invest 30:175–181.

29. Komi, P.V. 1984. Physiological and biomechanical correlates of muscle function: effects of muscle structure and stretch-shortening cycle on force and

speed. In: Terjung, R.L. (ed): Exercise and Sports Sciences Reviews (Vol. 12). Collamore Press, Lexington.

30. Clarkson, P.M., Kroll, W., et al. 1980. Plantar flexion fatigue and muscle fiber type in power and endurance athletes. Med Sci Sports Exer 12:262–267.

31. Elder, G.C.B., Bradbury, K., et al. 1982. Variability of fiber type distributions within human muscles. J Appl Physiol 53:1473–1480.

32. Komi, P.V., Vitasalo, J., et al. 1977. Skeletal muscle fibers and muscle enzyme activities in monozygous and dizygous twins of both sexes. Acta Physiol Scand 100:385–392.

33. Alen, M., Hakkinen, K., et al. 1984. Changes in neuromuscular performance and muscle fiber characteristics of elite power athletes self-administering androgenic and anabolic steroids. Acta Physiol Scand 122:535–544.

34. Gollnick, P., Armstrong, R., et al. 1973. Effect of training on enzyme activity and fiber composition of human skeletal muscle. J Appl Physiol 34:107–111.

35. Hakkinen, K., Komi, P.V., et al. 1981. Effect of combined concentric and eccentric strength training and detraining on force-time, muscle fiber, and metabolic characteristics of leg extensor muscles. Scand J Sports Sci 3:50–58.

36. Komi, P.V., Karlsson, J., et al. 1982. Effects of heavy resistance and explosive strength training methods on mechanical, functional, and metabolic aspects of performance. In: Komi, P.V. (ed): Exercise and Sport Biology. Human Kinetics, Champaign, IL.

37. Thorstensson, A., Hulten, B., et al. 1976. Effect of strength training on enzyme activities and fibre characteristics in human skeletal muscle. Acta Physiol Scand 96:392–398.

38. Tesch, P., Larsson, L. 1982. Muscle hypertrophy in body builders. Eur J Appl Physiol 49:301–306.

39. Schantz, P., Randall-Fox, E., et al. 1981. The relationship between the mean muscle fibre area and the muscle cross-sectional area of the thigh in subjects with large differences in thigh girth. Acta Physiol Scand 113:537–539.

40. MacDougall, J.D., Sale, D.G., et al. 1984. Muscle fiber number in biceps brachii in body builders and control subjects. J Appl Physiol 57:1399–1403.

41. Schantz, P., Randall-Fox, E., et al. 1983. Muscle fibre distribution, muscle cross-sectional area and maximal voluntary strength in humans. Acta Physiol Scand 117:219–226.

42. Clarkson, P.M., Kroll, W., et al. 1981. Age, isometric strength, rate of tension development and fiber type composition. J Gerontol 36:648–653.

43. Nimmo, M.A., Maughan, R.J. 1983. Influence of variations in muscle fiber composition on the ratio of strength to cross-sectional area of m. quadriceps femoris in man. Med Sci Sports Exerc 15:178.

44. Nygaard, E., Houston, M., et al. 1983. Morphology of the brachial biceps muscle and elbow flexion in man. Acta Physiol Scand 117:287–292.

45. Campbell, C.J., Bonen, A., et al. 1979. Muscle fiber composition and performance capacities of women. Med Sci Sports 11:260–265.

46. Bosco, C., Komi, P.V. 1979. Mechanical characteristics and fiber composition of human leg extensor muscles. Eur J Appl Physiol 41:275–284.

47. Nilsson, J., Tesch, P., et al. 1977. Fatigue and EMG of repeated fast voluntary contractions in man. Acta Physiol Scand 101:194–198.

48. Thorstensson, A., Karlsson, J. 1976. Fatiguability and fibre composition of human skeletal muscle. Acta Physiol Scand 98:318–322.

•24•

Massage and Sport

Carol Kresge

"Massage is a vital part of systematic training. It is a *must* in basic conditioning." Thus begins a 1979 article in *Track and Field News*; an accompanying article, by Bob Beeten, head of the United States Olympic Committee Sports Medicine program and a massage advocate, is entitled "But Not in U.S." (Nordqvist [1]). These articles aptly describe the state of massage in athletics in the United States and elsewhere. Until the early 1980s massage was extensively prescribed and researched in European countries, including those of the Communist bloc, while in the United States, it was replaced for a long period by technologic aids.

Massage is now reclaiming an important place in the U.S. athletic world, as evidenced by its availability at most major road races and its inclusion in the 1984 Olympics as a service available to all athletes, and the fact that the national American Massage and Therapy Association is now certifying therapists in the specialized field of sports massage.

In this chapter the role massage can play in the athlete's life is examined. Basically, massage can be an adjunct to training in three ways:

1. By enabling the athlete to recover from injury more rapidly and completely, with less likelihood of chronic problems;
2. By maintaining muscles in their best state of relaxation, flexibility, and nutrition; and
3. By reducing muscle soreness, enabling athletes to recover more quickly and to train at a higher level, thus pushing back that fine line between maximum training and overtraining.

An overview of the research into massage physiology as therapy is provided, as well as the athletic implications of such research. The reader should note that "massage" throughout refers to the technique of Swedish massage (including effleurage, pétrissage, friction, tapotement, and shaking) as well as sustained pressure on trigger points, compression in the form of muscle pumping, and cross-fiber massage on specific points, on injuries, or on entire muscle groups.

PHYSIOLOGY OF MASSAGE THERAPY

The therapeutic value of massage lies in its numerous and combined physiologic effects. These effects and their implications, as they apply to the systems important to athletic activity, are outlined in Table 24-1.

Table 24-1 Effects and Implications of Massage

Organ or Tissue	Effects of Massage	Implications/Applications

Vascular System	Manually increases blood flow
	Reflex vasodilation
	Increases diameter and
	  permeability of capillaries
	Increases red blood cell count
	Decreases blood pressure
	Increases systolic stroke
	  volume
	Decreases pulse
		Increases cellular-nutrition
		Decreases edema
		Increases toxin removal
		Decreases muscle soreness
		Decreases pain
		Decreases muscle fatigue
		Increases work capability
		Increases metabolism

Lymph	Manually empties	Decreases edema Decreases tendency toward fibrosis
Muscular System	Relaxes Manually separates fibers Can stimulate contraction	Increases flexibility Decreases spasm Decreases undesired adhesions Decreases atrophy Decreases pain Increases body awareness
Skeletal System	Increases retention of nitrogen, sulphur, and phosphorous	Aids fracture healing

Circulatory Effects of Massage

Massage produces two different circulatory effects. The first is a mechanical or manual pushing of the venous blood. The second is reflex, and this results from the release of acetylcholine and histamines that cause sustained vasodilation that can outlast the massage (Scull [2]; Meagher and Boughton [3]). The extent to which each of these effects operates is partly a product of which types of strokes are emphasized in the massage treatment.

Dubrovsky [4] injected tibialis anterior muscles with the radioisotope ^{133}Xe and recorded its clearance rate both before and after massage. Massage accelerated the clearance rate. He also found an increase in muscle blood flow from 4.5 ± 0.11 ml/100 g/min before massage to 6.4 ± 0.11 after massage. In another experiment with ^{133}Xe, Hansen and Kristensen [5] found massage to be more effective than shortwave diathermy or ultrasound in removing the ^{133}Xe from muscles. The increased clearance rate was attributed to an increase in blood flow. Similar experiments found no net increase in blood flow, and the increased disappearance rate of ^{133}Xe from muscles was attributed to the mechanical emptying and refilling of vascular beds (Hovind and Nielsen [6]).

Bell [7] found that blood volume and flow doubled and did not begin to drop until 40 min after completion of massage. Wakim et al. [8] found inconsistent increases in blood flow, but a definite decrease in edema in all subjects, indicating that lymph may play a greater role than blood in the physiologic effects of massage.

Wolfson [9] reported a great initial increase in blood flow with massage, and then a decrease while the treatment was still in progress. The total volume was no greater, but more complete emptying occurred associated with a greater influx of fresh blood. This suggests that more frequent, shorter duration massages may be more beneficial.

As can be seen, the research is contradictory as to which circulatory effect is the causative factor in the changes noted from massage. Regardless of whether the changes are due to increased blood flow, increased lymph, or simply from a more complete emptying and refilling of the vessels, the results in terms of decreased edema and increased muscle clearance rates are without doubt.

Increased blood flow and systolic stroke volume and decreased blood pressure and heart rate plus increased blood flow in the nontreated homologous limb have been reported in response to deep massage in athletes (Severini and Venerando [10]), suggesting possibilities for increasing blood flow through limbs in casts.

Wakim [11] cites other massage effects on circulation, including a study by Krogh that showed increased diameter and permeability of capillaries from mechanical stimulation. Experiments using "windows" in rabbit ears showed that massage increased the speed of circulating elements as well as the rate of exchange of substances between cells and circulating blood, thus improving metabolism (Wood [12]).

Massage raises the red blood cell count temporarily (Scull [2]) by mobilizing stagnant blood cells in the splanchnic circulation rather than by increased production (Schneider and Havens [13]). Dubrovsky [4] found increases in arterial blood saturation with oxygen of 1.6% after massage. This temporary increase in oxygen-carrying capacity supports increased metabolism.

Lymph Flow

Massage is more effective than passive motion or electrical muscle stimulation in increasing the lymph flow (Ladd et al. [14]). According to Paikov, the body contains 1200–1500 mm of lymphocytes moving at a speed of 4 mm/sec. Massage increased this eightfold (Paikov [15]).

Massage, Muscle Relaxation, and Performance

In a study utilizing the hamstring muscles, general massage was found to significantly increase range of motion (Crosman et al. [16]). The study was conducted on normal female subjects; however, the author noted, "Athletes may also benefit from massage treatments for prevention of injury associated with hamstring limitations. Massage to the hamstring muscle group is an effective means of increasing range of motion and should be an integral part of patient care" (p. 61).

Dubrovsky [4] found that massage decreases resting (plastic) muscle tone by 3.6 ± 0.1 myotones and decreases contractile muscle tone by 6.1 ± 0.1 myotones.

Generalized massage in which no special attention was given to specific tension areas palpable in 4 out of 5 subjects was found to consistently relax muscles and increase flexibility (Nordschow and Bierman [17]). The author noted, "The muscles of the back are kept at a tension beyond that required to hold the body in any plane, as judged by the fact that the reduction of this tension does not interfere with the function of the body, and indeed permits the performance of these functions with greater ease" (p. 656).

The implications of this for athletes for whom increased ease of movement can make the difference between winning and losing are important. It should be noted that in a clinical setting massage is not generalized but rather tailored to each individual's specific tension areas and this can create an even more profound effect.

Muscle Recovery and Efficiency

Massage of muscles tired from running or bicycle riding has been found to reduce recovery time, as shown by a faster decline in pulse rate and quicker recovery of muscle efficiency (Müller et al. [18]). Massage instead of rest periods enabled the subjects to almost triple their work capacity. At that point, inadequate "fuel" was thought to limit work, and massage effectiveness decreased. Quicker muscle recovery and greater work capacity were also achieved experimentally through massage by two other investigators (Wood [12]; Licht [19]).

A Soviet study of young gymnasts found both classical massage and point massage effective in promoting improved restoration between first and second training sessions. Both methods improved the latent period of motor response (LPMR) and the electrodermal resistance (EDR); however, point massage increased the EDR to a greater extent. Contractile ability increased with both methods, more so through classical massage (Peshkov [20]).

Skeletal System

Cuthbertson [21] showed that local massage in those with fractures of long bones increased significantly the retention of nitrogen, sulfur, and phosphorus necessary for tissue repair.

Myoglobin

Massage performed on areas of regional muscle tension and pain (known as fibrositis, interstitial myofibrositis, myofascial pain, and trigger points) increases plasma myoglobin. This increase is proportional to the degree of muscle tension and is not present when muscles without tension and pain are massaged. When multiple treatments are performed, there is a decrease from treatment to treatment in the degree of tension and pain and a corresponding decrease in the rise of plasma myoglobin until no significant rise is seen. This myoglobin effect does not appear to be due to mechanical muscle tissue destruction, since it decreases with repeated massage. Rather it suggests that muscle tension and pain are a disorder within the muscle, possibly related to a loss of oxidative metabolic capacity (Daneskiold-Samsøe et al. [22]).

Clinical Versus Experimental Results

It has been frequently noted that clinical results of massage are often more dramatic than experiments with massage would indicate. This is due to two factors: Massage tends to have a cumulative effect not generally shown in short-term experiments, and clinically, massage is individualized to suit what is found in a client and to emphasize the techniques most effective on that client, whereas scientific experiments must employ standardized, repeatable procedures.

MASSAGE AND THE INJURED ATHLETE

Massage can play an important role in the treatment of pain, edema, and decreased range of motion secondary to myofascial injury.

Pain

Massage is an effective treatment for the self-perpetuating pain cycle regardless of its cause (Fig. 24-1). A painful stimulus results in reflex muscle contraction and localized muscle splinting or guarding, which restricts movement and local circulation. The subsequent ischemia creates more pain. Muscle splinting is intensified and the cycle repeats itself (Jacobs [23]).

Experimental production of localized pain results in a more generalized secondary pain as splinting and the pain cycle begin, and the secondary, more generalized pain may

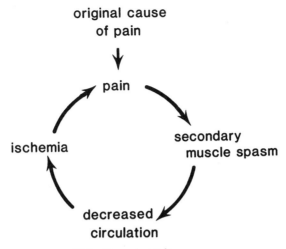

24-1 The pain cycle.

outlast or exceed the original discomfort (Jacobs [23]). Thus, it becomes important to treat the original cause and also the secondary muscle contraction. Massage effectively breaks the pain cycle by relaxing muscles (Nordschow and Bierman [17]), increasing circulation (Scull [2]; Wakim [11]), and removing metabolic wastes (Wakim [11]; Müller et al. [18]).

Anxiety and stress aggravate the secondary pain of muscle contraction (Jacobs [23]), and massage intervenes by promoting relaxation (Nordschow and Bierman [17]) and a sense of well-being (Nordschow and Bierman [17]; Jacobs [23]).

Edema

The localized swelling of soft-tissue injuries creates pain, pressure, stiffness, and impaired motion, and increases the tendency toward fibrosis (Scull [2]). It slows healing by reducing the metabolic circulation from the capillary across the interstitial space into the cell and back. As the distance from the cell to the capillaries is increased by excess extravascular fluid, diffusion time is increased by the square of the distance. Thus, with swelling doubling the distance, diffusion time is increased by four (Ladd et al. [14]). Massage is an effective means of reducing edema and thus speeding metabolic circulation.

Compensation

Muscle splinting secondary to pain not only causes localized spasm, but also may change the carriage of the body as a whole, resulting in distant compensatory problems. This is often the cause for chronic injuries in athletes who resume activity too soon with altered posture and create new areas of biomechanical stress. Massage can find and clear these areas before new injury occurs.

Limping, casting, and splinting likewise create compensatory muscle spasm in distant body parts. Foot casts create a functional long/short leg and may cause knee, hip, and lower back problems. These areas should be massaged while the cast is in place and afterward as gait and stance are changing.

Healing

The effects of massage on injured muscles was studied by producing crushing injury to animal muscle followed by massage to one group and no treatment to another group (Wood

[12]). Microscopic examination of the untreated muscle showed dissociation of the muscle fibers, hyperplasia, sometimes a swelling of the connective tissue, areas of increase in connective tissue nuclei, interstitial hemorrhages, and hyperplasia of adventitial layers of blood vessels. The sarcolemma was usually intact, but in one section, increased interstitial nuclei gave the appearance of myositis. In the massaged limbs, muscle fibers appeared normal. Fibrous thickening of vessel wall was not seen, muscle bulk was greater, and there were no hemorrhages. Thus, massage seems to promote healing of injured tissue.

Range of Motion

Early restoration of normal range of motion to an injured area is not only a therapeutic aim but is also excellent therapy. Motion decreases adhesion formation (Jacobs [23]), increases blood flow and nutrition to the area, and reduces healing time. Massage helps to increase range of motion by breaking the pain cycle and reducing edema. When active or passive motion is inappropriate, cross-fiber massage (Meagher and Boughton [3]; Cyriax [24, 25]) can create the necessary movement.

Cross-Fiber Massage

Longitudinal scars that parallel muscle fibers interfere less with normal contraction and strength and are less subject to reinjury and chronic pain than are transverse scars which may cause adherence of adjacent fibers or of muscle fibers to bony structures (Cyriax [24]). Adhesions between individual fibers limit contraction. Gross scarring across an entire muscle is often asymptomatic once healed, since equal tension is present on all parts of the muscle as it contracts. However, random adhesions within a muscle can cause chronic pain because of the variations of tension during contraction in the areas where normal tissue joins scar tissue.

To create strong scar tissue longitudinally and limit transverse adhesions, movement mimicking the muscle's normal use is most appropriate. This motion can be active (non-weight-bearing, or resisted), passive, or manual (as in deep cross-fiber massage).

During observation of scar tissue formation under the microscope, is was noted that the arrangement of fibrils was dependent on mechanical factors, especially movement (Cyriax [24]). Thus appropriate movement within the muscle as it is healing inhibits unwanted adhesion formation and creates a strong scar where it is needed.

Cross-fiber massage becomes a more important treatment modality the closer a muscle injury is to an immobile structure, since active movement is less effective in fiber spreading in this situation (Fig. 24-2).

Muscle tears heal best with cross-fiber friction massage followed by active movement, initially in a relaxed, non-weight-bearing isometric contraction (Cyriax [25]).

When ligaments at joints under voluntary control are injured, e.g., ankle sprains, chronic reinjury occurs as adhesions form between the ligament and bone. This limits the proper motion of the ligament over the bone and during later strenuous use predisposes the ligament to chronic injury. Appropriate rehabilitation includes cross-fiber massage, manually moving the ligament over the bone followed by passive motion under local anesthesia (Cyriax [25]).

Tendons with sheaths are subjected to tenosynovitis, a roughening between the surface of the tendon and its sheath, caused by longitudinal friction. Appropriate treatment is cross-fiber transverse friction with the tendon held taut. In this instance, passive and active movement should be avoided, since motion creates the longitudinal friction that caused the tenosynovitis (Cyriax [25]).

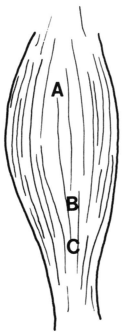

24-2 The closer a muscle lesion is to an immobile structure, the less effective is movement or local anesthesia, and the more effective is cross fiber massage. A, B, and C refer to lesions nearing the joint. The lesion in C would best be treated by cross-fiber massage. (Adapted from Cyriax [24].)

Cyriax, the orthopedic surgeon pioneering cross-fiber massage, maintains that there are a number of lesions in which cross-fiber friction massage is the *only* effective means of treatment. These lesions include injury of the following (Cyriax [25, 26]):

1. Subclavius belly
2. Supraspinatus, musculotendinous junction
3. Biceps brachii, longhead, belly, lower musculotendinous junction
4. Brachialis or supinator belly
5. Ligaments about carpal lunate bone
6. Interosseous belly and tendon of hand
7. Intercostal muscle
8. Oblique muscles of abdomen
9. Psoas, lower musculotendinous junction
10. Quadriceps expansion at patella
11. Coronary ligament at knee
12. Medial collateral ligament in athletes
13. Biceps femoris, lower musculotendinous junction
14. Musculotendinous junction of anterior tibial
15. Posterior or peronal tibial
16. Posterior tibiotalar ligament
17. Tendo Achilles in athletes
18. Anterior fascia of ankle joint
19. Interosseous belly of foot

For deep cross-fiber friction massage to be effective, the exact lesion site must be massaged and the friction must be at right angles to the fibers. It must be of sufficient depth and range to reach and separate the fibers. This author's experience using cross-fiber massage supports Cyriax's claims: Healing is rapid and appropriate.

Trigger Point Massage

Many myofascial pain syndromes can be attributed to trigger points, especially in the lower back, neck, and shoulder, although referred trigger point pain is possible anywhere in the body. Travel initiated the research in trigger points and their treatment through procaine injection (Travel [27]; Weeks and Travel [28]). Meagher with sports massage [3] and Prudden with pain erasure [29] have popularized this work for the athlete and general public by substituting sustained pressure, compression, massage, and cross-fiber massage on the points in place of injection. These massage techniques achieve comparable therapeutic results.

A trigger point is a small localized area of deep tenderness within a muscle. It is hypersensitive, with a lowered pain threshold (Bonica [30]; Travel [27]). Stimulation of the trigger point with mechanical pressure will elicit referred pain in the same remote area in different individuals. Thus, referred pain patterns are predictable and can be mapped and become easily recognized (Travel [27]).

This author's experience leads to the supposition that trigger points are primary or secondary causes of all myofascial pain. A trigger point mechanism may be suspected to be the primary cause of pain when there are no abnormal neurologic findings and when the pain distribution is neither segmental nor follows the peripheral nerve distribution (Bonica [30]). Even when neurologic findings are abnormal, trigger points may be a secondary cause and result in pain that outlasts the original pathology.

Many precipitating causes of trigger points are a part of everyday training for serious competitive and recreational athletes (Travel [27]; Weeks and Travel [28]; Bonica [30]). These include sudden trauma to muscle, tendon, ligament, and bone; unusual or excessive exercise; chilling; immobilization; and acute emotional stress. General fatigue, nutritional deficiencies, nervous tension, and chronic muscle strain produced by repetitive movements or poor posture predispose to precipitating causes of trigger points. To this list might be added muscular stiffness or lack of flexibility, and imbalances between antagonistic muscles.

An active trigger point may elicit enough pain to cause satellite trigger points to appear. Any intense pain can cause new trigger points. Once established, these points can be immediately activated or can lie dormant to be reactivated only when any of the above factors are present. This has important implications for injury prevention (Meagher and Boughton [3]). If an athlete is kept free of trigger points through massage, the chances of injury can be decreased.

Trigger points usually arise in areas of greatest biomechanical stress. The extremes of repetition inherent in athletic activities (1600 steps per mile) or the one-sided nature of many athletic activities, such as racquetball, subject the athlete's body to greater than normal mechanical stresses. The nature of the sport and the athlete's physical structure within that sport define the most common injuries and likewise the most common trigger areas for each sport (Fig. 24-3) (Meagher and Boughton [3]; Prudden [29]).

Overuse Injury

Athletic injury not attributable to accident is usually thought to result from overuse. The correlation of overuse with high intensity, such as high mileage in the runner, is a misunderstanding of the term. Overuse is essentially too much, too soon, before body structures have adapted to the stresses placed on them. Like massage, appropriate training is both a

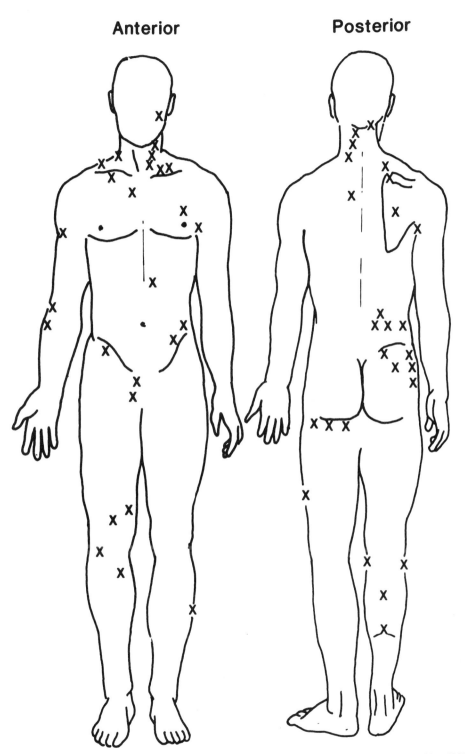

Anterior

Posterior

24-3 The most common trigger areas. (Adapted from Meagher and Boughton [3]; Prudden [29]; and Bonica [30].)

science and an art, which includes learning to individually recognize the fine line between appropriate stress and adequate time for adaptation (which builds an athlete's body) and excess stress with inadequate adaptation time (which breaks down tissue). Thus, overuse is not a cause of injury solely in athletes training at a high intensity. A study by Pagliano and Jackson [31] indicated that low-mileage runners most frequently sought injury evaluation and treatment (Table 24-2). This may be because less experienced runners lack understanding of training principles and body awareness. Massage enhances body awareness by "tuning in" the person to each part of his or her body. Those who are unaccustomed to massage usually comment that areas of soreness and tension exist that they were unaware of. Massage can aid in overuse injury prevention by making the person recognize problem areas and helping to alleviate them before they become serious.

MASSAGE AND THE HEALTHY ATHLETE

Massage for the healthy athlete prevents injury, improves function, and increases the recovery rate during a given period of time.

Muscle Soreness

Muscle soreness is a part of all athletic life. It arises when activity level is increased or activity is begun after an inactive lifestyle, when greater than usual effort is expended, or when activities utilize muscle groups in unaccustomed ways. Three theories exist concerning the cause of muscle soreness (Abraham [32]), and each probably plays a greater or lesser role depending on the situation. First is the spasm, metabolic waste theory, which holds that repeated strenuous activity overworks certain muscles, causing accumulation of metabolic wastes such as lactic acid that, in turn, affect muscle fiber osmotic pressure, water retention, and pressure. The wastes irritate nerve endings, resulting in pain, muscle contraction, and ischemia.

The second theory, the torn tissue hypothesis, suggests that untrained muscles worked for prolonged periods are especially susceptible to minute tears. Likewise, when metabolic wastes accumulate, muscle strength decreases and continued activity results in small tears in muscle fibers.

The third and most recent theory concerns connective tissue irritation, especially noted with eccentric, negative work, and associated with an increased inflammatory response in muscle components.

Massage can positively affect each of these processes by increasing circulation, increasing lymph flow, and relaxing muscles. It has been shown that massage is more effective than rest in removing the metabolic wastes produced by exercise (Müller et al. [18]). Massage is especially effective if administered shortly after the strenuous effort, although it decreases soreness at all stages. Athletes have noted that given an equal effort, recovery was greatly enhanced by massage.

Table 24-2   Weekly Distance of Injured Runners

Weekly Distance	% of Injured Runners
0–20 miles	48%
20–40 miles	32%
40–60 miles	13%
60–80 miles	5%
80 + miles	2%

Training Level

Training is based on repeated stressing of the system through specific overload, alternating with recovery and adaptation periods. Adaptation, and thus training, increase in a manner proportionate to the stress applied until maximum stress tolerance is reached, at which point the system begins to break down, causing stress or overuse injuries, fatigue, and decreased performance. Thus, establishing an optimum training program means continually reestablishing a delicate balance.

Massage can help an athlete become aware of and maintain balances between optimum training and overtraining. Massage decreases muscle soreness, and enables muscles to recover from work more rapidly and to perform more work or train at a higher level (Müller et al. [18]). Massage also identifies areas of tension and trigger points and relieves these, making the athlete more flexible, able to perform more easily, and less prone to injury (Meagher and Boughton [3]). Top-class European athletes will not train without regular massage and attribute the level of training they can handle to the use of massage (Nordqvist [1]).

Performance Improvement

Experiments concerning the effects of massage on performance have been contradictory. In one study, massage was shown to improve performance of both men and women in swimming 50 m, running 100 m, and riding the bicycle ergometer (Karpovich and Hale [33]). Other studies cited by Karpovich and Hale [33], however, found no effect on performance with massage; these were single experimental situations with standardized massage procedures. The effect of massage on performance, however, is cumulative and should be a regular part of athletic training individually designed for each athlete. With the use of cross-fiber massage and compression on trigger points, it has been said that one may improve performance, endurance, and athletic "lifetime" (Meagher and Boughton [3]).

Muscles work in antagonistic pairs; one pair must relax while the other contracts. Excess tension requires more work from the contracting muscle to overcome the resistance of its antagonist, resulting in loss of power, performance, and coordination (Meagher and Boughton [3]). The body is maintained at a tension level that affects ease of performance. Massage through muscle relaxation and relief of trigger points can reduce this tension and resistance (Nordschow and Bierman [17]).

INJURY PREVENTION

Prevention of injury is hard to document. Massage may help prevent injury by maintaining muscles in the best state of relaxation, flexibility, and nutrition, and by rapid removal of metabolic wastes. It may furthermore help by finding and alleviating problem areas before they become serious. Finally, it can help reduce chronic or repeated injury by aiding in appropriate healing, as discussed previously.

CATEGORIES OF MASSAGE

Massage treatments must be designed with the sport of the athlete, the timing of the treatment, and the specific effects of different techniques kept in mind. It must be individualized according to what is felt under the therapist's fingers and how the athlete is responding.

Athletes have different needs at different times. This is reflected in four general categories of sports massage:

Preevent—At this point the need is for a short treatment that will be an adjunct to warm-up by creating a durable hypermia, increasing flexibility, and leaving the athlete loose but not overly relaxed with his or her optimum reaction time capabilities. Strokes emphasized include compression and shaking with limited trigger point work and pétrissage (kneading).

Postevent—This calls for a massage whose intent is restorative. The aim is to increase the athlete's recovery rate by decreasing fatigue and soreness, speeding the removal of metabolic by-products and relieving spasms. This could be after competition, after a training session, or between two-a-day sessions. This massage is primarily a kneading (pétrissage) and effleurage massage with some shaking and limited trigger point work.

Regular Fine Tuning—These treatments are designed to search out the areas of biomechanical stress and relieve them before they become problems. In addition to all the elements of a postevent massage, compression, cross-fiber and trigger point work are included. This is the best time for trigger point or full body cross-fiber. It is more easily handled when it is not immediately postevent and an athlete new to this work can adapt to potential changes in timing in training rather than competition.

Injury Rehabilitation—These treatments are designed to speed healing, prevent compensatory problems, increase range of motion, and create a scar which is strong yet does not inhibit normal broadening of the muscle upon contraction. The stroke of most importance in appropriate scar formation is cross-fiber.

THE SOVIET SYSTEM

The Soviets have been perfecting sports massage through extensive use and research. It is an important part of the Soviet system of training for all athletes, and its usage is very specific with regard to frequency, intensity, technique, and duration. Their categories of massage are similar to those listed above, being preliminary, restorative, training, and medical massage. One indication of the level of usage and acceptance of sports massage is their recommendation of several repeated massage sessions 2–5 hr apart in the case of overworked "beat" muscles (Paikov [15]). This type of prescription denotes a system in which massage is well studied, well respected, and readily available. Little of the Soviet work has been translated. However, the following quotes from Paikov [15] give an indication of the depth and multifaceted nature of Soviet sports massage:

Preliminary massage is also used in the aim of regulating unfavorable starting states in the athlete. (p. 19)

In general fatigue it is especially effective to massage the body segments having great receptive fields (spine, thigh, etc.). (p. 16)

Where there is strong fatigue . . . the aim of the massage is to decrease the activity of the excitatory processes which were increased under the influence of the physical and psychological loads. (p. 17)

Sports massage to the Soviets is an integral part of training.

REFERENCES

1. Nordqvist, H. 1979. Massage: a training must. Track and Field News 32(5):50–51.

2. Scull, C.W. 1945. Massage—physiologic basis. Arch Phys Med 26:159–167.

3. Meagher, J., Boughton, P. 1980. Sportsmassage. Dolphin Books, Doubleday and Co., New York.

4. Dubrovsky, V.I. 1982. Changes in muscle and venous blood flow after massage. Teonya i Praktika Fizicheskoi Kultury 4:56–57.

5. Hansen, T.I., Kristensen, J.H. 1973. Effect of massage, shortwave diathermy and untrasound on the ^{133}Xe disappearance rate from muscle and subcutaneous tissue in the human calf. Scand J Rehab Med 5:179–182.

6. Hovind, H., Nielsen, S.L. 1973. The influence of massage on circulation in muscles. Ugeskr Laeger 135(39):2090–2092.

7. Bell, A.J. 1964. Massage and the physiotherapist. Physio-therapy 50:406–408.

8. Wakim, K.G., Martin, G.M., et al. 1955. Influence of centripetal rhythmic compression on localized edema of extremities. Arch Phys Med 36:98–103.

9. Wolfson, H. 1931. Studies on the effect of physical therapeutic procedures on function and structure. JAMA 96:2019–2021.

10. Severini, V., Venerando, A. 1967. Physiological effects of massage on the cardiovascular system. Europa Medicophysica 3:165–183.

11. Wakim, K.G. 1980. Physiologic effects of massage. In: Rogoff, J.B. (ed): Manipulations, Traction and Massage (2nd ed.). Williams & Wilkins, Baltimore.

12. Wood, E. 1974. Beard's Massage: Principles and Techniques. W.B. Saunders Co., Philadelphia.

13. Schneider, E.C., Havens, L.C. 1915. Changes in the blood after muscular activity and during training. Am J Phys 36:239–259.

14. Ladd, M.P., Kottke, F.J., et al. 1952. Studies on the effect of massage on the flow of lymph from the foreleg of a dog. Arch Phys Med 33:604–612.

15. Paikov, V.B. 1986. Means of restoration in the training of speed skaters. Sports Massage J 2(4):14–22.

16. Crosman, L.J., Chatauvert, S.R., et al. 1985. The effect of massage to the hamstring muscle group on the range of motion. Massage J, Fall:59–62.

XXXXXX XXXXXX

17. Nordschow, M., Bierman, W. 1962. Influence of manual massage on muscle relaxation: effect on trunk flexion. J Am Phys Ther Assoc 42(10):653–657.

18. Müller, E.A., et al. 1966. The effect of massage on the efficiency of muscles. Intz Agnew Physiol 22:240–257.

19. Licht, S. 1960. Massage, Manipulation and Traction. Physical Medicine Library (Vol. 5). Williams & Wilkins, Baltimore.

20. Peshkov, V.F. 1981. The effect of 10-minute restorative point massage on the functional state of young gymnasts. Teonya i Praktika Fizicheskoi Kultury 12:35.

21. Cuthbertson, D.P. 1933. Effect of massage on metabolism: a survey. Glasgow Med J 2:200–213.

22. Daneskiold-Samsøe, B., et al. 1983. Regional Muscle Tension and Pain ("Fibrositis"). Scand J Rehab Med 15:17–20.

23. Jacobs, M. 1960. Massage for the relief of pain: Anatomical and physiological considerations. Phys Ther Rev 40:2:93–98.

24. Cyriax, J. 1977. Textbook of Orthopoedic Medicine. 2. Treatment by Manipulation, Massage and Injection. Ballière Tindall, London.

25. Cyriax, J. 1980. Clinical applications of massage. In: Rogoff, J.B. (ed): Manipulations, Traction and Massage (2nd ed.). Williams & Wilkins, Baltimore.

26. Cyriax, J. 1955. Deep massage. Physiotherapy 63:2:60–61.

27. Travel, J. 1955. Referred pain from skeletal muscle. NY State J Med 55(2):331–340.

28. Weeks, V.D., Travel, J. 1955. Postural vertigo due to trigger areas in the sternocleido-mastoid muscle. J Pediatr 47:315–327.

29. Prudden, B. 1980. Pain Erasure. Ballantine Books, New York.

30. Bonica, J.J. 1959. The management of myofascial pain syndromes. Phys Ther Rev 39:6:389–395.

31. Pagliano, J., Jackson, D. 1980. The ultimate study of running injuries. Runner's World 15:42–50.

32. Abraham, W.M. 1979. Exercise-induced muscle soreness. Phys Sportsmed 7(10):57–60.

33. Karpovich, P.V., Hale, C.J. 1956. Effect of warming-up upon physical performance. JAMA 162:12:1117–1119.

.25.

Stretching and Sports

Bob Anderson

Few people stretch correctly. Stretching is generally thought of as a form of exercise, and is therefore subject to negative "exercise" jargon such as "the more it hurts, the better it is," or "no gain without pain." Only injuries and pain result from such a stretching philosophy, however.

Correct stretching is not exercise involving rhythmic extensions and contractions of muscles as in walking, running, swimming, hiking, and so on. It involves holding a comfortable stretched position for various lengths of time. There should be no bouncing or bobbing up or down or other movement. When stretching correctly, one is almost as still as a statue.

TENDENCY TO OVERSTRETCH

Most people stretch with the intention of becoming more "flexible." They therefore stretch as far as possible and, in so doing, constantly overstretch. This tightens the very muscles that they intend to stretch and causes microscopic tears of involved tissues and scar formation. As scars are nonelastic, muscle elasticity is therefore reduced, contributing to muscle pain. Muscle fibers replaced with nonelastic, dense scar tissue interfere with normal blood flow and disturb afferent nerve input, thereby leaving the intact muscle fibers and surrounding connective tissues vulnerable to further injury—a vicious cycle that is repeated each time overstretching occurs. Specifically, overstretching activates the stretch reflex, a monosynaptic reflex response that causes contraction of the muscle(s) that were intended to be stretched. Thus, when a person stretches too far, he or she defeats the purpose of the stretch. It bears repeating: *All overstretching is useless and injurious.*

STRETCHING CORRECTLY

When one stretches correctly, on the other hand, the stretch reflex is not activated and muscle tissues are not harmed. Proper stretching elongates the muscles slowly to a point where

Illustrations (by Jean E. Anderson) and text of exercises contained in this chapter are excerpted, with permission, from various *Stretching Charts,* © 1979–82 by Bob and Jean Anderson (Stretching Inc., P.O. Box 767, Palmer Lake, CO 80133) and the book *Stretching,* © 1980 by Bob Anderson (Shelter Publications, distributed by Random House, Inc.). No part may be reproduced in any form without prior written approval of both the author and the publisher.

mild tension is felt. For an easy stretch, the elongated position is held 10–30 sec, during which time the subject should not experience discomfort. The longer the easy stretch is held, the less it is felt. If the stretched feeling grows in intensity as the position is maintained, one is overstretching and should ease off into a more comfortable position. The easy stretch is important because it reduces muscle tension, maintains flexibility, and reduces or prevents soreness. The easy stretch does not activate the stretch reflex mechanism and should precede more vigorous stretching to increase flexibility.

After the easy stretch, a fraction of an inch more stretch may be added until a mild increase in tension is felt. This is the *developmental stretch,* which is held for 10–30 sec and should not be painful or increase in intensity. Increasing tension or pain indicates overstretching and stretch reflex activation. If this occurs, ease off slightly into a more comfortable position. If done correctly, the developmental stretch safely increases flexibility, reduces tension, and increases circulation to the stretched muscles.

This basic method of stretching can be learned regardless of age or flexibility. It is based on the "feel" method, which should be followed each time a person stretches. It allows one to adjust to daily fluctuations in muscle tension that affect flexibility.

Many people lose muscle elasticity, which adversely affects normal resting muscle length. This happens when the body assumes a rigid, fixed position, such as during sitting or standing for long periods of time and often resulting in muscle pain and excess tension. "Creeping rigor mortis," a slow, but continuous loss of flexibility over the years, describes this condition.

With the gradual loss in flexibility, our muscles become tighter, and we are less able to accomplish things we once did with ease. It has been said that we start losing flexibility by age 8. If this is true, then stretching should be taught in elementary school.

Preventive Stretching

Stretching is important in preventing muscular injuries, but unless a person has been injured, the motivation for stretching often does not exist. Enthusiasm for stretching usually comes after an injury and is maintained thereafter in an attempt to ward off further injury.

Preventive stretching combines the following:

1. Proper stretch and adequate warm-up
2. Regular strength activity
3. Aerobic conditioning through running, swimming, cycling, rope skipping, etc.
4. Proper rest (rest when you are tired)
5. Avoid overtraining (understand the law of diminishing returns)
6. Gradual increase in intensity and duration of exercise
7. Plenty of liquid thoughout each day (preferably cool, refreshing water)
8. Maintenance of proper body weight
9. Joyful attitude toward physical activity

Stretching after exercise is very important. Slight injuries can be detected during stretching by tightness or soreness of one muscle or another.

Ideally, stretching should be used in conjunction with weight training. Gently stretch the muscles to be used beforehand. Then load them and repeat the stretch. This gives better strength without loss of flexibility. The stretches should be held comfortably; there is absolutely no reason for straining.

This chapter describes 26 basic stretches explained as the physician, physical therapist, or trainer might teach them to an athlete. Regular practice of 8–10 stretches is enough to maintain flexibility. Since, as was stated, flexibility diminishes with age, maintaining one's current flexibility is the first goal of proper stretching.

The importance of not overstretching and of relaxing the muscles not being stretched cannot be over emphasized. Learning by doing is the best method—one learns to stretch by stretching.

HAMSTRING AND QUADRICEPS STRETCHES

Begin in this bent-knee position. This position contracts the quadriceps and relaxes the hamstrings. Hold for 30 sec. The primary function of the quadriceps is to straighten the leg. The basic function of the hamstrings is to bend the knee. Because these muscles have opposing actions, tightening the quadriceps will relax the hamstrings.

Now, as you hold this bent-knee position, feel the difference between the front of the thigh and the back of the thigh. The quadriceps should feel hard and tight while the hamstrings should feel soft and relaxed.

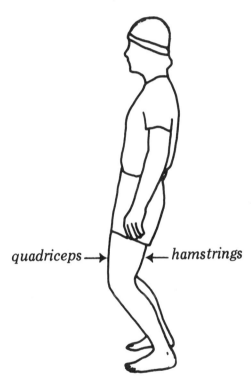

quadriceps → ← *hamstrings*

To stretch the upper hamstrings and hip (top of page 436), hold on to the outside of your ankle with one hand, with your other hand and forearm around your bent knee. Gently pull the leg *as one unit* toward your chest until you feel an easy stretch in the back of the upper leg. You may want to do this stretch while you rest your back against something for support. Hold for 30 sec. Make sure the leg is pulled as one unit so that no stress is felt in the knee.

Sit with your right leg bent, with your right heel just to the outside of your right hip. The left leg is bent and the sole of your left foot is next to the inside of your upper right leg. (Try not to let your right foot flare out to the side in this position.) Now slowly lean straight back until you feel an easy stretch in your right quadriceps. Use hands for balance and support. Hold an easy stretch for 30 sec. Do not hold any stretches that are painful to the knee.

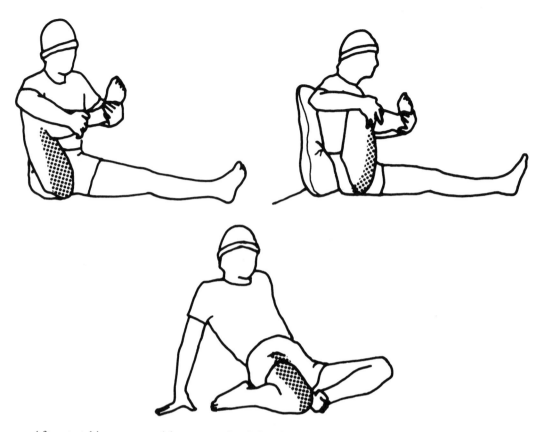

After stretching your quadriceps, practice tightening the buttocks on the side of the bent leg as you turn the hip over. This will help stretch the front of your hip and give a better overall stretch to upper thigh area. After contracting the buttocks muscles for 5–8 sec, let the buttocks relax. Then continue to stretch quad for another 15 sec.

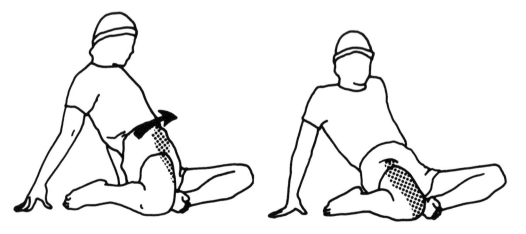

Next, straighten your right leg. The sole of your left foot will be resting next to the inside of your straightened leg. Lean slightly forward *from the hips* and stretch the hamstrings of your right leg. Find an easy stretch and relax. If you cannot touch your toes comfortably, use a towel to help you stretch. Hold for 50 sec. Do not lock your knee. Your right quadriceps should be soft and relaxed during the stretch. Keep your right foot upright with the ankle and toes relaxed.

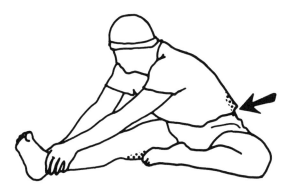

Opposite hand to opposite foot—quadriceps and knee stretch. Grab top of right foot (from inside of foot) with left hand and gently pull, heel moving toward buttocks. The knee bends at a natural angle in this position and creates a good stretch in knee and quad. This is especially good if you have had trouble or feel pain stretching in the hurdle stretch position leaning back, or when pulling the right heel to buttock with the right (same) hand. Pulling opposite hand to opposite foot does not create any adverse angles in the knee and is especially good in knee rehabilitation and with problem knees. Hold for 30 sec. Do both legs.

Hamstring pain after injury may last a long time. This can be due to *constant overstretching*, thus stressing the weakened area. An injured area can be stretched, but only *very, very gently*. Overstretching will simply prolong the injury.

The correct way to stretch an injured muscle is to stretch to the point where a slight stretch is felt first, then ease off slowly until no stretch is felt. This position should be held for 20–30 sec or longer. If is very helpful to use ice on the injured area while stretching.

If you can't find a position that does not give pain, the muscle should not be stretched. Prolonged hamstring injuries are helped by proper stretching, but forced overstretching can cause the injury to become chronic.

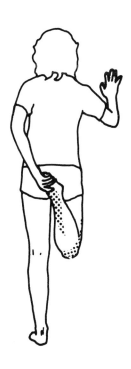

GROIN AND HIP STRETCHES

Relax with your knees bent and the soles of your feet together. This comfortable position will stretch your groin. Hold this for 60 sec.

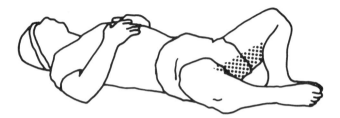

Put the soles of your feet together with your heels a comfortable distance from your groin. Now, put your hands around your feet and slowly pull yourself forward until you feel an easy stretch in the groin. Make your movement forward by bending from the hips and not from the shoulders. If possible, keep your elbows on the outside of your lower legs for greater stability during the stretch. Hold a comfortable stretch for 30–40 sec.

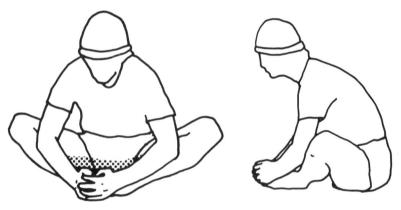

With hands supplying slight resistance on insides of opposite thighs, try to bring knees together, just enough to contract the muscles in the groin. Hold this stabilized tension for 5–8 sec, then relax and stretch the groin as in the preceding stretch. This will help relax a tight groin area. This technique of tension–relax–stretch is valuable for athletes who have had groin problems.

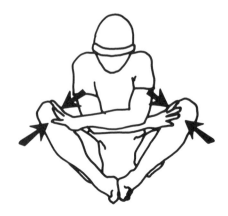

With your feet shoulder-width apart and pointed out to about a 15° angle, heels on the ground, bend your knees and squat down. If you have trouble staying in this position hold onto something for support. It is a great stretch for your ankles, Achilles tendons, groin, lower back, and hips. Hold stretch for 30 sec. *Be careful if you have had any knee problems. If pain is present, discontinue this stretch.*

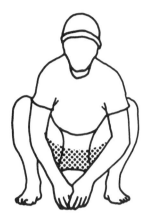 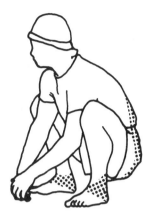

To increase the stretch in the groin, place your elbows on the inside of your upper legs, gently push outward with both elbows as you bend slightly forward from your hips. Your thumbs should be on the inside of your feet with your fingers along the outside border of the feet. Hold stretch for 20 sec. Do not overstretch. If you have trouble balancing, elevate your heels slightly.

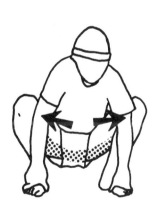 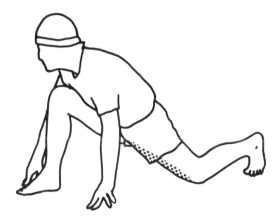

As in the above right drawing, move your leg forward *until the knee of the forward leg is directly over the ankle.* Your other knee should be resting on the floor. Lower the front of your hip downward until an easy stretch is felt in the front of the hip and possibly in your hamstrings and groin. Do this without changing position of the knee on the floor or the forward foot. Hold the stretch for 30 sec.

With your heels resting on the wall, slowly separate your legs until you feel an easy stretch in your groin. Be relaxed as you hold the stretch for 50–60 sec.

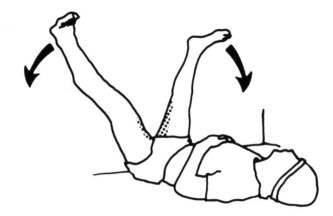

NECK AND LOWER BACK STRETCHES

Interlace your fingers behind your head and rest your arms on the mat. Using the power of your arms, *slowly* bring your head, neck, and shoulders forward until you feel a slight stretch. Hold an easy stretch for 5 sec. Repeat three times. Do not overstretch.

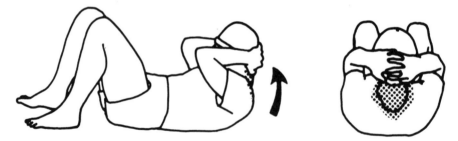

Shoulder Blade Pinch: From the bent-knee position, pull your shoulder blades together to create tension in the upper back area. (As you do this your chest should move upward.) Hold this controlled tension for 4–5 sec, then relax and gently pull your head forward as shown in previous stretch. This will help release tension and allow the neck to be stretched effectively.

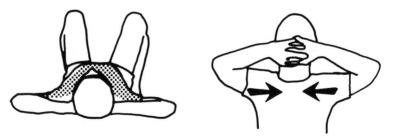

Next, straighten both legs and relax, then pull your left leg toward your chest. For this stretch keep the back of your head on the mat, if possible, but don't strain. Hold an easy stretch for 30 sec. Repeat, pulling your right leg toward your chest.

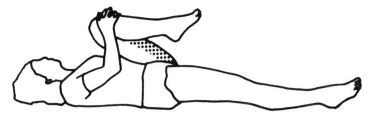

After pulling one leg at a time to your chest, pull both legs to your chest. This time concentrate on keeping the back of your head down and then curling your head up toward your knees.

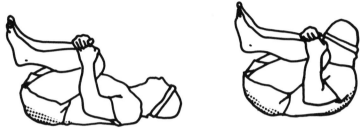

From a bent-knee position, interlace your fingers behind your head and lift the leg over the right leg. From here, use your left leg to pull your right leg toward the floor until you feel a stretch along the side of your hip and lower back. Stretch and relax. Keep the upper back, shoulders, and elbows flat on the floor. The idea is not to touch the floor with your right knee, but to stretch within *your* limits. Hold for 30 sec. Repeat stretch for other side.

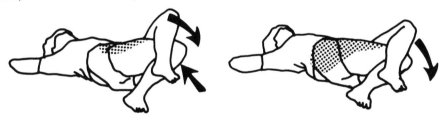

Variation: Some people, especially women, will not feel a stretch. If that is the case with you, use opposite tension to create a stretch:

To do this, hold down the right leg with the left leg, as you try to pull the right leg back to an upright position (but, because you are holding the right leg down with the left leg, the right leg won't move). You will get a stretch on the side of the hip area. This technique is good for people who are tense as well as for those who are extremely limber in this area. A possible way to incorporate this variation in a series of stretches is to first do the previous stretch shown in this section, then use opposite tension, relax, and do the previous stretch again.

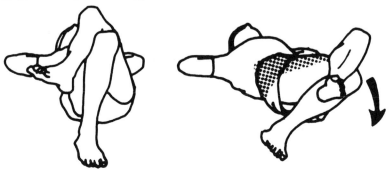

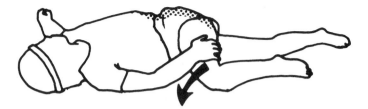

Next, straighten your right leg, and with your right hand pull your bent leg up and over your other leg as shown in the drawing above. Make sure that both of your shoulders and your head are on the floor. Turn your head to look toward your left. Now with your other hand on your thigh (resting just above the knee), control the stretch in your lower back and buttock muscles by pulling your upper leg down toward the floor. Repeat the stretch to your other side. Hold stretch for 30 sec, each side.

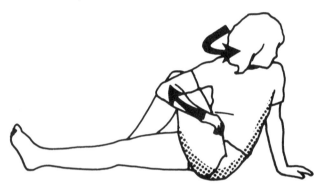

Sit with your right leg straight. Bend your left leg, cross your left foot over and rest it to the outside of your right knee. Then bend your right elbow and rest it on the outside of your upper left thigh, just above the knee. During the stretch use the elbow to keep this leg stationary with controlled pressure to the inside. Now, with your left hand resting behind you, slowly turn your head to look over your left shoulder, and at the same time rotate your upper body toward your left hand and arm. As you turn your upper body, think of turning your hips in the same direction (though your hips will not move because your right elbow is keeping the left leg stationary). This should give you a stretch in your lower back and side of hip. Hold for 15 sec. Do both sides. Do not hold your breath; breathe easily.

CALF, ACHILLES, AND ILIOTIBIAL BAND STRETCHES

To stretch your calf, stand a little away from a solid support and lean on it with your forearms, your head resting on your hands. Bend one leg and place your foot on the ground in front of you, leaving the other leg straight, behind you. Slowly move your hips forward until you feel a stretch in the calf of your straight leg. Be sure to keep the heel of the foot of the straight leg on the ground and *your toes pointed straight ahead*. Hold an easy stretch for 30 sec. Do not bounce. Stretch both legs.

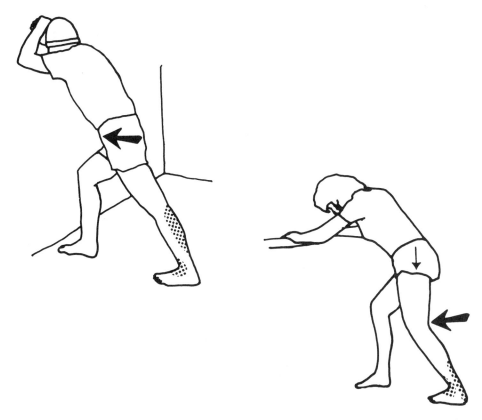

Now, to stretch the soleus and Achilles tendon, slightly bend the back knee, keeping the foot flat. This gives you a much lower stretch, which is also good for maintaining or regaining ankle flexibility. Hold 15 sec, each leg. This area needs only a *slight feeling of stretch*.

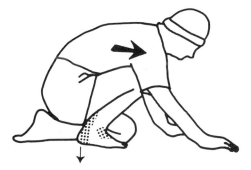

As shown, place your big toe even with your opposite knee. Start with your foot flat and use your shoulder to push forward on your knee until your heel comes off the floor about one-fourth to one-half of an inch. Then think of making your heel go flat as you lean forward with your shoulder against your knee. This should stretch your Achilles tendon. Hold only a slight, easy stretch for 20 sec.

To stretch the outside of the hips and upper leg, start from the same position as in the calf stretch. Stretch the right side of your hip by slightly turning your right hip to the inside. Project the side of your hip to the side as you lean your shoulders very slightly in the opposite direction of your hips. Hold an even stretch for 25 sec. Do both sides. Keep foot of back leg pointed straight ahead with heel flat on ground.

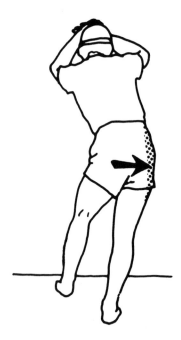

While lying on your back, pull your knee to your chest, then think of pulling the knee across your body toward your opposite shoulder to create a stretch on the outside of your right hip. Hold an easy stretch for 20 sec. Do both sides.

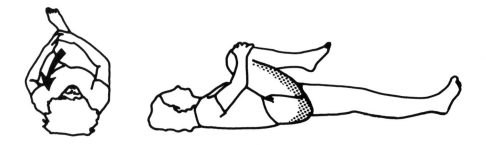

ARM AND SHOULDER STRETCHES

A stretch for the arms, shoulders, and back. Hold onto something that is about shoulder height. With your hands shoulder-width apart on this support, relax, keeping your arms straight and your chest moving downward, and *your feet remaining directly under your hips*. Keep your knees slightly bent (1 inch). Hold this stretch 30 sec. This is a good stretch to do anywhere, at anytime.

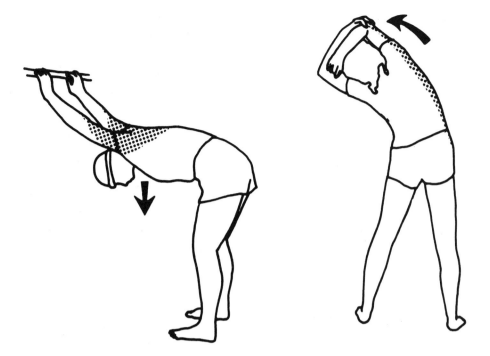

With arms overhead, hold the elbow of one arm with the hand of the other arm. Keeping knees slight bent (1 inch), gently pull your elbow behind your head as you bend from your hips to the side. Hold an easy stretch for 10 sec. Do both sides. Keeping your knees slightly bent will give you better balance.

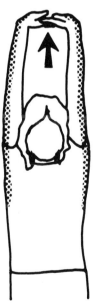

In a standing or sitting position, interlace your fingers above your head. Now, with your palms facing upward, push your arms slightly back and up. Fell the stretch in arms, shoulders, and upper back. Hold stretch for 15 sec. Do not hold your breath. This stretch is good to do anywhere, anytime. Excellent for slumping shoulders.

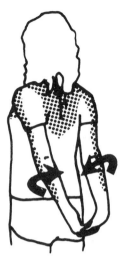

The next stretch is done with your fingers interlaced behind your back. Slowly turn your elbows inward while straightening your arms. An excellent stretch for shoulders and arms. This is good to do when you find yourself slumping from your shoulders. This stretch can be done at any time. Hold for 5–15 sec. *Do twice.*

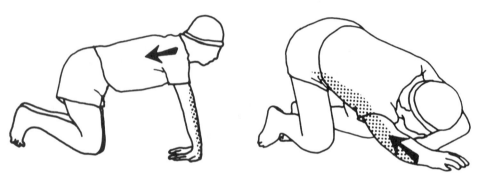

From the position illustrated on the left above, with your palms flat and fingers pointed back toward your knees, slowly lean backwards to stretch the forearms and wrists. Be sure to keep your palms flat. Hold a comfortable stretch for 20–25 sec. *Do not overstretch.* Stretch for a good feeling. Enjoy stretching.

With legs bent under you, reach forward with one arm and grab the end of the mat, carpet, or anything you can hold onto. If you cannot grab onto something, just pull back with your arm straight while pressing down slightly with your hand. Do likewise pulling on end of mat. Hold stretch for 20 sec. Stretch each side. Do not strain. You should feel the stretch in your shoulders, arms, sides, upper back, or even in your lower back.

.26.

Cryotherapy—Using Cold to Treat Injuries

Stephen R. Loane

Cryotherapy is the therapeutic application of ice or cold and a proven modality for use in the initial treatment and successful rehabilitation of musculoskeletal injuries. The safety, simplicity, and economy of cryotherapy contribute to its usefulness, and when used properly it can save days and weeks in rehabilitation (Barnes [1]).

In this chapter the beneficial effects of cold application and the role of cryotherapy in acute and rehabilitative care are discussed. Techniques of cryotherapy are presented, and indications, precautions, and contraindications for its use are reviewed.

PHYSIOLOGIC EFFECTS OF COLD

An understanding of the physiologic responses to applications of cold is necessary for properly treating musculoskeletal injuries with cryotherapy. An important distinction should be made between the use of cryotherapy during the acute and the rehabilitative phases of care (Barnes [1]).

The goals for using cryotherapy in the acute stage of injury are to limit the formation of edema and to reduce pain and muscular spasm. The objectives for cryotherapy during the rehabilitative phase of treatment are to reduce pain and spasm prior to and during therapeutic exercise.

The physiologic responses to cold are varied, and the mechanisms not clearly understood. There is disagreement as to whether some responses occur at all.

From an extensive review of the literature on cryotherapy, Kowal [2] found these consistent results: The application of cold results in a reduction of musculoskeletal pain, reduction in muscular spasm, a decrease in intramuscular temperature, a slowing of nerve conduction velocity, a decrease in connective tissue distensibility, and a decrease in spasm (except upon initial contact with cold). The inconsistent findings were the effects of cold on swelling, blood flow, heart rate, blood pressure, intraarticular temperature, rheumatoid arthritis, the monosynaptic reflex, and the muscle spindle.

Reduced cellular metabolism is cited as the beneficial effect of cryotherapy in reducing swelling and edema formation during the acute phase of injury (Knight [3]; Warren [4]; Barnes [1]). The reduced metabolism and oxygen consumption allow uninjured tissue peripheral to the trauma to survive longer periods of ischemia. This limits the extent of edema caused by the injury and results in a decrease of "secondary hypoxic injury." (Knight [5]). By controlling the extent of tissue damage, fewer waste products will need to be removed and resolution of the injury can begin earlier.

The effect of cold in reducing the pain response is well documented, though there is speculation about the actual mechanisms involved. A reduction in transmission of nervous impulses (Gieck [6]), the action of cold as a counterirritant (Mennell [7]), and the release of opioids (Raethar [8]) have been proposed. Initial contact with cold tends to elicit a pain response, though most individuals will adapt to this pain (Knight [3]).

Cryotherapy is effective in reducing muscle spasm (Lee and Warren [9]), though there is confusion as to how this occurs. Spasm may be relieved by decreasing muscle activity and muscle spindle firing (Gieck [6]) or through a reflex response of sensory nerves overlying the muscle (Mennell [7]).

Cold applications increase muscle viscosity (Gieck [6]) and decrease elasticity in muscle and connective tissue (Knight [3]).

The effect of cold on the circulatory system is vasoconstriction (Warren [4]; Barnes [1]; Knight [3]). This is apparently followed by a secondary reflex vasodilation (Warren [4]; Barnes [1]; Ork [10]). These effects alternate and are termed the "hunting reaction." However, recent research by Knight [3] has shown that cold-induced vasodilation does not occur.

Cold increases blood viscosity (Barnes [1]) and decreases capillary permeability, which slows continued fluid leakage from ruptured blood vessels (Griffin and Karselis [11]). Applications of cold decrease local tissue temperature (Gieck [6]), though temperature depression is dependent on the thickness of overlying tissue layers and the length of time that cold is applied.

CRYOTHERAPY IN THE ACUTE CARE OF INJURY

The protocol for treatment of acute musculoskeletal injury should begin with a thorough examination by a physician or athletic trainer. X rays may be necessary to determine the severity of the injury (Barnes [1]).

The injury should be protected and rested, and the application of ice or cold should begin immediately. The sooner ice is applied the more effective it will be in reducing secondary hypoxic injury. Ice should be made readily available at all sporting events for immediate use (Knight [3]). An ice pack should be applied to the injury, compression with an elastic wrap should be initiated, and the injured limb should be elevated (Warren [4]); Barnes [1]; Gieck [6]; Knight [5]).

Ice will lower the metabolism of the tissue and thereby decrease the extent of secondary hypoxic injury. Compression increases external pressure, and elevation decreases capillary hydrostatic pressure; these limit the formation of edema (Knight [3]). Ice is beneficial in reducing swelling so that a better fitting cast may be applied if a fracture is present (Gieck [6]).

Ice should be applied for 30 min every 2 hr for the first 24–48 hr following the injury (Barnes [1]; Gieck [6]; Knight [3]). Compression and elevation should be used continuously (Knight [3]). The use of cold during the acute phase of injury lessens or prevents edema and hematoma formation (Ork [10]) and provides relief from pain and muscle spasm. The important principle in using cold for treating acute injury is early and prolonged application (McMaster [12]).

In a study comparing the effectiveness of cryotherapy and heat therapy for treating ankle sprains, Hocutt et al. [13] found that early application of cryotherapy (begun within 1 hr after injury), combined with adhesive compression, was more effective than delayed cryotherapy (begun from 1 to 36 hr after injury) or heat therapy (begun 36 hr after injury). Early use of cryotherapy allowed patients to resume full activity on the average of 15 days sooner compared to delayed cryotherapy or heat therapy (Hocutt et al. [13]).

CRYOTHERAPY IN THE REHABILITATIVE CARE OF INJURY

Cryotherapy may be used in the rehabilitative care of musculoskeletal injuries to provide relieve from pain and muscular spasm in order to allow remedial exercise of the injured limb. Applications of cold are used in conjunction with active exercise for acute injury rehabilitation (Knight [3]).

Initially upon application of cold, a perception of cold or pain is experienced. This is followed by a feeling of warming or burning. Gradually an aching or throbbing sensation is felt. In the final stage, a state of numbness is reached ([Barnes [1]). Once numbness is achieved, which usually occurs after 10–15 min, cold application is stopped.

Active exercise is then begun. Exercise should be simple at first, and it is important that all motions are performed without pain. Exercises that include rotary, spiral, and diagonal movement are encouraged (Barnes [1]). Exercise is continued until numbness wears off, and then the injured area is iced again until numbness returns; the cycle is repeated.

Exercise is the key to rehabilitation with cryotherapy. Without properly executed therapeutic exercise, cold applications will hinder rather than promote rehabilitation (Knight [3]). Applications of ice facilitate exercise by decreasing pain and muscular spasm, thus allowing exercise to begin earlier and progress at a faster rate. Active exercise increases blood flow to the injured area and is beneficial for repair (Knight [3]).

In treating over 7000 patients with various acute and chronic painful conditions of musculoskeletal origin, Grant [14] achieved satisfactory results with over 80% of the group with no more than three formal treatments. He used the term "cryokinetics" to describe his ice and exercise program.

Ice should be used until there is no further hemorrhage or edema and until range of motion is full and pain free (Gieck [6]).

"Cryostretch" is a technique developed by Knight [5] for relieving muscular spasm associated with acute injury. Cryostretch combines intermittent applications of cold, static stretching, and isometric contractions of the affected muscle in order to relieve muscular spasm and increase range of motion.

INDICATIONS FOR THE USE OF CRYOTHERAPY

Cryotherapy is indicated in the treatment of muscle spasm (Griffin and Karselis [11]), relief of pain (Mennell [7]), and reduction of inflammation (McMaster [12]) for a variety of musculoskeletal injuries, including sprains, strains, contusions, and fractures (McMaster [12]). It is recommended for treating the acute phase of inflammatory conditions of bursitis, tenosynovitis, and tendonitis (McMaster [12]). Applications of cold can be useful for treating heat illness, minor burns (Gieck [6]), and contractures, and in postoperative treatment (Ork [10]). It is also indicated in the rehabilitation of injuries by providing relief of muscle spasm and pain, which allows therapeutic exercise to commence earlier (Knight [3]).

PRECAUTIONS AND
CONTRAINDICATIONS FOR THE USE OF CRYOTHERAPY

The use of cryotherapy is contraindicated for patients with Raynaud's phenomenon, cold allergy, cold hypersensitivity, compromised local circulation, and cardiac disorder (Knight [3]). Cryotherapy should not be used for those with impaired sensation, with paralysis, or in a coma (McMaster [12]; Barnes [1]; Knight [3]). Cryotherapy is contraindicated for rheumatoid conditions (McMaster [12]; Barnes [1]; Knight [3]), though Packman [15] has used ice massage in treating painful conditions of rheumatoid arthritis.

Caution should be used when edema is due to cardiac, renal, and/or pulmonary pathology (Griffin and Karselis [11]). Cryotherapy should not be used directly over a superficial nerve. A sharp transient rise in systolic pressure, apparently due to massive reflex vasoconstriction, has been noted, and caution should be observed when treating persons with a history of high blood pressure (Griffin and Karselis [11]).

Cryotherapy should not be used directly on the skin for longer than ½ hr continuously. Frostbite apparently does not occur from short-term application directly to the skin, though using a frozen gel pack (which can be cooled below 32° F) directly on the skin for longer than 15–20 min may cause cold injury (Knight [3]).

Performing exercises that cause pain following cold applications should be avoided (Knight [3]). It should be noted that one should never return to full activity on a limb numbed by the use of ice, since the protective pain mechanism will be compromised and further injury and damage may result (Warren [4]; Barnes [1]).

METHODS OF APPLICATION OF CRYOTHERAPY

Ice Massage

Ice massage may be accomplished with ice cubes or blocks held in a towel, water frozen in styrofoam cups with the edges torn away to expose the ice, or a wooden stick frozen in a cup of water to make an ice "popsicle." Ice is gently massaged over the injured area by using overlapping strokes so that the entire area is covered. Ice massage stimulates mechanoreceptors (Knight [3]) and provides a superficial cooling effect that decreases surface tissue temperature and produces local anesthesia (Warren [4]). As a state of numbness is achieved, this is followed by an exercise program to achieve full mobility (Grant [14]).

Ice Packs

Ice packs are made by placing cubed, chipped, or crushed ice in plastic bags, towels, or caps. Ice may be applied directly to the skin and seems to be most effective in reducing deep tissue temperature (Warren [4]). Ice packs can be made in different sizes depending on the area to be treated. These are indicated for the immediate care of musculoskeletal injury to limit the formation of edema.

Ice Immersion

Ice immersion is a technique in which ice is added to a container filled with water to lower the temperature. The optimal temperature is not known (Knight [3]), though Barnes [1] recommends 40°F for ice immersion. Ice immersion tends to be more uncomfortable than ice massage and should be discontinued once a state of numbness is reached. This is followed by range-of-motion and mobility exercises (Grant [14]). This method is suitable for treating feet, ankles, hands, arms, and elbows.

Cold Whirlpools

Cold whirlpools combine the massage action of the whirlpool agitator with the effect of cold water. Cold whirlpools are useful for treating larger body area such as knees and the lower back (Knight [3]).

Cold Towels

Cold towels are made by wringing towels in 40°F water and then applying them directly to the body (Barnes [1]).

Cold Gel Packs

Cold gel packs consist of a gelatinous substance enclosed in a heavy vinyl cover that may be chilled in a refrigerator and may be used over again. Caution must be used since cold gel packs can be chilled below 32°F and may cause cold injury if applied too long. They should not be used for more than 15–20 min at a time and may need to be applied over a damp towel (Knight [3]).

Cold Chemical Packs

Cold chemical packs consist of two separate chemical substances enclosed in a vinyl pouch. When these substances are combined they produce a chemical reaction that has the effect of lowering the temperature of the pouch. They are convenient for short-term emergency use, but are not reusable, could cause chemical burns if they leak, and may not lower the body temperature enough to be effective (Knight [3]).

Vapocoolant Spray

Vapocoolant spray is a cryotherapy technique that is used for localized cooling of tissue. Ethyl chloride (highly flammable) or fluoromethane (preferred) is sprayed over the affected body part from a distance of 2 ft at a rate of 4 in per second and in a single direction so that the area can be covered twice. Caution is required so that the skin is not frosted (Knight [3]). In treating painful spasms, the use of fluoromethane spray in combination with gentle stretching has been successful in relieving pain and spasm and restoring function (Mennell [7]).

Cryomatic

Cryomatic is a refrigeration unit that circulates freon through enclosed coils in a protective pad. The temperature may be set between −6°C and 27°C. It may be wrapped around a limb or joint or placed upon the back or abdomen. Cryomatic is relatively untried on humans, though it is established at race tracks for treating musculoskeletal injuries of thoroughbred race horses (Knight [3]).

SUMMARY

The use of cold or ice in treating musculoskeletal injuries is simple, inexpensive, and effective. Cryotherapy is beneficial in reducing pain and muscular spasm. Cryotherapy in conjunction with compression and elevation is indicated for treating the swelling associated with acute injuries. For rehabilitation of injuries, cryotherapy is used to provide anesthesia so that exercise and range of motion can commence sooner. A variety of methods are used and may be adapted for the situation at hand. Contraindications are few, though caution should be observed, in nonathletes particularly, so that cryotherapy is applied properly and effectively.

REFERENCES

1. Barnes, L. 1979. Cryotherapy—putting injury on ice. Phys Sportsmed 6:130–136.
2. Kowal, M.A. 1983. Review of physiological effects of cryotherapy. J Orthop Sports Phys Ther 5:66–73.
3. Knight, K.L. 1985. Cryotherapy: Theory, Technique, and Physiology (1st ed.) Chattanooga Corp., Chattanooga, TN.
4. Warren, C.G. 1983. The use of heat and cold in treatment of common musculoskeletal disorders. In: Kessler, R.M., Hertling, B. (eds): Management of Common Musculoskeletal Disorders. Harper & Row, New York.
5. Knight, K.L. 1978. Cryotherapy in sports medicine. In: Schriber, K., Burke, E.J. (eds): Relevant Topics in Athletic Training. Mouvement Publications, Ithaca, NY.
6. Gieck, J.H. 1982. The athletic trainer and rehabilitation. In: Kunlund, D.N. (ed): The Injured Athlete. Lippincott, Philadelphia.
7. Mennell, J.M. 1975. The therapeutic use of cold. J Am Orthop Assoc 74:1146–1158.
8. Raethar, P.R. 1983. The cold treatment—putting injuries on ice can be more complicated than it sounds. The Runner 6:14.
9. Lee, J.M., Warren, M.P. 1974. Ice, relaxation, and exercise in reduction of muscle spasticity. Physiotherapy 10:296–301.
10. Ork, H. 1981. Uses of cold. In: Kuprian, W. (ed): Physical Therapy for Sports. W.B. Saunders, Philadelphia.
11. Griffin, J.E., Karselis, T.C. (eds). 1982. Physical Agents for Physical Therapists (2nd ed.). Charles C Thomas, Springfield, IL.
12. McMaster, W.C. 1977. A literary review on ice therapy in injuries. Am J Sports Med 3:124–126.
13. Hocutt, J.E., Jaffe, R., et al. 1982. Cryotherapy in ankle sprains. Am J Sports Med 10:316–319.
14. Grant, A.E. 1964. Massage with ice (cryokinetics) in the treatment of painful conditions of the musculoskeletal system. Arch Phys Med Rehabil 45:233–238.
15. Packman, H. 1977. Ice Therapy. Packman, Bayside, NY.

•27•

Biomechanics of the Foot
and Lower Extremity

Robert M. Parks

The clinical application of lower extremity biomechanics has received increased attention in recent years, partly because of computer availability, refinements in photography, and the search for ways to improve athletic performance. The axiom "structure dictates function" is now more clearly appreciated by sports physicians. Normal structure often results in superior performance, and abnormal body mechanics frequently correlate with poor performance and athletic injuries. The coach, trainer, and medical clinician who understand the musculoskeletal system in motion will be more effective in their respective roles.

HISTORY

Investigation of lower-extremity biomechanics arose from the need to treat post-World War II amputees more effectively. Thorough understanding of joint motion and function was necessary in order to build better limb prostheses. Researchers at the University of California established normal values for ranges of motion in the major joints of the foot and ankle. Podiatric physicians (Root et al. [1–3]; Sgarlato [4, 5]) confirmed these findings clinically and have found them to be of value in treating common foot and leg disorders. Practitioners can now distinguish normal from abnormal function and can determine the degree of deviation from normal by basic measurements. Many developmental osseous and soft-tissue disorders of the foot and leg benefit by biomechanical evaluation and treatment.

BIOMECHANICS IN SPORTS AND MEDICINE

The ability to categorize extremity types through quantitative biomechanical assessment is invaluable in sports research and clinical medicine. The researcher can roughly predict an athlete's maximum potential and can more effectively help him or her overcome problems. Sports medicine practitioners can now uncover the athlete's "weak link" during the stress of athletic participation. The cause of injury is identified and corrected rather than the practitioner's providing treatment based on symptoms. Prediction of future injury is also possible through biomechanical analysis. Preventive medicine can then be practiced by altering variables of training, environment, exercise, and equipment.

The study of lower extremity biomechanics is not a concrete science, and accepted principles should be evaluated critically. The intent of this chapter is to help the reader understand mechanics of the lower extremity and foot.

ANATOMIC CONSIDERATIONS

The bony anatomy of the foot is complex, and each part allows many movements (Fig. 27-1). From proximal to distal, bones of the foot can be categorized as the greater tarsus, lesser tarsals, metatarsals, and phalanges (Figs. 27-2, 27-3). The greater tarsus includes the

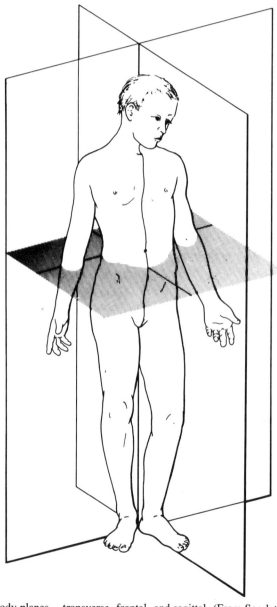

27-1 Cardinal body planes—transverse, frontal, and sagittal. (From Sgarlato, T.E. 1971. A Compendium of Podiatric Biomechanics. College of Podiatric Medicine Corp., San Francisco. Reprinted with permission.)

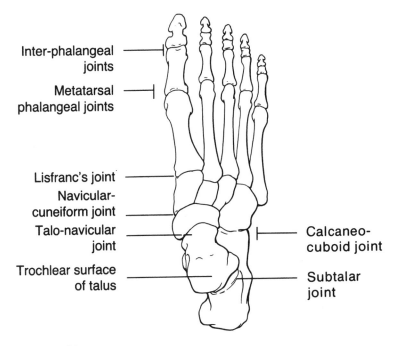

27-2 Dorsal view of foot.

talus and calcaneus; the lesser tarsals are the navicular, cuboid, and the first, second, and third cuneiforms. There are five metatarsals. Each digit has three phalanges, proximal, intermediate, and distal, except for the hallux, which has two. The metatarsals and phalanges are long bones; the tarsal and lesser tarsal bones are not long bones and, in contrast, have multifaceted articulations supported by interconnecting ligaments.

The talus is one of three bones of the ankle joint. Its superior articulating surface forms an arc, which permits flexion and extension of the ankle. Its medial and lateral borders form angles of approximately 90° to its superior surface and articulate with the tibial and fibular malleoli, respectively. This architecture does not permit transverse and frontal plane motion within the ankle joint. Transverse plane movement of the talus at the subtalar joints is transmitted directly into transverse plane leg rotation. The bony architecture of the ankle joint and weight bearing prevent ankle inversion and eversion. Medial and lateral collateral ligaments function only when a subluxatory force is present and, therefore, do not provide

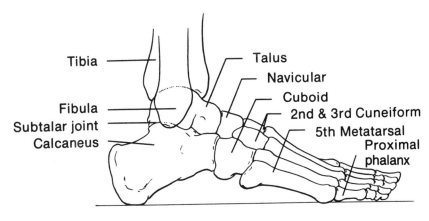

27-3 Lateral view of foot.

frontal plane stability. The inferior surface of the talus articulates with the calcaneus to form the subtalar joint. This joint consists of three facets, the surfaces of which lie near the transverse plane of the body. When the subtalar joint moves, all facets glide simultaneously. This motion, although derived from a common axis, lies oblique to the three cardinal planes of the body and is termed triplane. The two movements of the subtalar joint are supination (turning-in of the foot) and pronation (outturning of the foot) and will be discussed in more detail later.

The calcaneus articulates with the talus on its superior surface; the plantar aspect is the surface of the heel that strikes the ground. The distal part of the calcaneus articulates with the cuboid bone to form the calcaneocuboid joint. The articulating surface of the cuboid is somewhat egg-shaped and lies on the frontal plane of the body with greatest dimensions running in a dorsoplantar direction. The calcaneocuboid joint forms the apex of the lateral arch of the foot and functions in unison with the talonavicular joint. The two joints combined form the midtarsal joint, which moves around two separate axes. The longitudinal axis of the midtarsal joint, although providing triplane motion, functions maximally in the frontal plan. The oblique axis of the midtarsal joint, also triplane, allows for a predominance of sagittal plane motion.

The distal aspect of the talus articulates with the navicular (boat-shaped) bone. This joint is similar to the calcaneocuboid joint and, as previously mentioned, the two together comprise the midtarsal joint.

The three cuneiform (wedge-shaped) bones lie adjacent to one another from medial to lateral and articulate proximally with the navicular bone. The external cuneiform articulates laterally with the cuboid bone. In a normal foot, the shape and close proximity of the bones of the lesser tarsal joints permit only minimal movement. In cases of altered foot mechanics, increased sagittal plane motion may occur. The distal surfaces of the medial, middle, and external cuneiforms and the cuboid articulate with the five metatarsals to form the Lisfranc's joint. Motion at this location results in sagittal plane movement of the metatarsals. The second, third, and fourth metatarsals function around a common axis, while the first and fifth metatarsals function independently. Ground reactive forces tend to dorsiflex and invert the first metatarsal. The fifth metatarsal responds to plantar pressure by dorsiflexing and everting. The metatarsal heads articulate with the proximal phalangeal bases to form the five metatarsal-phalangeal joints. These joints are condyloid in nature, permitting primarily sagittal plane motion (flexion, extension) with lesser degrees of transverse and frontal plane motion. The interphalangeal joints are hinge-like, permitting only sagittal plane motion (flexion, extension).

PHYSICAL PRINCIPLES OF JOINT FUNCTION

To understand the mechanics of weight-bearing joints, one must appreciate basic physical principles that govern their function. Body movement abides by the Newtonian laws of motion and modern physics. Weight-bearing joints of the body have a dual function: They allow movement and provide support and stability. Stability is necessary for upright posture and locomotion. It is generally accepted that more mobile joints are also more unstable. Lack of stability arises from intrinsic or extrinsic forces. What, then, allows a weight-bearing joint to be both mobile and stable simultaneously?

First consider the angle that joint surfaces form in respect to the ground. In the knee, for example, forces acting when the extremity strikes the ground are the result of body mass multiplied by body acceleration (force = mass × acceleration). This force is equalized at heel contact by an equal and opposite force of ground resistance, termed *ground-reactive force,* which enters the knee perpendicular to the joint surfaces and compresses them together. This *joint compressional force,* applicable only during weight bearing, maintains joint congruity by bone-on-bone compression.

When joint alignment is oblique to ground-reactive forces, the resulting stress may produce joint subluxation. This is successfully resisted when body function is normal. A force producing joint instability is termed *joint rotational force.* Factors other than joint compression help maintain joint stability. These include articular surface configuration and the axis on which it functions. A joint surface with a deep socket or curves and irregularities has greater ability to resist rotational forces. Abnormal ranges of joint motion result in a jamming effect on the opposing joint surfaces. This locking mechanism can be overcome only if rational forces exceed joint compressional forces.

The axis of joint motion not only indicates its direction of movement but also the direction of force from which the joint can maintain stability. Joint motion occurs at 90° to a joint axis (examine the mechanics of a door and note that movement occurs 90° to the supporting hinge) (Fig. 27-4). Forces directed obliquely to a joint must increase as the angle of applied force decreases from 90°. No force parallel to an axis can produce motion.

Soft tissue, as well as bone, help maintain joint stability. Tendons crossing joints serve a dual function in providing both motion and stability. A tendon's ability to resist rotational forces and provide motion depends upon the lever arm length and direction in relation to a joint axis. A tendon with a long lever arm coursing perpendicular to a joint axis provides maximum stability. Ligaments do not stabilize joints moving within their normal range. When a normal range of motion is exceeded, ligaments become taut and help resist subluxation and possible dislocation.

Gait Cycle

Upright locomotion in humans results from functional integration of many body segments. Walking requires corresponding movement from the head, arms, torso, and lower extremities. The apparent fluidity of forward progression is actually the result of movement in all body plans simultaneously. Muscles accelerate, decelerate and stabilize at the same time. It is only through this mechanical complexity that human beings can propel and maneuver with such great precision.

Observation of gait is the clinician's way of assessing segmental body locomotion. A full gait cycle is the period beginning with heel contact of one foot and ending with heel contact of the same foot. This includes the entire interval of foot support (stance phase of gait) and also the period when the extremity is swinging forward in preparation for heel strike (swing phase of gait). The gait cycle is further divided by percentages, so that muscle function and joint motion can be assessed in relation to a specific time within the gait cycle.

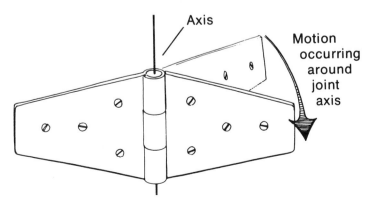

27-4 Axis of motion around hinge.

Swing Phase of Gait

The swing phase of gait begins immediately after toe-off and ends with heel contact of the same foot. This phase of gait carries the extremity from one step to the next and is also referred to as the stride. The hip and knee joint flex during this period, allowing for ground clearance of the swinging limb. The ankle and subtalar joints dorsiflex and pronate, respectively, to assure forefoot and digital ground clearance. The stride length in walking or running is influenced by the degree of hip flexion, speed of progression, and limb length. When a person walks, body weight transfers from limb to limb with a corresponding shift in the center of gravity. In running, a double-float phase or period occurs, during which both limbs are off the ground. When heel contact ensues, the runner's center of gravity must be balanced above one limb to prevent falling toward the non-weight-bearing side. The center of gravity for the runner is nearly, therefore, a straight line of progression, and shifts forward (anterior) according to speed of progression.

As a runner attains greater speeds, the upper extremity swings forward with hip flexion. Acceleration of swing phase requires increasing hip flexion for adequate extremity ground clearance. Just prior to heel contact, the forward-progressing limb extends to approximately 175° at the knee joint, and the foot supinates in preparation for body support.

Stance Phase of Gait

The stance phase of gait is subdivided into contact, midstance, and propulsive phases (Fig. 27-5). The three phases are analyzed sequentially below.

Contact Phase of Gait   The contact phase of gait, which comprises 25% of the stance phase, begins with heel contact and lasts until the forefoot meets the ground. Two important functions of the foot during this period are to dissipate shock resulting from heel strike and to adapt to variations in terrain.

The lower extremity absorbs heel-contact shock by slight knee flexion, ankle plantar flexion, and subtalar joint pronation. The unweighting effect of these movements dissipates shock. Vertical ground-reactive forces during walking do not approach the force of body weight until the midstance phase of gait. During the contact phase of gait, the foot functions much like a universal joint, to accommodate for variations in ground terrain. This is achieved through subtalar joint pronation, which is associated with calcaneal eversion, plantar flexion, and adduction of the talus.

As indicated previously, adduction of the talus cannot occur without simultaneous internal rotation of the leg. The tibia and fibula, therefore, rotate internally throughout the contact phase of the gait. Internal rotation of the leg is transmitted to the femur and hip joint since the knee does not permit transverse plane motion. Excessive internal rotation of the limb can be assessed by examining the transverse plane rotation of the patella. Normally, the patella rotates inward during the contact phase of gait to the same degree that it externally rotates during propulsion. If inward rotation is favored over external rotation, the cause is likely to be excessive subtalar joint pronation, if it may be assumed that there are no abnormalities at the hip or knee.

Midstance Phase of Gait   The midstance phase of gait normally comprises 40% of the stance phase and begins with cessation of contact and ends with heel-off. At the beginning of midstance, the weight-bearing limb begins to externally rotate and the foot to supinate. In contrast to the foot's function as a mobile adapter during the contact phase, at midstance the foot must now be ready for full weight bearing, so propulsion muscles can function around stable bony segments. Stress-related injuries of the foot and leg occur when

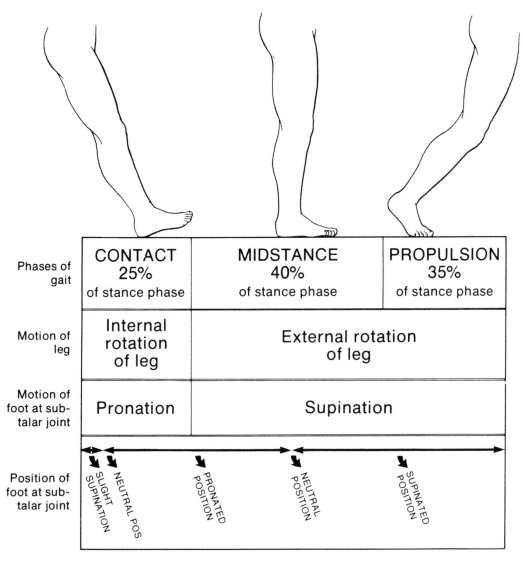

27-5 Stance phase of gait. (From Sgarlato, T.E. 1971. A Compendium of Podiatric Biomechanics. College of Podiatric Medicine Corp., San Francisco. Reprinted with permission.)

muscles are required to stabilize an otherwise unstable foot and also function as prime movers.

Supination of the foot is initiated by external rotation of the hip. Again, the closed-chain effect of transverse plane rotation is transmitted distally into the foot, producing external rotation and dorsiflexion of the talus. The calcaneus inverts simultaneously with rearfoot supination. Muscular contraction also plays an important role in foot supination. All posterior leg muscles with a supinating action at the subtalar joint, particularly the gastrosoleus group and the tibialis posterior, assist in foot supination. This reversal of motion can be visualized by external rotation of the patella and inversion of the heel.

The foot actively supinates from its pronated position, achieving joint neutrality halfway through the midstance phase of gait. It must be noted that the terms *supination* and *pronation* refer to motion, and *supinated* and *pronated* refer to position. With the "rearfoot" in a functionally stable position, the ball of the foot accepts greater amounts of body weight.

For maximum stability, body weight rests on a triangle of support, the heel posteriorly and the first and fifth metatarsals distally. Weight transference continues from heel to "forefoot" as the tibia moves anteriorly over the foot and the posterior leg muscles continue to fire.

Propulsive Phase of Gait   The propulsive phase comprises the last 35% of the stance phase of gait. This begins at the instance of heel elevation and terminates with toe-off.

Efficient foot propulsion depends upon osseous stability and normal muscular function. Most of the foot's propulsive stability is due to the extremities' preparation during midstance. Dynamic balance and stability is, therefore, necessary during contact and, particularly, during midstance for normal propulsion to occur.

Subtalar joint supination continues throughout the propulsive phase of gait. Although the subtalar joint no longer directly contacts the ground by means of the calcaneus, its position continues to account for distal stability. The midtarsal and lesser tarsal joints are subjected to the greatest load during propulsion. As the foot plantarflexes at the ankle for forward acceleration, weight transmitted through the forefoot clearly exceeds body weight. Osseous restraint and stability are, therefore, essential to prevent subluxation of the lesser tarsal joints.

During the propulsive phase of gait, weight is transferred from the lateral metatarsals medially (Fig. 27-6). This medial shift in weight is necessary for the foot to obtain its most efficient propulsive lever, the first metatarsal phalangeal joint. The metatarsal parabola (length pattern) and the peroneal muscles are responsible for this weight shift. The peroneus

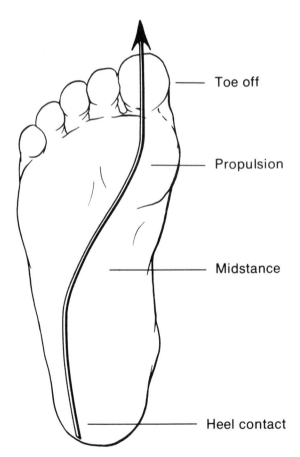

27-6   Force curve: Weight-bearing forces as they occur from heel contact to toe-off.

longus muscle stabilizes the first metatarsal until the final moments of toe-off. Efficient propulsion from the hallux, as stabilized by the first metatarsal, is then possible. Most extrinsic muscles attaching to the mid- or rearfoot that coordinate foot position during contact and midstance cease to function midway through the propulsive phase of gait. The majority of extrinsic and intrinsic muscles that have digital insertions function until toe-off. The completion of stance phase propulsion initiates swing phase of the same limb and weight bearing of the opposite limb.

BIOMECHANICAL DETERMINANTS OF FOOT AND LEG STABILITY

"Chain-Reaction Principle"

Early investigators believed that ligamentous and muscular tension were largely responsible for maintenance of a normal arch and efficient foot function. Today, we understand that the precise function of each segment of the lower extremity and foot determines effciency of motion. Root et al. [3] state: "No bone can be stabilized at a joint if the bones proximal to it are unstable." This phenomenon of joint mechanics relates to the absolute dependence of one foot segment's stability on another segment's function, a principle this author refers to as the "chain-reaction principle."

Subtalar Joint Function The largest and most proximal joint in the foot is the subtalar joint. This joint is sometimes called the "universal joint" of the foot, since it allows the plantar aspect of the foot to accommodate for variations in terrain. The motion in this joint, termed *triplane,* is oblique to all body planes. The collective triplane motions are called supination (turning in of the rearfoot) and pronation (turning out of the rearfoot) (Fig. 27-7). Subtalar joint motion can be assessed by measuring frontal plane excursion of the heel bone in relation to the distal leg. Although the total range of motion of the subtalar joint is approximately 30°–40° (measured on the frontal plane), the normal range used during gait is only about one-fourth of this. The subtalar joint range of motion must be maintained within this narrow range to assure maximum foot efficiency. This joint must unlock itself by pronating during the contact phase of gait and then quickly begin supinating prior to heel-off so the foot may become a solid foundation from which to propel. The posterior aspect of the heel should remain nearly vertical during stance and ambulation. Structural abnormalities, such as tibial vara, genu valgum, or frontal plane deformities of the forefoot and rearfoot that require subtalar joint compensation, excessively pronate or supinate this joint.

Midtarsal Joint Function The midtarsal joint is important in allowing independent movement of the forefoot and the rearfoot in all three body planes. Motion available at the midtarsal joint is derived from two independent axes. The oblique axis allows the forefoot to dorsiflex and plantarflex on the rearfoot. (This motion is actually triplanar, but the greatest movement occurs in the sagittal plane.) The longitudinal axis allows the forefoot to invert and evert in relation to the rearfoot. Longitudinal axis motion is also triplanar, but its greatest movement is in the frontal plane.

The articular surfaces of the midtarsal joint, like almost all other lesser tarsal joints, are at near right angles to ground reactive forces. The midtarsal joint depends mainly on muscular and ligamentous tension to withstand rotation forces, unlike the subtalar and ankle joints, where compressional forces are great. Chronic subluxations, therefore, frequently occur in the lesser tarsal joint as a result of ineffective bone and soft-tissue support.

Like the subtalar joint, the midtarsal joint locks and unlocks, depending on the phase

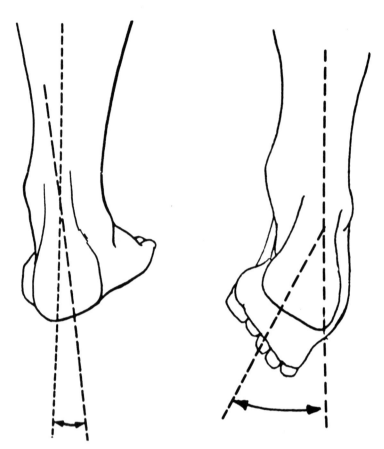

27-7 Non-weight-bearing subtalar joint, total range of movement. (From Root, M.L., Orien, W.P., et al. 1977. Normal and Abnormal Function of the Foot. Clinical Biomechanics Corp., Los Angeles. Reprinted with permission.)

of gait and compensatory requirements. The midtarsal joint must be mobile during initial ground contact and become rigid or locked prior to heel-off. If the oblique axis is mobile at midstance, the midtarsal joint or instep sags with body weight. This presents clinically as a low instep or an abducted forefoot in relation to the rearfoot.

Midtarsal joint stability depends on the position of the subtalar joint. When the subtalar joint is neutral or supinated, the talonavicular joint is superior to the calcaneocuboid joint. (These two joints make up the midtarsal joint [Fig. 27-8].) If the subtalar joint pronates, the two joints are almost side by side. In the first instance, the oblique midtarsal joint axis is almost parallel to ground reactive forces. Weight bearing is thereby met with osseous resistance. In the second case, ground reactive force during gait is sufficient to dorsiflex the forefoot on the rearfoot. This results in skeletal imbalance and hypermobility.

It is then clear that the positions of the talus and calcaneous are determined by the subtalar joint, and their relationship determines the longitudinal and oblique axes of the midtarsal joint, which in turn determine the midtarsal joint's stability. Midtarsal joint stability therefore depends upon subtalar joint stability.

A second means of attaining osseous stability of the midtarsal joint is based upon differences in joint congruity existent with varying positions of the talonavicular and the calcaneocuboid articulations (Elftman [6]) (Fig. 27-9). The articulating surfaces of both joints are egg-shaped. When the subtalar joint is neutral or supinated, the long axes of the joint surfaces are oblique to each other. Weight bearing results in stability based on joint

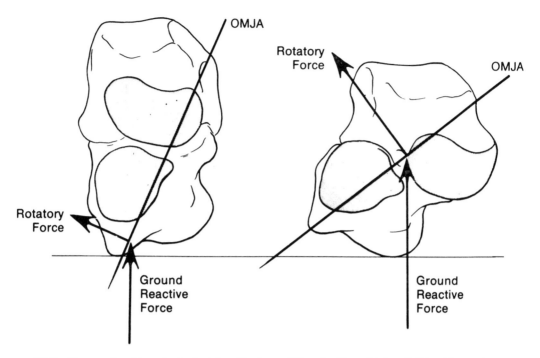

27-8 Change of position of subtalar joint affecting stability of midtarsal joint. OMJA, oblique mid-tarsal joint axis. (From Root, M.L., Orien, W.P., et al. 1977. Normal and Abnormal Function of the Foot. Clinical Biomechanics Corp., Los Angeles. Reprinted with permission.)

incongruity. If the subtalar joint pronates, the long axes of the joints become more parallel, creating a common axis for movement. Motion and the tendency for joint instability are, therefore, increased.

Lesser Tarsal Joint Function The lesser tarsal bones are wedge- or cube-shaped. Their articulating surfaces are subjected to large rotational forces during weight bearing, which must be resisted by both osseous and soft-tissue structures. The lack of motion between the lesser tarsal bones allows them to function as a unit, and their position is determined by the subtalar and midtarsal joints. Protection against subluxation in the lesser tarsal region depends on the multifaceted nature of the articular surfaces and the strength with which the joints are held together by muscles and ligaments.

A second osseous locking mechanism is responsible for lesser tarsal joint stability as well as for metatarsal-tarsal joint (Lisfranc's joint) stability. This is derived from the midtarsal joint's position. When the midtarsal joint is neutral or supinated, the lesser tarsal region becomes dorsally convex from medial to lateral. The bones move closer together and ground-reactive forces are resisted. If the midtarsal joint pronates, the lesser tarsal bones are more parallel to the ground, joint compressional forces are reduced, and ground-reactive forces result in saggital plane hypermobility of the forefoot.

The ligaments of the lesser tarsus, normal muscular function, and bony restraints provide local stability. Muscular support is from the medial pull of the tibialis posterior and the lateral pull of the peroneus longus and brevis; retrograde stability is assisted by intrinsic foot muscles.

Metatarsal Function The greatest motion of the metatarsals occurs on the sagittal plane, with lesser movement occuring on the transverse plane. Stability of the second,

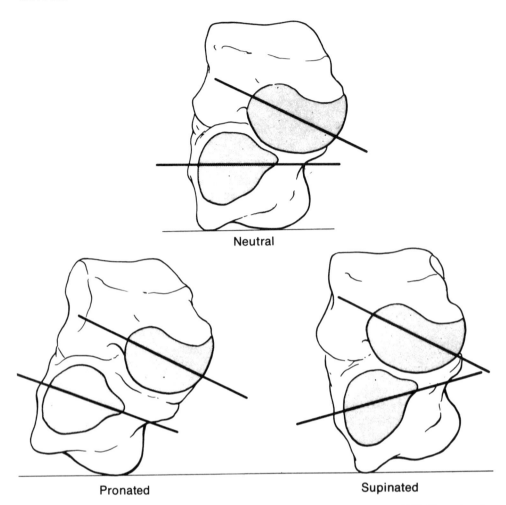

Neutral

Pronated

Supinated

27-9 Axial locking of midtarsal joint. (From Root, M.L., Orien, W.P., et al. 1977. Normal and Abnormal Function of the Foot. Clinical Biomechanics Corp., Los Angeles. Reprinted with permission.)

third, and fourth metatarsals is derived from osseous resistance and normal muscular function. Proximal bony stability is necessary for metatarsal stability with each muscle contraction.

The first metatarsal functions independently of other metatarsal bones. It is the largest of the metatarsals and carries approximately twice the weight of the lesser metatarsals. The first metatarsal and first cuneiform normally move as a unit called the first ray. First ray motion is triplanar, although the largest movement is in the sagittal plane (dorsiflexion, plantarflexion). During the propulsive phase of gait, weight is transferred from the lateral metatasals medially. The first metatarsal must be stable when weight is borne on the first metatarsal phalangeal joint; otherwise the foot pronates as the medial aspect of the foot collapses.

First metatarsal stability depends upon the function of the peroneus longus muscle (Fig. 27-10). The peroneus longus enters the foot laterally, goes below the cuboid on the plantar surface of the foot, making a near right-angle turn to insert medially at the base of the first metatarsal and cuneiform. The stability of the cuboid allows the peroneus longus to function like a pulley to increase its effective force from medial to lateral. The peroneus longus abducts the foot and plantar-flexes the first ray, and the position of the rearfoot (sub-

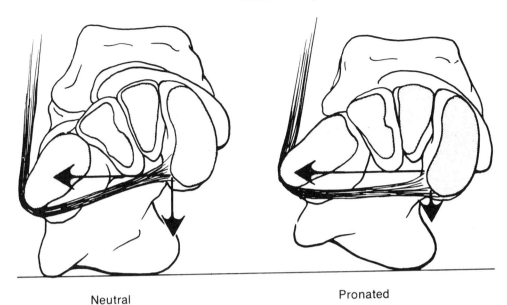

27-10 Changes of peroneus longus force vectors at insertion into first ray. (From Root, M.L., Orien, W.P., et al. 1977. Normal and Abnormal Function of the Foot. Clinical Biomechanics Corp., Los Angeles. Reprinted with permission.)

talar joint) determines which function predominates. Stability of the first ray depends on the ability of the peroneus longus to plantar-flex the first ray (not its ability to abduct). When the subtalar joint pronates, the medial arch of the foot approaches the supporting surface. As the first metatarsal and cuneiform descend, the peroneus longus approaches the transverse plane. Muscular contraction under these circumstances results in transverse plane motion or abduction of the foot. Supination of the subtalar joint allows the base of the first metatarsal and cuneiform to rise above the cuboid. Contraction of the peroneus longus pulls downward on the first ray to plantar-flex and stabilize the first metatarsal. It is, therefore, necessary that the subtalar joint cease contact phase pronation and reverse into a neutral or supinated position prior to midstance and foot propulsion. Only under these circumstances is the medial column of the foot prepared for weight bearing and toe-off.

The fifth metatarsal functions around an independent axis much like the first metatarsal. As the fifth metatarsal dorsiflexes, it simultaneously everts and abducts; as it plantarflexes, it inverts and adducts. The fifth matatarsal articulates proximally with the fourth metatarsal base and cuboid. This bony segment, like other bones of the lesser tarsus and forefoot, depends on subtalar joint position for stability. The fifth metatarsal is the first bone of the forefoot to make ground contact during gait. Stability of the fifth metatarsal depends largely upon subtalar joint position, which, in turn, determines midtarsal joint stability and the degree of frontal plane rotation of the cuboid. As the midtarsal joint pronates around its oblique and longitudinal axis, the cuboid abducts, dorsiflexes, and everts. This author believes that the change in position of the cuboid flattens the transverse metatarsal arch and causes the fourth metatarsal to descend in relation to the fifth. The osseous restraint between the fourth and fifth metatarsals diminishes, allowing greater freedom of movement of the fifth ray. Midtarsal joint pronation permits hypermobility at the calcaneocuboid joint and is another means for sagittal plane compensation of the lateral forefoot. Joint resistance and stability of the fifth metatarsal is attained in converse fashion as the subtalar joint supinates. Soft tissue assists fifth metatarsal stability in a way similar to that mentioned for the second, third, or fourth metatarsals.

CONCLUSION

The foot is the foundation of body support. Its two major functions are to provide stability and to aid in body propulsion. The subtalar joint of the rearfoot determines the way in which forces are transmitted through the foot and lower extremity. Subtalar joint function is responsible for frontal plane stability of the ankle and mechanical efficiency of the knee and hip, as determined by transverse plane position. Sagittal plane positioning of the pelvis and its effect on the lumbosacral angle are also influenced by subtalar joint position. In the foot, subtalar joint alignment directly or indirectly determines tarsal and lesser tarsal stability as well as efficiency of muscle function. Osseous instability resulting in biomechanical imbalances is the major cause of injuries to the endurance athlete. Clinicians must be aware of the important role improper body mechanics play in injury processes and learn to alter mechanical imbalances whenever necessary.

REFERENCES

1. Root, M.L., Weed, H.H., et al. 1966. Axis of motion of the subtalar joint. J Am Podiatry Assoc 56b(4):149–155.
2. Root, M.L., Orien, W.P., et al. 1971. Biomechanical Examination of the Foot. Clinical Biomechanics Corp., Los Angeles.
3. Root, M.L., Orien, W.P., et al. 1977. Normal and Abnormal Function of the Foot. Clinical Biomechanics Corp., Los Angeles.
4. Sgarlato, T.E. 1965. The angle of gait. J Am Podiatry Assoc 55(9):645–650.
5. Sgarlato, T.E. 1971. A Compendium of Podiatric Biomechanics. College of Podiatric Medicine Corp., San Francisco.
6. Elftman, H. 1960. Transverse tarsal joint and its control. Clin Orthop 16:41–44.

·28·

Biomechanics and Sports
Injury Treatment

Robert M. Parks

The sports physician must differentiate between injury cause and effect. The success of treating the effects of overuse injury, such as pain and swelling, may be dramatic, but is ultimately short lived. Successful overuse injury treatment may require altering the participant's body mechanics and style of movement, in addition to weight and flexibility training, changes in equipment or shoes, and modifications of training technique.

This chapter deals with treatment of sports injury based on the biomechanical principles discussed in Chapter 27.

The clinical application of biomechanics in treating sports injuries does not require a full understanding of anatomy or the concepts presented in Chapter 27. Coaches, trainers, and athletes themselves can administer successful biomechanical treatment. Unfortunately, the recent marketing of biomechanical paraphernalia, such as runner's shoe wedges and instant orthotic devices, and the overuse of rigid orthotic appliances may have distorted the value of biomechanics as applied to sports injury. The effective "sports biomechanist" appreciates the indications and limits of biomechanics and can integrate this treatment into a multifaceted therapeutic program.

The following discussion of common overuse injuries provides examples of how biomechanics may be important in sports injuries and their prevention. Treatment modalities presented are biomechanically oriented only and are not intended to be complete.

FOREFOOT PAIN

A number of overuse injuries occur in the area of the forefoot. The metatarsals and metatarsal phalangeal joint regions are most vulnerable to repetitive trauma seen in running and jumping sports. A larger number of forefoot injuries are seen in conjunction with the jumping activities of aerobics and "jazzercise." The toes of the feet are nearly always spared injury since they carry essentially no body weight during exercise and, with the exception of the big toe, function in a passive manner. Instability or hypermobility of the foot's structure, particularly the metatarsals, is the common denominator with most forefoot injuries occurring in athletics.

Chronic capsulitis of the second metatarsal phalangeal joint (MPJ) is the most frequent forefoot injury seen in this author's sports medicine practice. The signs and symptoms of this condition are quite specific (Fig. 28-1). The examiner must differentiate this condition from metatarsal stress fractures and intermetatarsal neuromas.

There are two common mechanical etiologies that may lead to second MPJ capsulitis. Mechanical weakness leading to capsulitis occurs when the foot is seen to be excessively pronated throughout the midstance and propulsive phases of gait. Excessive subtalor joint pronation indirectly renders the metatarsals unstable when subjected to ground reactive forces. In addition, the muscles governing the stability of the forefoot are put at a mechanical disadvantage when the foot remains pronated throughout the gait cycle. In this instance, as the heel elevates from the ground preparing the foot for propulsion, the first and fifth metatarsals elevate from their position adjacent to the middle three metatarsals. As the body guides its weight forward over the big toe joint in preparation for toe-off, it finds the first metatarsal (in its elevated position) unwilling to accept normal amounts of body weight. Weight is therefore transferred disproportionately onto the second metatarsal head prior to toe-off. The loading forces that occur in the second MPJ are apt to cause capsulitis, stress fractures, or a cortical thickening of the second metatarsal that is visible on X ray.

The second structural abnormality leading to capsulitis is seen with an abnormally long second metatarsal. This structural anomaly is termed *Morton's foot* and is clinically visible when the second digit is longer than the big toe when standing. The relative length of the digits is inconsequential, but this finding corresponds directly to the relative lengths of the metatarsals. Athletes possessing a Morton's foot may also display a callus or thickened tissue under the second metatarsal head. This finding is the skin's way of protecting itself from excessive pressure. Injury occurs in the Morton's foot type irrespective of the foot's mechanics. Any time the heel is off the ground and the metatarsal heads are "loaded" in preparation for propulsion, whether it be walking, running, or jumping, the second metatarsal will be overstressed.

Clinically, athletes presenting with capsulitis will display pain to pressure on the plantar aspect of the metatarsal head. If the condition is acute, swelling may be seen around the

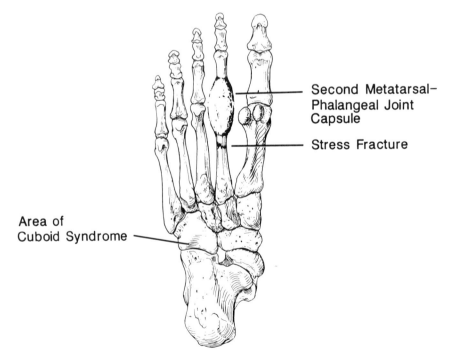

Second Metatarsal–
Phalangeal Joint
Capsule

Stress Fracture

Area of
Cuboid Syndrome

28-1 Top view of foot.

joint or even at the base of the second toe. Pain may also be elicited on the dorsal surface of the joint or by moving the second digit up and down. Pain elicited plantarly, just proximal to the metatarsal head, would indicate a distal fascial strain at the insertion into the metatarsal head. This condition should be treated as a fasciitis. Pain is described as dull and deep in nature. It is often described as a stone bruise sensation. Capsulitis is aggravated by going barefoot, wearing shoes with inadequate soles, or stepping on rocks or irregularities. Running or jumping activities may be particularly painful.

Treatment should consist of specific recommendations for athletic shoes. Running shoes should provide good shock absorption under the ball of the foot and be cardboard lasted from heel to toe if possible. Cardboard lasting as opposed to slip lasting will stiffen the shoe under the ball of the foot and therefore reduce digital flexion. Accommodative padding under the ball of the foot is particularly beneficial in treating capsulitis. This author prefers to place 1/8-in felt or cork under the first metatarsal head and laterally under the third, fourth, and fifth metatarsal heads. This treatment lessens the direct weight bearing under the second metatarsal head. Metatarsal cookie pads are also helpful if properly placed proximal to the metatarsal heads to support the transverse metatarsal arch. For resistant cases, quality arch supports or functional orthoses are helpful in stabilizing the entire foot structure and metatarsals.

Stress fractures of the metatarsals are seen most commonly in those athletes pursuing high levels of running or jumping activities. The metatarsal most vulnerable to injury is the second metatarsal with fractures occurring less frequently in the third and fourth metatarsals (Fig. 28-2). Abnormal weight distribution across the ball of the foot when bearing weight is the most frequent cause of injury. The mechanical etiology resulting in metatarsal fractures is the same as that described for capsulitis. It is unclear why one foot will develop joint swelling at the end of the metatarsal while another foot will simply fracture. It is generally accepted that more repetitive stress is necessary for stress fractures to occur.

Examination of the foot usually reveals a localized area of swelling and pain at the midshaft of a metatarsal. If fracture healing is far enough advanced, the swelling will be quite firm. Clinicians should remember that it takes approximately 3 weeks of having clinical symptoms before a metatarsal stress fracture will appear on X ray. Bone scans may be useful in high-level athletes when an accurate determination is needed quickly. Generally, pain prevents any reasonable participation in sports, and the clinical symptoms and findings are quite conclusive even without X-ray findings. Radiographic verification would therefore have little impact on the initial treatment plan. Most athletes with stress fractures should cease all running activities for 6 weeks after the diagnosis of a fracture has been made. Bicycling and swimming are allowed as well as required walking. Accommodative cork or

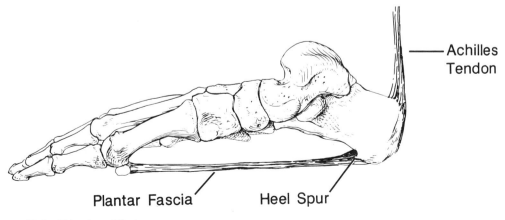

Achilles Tendon

Plantar Fascia   Heel Spur

28-2 Side view of foot.

felt padding placed under a full-length Spenco® insole (as described for capsulitis) provides sufficient relief and allows for an uncomplicated recovery. This padding should be worn for 3–4 months. Casting is not necessary unless the metatarsal head is significantly dorsiflexed as a result of injury. The postfracture position of the involved bone will nearly always prevent recurrent fractures. Adjacent metatarsal fracture, however, could occur if the postfracture weight-bearing surface of the foot is affected.

Intermetatarsal neuromas or Morton's neuromas occur most frequently between the third and fourth metatarsal heads. This condition presents clinically as a nerve-like pain between the metatarsals and often radiating into the corresponding toes. Digital numbness or paresthesias may also be described. Deep palpation between the involved metatarsals often elicits the symptoms described by the patient. A neuroma is an enlarged and inflamed nerve, usually aggravated by adjacent bony compression. Attempts have been made to categorize foot types that may predispose to neuroma pain. Many investigators feel an excessively mobile or flat foot will more likely precipitate injury. Arch supports and functional orthoses are therefore a form of treatment recommended in some cases. It is this author's experience that neuromas are equally prone to occur in any foot type.

THE SUBLUXED CUBOID

Lateral instep or lateral arch pain occurs frequently in running sports and may also be associated with inversion-type ankle sprains, a condition often misdiagnosed and mistreated. Pain from this syndrome may be located on the dorsal aspect of the calcaneocuboid joint, the lateral surface of the cuboid, or around the fifth metatarsal-cuboid joint. This syndrome most commonly occurs during long runs on asphalt or concrete surfaces or in runners with poorly maintained shoes. Quick movement sports may also precipitate "cuboid" pain if the heel twists (inverts or everts) in relation to the forefoot.

The "cuboid syndrome" is caused by ligamentous or capsular sprain of the above-mentioned joints due to bony instability. Any acute or chronic joint movement beyond the normal range places excessive strain on soft-tissue supporting structures in the area. The cuboid syndrome, also called "subluxed cuboid," refers to a positional change between the cuboid and calcaneus, and an important method of treatment involves manipulation. The cuboid and the attaching fifth metatarsal bone dorsiflexes, abducts and everts in relation to the calcaneus, and an important method of treatment involves manipulation. The manipulative technique for correction, therefore, involves quick plantar flexion and inversion of the forefoot on the heel. An audible click occurs when the manipulation is successful, and the patient experiences sudden pain relief. Other investigators believe the pathology of the cuboid syndrome involves slippage of the peroneus longus tendon from its groove under the cuboid, and the click during manipulation occurs when the tendon moves into place. Whether the pathology of the cuboid syndrome results from joint subluxation and subsequent inflammation or abnormal tendon position, the abnormal foot mechanics are often the same and the above treatment is usually successful.

The lateral column of the foot, or lateral arch, composed of the calcaneus, cuboid, and fifth metatarsal, normally forms a concave arch laterally. This is high in the high-arched foot (pes cavus) and low in the flat or pronated foot. It is not clear why the lateral column often becomes progressively higher in severe pes cavus, but the cause of breakdown and associated pain within the lateral column is well accepted.

Stability of the calcaneocuboid joint (the outer half of the midtarsal joint) is determined by factors described in Chapter 27, the most important being heel position as dictated by subtalar joint position. If the foot is pronated during gait, calcaneocuboid joint stability is lost, allowing the lateral column to dorsiflex, evert, and abduct on the rearfoot. If the fourth and fifth metatarsals are unstable, similar movement occurs and the result is strain of the capsules and ligaments on top of these joints. The cause of the cuboid syndrome is inherent biomechanical weakness of the foot. If the foot is highly unstable, normal walking may bring about symptoms. If the foot is more stable, worn shoes, severe jarring of the lateral column from running on hard surfaces, or trauma may instigate pain.

Pain of the cuboid syndrome is dull and deep and interferes with running and sometimes walking, but little pain is felt during non-weight-bearing times, unless swelling is present. A crippling type of pain occurs when the patient arises from bed; such pain usually dissipates with ambulation. Pain becomes progressively worse with persistence of running.

On physical examination, palpation produces pain directly below the extensor digitorum brevis muscle belly on the dorsolateral aspect of the foot and more distally along the lateral column. This should not be mistaken for pain arising from the sinus tarsi or from a previous ankle sprain with injury to the anterior talofibular ligament. Pain occasionally spreads distally as far as the fifth toe. Joint movement through a full range is pain free, and weight bearing is necessary to bring about symptoms. Fractures should be ruled out radiographically. The subluxation of the cuboid is usually not apparent on X rays. One should attempt to alleviate symptoms and then assess the mechanical causes. Runners should train to tolerance on soft surfaces and apply ice as necessary. Running shoes with superior heel counter-stability and good shock absorption are important. A $^1/_8$- to $^1/_4$-in heel lift in both shoes that artificially heightens the lateral column and reduces plantar fascia and Achilles tendon stress may be surprisingly effective. A tight Achilles tendon can strongly pronate the foot, so this should be stretched daily. Manipulation by trained personnel is worth trying. The patient should massage the painful site daily, and foot strapping may be used to stabilize the rearfoot and plantar fascia. If these measures relieve early symptoms, it is of diagnostic significance. If progress does not occur, other means to enhance foot stability may be required. A varus wedge or over-the-counter arch supports help control subtalar joint pronation and heel position. Some clinicians find that a silver dollar-sized $^3/_8$-in pad under the lateral arch reduces discomfort. If the latter modalities are employed, the heel lifts should be removed. When the therapeutic response continues to be less than optimal, and nonbiomechanical causes have been ruled out, functional orthotic devices made from neutral foot casts should prove successful. Rigid foot orthotics worn during sport and nonsport activities will establish dynamic foot stability that is often difficult to obtain by other means.

HEEL SPUR SYNDROME AND PLANTAR FASCIITIS

Heel and plantar fascial injuries are common complaints of endurance athletes as well as those involved with sports requiring quick body movements. The high frequency of fascial injuries is related to its important weight-bearing role. The heel accepts the largest and most direct impact at heel contact, and the plantar fascia aids in maintaining the foot's arch during stance. Since running and jumping sports increase the foot's load three to five times that of walking, it is no wonder that injuries develop. Heel spur syndromes occur at the medial plantar tubercle of the calcaneus, where the plantar fascia originates (Fig. 28-2). The cause of heel spur syndrome has been attributed to tension or pull of the plantar fascia on the calcaneus. The continual pull causes the periosteum to become inflamed (periostitis), and subsequent calcification produces the radiologically evident heel spur. A bony spur does not have to be present to produce pain or heel spur syndrome.

The same strain or pulling force within the fascia that causes the heel spur syndrome produces plantar fasciitis. Patients often describe fasciitis-type pain just previous to the onset of heel pain. Plantar fasciitis pain is usually in the center of the medial longitudinal arch but can occur in any area of the fascia. The mechanisms of injury to the heel and the plantar fascia appear similar. In this author's practice, heel pain is more prevalent than fascial pain. Some athletes may associate plantar fasciitis pain with fallen arches or arch fatigue and not seek medical advice. Excessive foot pronation during gait predisposes to symptoms of fasciitis or heel spur. This foot type has a normal arch during non-weight-bearing times, but flattens out when the subject stands or walks. Excessive mobility seen with the pronated foot appears to be the most significant factor predisposing toward injury. The congenital flat foot, by comparison, with little or no arch when the subject is sitting or standing, is less likely to develop heel and arch symptoms.

The mechanics of foot pronation that precipitate plantar fasciitis begin at the subtalar joint. Subtalar joint pronation unlocks the midtarsal joint, causing the arch to sag and the foot to elongate. Elongation of the foot stretches the plantar fascia at the center of the arch or at its origin on the heel. This stretching eventually leads to tissue overuse, producing inflammation and pain. Examination for plantar fasciitis and heel spur syndrome shows tenderness to palpation in the arch or on the undersurface of the heel. Clinical signs of inflammation are generally not seen with either complaint. Visible or palpable swelling indicates more significant tearing within the tissues. Practitioners treating these injuries should strongly advise physical therapy, tape immobilization, and cessation of sports that may aggravate this condition.

Treatment for plantar fasciitis and heel spur syndrome is similar, since they both share a common cause. If attention is sought soon after the onset of symptoms, simple measures are likely to alleviate the complaint. If the condition is long-standing, however, quick recovery is less likely. Initial care should be directed at reducing inflammation in the acute stage.

Tape strapping of the foot to support the plantar fascia, if applied correctly, reduces symptoms immediately. A ¼-in shock-absorbing heel lift in both shoes reduces plantar fascia tension and dissipates heel contact shock. This author prefers lifts fabricated from rubberized cork, Spenco®, or ¼-in Sorbathane®, and has not found that heel cups or heel pads with central cutouts significantly reduce heel or arch pain. Street shoes with rigid shanks and firm heel counters should be worn during daily activities. If sports activities are allowed, cardboard-last shoes with good heel counter-control are preferred. Achilles stretches should be recommended twice daily since they therapeutically stretch the plantar fascia. If heel lifts are ineffective, attempts should be made to control foot pronation, using the same criteria for foot supports as with the cuboid syndrome. When abnormal foot mechanics are present in conjunction with chronic fasciitis or heel spur syndrome, the use of functional foot orthotics is mandatory. In this author's experience, the use of orthotic devices for symptoms of chronic fasciitis is nearly 95% effective, and with heel spur syndrome, almost 85% effective.

ACHILLES TENDONITIS

The Achilles tendon and calf muscles provide foot plantar flexion and body propulsion, and are frequently injured in running and ballistic movement sports (Fig. 28–2). Runners are especially prone to Achilles tendonitis, since their sport is unidirectional, requiring continuous propulsion from the calf and hamstring muscles. The ensuing muscular imbalance from tight calf muscles is the major cause of overuse Achilles injuries. Daily stretching of the calves and hamstrings for all athletes engaged in running activities is imperative to avoid injury. Quantitative testing for calf and hamstring flexibility can identify athletes who may be prone to Achilles injury. Athletes with tight Achilles tendons, whether acquired or congenital, additionally display early heel-off or bouncy gait. When these athletes are injured, heel lifts should be placed in the shoes to reduce the tension within the muscle-tendon complex.

Abnormal foot pronation may also precipitate Achilles tendonitis. Abnormal foot mechanics were not appreciated as a contributing cause of Achilles tendonitis until slow-motion photography. Films revealed how the Achilles tendon near its insertion onto the heal actually moved on the frontal plane to a lesser or greater degree dependent on the corresponding movement of the heel. The Achilles attachment on the heel tolerates an unlimited range of sagittal plane motion (caused by contraction of the tendon and its antagonist) but only a small amount of frontal plane motion when the foot pronates and supinates. If the heel everts past normal ranges, as seen with pronatory deformities of the foot, it subjects the Achilles tendon to excessive frontal plane motion (in addition to its sagittal plane requirements), often leading to overuse and subsequent injury.

The treatment for Achilles tendonitis should begin with calf muscle stretching exercises. It will be helpful to measure the degree of flexibility in the calf and Achilles at the onset of the treatment program. Contractures of the gastrosoleus muscle group and Achilles tendon may be divided into hereditary and acquired categories. This can be done by testing ankle dorsiflexion with the knee both extended and flexed. Athletes who display limited flexibility with the knee extended but normal values with the knee flexed should expect greater flexibility after an intensive stretching program. Normal values for ankle dorsiflexion with the knee fully extended are 10° or greater, and values of 15° or greater are considered normal in a flexed knee position. Hereditary deformities are usually associated with lack of dorsiflexion in both knee positions and result from contractures of both the soleus and gastrocnemius muscles. Although hereditary contractures respond poorly to stretching exercises, they should be recommended. These athletes may perform more efficiently with heel lifts, whether or not they are injured. Clinicians should recommend icing and other physical therapy modalities as indicated. Shoes with good shock absorption and heel counter-control to lessen the shock of heel contact are recommended. If heel lifts, appropriate shoes, and other necessary modalities do not bring relief, practitioners should seriously consider abnormal foot function as a possible cause. Abnormal frontal plane motion of the heel can be controlled with appropriate wedging, arch supports, and functional orthotic devices.

SHIN SPLINTS

Historically, any athlete with pain between the knee and ankle was thought to have shin splints. The cause of shin splints was unknown and treatment was usually unsuccessful. Many running careers were interrupted or terminated because of this problem. Today, sports physicians can classify leg injuries anatomically and often are able to treat them successfully without interruption of training.

Each muscle compartment in the leg is separated by thick fascia and serves a specific locomotive function. If muscle balance is not maintained by proper training, strength building, and stretching, one compartment may overpower another, resulting in overstress and injury. Shin splints may occur in either the anterior or posterior compartment of the leg. Either type results from pulling of the involved muscle away from its tibial origin. Anterior shin splints, an injury seen most often in beginning runners, affect the front of the leg on the outer side of the tibia (Fig. 28-3). Posterior shin splints, the more common of the two injuries, occur along the inside border of the tibia and affect more seasoned athletes.

The injured muscle responsible for posterior shin splints is generally the tibialis posterior. This muscle originates on the medial side of the tibia and becomes tendon above the inside ankle bone (medial malleolus), making a near 90° deviation around the medial longitudinal arch. The tibialis posterior muscle supports the arch and supinates the foot. Abnormal biomechanics leading to injury occur if the foot pronates excessively during gait. This

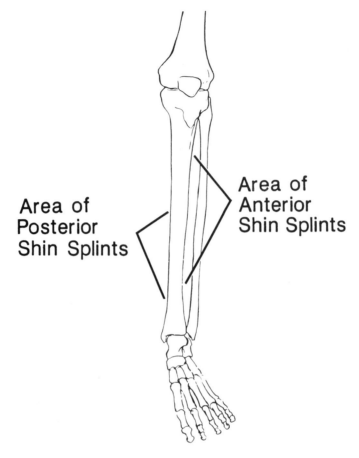

Area of Posterior Shin Splints

Area of Anterior Shin Splints

28-3 Front view of foot.

motion places undue stretch on the muscle tendon near its insertion. As the strain continues, the pull is transmitted to the ankle bone (functioning as a pully) and into the muscle bell where it pulls at its origin, the tibia. The tibial periosteum becomes inflamed from chronic tension and posterior shin splint pain ensues. Posterior shin splints are also thought to occur when the foot fails to adequately dissipate ground reactive forces or shock. Remember, in the running gait the foot must pronate within normal limits to act as a shock absorber at heel contact. Feet that have excessively high arches or that oversupinate during gait may produce this effect. This particular foot type and problem is also largely responsible for tibial stress fractures. If the possible cause of posterior shin splints is thought to be an oversupinated foot, steps should be taken to control foot mechanics within the shoe with appropriate foot orthoses. Running shoes should provide a high degree of shock absorption at heel contact and under the forefoot. Heel lifts may be recommended in all athletic shoes to lessen heel contact shock. Posterior shin splints also occur if the posterior compartment muscles are not stretched regularly. Participation in running sports without stretching results in increasingly tighter and more inflexible muscles. Fast running on hard surfaces and poor footwear are therefore more likely to cause injury when the tightened muscles are strained.

Posterior shin splint pain occurs along the lower midportion of the tibia starting 3–4 in above the medial malleolus. When the leg is straightened and the belly of the calf hangs freely, palpation along the tibia produces exquisite pain. Swelling may also be found. The swelling will be dispersed and boggy if the injury is acute or subacute. If nodular formation is felt, the injury is typically of a more chronic nature. Tibial stress fracture must not be mistaken for shin splints. Tibial stress fractures usually occur in the lower or upper one-third of the tibia and are associated with circumferential bone swelling and more localized pain that does not "warm up" with sports activity.

Early treatment for posterior shin splints should include ice massage. A good method for application is freezing water in a styrofoam cup. The top inch of the cup is then peeled away and the denuded ice is used to massage along the length of painful bone. Ten to fifteen minutes of ice massage applied twice daily, and especially after sports activity, is recommended. Athletes should stretch the posterior leg compartment (calf stretch), which contains the tibialis posterior muscle, three times per day. Ankle dorsiflexion exercises should be performed to strengthen the anterior compartment muscles and maintain equilibrium between compartments.

The foot structure of athletes with posterior shin splints should be evaluated, and structural deformities that result in abnormal pronation or supination should be supported. Varus wedges could be used to lessen the stress on the tibialis posterior muscle at heel contact, and a Morton's pad under the first metatarsal will help control pronation during the propulsive phase of gait. Appropriate taping to support the arch may reduce the pronatory stretch on the affected muscle. Taping of the leg in the vacinity of pain may be helpful if other methods of treatment prove unsuccessful. Leg taping, although having no significant biomechanical merit, tends to disperse ascending shock entering the leg. If the structural abnormality of the foot and its relationship to injury is not clear, the above treatment may be used for diagnostic purposes. If foot support improves symptoms, the mechanical etiology is verified. Heel lifts can also reduce stress within the posterior compartment that occurs during walking or running. If heel lifts and arch supports or varus wedges are used together, the lifts should be placed under the supports or on top of any wedging. Running shoes should have superior heel counter-stability. If biomechanical therapy fails and functional foot control is needed, rigid or semirigid orthotic devices are the next step. These offer a favorable prognosis in selected patients.

Anterior shin splints result from overuse of the tibialis anterior muscle. This muscle originates laterally on the tibia, crosses the front of the ankle, and attaches to the medial side of the foot. The function of the tibialis anterior muscle is to dorsiflex the foot at the ankle joint. During gait, the tibialis anterior muscle raises the foot during swing phase to alow toe clearance, and at heel contact, to slowly lower the forefoot to the ground, preventing foot-slap.

In most cases, the cause of anterior shin splints is strictly overuse and not biomechanical abnormalities. Sports that involve running, as well as bicycling and types of Nordic skiing, place high demands on the tibialis anterior muscle. The muscle subsequently weakens with fatigue and therefore loses its ability to withstand injury. Tight calf muscles may contribute to anterior shin splint injury. The calf's antagonistic function opposes the tibialis anterior muscle's ability to dorsiflex the foot. When more muscular effort is needed to resist the opposing pull of the calf muscle, the anterior leg muscles fatigue prematurely and injury results. Pain from anterior shin splints is felt along the lateral aspect of the tibia. Nodule formation may be present with anterior shin splints but is less dramatic than that seen with posterior shin splints.

Pain and stiffness within the entire anterior compartment, but not necessarily along the bone, compose a separate entity called "anterior compartment syndrome." The cause of this injury is similar to anterior shin splints, although the pain results from muscle swelling in response to exercise instead of the pulling of muscle from bone.

Treatment for anterior shin splints includes icing, stretching, and strengthening similar to that used for posterior shin splints. The anterior leg muscles should be stretched, with forced plantar flexion of the foot. Running speed and stride length should be reduced, and during the rehabilitative period training should be on natural surfaces. Running shoes should be those that provide good midfoot shock absorption.

KNEE INJURIES

Athletic knee injuries occur frequently, due to the knee's principle role in providing body support and locomotion. Each knee must individually support and dissipate ascending forces from heel strike that may reach three to five times body weight. Structural deviations around the knee joint or faulty lower extremity mechanics most frequently contribute to injury. Knee injuries can be either traumatic or overuse in nature. Acute traumatic injuries are not discussed here.

Overuse knee injuries may involve the medial, anterior, lateral, and, less often, posterior aspects of the knee (Fig. 28-4). Soft-tissue structures that cross the knee to lend support or provide motion may be injured, with the exception of the collateral ligaments, which require a subluxatory force for damage to result. Knee ligament injury is the primary etiology. Bony structures, particularly involving the patellofemoral joint and its cartilaginous surfaces, are subject to overuse when abnormal form and function exist over prolonged periods of time. Biomechanical treatment of overuse knee injuries may be initiated based on the generalized location of pain without arriving at a specific diagnosis. It is preferable, however, to define the structure involved whenever possible.

Medial Knee Injuries

Overuse injuries involving the medial aspect of the knee most frequently involve the tendons making up the pes anserinus, which include the sartorius, semitendinosus, and gracilis. The injury is typically a tendonitis near the tendon's common insertion or a bursitis underlying these tendons. Repetitive valgus and rotatory stress from abnormal foot pronation and flat feet are most frequently attributed as the cause. Foot deformities that cause compensatory foot pronation always result in simultaneous internal knee rotation (see Chapter 27). Excessive internal knee rotation during gait imposes a rotatory torque that pulls on the medial knee tendons with each foot strike. The knee that has a structural valgus genu valgum may sustain a similar injury. This knee type directs the body's center of mass to the inside of the feet, causing compensatory foot pronation that, in turn, further rotates the knee. Individuals possessing a structural genu valgum when lying supine will exhibit a more extreme deformity when bearing weight due to this functional component. It is important to recognize and treat the primary deformity causing abnormal knee function. Athletes must be evaluated while bearing weight, during non-weight-bearing times, standing still, and in motion to fully appreciate any abnormal structure and function. Medial knee tendonitis, as discussed, presents with pain to palpation at the insertion of the pes anserinus onto the medial tibial condyle or very near the medial joint margin. Injuries to the medial collateral ligament, medial joint capsule, and medial meniscus must be ruled out in these cases. If pain is exquisite on palpation, bursal inflammation may be involved.

Range-of-motion testing of the knee is usually pain free with medial knee pain. Forced adduction of the leg against resistance may produce pain in these patients. Pes anserinus tendonitis, in both acute and subacute stages, is cared for by icing and stretching. Biomechanical therapy should be aimed at reducing rotational or valgus torque in the knee. Shoes with good torsional stability and heel counter-control are mandatory in these individuals to help stabilize subtalor joint motion. Varus heel wedges and Morton's pads under the

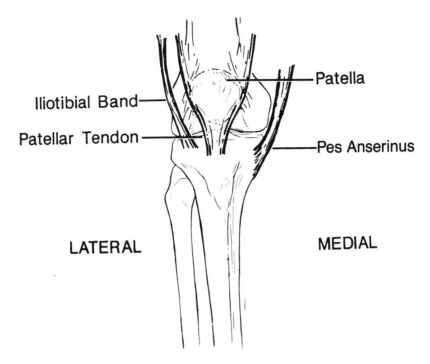

28-4 Front view of knee.

forefoot should help control foot pronation and thereby alleviate medial knee tendonitis. If symptoms persist and foot pronation is significant, arch supports or functional orthotic devices should be attempted. The results of even the most basic mechancial therapy should be rewarding when treating medial knee pain.

ANTERIOR KNEE PAIN

Injuries resulting in anterior knee pain may involve the quadriceps and its retinacula, the patella, or patellar tendon. Since these structures function as a unit, injuries to them may be classified as extensor mechanism disorders. The patella enhances the power of the quadriceps by increasing the distance of the tendon from the knee's axis of motion, creating a greater lever arm and more efficiency in extending the knee. The V-shaped articulation between the patella and the femoral condyle prevents subluxation and controls patellar tracking within its groove. The quadriceps muscle extends the knee from a flexed position during the swing phase of gait and supports the knee in an extended position during heel contact. The four individual muscles that make up the quadriceps attach into the patella by retinacular fibers, and the patella attaches to the tibial tuberosity via the patella tendon.

The quadriceps mechanism, particularly the patellofemoral joint, is highly susceptible to injury at heel contact. Ground-reactive forces tend to buckle the knee and must be adequately countered by the extensor mechanism. The quadriceps contracts firmly, driving the patella against the femur and resulting in strong compressive forces between the two bones. If the gliding function of the patella (or patellar tracking) is altered by anatomic variants or by faulty extremity mechanics, injuries are apt to occur.

The most common athletic injury to the anterior knee is patellofemoral syndrome, characterized by pain and swelling within the patellofemoral joint. Bone or cartilaginous changes are not visible on X ray or by arthroscopic examination in this early stage of injury. As this injury progresses, cartilage erosion develops on the undersurface of the patella, resulting in chondromalacia patellae. Treatment is more effective during the early stages of injury. Pain within the patellofemoral joint may be due to structural deformities of the knee such as patella alta, patella baja, or an abnormally high Q angle. All of these deformities adversely affect patellar tracking within the femoral condylar grooves. Structural deformities either extrinsic or instrinsic to the foot, resulting in abnormal foot pronation, may contribute to patellofemoral disorders. Internal rotation of the knee initiated by foot pronation shifts the patella laterally in the femoral groove and may produce articular irritation. Knee alignment and Q angle should be examined during weight-bearing and non-weight-bearing times, since functional disorders from biomechanical causes are not evident at non-weight-bearing times. Related injuries may affect the extensor retinaculum or patellar tendon. These injuries may result from similar causes and respond to similar therapy. Pain within the quadriceps muscle may occur in those participating in ballistic sports and should be treated as a muscular injury. Pain at the tibial tuberosity in adolescents, consistent with Osgood-Schlatter disease, should be differentiated from overuse injuries and treated accordingly.

Patellofemoral pain should be evaluated with the athlete supine. The ankle is grasped and the knee is taken through a full range of motion while lightly compressing the patella with the opposite hand and checking for crepitation throughout the range of motion. Next, the patella is compressed firmly with the knee in 160° of extension. The patient is asked to contract the quadriceps, and the examiner feels for crepitation and determines whether or not the patient feels pain. The examiner should palpate around the patella carefully, checking for discomfort. With the aid of appropriate testing to rule out the presence of other knee pathology and a thorough history, the diagnosis of a patellofemoral disorder should be established.

Treatment includes reduction of sports activities to tolerance. Strength-building exercises for the quadriceps is the hallmark of therapy and should begin at once. The athlete should start with straight leg raisers using a tolerated amount of weight (typically 0–5 lbs) and performing about 30 repetitions. These exercises then progress into tolerated leg extensions using only the last 20°–30° of motion prior to full extension. When the athlete is back to normal activities and is considered well, leg extensions using relatively light weight and high repetitions can begin. This phase should be implemented carefully and under supervision so as not to aggravate the joint. Deep squats should be eliminated from any weight program. Cybex testing is of particular value during each phase of rehabilitation to evaluate strength and progress. Hamstring stretching is helpful in reestablishing muscular equilibrium between the posterior and anterior thigh muscles. The patella should be examined during static stance and throughout gait for internal positioning caused by excessive foot pronation. Abnormal foot pronation will cause a very sudden internal rotation of the knee that is visible only during the heel contact phase of gait and will then reverse itself by midstance. If abnormal pronation is present or excessive internal rotation of the knee is visible during gait, proper shoes, varus wedges, and orthotic therapy are indicated. If abnormal extremity mechanics are questionable, the use of appropriate wedging or suitable arch supports may be helpful therapeutically as well as in establishing a mechanically oriented diagnosis.

Lateral Knee Injuries

Overuse injuries to the lateral knee may affect the iliotibial band, popliteus tendon, or long head of the biceps femoris. Injuries near the insertion of the iliotibial band are clearly most common in runners. The popliteus tendon is near the iliotibial band, so the differentiation of these structures may be difficult. Fortunately, much of the conservative treatment for popliteus tendonitis and iliotibial band syndrome is similar. Tendonitis of the biceps femoris insertion at the head of the fibula, although located laterally, is best discussed with posterior knee complaints.

Mechanical stresses adversely affecting the lateral knee may result from structural deformities such as rigid pes cavus (high-arched feet), uncompensated rearfoot varus, and tibial varum (inverted positioning of the heel or leg, respectively). The shock of weight bearing occurring with these conditions is directed laterally at the knee joint. Deformities of this nature will either cause increased compressional forces or grinding to occur within the lateral knee, or, if severe, may cause a frontal plane distraction or visible bowing to occur at the lateral joint margin. Both possibilities result in repetitive stress to all lateral soft-tissue structures. Individuals possessing these deformities appear clinically as having bowed legs, and if viewed from behind, the lower leg and heel appear to be grossly inverted in relation to the floor. Gait analysis shows jarring at the knee and within the quadriceps musculature, and an abrupt heel contact. When the above-mentioned deformities are flexible and allow the foot to compensate with pronation, an internal rotatory torque is applied to the knee joint. The transverse plane torque resulting from excessive pronation of the foot twists the knee-supporting structures and promotes injury with each step. Twisting and poor shock dissipation are therefore two components of injury that must be considered when treating lateral knee pain.

The iliotibial band is a fascial structure that helps stabilize the hip, thigh, and knee during heel contact. It originates proximally from the iliac crest, where it is called the tensor fascia lata. The iliotibial band descends along the lateral thigh to become tendon-like just above the knee, where it attaches on the anterolateral aspect of the tibia, called Gerdes tubercle. The iliotibial band is made visible by having the athlete extend the involved extremity. Injury occurs most often over the lateral femoral epicondyle, a bony prominence that may rub the iliotibial band during knee flexion and extension, producing inflammation and pain. So the examiner can palpate this structure, the patient is asked to flex the knee joint approximately 20° and the examiner then compresses the epicondyle. In this position, the iliotibial band lies directly over the epicondyle and is usually painful. Palpation may also induce pain at its tibial insertion, although this is less frequently seen. Iliotibial band syndrome of the knee should be distinguished from pain within the lateral collateral ligament and other conditions involving internal knee derangement. Primary pain in the tensor fascia lata is seen also as a primary complaint. Pain in the tensor fascia lata may stay localized or tend to radiate distally. This injury is seen more frequently in females and may be related to leg length discrepancy or attempting to progress too rapidly with training.

Iliotibial band syndrome responds well to icing. Specific stretches for the lateral thigh and hip and strengthening exercises for thigh abductors are recommended. Examiners should attempt to differentiate the mechanical cause of iliotibial band syndrome. The two common causes should be categorized as either rigid uncompensated pes cavus with lateral knee joint jamming and bowing or pronatory compensation of the foot with excess transverse plane motion occurring at the knee joint. The former is treated more specifically with soft shoes that encourage foot motion within the shoe, and the latter case requires a shoe that provides motion control of the foot. Running should be reduced to tolerance, and speed and stride length should be decreased. Athletes with rigid, high-arched feet should therefore purchase running shoes with good heel and midsole shock absorption, and those who pronate excessively should use wedges, Morton's pads, or arch supports as necessary. Functional orthoses tend to work well for the overpronator but should be avoided by those with a rigid foot type.

Posterior Knee Injuries

Injuries to the posterior aspect of the knee largely result from ballistic sports and sprinting. Muscle strains and tears are the most common injuries to the hamstrings. Tendonitis at the knee is common in distance runners and is nearly always related to poor flexibility or improper training methods. Therapeutic measures for these injuries include ice massage and stretching. Fast running and sprinting should be restricted. Biomechanical faults are rarely implicated in hamstring injuries. If pain cannot be palpated at a tendonous insertion behind the knee, careful examination should be employed to rule out intrinsic knee pathology.

.29.

Physical Therapy in Maintenance of Athletic Performance

William J. O'Brien

The weekend athlete, the serious competitor, and the professional athlete all have one thing in common: the biomechanical and physiologic characteristics of their bodies. In the resting state, the body displays certain biomechanical and physiologic adaptations. Exercise by definition is a perturbation of the resting state, accompanied by its own physiologic and biomechanical adaptations to that perturbation.

STRETCHING AND WARM-UP

Since exercise is a form of stress, one must prepare the body for it. This requires a gradual warm-up of 5 to 10 min that includes stretching of muscles to be exercised. Joint movement allows stretching of soft tissues—joint capsules, ligaments, and muscle—and spreads synovial fluid over the cartilage for lubrication to maintain it as a shock absorber during impact. Stretching muscles and tendons facilitates blood flow into the area, which "warms up" the peripheral nerves for better impulse conduction. The muscle spindles and joint receptors provide feedback information on muscle length and movement to the spinal cord and are "biased" to expect the changes in length and tension that accompany exercise.

The type of exercise dictates the style of warm-up and stretching. A jogger or runner will place great demands on the hamstrings for deceleration. Therefore, emphasis must be placed on stretching the hamstrings.

Physical differences among individuals are expressed by the person's stance, gait, and sleeping posture. A person's unique posture predetermines the muscle groups that will be tight. If one sits most of the day, one will have tight hip flexors and hamstrings; special attention should, therefore, be given to stretching those muscles. Flexibility requires a stretching program based on knowledge of biomechanics and anatomy. No universal formula can be applied uniformly to all body types for all exercises.

After exercise, the body must cool off and return to its resting state gradually. Adequate cardiac output depends upon venous filling of the heart. During exercise, extremity muscular contraction and abdominal and thoracic movements facilitate venous return mechanically. When exercise stops, mechanical compression ceases abruptly while peripheral vasodilation persists. Therefore, the venous return and, hence, cardiac output may fall to dangerously low levels. This usually causes "dizziness" and the person lies down which increases venous return and the "dizziness" clears. For similar reasons, one should not take a hot shower immediately after exercise.

Training specificity is well documented (Morehouse and Miller [1]); a sprinter trains by sprinting and a swimmer by swimming. An athlete's physical prowess is, however, determined by his or her vascular, biochemical, and muscular makeup, which is genetically determined. By training, optimum performance based on genetic potential can be achieved (Al-Amound et al. [2]; Peckham et al. [3]; Pette et al. [4]; Riley and Allin [5]; Salmons [6]; Salmons and Henriksson [7]). Most individuals have muscles that are heterogenous in fiber type, but are capable of adaptations in response to training (Salmons and Henriksson [7]).

TRAINING AND MUSCLE FIBER ADAPTATIONS

A specific training program can be designed to stress and cause adaptation of the appropriate muscle fiber type. Rapid, large increases in tension require maximum effort for short time periods. This favors Type II or fast-twitch muscle fibers. An intense effort is needed to activate these fibers, a process that can be explained by Henneman's spinal neuron recruitment theory (Henneman et al. [8]). According to that theory, big motor units are innervated by large anterior horn cells that require a large excitatory input before they fire. These large motor units contain many muscle fibers that can rapidly increase tension with maximum effort. Because the smaller, slower motor units are already active, explosive anaerobic exercise stresses the fast-twitch motor units and are appropriate for weight lifting, sprinting, or similar activities.

Regular exercise increases oxidative enzymes and skeletal muscle mass. The former is evidenced histologically by increased numbers of mitochondria and greater capillary density, changes that facilitate oxygen delivery. Increased muscle fiber diameter that depends on the type of exercise program also occurs. Heavy resistance anaerobic exercises result in the greatest hypertrophy (Salmons and Henriksson [7]). Weight lifting is not only anaerobic exercise, but can also be a useful aerobic program.

APPLICATION OF MODALITIES

The physical therapist is often called upon to treat athletic injuries with heat or cold application or special exercises. During the acute phase of injury, cold is the modality of choice, since it slows local metabolic activity, decreases inflammation, and minimizes vasodilation (Grant [9]; Gucker [10]). Reduced venous dilation limits edema since the capillary bed hydrostatic pressure is influenced by venous pressure. Swelling can hide bony and ligamentous injuries; therefore, it is important to minimize it, using cold, early. Cold also slows peripheral nerve conduction and decreases pain. A basic rule for modality application is that the area to which it is applied should have normal sensation and the patient should be capable of communicating his or her sensations to the person applying the modality.

Generalized soreness after exercise often improves with heat (Gucker [10]). Whirlpool therapy is relaxing and comfortable, but the high temperature can cause significant peripheral vasodilation that may interfere with adequate cardiac filling and hence cardiac output. A person going into the whirlpool must have recovered fully from exercise, e.g., have resting respiratory and heart rates.

Heat facilitates edema formation in dependent extremities and may make examination of an injured joint or bone difficult, but during healing, the vasodilatory effects of heat are beneficial. In chronic, noninflammatory athletic injury, heat is often used to increase local circulation (Gucker [10]) and tissue healing. Local heating modalities include whirlpool, hot packs, short-wave diathermy, microwave, and ultrasound (Grant [9]; Gucker [10]; Griffin and Karselis [11]; McCluskey et al. [12]).

On occasion, an injured extremity must be immobilized prior to moving the patient (McCluskey et al. [12]; Malone et al. [13]). This can be achieved by using prefabricated or air splints or even rolled magazines. Immobilization is important in fractures to prevent pain and vascular tears by bony fragments, or nerve injury from compression or laceration. The injured extremity should be immobilized without compromising body supply and should be kept elevated until examined by a physician. If a physician is not immediately available, the immobilized extremity can be cooled with ice packs. One should remember to inspect the injured limb periodically.

Physical therapy of athletic injuries requires understanding of the principles stated earlier: cold application, inflammation, and the associated pain and edema. Cold should not be used after the acute stage of injury. A good rule of thumb is if the injured part is warm, red, or swollen, elevate and cool. Once the injured area has passed through the acute warm, red, and swollen stage, circulation can be improved by warming (Gucker [10]).

Injuries are cooled by ice and water applied in plastic bags held in place with an elastic bandage. Elevation decreases pain, edema, and inflammation. The injured area should be examined periodically to prevent additional damage by the modality itself, and ice should be removed if the area becomes completely anesthetic. It should warm up until sensation returns. Generally, ice packs are applied for 15–20 min. Other means of applying cold include chemical cold generation packs, or fluoromethane spray.

Heat applications can be provided by a variety of modalities, from hot towels to pulsed short-wave diathermy. The depth of penetration ranges from superficial infrared and hot packs to microwave, short-wave, pulsed-short-wave diathermies, and ultrasound, which provides the greatest depth of penetration (Griffin and Karselis [11]). The modality selected for heat application should be based on the area to be treated and patient comfort. Contraindications for various modalities are shown in Table 29-1.

The most common sports injuries referred to physical therapists involve the ankle, knee, elbow, and foot, and occasionally, the shoulder and back.

ANKLE INJURIES

Ankle injuries are often seen first by orthopaedists or emergency room physicians. Physical therapy of ankle sprains depends upon the grade of the sprain. The basic management includes ice and elevation initially, followed by a graded exercise program. Grade I sprains should be taped to limit subtalar motion, inversion, and eversion. The patient should be taught a partial weight-bearing gait with the aid of crutches, and the ankle should be elevated and iced, when the patient is not walking, for 3–5 days (McCluskey et al. [12]; Connolly [14]; Starkey [15]).

Grade II sprains should be taped, iced, elevated, and the patient mobilized with a partial weight-bearing gait and crutches (McCluskey et al. [12]; Connolly [14]; Starkey [15]).

Grade III sprains require cold, compression, elevation, and massage and, occasionally, surgical repair of ruptured ligaments. The patient is often fitted with a below-knee, short-leg cast. Partial weight-bearing ambulation with crutches is permitted (McCluskey et al. [12]; Connolly [14]; Starkey [15]).

Nonoperated cases are treated with ankle exercises alternating with elevation and icing. The exercises for eversion, inversion, dorsiflexion, and extension are at first isometric and progress to full resistive exercises as the patient's condition improves. Commercial

Table 29-1 Heat Modalities

Modality	Contraindications
Infrared	Do not administer over "artificial hair" wigs
Hot Packs	Diabetes or peripheral vascular disease Areas of abnormal sensation
Microwave Diathermy (2450 Megacycles [Mc])	Areas of abnormal sensation Diabetes or peripheral vascular disease Metastatic disease Obesity
Short-Wave Diathermies (13.56 and 27.12 Mc)	Areas of abnormal sensation Diabetes or peripheral vascular disease Metastatic disease Metal in or on field
Ultrasound (1 Mc)	Growth plates in bones of children Do not administer directly over bone Do not apply over stellate ganglion Diabetes or peripheral vascular disease

exercise devices are available to strengthen the muscles that move the ankle joint. An inner tube can be cut to shape to be used throughout the day. The uninjured foot anchors one end of the rubber loop and the injured foot inserted into the other end pushes, pulls, inverts, or everts against the resistance of the rubber.

Complete rehabilitation of a severe ankle sprain can take 4–8 months and requires motivation of the patient to achieve full range of motion (McCluskey et al. [12]; Connolly [14]; Starkey [15]). Rehabilitation consists of an ankle range-of-motion exercise against resistance followed by elevation and icing if postexercise swelling occurs (McCluskey et al. [12]; Connolly [14]; Starkey [15]).

Isokinetic testing on a Cybex® machine allows comparison of work performance of the muscles of the injured ankle with those of the uninjured side and objectively measures progress before permitting the patient to return to athletics.

KNEE INJURIES

Knee injuries are common in contact sports like football. However, significant knee damage can also occur in dancers and runners, is often accompanied by pain and swelling, and accounts for many referrals to physical therapists (Davies et al. [16]).

The biomechanical complexity of the knee joint leads to significant problems when the joint is unstable (Derscheid and Malone [17]; McLeod and Hunter [18]).

The basic management of acute knee injuries includes elevation, icing, compression, and ambulation with use of crutches and partial weight bearing. After surgical procedures, 6–8 weeks of immobilization with a cylinder cast or cast brace and nonweight-bearing walking with the aid of crutches may be necessary followed by graded institution of a full resistive exercise program. To permit active knee motion is a difficult decision because the longer the joint is immobilized, the more difficult it is to obtain full range of motion.

Knee sprains accompanied by pain and joint effusion should be elevated, compression-wrapped, and iced for 3–5 days or until the knee is no longer warm or swollen (Connolly [14]; Derscheid and Malone [17]). During this time, patients should perform isometric quadriceps exercises and straight-leg raising throughout the day. Following the acute phase, if significant joint damage has not occurred, active range of motion exercises on a stationary bicycle and/or exercise table may be started. Initially after each bout of exercise, the knee is elevated and iced; later it is elevated and iced only if the exercise causes pain and edema. If active range of motion is tolerated, the patient may then progress on an exercise table, bicycle, or isokinetic exercise device like the Orthotron® or Fitron®. Joint instability may be increased by the use of free weights.

Patients with surgically treated knee injuries should be instructed preoperatively in isometric quadriceps exercises, and these should be done for 5–10 min every hour postoperatively (Connolly [14]).

Patients should then be taught partial or nonweight-bearing ambulation with crutches depending on operative procedure. The postoperative knee can also be elevated and iced. Gentle active range of motion exercises are in order about 10 days postoperatively, depending on the surgical procedure. Active knee exercises followed by icing, if necessary, may then progress to full resistive exercises with the above-mentioned equipment. Maximum exercise with minimum pain and edema is a measure of progress. Knee function can be evaluated objectively by Cybex® testing and comparison with the contralateral healthy side. The power output ratio of the quadriceps to the hamstrings is an important guide for return to active sports. When this is favorable and range of motion is full, the patient should again be able to participate successfully in athletic activities.

The reestablishment of quadriceps and hamstring power is often the major goal of rehabilitation. Joint flexibility of both the knee and proximal and distal joints must be maintained by stretching exercises. The hip flexors, abductors, extensors, and adductors are best gently stretched by using positions that isolate these muscles. Special attention should be paid to obtaining a full range of motion at the ankle, and the gastrocnemius group may be stretched by passive foot dorsiflexion; i.e., face a wall and place the palms against the wall, back away with knees and hips straight so that by leaning against the wall, body weight stretches the posterior calf muscles.

ELBOW INJURIES

Elbow injuries have escalated with the increase in popularity of racquetball, tennis, and golf. Previously, most elbow injuries occurred in baseball players.

The typical elbow injury is from overuse. In baseball pitching, a valgus thrust to the arm results in medial collateral ligament stress and injury (Connolly [14]). A topspin forehand in tennis places great demand on the forearm extensors to decelerate forearm pronation, and the racket weight stresses wrist extensors as the follow-through tends to flex the wrist.

Acute overuse elbow injuries are treated with elevation, ice, compression, and rest. Active elbow motion may be resumed as the pain, swelling, and heat subside.

Nonoperative management of elbow overuse also includes taping to restrict wrist movement, and support of the medial and lateral collateral ligaments with tape or special elastic bands.

Resistive exercises followed by icing for the first few weeks strengthen the muscles originating from both medial and lateral epicondyles. Specific resistive exercises for the forearm pronators (pronator teres and quadratus) and supinator include use of a hammer or a rotational exercise device. Most elbows nonsurgically treated for overuse improve within 6–8 weeks.

FOOT INJURIES

Injuries to ligaments and muscles of the feet occur more often today because of the increased popularity of running. A common problem is calcaneus spurs. These bony elongations of the calcaneus resemble a bird's beak, and mark the origin of the long plantar ligament of the foot. They are acutely painful to palpation, and may be treated with phonophoresis of 5–10% hydrocortisone cream. Ultrasound is less painful, and a good response can be expected after six to eight 10-min treatments. Arch support with padding over the painful area and stretching exercises for the gastrocnemius soleus muscle group are recommended.

SHOULDER INJURIES

Common shoulder injuries result from falling on the outstretched arm or from an acute exacerbation of bursitis. Acromial separations can be managed with ice and a figure-eight bandage and/or an arm sling. Ice is applied when the shoulder is swollen and hot. After the acute inflammation subsides, simple active range of motion exercises can be done. Initially, the patient can let the arm hang and gently swing it to and fro ("Codman's" exercises), and then should progress to active shoulder motion using a shoulder wheel, wall ladder or simple overhead pulleys. If the shoulder remains painful after exercise, icing may be necessary. Resistive shoulder exercises using weights, pulleys, or isokinetic apparatus are the next step. Resistance is applied to the internal and external rotators, the shoulder abductors, flexors, and extensors. When the patient performs these exercises without pain, he or she may return to previous activities. Power can be measured with a Cybex® isokinetic testing unit and compared with power output curves of the uninjured side.

BACK INJURIES

Most acute back injuries result from occupational activities superimposed upon bad postural habits, and rarely occur in athletes. The lumbosacral fascia and paravertebral muscles shorten with longstanding lordosis and failure to stretch them. In this situation, even a minor twist may cause severe and long-lasting pain.

Application of ice packs or ice massage usually relieves acute muscle spasm, but to correct the long-standing problem, education of the patient is needed. Once the spasm, swelling, and pain resolve, gentle exercises to increase back flexibility are in order. These include classic Williams flexion exercises to stretch paravertebral and hamstring muscles, along with strengthening of abdominal muscles. Obesity aggravates back pain by perpetuating poor posture; proper body weight minimizes the stress placed on the back. Heat modalities such as whirlpool, hot packs, diathermy, and/or ultrasound can be used after the acute phase in conjunction with massage to gently stretch and relax the paravertebral muscles. Combined electric stimulation and ultrasound Medco-sonlator® are often relaxing during recovery.

Paravertebral muscles should be stengthened to support the vertebral column. Situps with knees and hips flexed are good abdominal stengthening exercises; half a twist can be added as the patient progresses. Back extension exercises are as follows: the patient lies across several tightly rolled pillows and extends the upper trunk. Hip extensors can be strengthened by extending one leg at a time with progression to extension of both legs as they get stronger.

PREVENTING INJURY

The key to prevention of injuries is flexibility and balanced power between opposing muscle groups. If the body is structurally sound, it will work well as long as it is in balance with the forces acting on it. It is that balance that physical therapy endeavors to maintain or restore.

REFERENCES

1. Morehouse, L.E., Miller, A.T. 1976. Skill development. In: Physiology of Exercise, 7th Ed. C.V. Mosby Co., St. Louis, pp 287–288.
2. Al-Amound, W.S., Buller, A.J., et al. 1973. Long-term stimulation of cat fast-twitch skeletal muscle. Nature 244:225–227.
3. Peckham, P.H., Mortimer, J.T., et al. 1973. Physiologic and metabolic changes in white muscle of cat following induced exercise. Brain Res 50:424–429.
4. Pette, D., Smith, M.E., et al. 1973. Effects of long-term electrical stimulation on some contractile and metabolic characteristics of fast rabbit muscles. Pfleugers Arch 338:257–272.
5. Riley, D.A., Allin, E.F. 1973. The effects of inactivity, programmed stimulation and denervation on the histochemistry of skeletal muscle fibre types. Exp Neurol 40:391–413.
6. Salmons, S. 1967. An implantable muscle stimulator. J Physiol (Lond) 188:13.
7. Salmons, S., Henriksson, J. 1981. The adaptive response of skeletal muscle to increased use. Muscle Nerve 4:94.
8. Henneman, E., Somjen, G., et al. 1965. Functional significance of cell size in spinal motoneurons. J Neurophysiol 28:560–580.
9. Grant, A.E. 1964. Cold: Massage with ice (cryokinetics). Arch Phys Med 45:233–238.
10. Gucker, T. 1965. Heat: The use of heat and cold in orthopaedics. In: Licht, S. (ed): Therapeutic Heat and Cold. Elizabeth Licht, New Haven, pp 398–406.
11. Griffin, J.E., Karselis, T.C. 1982. The infra red energies; ultraviolet light; ultrasound energy. In: Physical Agents for Physical Therapists, 2nd Ed. Charles C Thomas, Springfield, IL, pp 177–309.
12. McCluskey, G.M., Blackburn, T.A., Jr., et al. 1976. A treatment for ankle sprains. Am J Sports Med 4:158–161.
13. Malone, T.R., Blackburn, T.A., et al. 1980. Knee rehabilitation. Phys Ther 60(12):1602–1609.
14. Connolly, J.F. 1981. Mechanisms of Injuries: The Management of Fractures and Dislocations. W.B. Saunders Co., Philadelphia, pp 1802–1808.
15. Starkey, J.A. 1976. Treatment of ankle injuries by simultaneous use of intermittent compression and ice packs. Am J Sports Med 4:142–144.
16. Davies, G.J., Wallace, L.A., et al. 1980. Mechanisms of selected knee injuries. Phys Ther 60(12):1590–1595.
17. Derscheid, G.L., Malone, T.R. 1980. Knee disorders. Phys Ther 60(12):1582–1589.
18. McLeod, W.D., Hunter, S. 1980. Biomechanical analysis of the knee: Primary functions as elucidated by anatomy. Phys Ther 60(12):1561–1565.

•30•

Investigation of Sports-Related Deaths

John E. Smialek

The death of an athlete, whether the person is engaged in a sport or not, is an uncommon event (Thompson et al. [1].) Since such individuals are generally considered healthy, death is clearly unexpected. Sudden and unexpected deaths which result from unknown or obscure causes are required by most state laws to be investigated by the local medical examiner or coroner (Kornblum and Fisher [2]; Spitz and Fisher [3]; Curran et al. [4]; DHEW [5]). This public official, usually a physician, is responsible for the investigation of the circumstances of such deaths. Part of this type of investigation is an examination of the body, that will include a careful search for alcohol and drugs, and, finally, developing a report identifying the cause and manner of death.

In the United States, boxing has received the most medical attention as a dangerous sport, since it has been responsible for several highly publicized deaths. However, an analysis of mortality data related to all types of sporting activities reveals that boxing ranks ninth behind horse racing, sport parachuting, hang gliding, mountaineering, and scuba diving (Ward [6]).

A thorough investigation of the circumstances of a death is necessary for the reconstruction of the fatal event. It can provide valuable information related to the inadequacy of safety measures such as available medical facilities, as well as to failure of protective equipment such as helmets.

A forensic autopsy is essential in the identification of subtle abnormalities that may have contributed to or caused an athlete to lose consciousness and die.

FORENSIC AUTOPSY

The forensic autopsy is similar to a hospital autopsy in that it involves a thorough examination of both the internal and external aspects of the body and a written description of all the factual findings observed during the examination. However, the forensic autopsy differs from the hospital autopsy by the inclusion of an expert opinion at the end of the report which should incorporate all the medical facts noted during the examination: the results of auxiliary tests on various organs, body tissues, and fluids, and the circumstances under which the death occurred. Thus, the forensic autopsy ascertains both the cause and manner of death.

While the cause of death may be determined to be a cardiac arrhythmia (irregular heartbeat), it could be classified as natural, accidental, homicidal, or undeterminable. For example, say that a baseball player collapses, during or following a game, from such a cardiac arrhythmia, which might be the result of an underlying medical condition such as arteriosclerotic cardiovascular disease. The manner of death in this case would be classified as natural. However, if the player were struck severely in the chest with a baseball prior to collapse, then this injury could have precipitated a sudden cardiac arrhythmia resulting in death. The key role of the injury in initiating the fatal event would result in the death being ruled accidental in manner. If a violent physical altercation occurred during the sports event, and the player collapsed during such an altercation, then the manner of death would be ruled homicidal.

Defining the Role of Drugs Through Autopsy

Similarly, if it were determined at autopsy that drugs were present in the blood of the athlete and were significantly involved as the cause of death, then the manner would be classified as either accidental, homicidal, or undeterminable, depending on whether the drugs had been taken voluntarily or whether they had been administered by another person without the athlete's awareness. Robert Goldman [7] related in *Death in the Locker Room* documented examples of drug use in athletes from as far back as 1865, when swimmers in canal races were charged with taking dope. He further states that, "In November 1968, Yves Moltin won a cross-country bicycle race in Grenoble, France. Two days later, he collapsed and died. In the following year, two of his friends, both French cyclists, were indicted on a charge of having given Moltin the amphetamines that caused his death" (p. 28).

The drug issue arose during the investigation of the 1986 death of Len Bias, the star basketball player for the University of Maryland Terrapins. The initial death investigation in this case revealed that Bias had died as a result of the administration of a large amount of cocaine. His college friends had "cleaned up" his room following the death and refused, on advice of their attorneys, to discuss the circumstances of his collapse with the police. The Bias family maintained that their son would not have voluntarily taken cocaine and claimed that the residue of cocaine found in the stomach contents meant that this drug had been put into a drink and consumed by Bias unknowingly.

The Assistant Medical Examiner who performed the autopsy failed to take nasal swabs to ascertain positively that snorting had been the route of administration. Scene evidence, including straws that tested positive for cocaine and a small amount of cocaine in the stomach, was consistent with cocaine having been snorted, since a certain percentage of snorted cocaine is swallowed and can later be found in stomach contents. Thus it was determined that, under the circumstances, the most reasonable route of administration was by snorting. As in most other drug-related deaths, the manner of death in the Bias case was considered to be undeterminable because of unanswered questions of whether the drug had been provided, without the victim's knowledge, in an unadulterated and unexpectedly pure form.

Identifying Underlying Heart Disease Through Autopsy

The role of underlying heart disease as a major cause of athletes dying suddenly has been the subject of extensive analysis (Ward [6]; Bharati and Lev [8]; Jokl and Thomas [9]). It is not the purpose of this chapter to report the information contained in these articles. However, there are certain positive cardiac findings identifiable at autopsy that can raise legal questions as to the mechanism of death. Several of these are discussed below.

In the Len Bias case, initial gross examination of the heart did not reveal any apparent abnormality. However, after intensive microscopic examination was carried out, focal areas of myocardial fiber necrosis were identified. Such findings are characteristic of the now recognized cocaine-related cardiomyopathy (Tagelaar et al. [10]; Isner et al. [11]; also see Ch. 13) and provided evidence that Len Bias had used cocaine at least weeks prior to the fatal episode. Subsequent grand jury testimony confirmed this conclusion and revealed that the abuse had occurred over an extended period.

In another case, a relatively young physician died while swimming laps in the shallow end (4 ft) of a hotel pool. He had been observed to stand up after having completed several laps, raise his hands above his head as if to dive in again, and fall forward face down in the water. He was pulled out of the water almost immediately and resuscitation was performed by a nurse who was a witness at the scene. This continued for several minutes until an emergency rescue unit arrived and transported the victim to the hospital. Resuscitation attempts were unsuccessful and the swimmer was pronounced dead in the emergency room.

The family maintained that the physician had died as a result of drowning and the owners of the pool were therefore responsible for his death because they provided inadequately for rescue and resuscitation. Subsequent examination of the heart, however, revealed an abnormality of a coronary vessel that could have accounted for his sudden death. The physician had stenosis of an abnormally placed coronary ostium surrounded by atheromatous "ridges." While the abnormality was not a common type usually identified with sudden death, recent medical literature has described several cases of such rare abnormalities (Virmani et al. [12]).

Several years ago, the author studied deaths that occurred while people were jogging in Wayne County, Michigan. Within a population of approximately 2.3 million, nine such deaths were identified over a 3-year period (1978–1980). Six of the deaths occurred in low distance runners and were due to arteriosclerotic cardiovascular disease. Two deaths were the result of collision with automobiles. Both runners were running with, instead of against, the flow of traffic and thus were unsuspectingly struck from the rear and killed. One running victim was a well-conditioned athlete who collapsed in the middle of a 10-kilometer race. Investigation of his death revealed that he was recovering from the flu and did not want to prolong his convalescence. His heart exhibited evidence of myocarditis indicating that the flu had involved his myocardium, rendering him susceptible to a fatal cardiac arrythmia during the race.

This mechanism of a fatal spontaneous cardiac arrythmia seems to be the culprit in deaths of individuals who collapse and die despite considerable running endurance. When, on occasion, one reads of a death occurring during a running competition, a common explanation provided is heat stroke. This diagnosis is overused and undersupported by medical evidence. Heat exhaustion can certainly contribute to induction of a cardiac arrythmia, resulting in cerebral hypoxia and uncoordinated activity. The eventual outcome might be sudden death. On the other hand, a victim might survive complications of hypotension associated with peripheral vascular collapse. In either case it is the disruption of normal cardiac activity that results in serious pathologic changes in heat-related collapse of runners.

FORENSIC INVESTIGATION OF DELAYED DEATHS RELATED TO SPORTS ACTIVITIES

Although many of the deaths investigated by medical examiners or coroners can be described as sudden, this factor is not essential to the requirement for medicolegal investigation. Indeed, deaths as a result of injuries sustained during certain sporting events such as boxing, football, or rodeo events might not occur for days or weeks following the injury. Even in heart-related deaths, resuscitation is sometimes successful but only after brain damage has occurred, and the individual can die weeks later.

In those cases where the individual is maintained in hospital for an extended period of time before dying, the cause and manner of death can be obscured. For example, unless the hospital is diligent in taking blood and urine samples for toxicological testing, the presence or absence of drugs that may have been implicated in the death might never be ascertained. When complications occur as a result of medical therapy, such as a comatose patient being maintained on life support systems, the death certificate might be completed incorrectly to reflect that death was due to natural causes such as bronchopneumonia, obscuring the role of the accidental injury which initiated the sequence of fatal events. Such inaccurate determinations of manner of death can have significance for the beneficiaries of life insurance policies which pay increased benefits for accidental deaths.

While many sports-related deaths are due to a manifestation of some unrecognized abnormality of the athlete, other types of deaths are related directly to injury received during the event itself. A common injury sustained by boxers is subdural hematoma. This is a blood clot that results from bleeding beneath a thick membrane (the dura mater) which surrounds the brain. It occurs when certain blood vessels (bridging veins) tear as the result of a sudden rapid movement of the brain produced by the blow. The accumulation of blood causes pressure on the brain and, if unrelieved, can result in coma and death. However, if the blood clot is drained surgically, the intracranial pressure will be reduced and survival will depend on the associated injuries suffered by the brain. Often boxers survive several days before they die of brain injuries. Nevertheless, the death must still be reported to the medical examiner or coroner, who can then conduct an official investigation before the death certificate is completed.

The death of a boxer raises an interesting question as to the manner of death. Is it a homicide, since another person inflicted the fatal injuries, or should it be considered accidental, since the damage was not predictable or anticipated and safety measures had been instituted to protect the boxer against such a possibility? In such a case, an important consideration would be the personal motivation and willingness of the contestants to participate in such a dangerous sport.

COMPONENTS OF THE FORENSIC
INVESTIGATION OF SPORTS-RELATED DEATHS

A proper forensic investigation of a sports-related death will have the following components:

1. A thorough investigation of the circumstances of the death
2. A careful postmortem examination or autopsy that will include detailed studies of critical structures that can cause sudden death
3. A comprehensive toxicological study to determine the presence of alcohol or drugs in the body of the victim at the time of death

When the above steps have been completed, an official opinion can be generated that will explain how the death occurred. Each of the steps will be described in more detail below.

Investigation

If an appropriate diagnosis is to be reached after considering the anatomical findings in an autopsy, as complete a picture as possible of the events surrounding the collapse or death must be provided. In the case described earlier, in which the physician collapsed and died of a cardiac arrhythmia while swimming in a hotel pool, the information initially given the pathologist was cursory, indicating only that the victim had drowned in the pool. If the pathologist had known that the relatively young physician had been swimming actively in relatively shallow water when he suddenly stopped without a struggle or sign of distress, an intensive examination of the heart could have been carried out. Instead, the initial examination was relatively superficial and the role of the abnormal coronary artery was thought to be clinically insignificant. If the investigation of sports related death is to be complete, the following information must be obtained in addition to the regular data:

1. In what type of activity was the victim engaged?
2. Were there witnesses to the collapse?
3. Had the victim ceased this activity before the collapse?
4. What was the time interval between activity and collapse?
5. What were the climatic conditions, such as temperature, at the time of the collapse?
6. Did the victim exhibit any signs or symptoms before the collapse, such as nausea, vomiting, syncope, dizziness, chest pain, headache, difficulty breathing, or convulsions?
7. Did the victim have a medical history, e.g., congenital heart disease, sickle cell anemia?
8. Was the victim on any medication?
9. Was there a family history of sudden death, death at a young age, or familial disorder, e.g., hypertension?
10. Was the victim suspected of abusing alcohol and/or drugs?
11. Did the victim strike the head or chest during the collapse?
12. What emergency treatment was administered?
13. Was this treatment provided by laypersons, paramedics, or hospital personnel?
14. What observations were made by the initial medical responders about signs of injury?
15. Was any equipment being used at the time of the collapse, e.g., air tanks in a scuba diving death, and is this being evaluated?

Autopsy

Assisted by the information regarding the circumstances of the death, the pathologist can conduct a complete postmortem study that might provide immediate answers to the next of kin. However, the sudden death of an athlete often requires more intensive study of the neurological and cardiovascular systems before a final determination of the cause can be made. A forensic autopsy begins with the external examination and documents the following:

1. Physical abnormalities (e.g., "spider fingers" of Marfan's syndrome)
2. Signs of injury (e.g., fall, electrical burns)
3. Evidence of drug use (e.g., powder residue in nose)
4. Signs of emergency medical treatment

The internal examination must include a thorough review of all systems that documents evidence of acute and chronic illness, e.g., myocarditis, and sites of injury, e.g., fracture sites, which can indicate the original point of impact.

Specialized procedures for testing for air embolism in a scuba death should be carried out when the body is first opened. Samples of blood, bile, urine, and vitreous humor should be obtained for alcohol and drug studies. The heart should be carefully examined for:

1. Abnormal size or configuration, which may be local (tumor) generalized (cardiomyopathy) or regional (subaortic) stenosis
2. Valvular abnormalities

3. Coronary artery abnormalities
4. Myocardial disease

When such abnormalities are detected, microscopic evaluation of the lesion is indicated. If no gross abnormality can be identified, extensive sampling of the myocardium, including the conduction system, should be carried out.

Central Nervous System

Signs of brain injury, such as cerebral contusion, epidural or subdural hematoma, or cerebral edema, may be evident. However, if there was an interval between the collapse and death, the sites of injury should be studied microscopically. This might help resolve questions as to whether the hemorrhage occurred at the time of collapse or during medical treatment. Underlying brain disease, such as healed cerebral contusions due to previous injury, might be apparent.

Peripheral Nervous System

Tumors of the peripheral nervous system can occur and precipitate cardiac arrhythmia leading to death. The author recently identified such a lesion in a skier who collapsed and died after coming down from the ski hill (Sperry and Smialek [13]). If hypothermia is considered a possible factor in the death, microscopic examination of the renal system should be carried out.

Toxicological Studies

As stated above, appropriate sampling of body fluids should be carried out which will allow testing that will determine if alcohol and/or drugs caused or contributed to the death. Nasal swabs to identify the site of entry of snorted drugs—cocaine, heroin, phencyclidine (PCP)—should be carried out in any apparently healthy individual dying under suspicious circumstances.

The approach to drug testing should be adapted to ensure that the presence of prescribed or illicit drugs is properly established or ruled out. It is not adequate to request a drug screen from a hospital or commercial laboratory. Drug screens vary in their comprehensiveness. If the victim was known to have been using prescribed medication, the laboratory should be informed of this and appropriate evaluation of levels of the drug requested. Also, a search for illicit drugs known to exist in the area should be conducted, with quantitation of positive results.

DISCUSSION

The medicolegal investigation of a sports-related death requires a thorough search for information regarding the circumstances of the death, and usually requires the assistance of law enforcement agencies. However, when the victim is rushed to the hospital, such information regarding the scene of the collapse is usually lacking and, unfortunately, might never be sought. Furthermore, an athlete might die in circumstances far removed from competitive events and the need for in-depth studies to identify the cause and manner of death might not be recognized because of inadequate information. If the local death investigation system is functioning efficiently, proper handling of such cases will usually result.

REFERENCES

1. Thompson, P.D., Stein, M.P., Williams, P., et al. 1979. Death during jogging or running. JAMA 242:1265–1267.

2. Kornblum, R.N., Fisher, R.S. 1972. A Compendium of State Medico-Legal Investigative Systems. Maryland Medical-Legal Foundation, Baltimore.

3. Spitz, W.V., Fisher, R.S. 1980. Medicolegal Investigation of Death. Charles C Thomas, Springfield, IL.

4. Curran, W.J., McGarry, A.L., Petty, C.S. 1980. Modern Legal Medicine. F.A. Davis Co., Philadelphia.

5. U.S. Department of Health, Education, and Welfare. 1978. Death Investigation: An Analysis of Laws and Policies of the United States, Each State and Jurisdiction. DHEW Publication no. 78–5252. U.S. Government Printing Office, Washington, D.C.

6. Ward, S. 1986. Sports medicine. USA Today.

7. Goldman, R. 1987. Death in the Locker Room. H.P. Books, Tucson, AZ.

8. Bharati, S., Lev, M. 1985. Cardiovascular clinics—Sudden cardiac death. In: Brent, A.N. (ed): The Pathology of Sudden Death, F.A. Davis, Philadelphia.

9. Jokl, E., Thomas, C.C. 1985. Sudden Death of Athletes. Charles C Thomas, Springfield, IL.

10. Tagelaar, H.D., et al. 1987. Cocaine and the heart. Hum Pathol 18:195–199.

11. Isner, J.M., et al. 1986. Acute cardiac event temporally related to cocaine abuse. N Engl J Med 315:1438–1443.

12. Virmani, R., et al. 1984. Acute takeoffs of the coronary arteries along the aortic wall and congenital coronary ostial valve-like ridge: Association with sudden death. JACC 3:766–71.

13. Sperry, K., Smialek, J.E. 1986. Sudden death due to a paraganglioma of the organs of Zuckerkandl. Am J For Med Pathol 7:23–29.

Index